SECOND EDITION

Office SPORTS MEDICINE

SECOND EDITION

Office SPORTS MEDICINE

Edited by

MORRIS B. MELLION, MD

Medical Director
Sports Medicine Center
Omaha, Nebraska
Clinical Associate Professor
Departments of Family Practice and
Orthopaedic Surgery (Sports Medicine)
University of Nebraska Medical Center
Omaha, Nebraska
Adjunct Associate Professor
School of Health, Physical Education and Recreation
University of Nebraska at Omaha
Omaha, Nebraska
Team Physician, Men's and Women's Sports
University of Nebraska at Omaha
Omaha, Nebraska

HANLEY & BELFUS, INC./ Philadelphia
MOSBY/ St. Louis • Baltimore • Boston • Carlsbad • Chicago • London
Madrid • Naples • New York • Philadelphia • Sydney • Tokyo • Toronto

Publisher: HANLEY & BELFUS, INC.
210 S. 13th Street
Philadelphia, PA 19107
(215) 546-7293
FAX (215) 790-9330

North American and worldwide sales and distribution:

MOSBY
11830 Westline Industrial Drive
St. Louis, MO 63146

In Canada: Times Mirror Professional Publishing, Ltd.
130 Flaska Drive
Markham, Ontario L6G 1B8
Canada

Library of Congress Cataloging-in-Publication Data

Office sports medicine / [edited by] Morris B. Mellion. — 2nd ed.
p. cm.
Rev ed. of: Office management of sports injuries & athletic problems. ©1988.
Includes bibliographical references and index.
ISBN 1-56053-120-7 (hard cover : alk. paper)
1. Sports medicine. 2. Sports injuries. I. Mellion, Morris B. II. Office management of sports injuries & athletic problems.
[DNLM: 1. Athletic Injuries. 2. Sports Medicine. QT 261 032 1995]
RC1210.034 1995
617.1′027—dc20
DNLM/DLC
for Library of Congress 95-35462
CIP

OFFICE SPORTS MEDICINE, 2nd edition ISBN 1-56053-120-7

Last digit is the print number: 9 8 7 6 5 4 3 2 1

Dedication

To Irene, Rosie, and Frank,

who make it all worthwhile.

Contents

Contributors

Loren H. Amundson, M.D.
Professor, Department of Family Medicine, University of South Dakota School of Medicine, Sioux Falls, South Dakota

Kris Berg, Ed.D.
Professor, Department of Physical Education, School of Health, Physical Education, and Recreation, University of Nebraska at Omaha, Omaha, Nebraska

David E. Brown, M.D.
Clinical Assistant Professor, Department of Orthopaedic Surgery, University of Nebraska Medical Center, Omaha, Nebraska; Team Orthopaedist, Wayne State College

Gene F. Burrish, M.D.
Clinical Assistant Professor, Department of Dermatology, University of South Dakota School of Medicine, Sioux Falls, South Dakota

David R. Burton, C. Ped.
Certified Pedorthist, Midwest Orthotic and Prosthetics, Omaha, Nebraska

Loren A. Crown, M.D.
Assistant Professor, Director of Sports Medicine Section, Department of Family Medicine, University of Tennessee, Memphis, Tennessee

Denise M. Fandel, M.S., A.T.C.
Head Athletic Trainer, and Instructor, School of Health, Physical Education, and Recreation, University of Nebraska at Omaha, Omaha, Nebraska

Timothy C. Fitzgibbons, M.D.
Assistant Clinical Professor, Department of Orthopedic Surgery, Creighton University School of Medicine; Clinical Instructor, Department of Orthopedics, University of Nebraska Medical Center, Omaha, Nebraska

Walter B. Franz, III, M.D.
Associate Professor, Mayo Medical School; Staff Physician, Department of Family Practice, Mayo Clinic, Rochester, Minnesota

Ann C. Grandjean, Ed.D.
Director, International Center for Sports Nutrition, Omaha; Clinical Assistant Professor, Sports Medicine Program, Department of Orthopedic Surgery and Rehabilitation, University of Nebraska Medical Center, Omaha, Nebraska

Ronnie D. Hald, R.P.T., A.T.C.
Sports Physical Therapist, HealthSouth Sports Medicine and Rehabilitation Center, Omaha, Nebraska

Brian Halpern, M.D.
Assistant Attending and Medical Director, Department of Sports Medicine, Hospital for Special Surgery; Assistant Attending, Department of Sports Medicine, New York Hospital–Cornell Medical Center; Clinical Assistant Professor and Fellowship Director, Department of Sports Medicine, UMDNJ Robert Wood Johnson Medical School; Assistant Team Physician, New York Mets; Team Physician, Georgian Court College, Marlboro High School, Freehold Township High School, New Jersey

Michele Helzer-Julin, M.S., P.A.
Physician Assistant, Exercise Physiologist, Sports Medicine Center, Omaha, Nebraska

Todd Paul Hendrickson, M.D.
Assistant Professor, Department of Psychiatry, Director, Medical Student Education, Creighton-Nebraska Combined Department of Psychiatry, Omaha, Nebraska

Timothy P. Huston, M.D.
Laguna Niguel, California

Walter W. Huurman, M.D.
Professor, Department of Orthopaedic Surgery and Pediatrics, University of Nebraska, Omaha, Nebraska

Brian R. Incremona, M.D.
Director, Department of Sports Medicine, Rutgers The State University of New Jersey; Clinical Instructor, Department of Internal Medicine, Robert Wood Johnson Medical School, Piscataway, New Jersey

Bernard Keown, M.D.
Medical Director, Sports Medicine Center West; Associate Professor, Department of Family Practice, University of Nebraska Medical Center, Omaha, Nebraska

J. B. Ketner, M.D.
Department of Family Practice, Lincoln Family Practice Program, Lincoln, Nebraska

Roger H. Kobayashi, M.D.
Associate Clinical Professor, Department of Pediatrics, UCLA School of Medicine, Los Angeles, California

Morris B. Mellion, M.D.
Medical Director, Sports Medicine Center; Clinical Associate Professor, Departments of Family Practice and Orthopaedic Surgery (Sports Medicine), University of Nebraska Medical Center; Adjunct Associate Professor, School of Health, Physical Education and Recreation, University of Nebraska at Omaha; Team Physician, Men's and Women's Sports, University of Nebraska at Omaha, Omaha, Nebraska

Randall D. Neumann, M.D.
Orthopaedic Surgeon, Sports Medicine Center, Omaha, Nebraska

James C. Puffer, M.D.
Professor and Chief, Division of Family Medicine, UCLA School of Medicine, Los Angeles, California

Margot Putukian, M.D.
Assistant Professor, Departments of Internal Medicine and Orthopedics, Hershey Medical Center, Hershey, Pennsylvania; Team Physician, Penn State University, University Park, Pennsylvania

Kristin J. Reimers, M.S., R.D.
Programs Coordinator, International Center for Sports Nutrition, Omaha, Nebraska

William MacMillan Rodney, M.D.
Chairman and Professor, Department of Family Medicine, University of Tennessee, Memphis, Tennessee

Jaime S. Ruud, M.S., R.D.
Nutrition Consultant for Sports Nutrition, International Center for Sports Nutrition, Omaha, Nebraska

Colleen R. Sampson, L.P.N.
Orthopedic Foot and Ankle Nurse, Omaha, Nebraska

Guy L. Shelton, M.A., P.T., A.T.C.
Administrator and Sports Physical Therapist, HealthSouth Sports Medicine and Rehabilitation Center of Omaha, Omaha, Nebraska; Clinical Instructor, Division of Physical Therapy Education, School of Allied Health Professions, University of Nebraska Medical Center, Omaha, Nebraska

David M. Smith, M.D.
Co-Medical Director, Sports Care, Shawnee Mission Medical Center; Clinical Assistant Professor, Department of Family Practice, University of Kansas Medical Center, Shawnee Mission, Kansas

Jeffrey L. Tanji, M.D.
Associate Professor, Department of Family Practice and Exercise Science, University of California at Davis, Davis, California

W. Michael Walsh, M.D.
Clinical Associate Professor, Department of Orthopaedic Surgery; Adjunct Graduate Associate Professor, School of Health, Physical Education, and Recreation, University of Nebraska Medical Center, Omaha, Nebraska

Michael J. Whalen, PA-C
Sports Medicine Center, Omaha, Nebraska

Glenda R. Woscyna, M.S., R.D.
University of Nebraska Medical Center, Omaha, Nebraska

Frank G. Yanowitz, M.D.
Associate Professor, Department of Internal Medicine, University of Utah School of Medicine; Medical Director, The Fitness Institute, LDS Hospital, Salt Lake City, Utah

Preface to First Edition

Although sports medicine has historical roots that date back to the ancient Greek Olympics, it is also a very young area of medicine in the modern sense. The term "sports medicine" was probably coined at the 1928 San Moritz Winter Olympics, when 33 team physicians from 11 nations met and formed a committee to plan the First International Congress of Sports Medicine, to be held that summer at the Amsterdam Summer Olympics. The first book using the term "sports medicine" in its title was published in German in 1932, but the term was not used in the title of an English-language book until 30 years later.

Sports medicine has not been a specific medical discipline such as general surgery or cardiology or family practice. It has been an area of interest and concentration for physicians, other health care professionals, researchers, and educators in a wide variety of disciplines.

Ideally, sports medicine is practiced by a "team" consisting of athlete, physician, and coach, each of whom has a support system to draw upon (Fig. 1). For the athlete, the support system consists primarily of family, with friends and teammates also playing nurturing roles. The coach is backed up by the administration of the school, team, or league. The physician can draw upon two major support groups. For clinical support, the physician may turn to specialist colleagues, physical therapists, nutritionists, sports psychologists, podiatrists, and health educators. For a better understanding of the performance capabilities of the athlete, the physician may turn to medical researchers, exercise physiologists, kinesiologists, and a variety of physical educators and other researchers.

The athletic trainer plays a special role on the sports medicine team, since he or she is in an ideal position to maintain open and free communication with athlete, physician, and coach alike. The athletic trainer is therapist and counsellor for the athlete, advisor and friend to the coach, and eyes and ears for the physician. The importance of the athletic trainer as a key member of the sports medicine team has become so obvious in high level competition that it is now becoming clear that every high school should have an athletic trainer on its staff.

In spite of the fact that the ideal delivery of health care to the athlete would take place in a team or school facility, such as an athletic training room, the vast majority of sports medicine is practiced in the physician's office. The editor has surveyed family physicians in Nebraska to determine the sports medicine content of their practices; 216 responded. One hundred forty-one (65%) perform "organized team or league physical examinations" for school sports or community leagues, and 200 (93%) routinely perform preparticipation physical examinations in their offices for their own patients participating in school or community league sports. Ninety-seven (45%) of the family physicians responding indicated that they serve as team physicians in one or more sports, with 76 of these indicating that they are team physicians for both male and female sports teams.[1] These data only begin to suggest the depth of involvement in sports medicine of the practicing family physician, pediatrician, general internist, and general practitioner.

It is axiomatic that, in order to supervise the health care of athletes, the physician practicing sports medicine must function as a generalist. There are many specialists and subspecialists with strong interests in the care of the athlete, but their success in the long run will depend on their being versatile enough to take the generalist approach, which is so important for the athlete's physical and emotional well-being.

This book is written for the office-based physician, generalist and specialist alike, who finds that he or she is caring for competitive or recreational athletes. It focuses on the issues, injuries, and medical problems faced by people of all ages who incorporate athletics as a part of their basic life-style. It is not meant to be a comprehensive, encyclopedic reference but rather a readable, informative text for the practicing physician, resident, and medical student. Many sections are orthopedically oriented in order to deal with the common overuse problems in athletic injuries, but these sections are not designed to go into surgical management or fracture reduction in any depth.

Two chapters deserve special mention. "Tracking Problems of the Kneecap," by Dr. W. Michael Walsh, is a separate chapter with its own identity because it is the editor's belief that, while these problems are one of the most commonly encountered groups of musculoskeletal syndromes, they are also the most commonly misdiagnosed and inadequately treated. "Bicycle Injuries: Prevention, Diagnosis, and Management," by Drs. Jeffrey W. Hill and Morris B. Mellion, is included because most bicycle in-

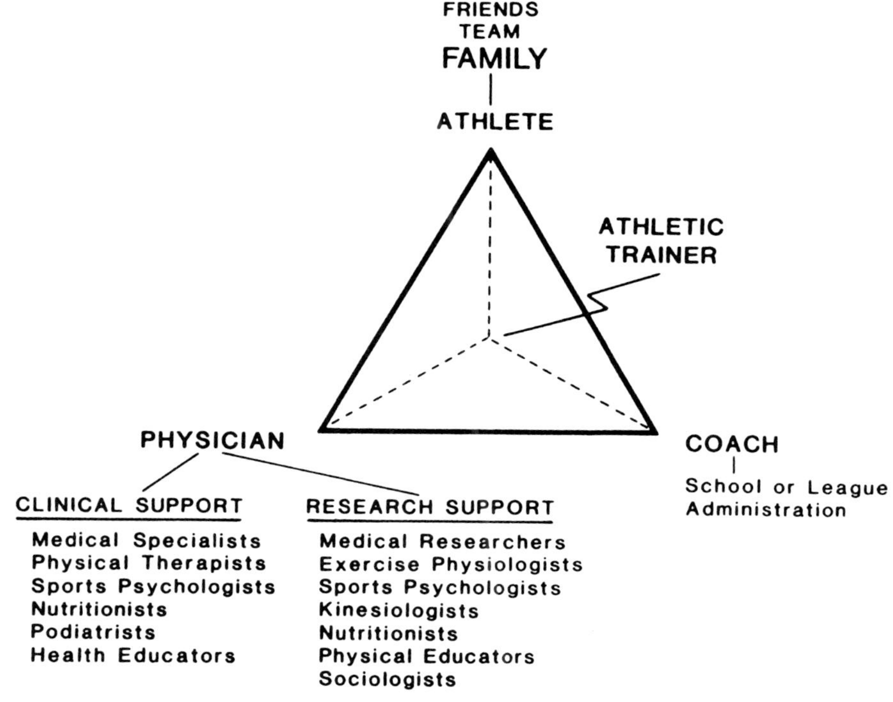

FIGURE 1. The Sports Medicine Team.

juries and overuse syndromes require that the physician have a reasonably in-depth understanding of the mechanics and fit of the modern bicycle in order to provide proper diagnosis and treatment.

REFERENCE

1. Mellion MB: The sports medicine content of family practice. J Fam Pract 21:473–474; 1985

Preface to Second Edition

Offfice Sports Medicine is the 2nd edition of a volume originally published as *Office Management of Sports Injuries & Athletic Problems*. My wife, Irene, felt that the original name was long and cumbersome. After offering several humorous substitutes, she proposed the new title, which is more concise and equally descriptive.

The old chapters have been completely rewritten, some by new authors. New chapters on Eating Disorders in Athletes, Sports Psychiatry/Psychology, Forearm, Wrist and Hand Injuries, and Foot Injuries have been added in an attempt to make the book more comprehensive.

I would like to express my personal thanks to those who have contributed to the success of this book. First, I want to thank Robert Gibson, David Cox, and Connie J. Claussen, Athletic Directors, Denise M. Fandel and Thomas A. Frette, Athletic Trainers, and the entire coaching staff at the University of Nebraska at Omaha for providing the opportunity for me to work as team physician with an excellent group of college athletes competing in a variety of men's and women's sports.

Special thanks go to Mary Parnick and Marilyn Novak for tireless devotion to this project.

Finally, I want to express my deepest appreciation to a very talented group of sports medicine colleagues—the authors and co-authors who made this book possible. It has been a wonderful treat to work with these bright, articulate men and women.

Morris B. Mellion, M.D.
Omaha, Nebraska

1

The Preparticipation Evaluation of Young Athletes

David M. Smith, M.D.

Primary care physicians serve an important role in the sports medical team in regard to maintaining the health and safety of athletes. Physicians involved in the care of athletes determine each athlete's readiness for training and competition by performing a comprehensive preparticipation evaluation (PPE). Whereas athletes may look upon this evaluation as simply a requirement with the potential to limit or restrict participation, physicians must consider the PPE as a positive intervention that ensures safe participation in sports.

Those who read a newspaper sports section on a regular basis commonly see accounts of the tragic death of young athletes that occurred during practice or competition. The question frequently asked following these tragedies is, Could this death have been prevented? Likewise, when a serious injury occurs as a result of sports participation, the question may arise: Was the athlete predisposed and could the injury have been prevented? These questions are frequently directed toward the sports medical team, and unfortunately, the answers are not always clear. However, the physician responsible for clearing athletes for sport may have the media seriously questioning the validity of the PPE and whether more comprehensive preparticipation screening is necessary.[4]

Up until recently there was no standard approach to the PPE, which carried wide variability in its recommendations and requirements.[6,10,12,16,20,28] Fortunately, with the December 1992 publication of an educational monograph[17] endorsed by the American Academy of Family Physicians, American Academy of Pediatrics, American Medical Society for Sports Medicine, American Orthopaedic Society for Sports Medicine, and American Osteopathic Academy of Sports Medicine there now exist more uniform guidelines for the PPE. It should be kept in mind that these guidelines are a foundation that the primary care physician may expand and tailor to the individual athlete and setting in which the PPE is performed

The goal of this chapter is not to critically review the aforementioned guidelines but rather to present a practical approach for the primary care physician who evaluates young athletes in the office prior to sports participation.

GOALS AND OBJECTIVES

Whereas the athlete generally presents for the PPE because it is a requirement for clearance to participate, the physician must remember that the main goal of the PPE is to ensure the health and safety of the athlete. The foundation, then, for a comprehensive PPE may be established by fulfilling the following primary objectives.

1. *Identify medical conditions that may limit athletic participation.* Such cardiovascular conditions as hypertrophic cardiomyopathy, aortic stenosis, and poorly controlled hypertension are examples of screenable conditions that may be absolute or relative contraindications to certain activities.

2. *Identify medical conditions that may predispose to injury or illness.* Such orthopedic conditions as an anterior cruciate ligament–deficient knee, an unstable shoulder, and an inadequately rehabilitated remote ankle sprain are examples of conditions that may be identified and would require further treatment prior to participation. Identifying the obese athlete who may be at risk for heat illness and the athlete with exercise-induced asthma who may have exacerbations in the cold or with exposure to extrinsic allergens are examples of nonorthopedic conditions.

3. *Comply with all legal and insurance requirements.* This objective may seem self-explanatory, but confusion may exist because of the wide variety of state guidelines and forms.[10]

Because young athletes usually seek medical attention only for acute medical illnesses and injuries, their visits with a primary care physician may be sporadic at best. However, more than 78% of athletes view the PPE as their annual health examination,[12,24] and thus the primary care physician has a unique opportunity to fulfill a secondary objective.

1. *Evaluate health risk behaviors and counsel on health-related issues.* Questioning and counseling an athlete regarding health risk behaviors such as alcohol and tobacco use, illicit drug and ergogenic aid use, pathogenic weight control behaviors, sexually transmitted diseases, and unwanted pregnancies are highly recommended[6,7,17] if time permits and the athlete is receptive. Furthermore, discussion of preventive measures such as breast and testicular self-examination and routine Pap smears may be included.

And finally, in the ideal setting, if the physician has either the expertise or access to well-trained ancillary personnel, another secondary objective may be fulfilled.

2. *Evaluate fitness level and assess performance.* Although testing of the components of fitness and performance such as body fat composition, flexibility, strength, power, and endurance is generally more practical in a mass-screening-station-type evaluation, adapting all or a portion of such tests to an office setting is possible. Information gained from the inclusion of these tests may assist the physician in identifying potential risk factors for injury or illness and may assist the athlete and coach in designing training programs. This approach is advocated by some who believe the PPE needs to be as sport specific as possible.[13]

TIMING AND FREQUENCY

Most primary care physicians who have performed PPEs are familiar with that frantic phone call from the athlete, the parent, or the coach begging for an appointment time on the day prior to the start of the competitive season in order to "have the form signed" providing clearance to begin practice. How frustrating it is to all involved when a medical condition is identified that requires further evaluation, treatment, or rehabilitation prior to clearing the athlete to participate. To prevent this from happening, the current recommendation is to perform the PPE at least six weeks prior to the start of the season. The risk of performing the evaluation this far in advance of the season is that illness or injury may occur in the interim; however, this can be circumvented by encouraging the athlete to report any illness or injury that required medical attention so that specific follow-up may be provided. Six weeks prior to a fall season occurs midsummer, so it may be more practical to perform PPEs on the fall competitive athletes at the end of the previous school year.

Although there have been differing opinions regarding recommended frequency of the PPE, the most current recommendation is to perform a complete evaluation prior to entry into a new level of sport (i.e., middle school, high school, college), with annual, limited reevaluations thereafter.[17] This system works especially well when continuity of care is provided by the same primary care physician, and medical records are available from the previous year's exam. As discussed in a subsequent section of this chapter, the recommended history and physical form lends itself well to this system.

FORMAT OF THE EVALUATION

The majority of primary care physicians perform PPEs in their medical office, but it is not uncommon for physicians to help schools organize mass screening station examinations, especially if the physician serves as that school's team physician. Although neither format has been proven to be superior, distinct advantages and disadvantages accrue to each, as outlined in Table 1. Perhaps the ideal situation would be one in which a physician who has a special interest and expertise in sports medicine problems and who serves as both the athletes' primary care physician and the team physician for the athletes' school would have adequate time in the office to perform a thorough PPE fulfilling the previously discussed primary and secondary objectives of the PPE. Since that ideal situation rarely exists, it is recommended that physicians evaluate their practice

***TABLE 1.* Office-Based versus Station-Screening PPEs**

Office-Based PPE	Station-Screening PPE
Advantages	*Advantages*
Familiarity with patient (athlete)	Specialized personnel
Continuity of care	Efficient
Counseling opportunity	Less costly
Better record keeping	Better communication with school athletic staff
	Performance testing opportunity
Disadvantages	*Disadvantages*
Lack of primary care physician for some athletes	Potential for noisy and hurried environment with lack of privacy
Limited appointment time	Difficulty following up medical problems and recommendations
More costly	Less communication with parents
Less communication with school athletic staff	
Varying physician knowledge and interest in sports medicine problems	

Adapted from *Preparticipation Physical Evaluation* monograph, AAFP, AAP, AMSSM, AOSSM, AOASM, p. 9, 1992, with permission.

setting individually to decide which format—office based versus mass screening station based—would be most effective. For physicians interested in organizing a mass screening station evaluation, Table 2 outlines an efficient method with suggested personnel if resources allow.

MEDICAL HISTORY AND PHYSICAL EXAMINATION

What questions to ask and what things to include in a physical exam of an athlete preparing to participate in sport have been debated by physicians for years. Multiple forms have been proposed,[3,5,6] and individual states have experienced wide variability in recommendations.[10] The recently published form seen in Figures 1 and 2 serves as a practical tool to assist physicians in effectively screening athletes for sports participation and is currently under review to ensure that it indeed is both effective in fulfilling the objectives of the PPE and user-friendly for both physicians and athletes.

All primary care physicians know that a comprehensive history is the cornerstone of any medical evaluation. With regard to the PPE history, it has been shown that up to 75% of problems affecting athletes may be identified by history alone.[12,24] However, less than 40% of histories reported by athletes agreed with information provided by parents.[24] Therefore, it is recommended that the medical history be completed by the athletes and reviewed by their parents to enhance the accuracy of the history.[17] The physician should then discuss with the athlete prior to the physical examination any pertinent history findings.

Noticeably lacking from the recommended history form (Fig. 1) are questions regarding health-risk behaviors such as alcohol and tobacco use, illicit drug and ergogenic aid use, pathogenic weight control behaviors, sexually transmitted diseases, and unwanted pregnancies. Opinions vary on how to question young athletes regarding these sensitive issues in order to obtain honest answers and ensure confidentially. Most agree that if questions are included on the history form, they should be carefully worded so as to ensure accurate responses the athlete would not consider incriminating. As an example, asking an athlete, "Are you happy with your current weight?" and "What methods do you use to control your weight?" may assist in identifying an athlete with pathogenic weight control behavior. Although this area is currently under review[26] in order to establish more specific guidelines, primary care physicians involved with PPEs may need to individualize their approach to eliciting a history of health-risk behaviors depending on the setting in which they practice.

Recalling the first two objectives of the PPE to "identify medical conditions that may limit athletic participation" and "identify medical conditions that may predispose to injury or illness," practitioners should ensure that the physical examination is comprehensive yet focused on salient findings from the medical history. For example, a complete head, eyes, ears, nose, and throat (HEENT) exam is not absolutely necessary, because vision screening and pupil exam (for anisocoria) will suffice in the athlete whose history is unremarkable for HEENT problems. However, in an athlete who complains of headaches, seasonal allergies or other HEENT symptoms or who has health-risk behaviors such as the use of smokeless tobacco—which would indicate more extensive exam of the HEENT—or in an athlete who will be participating in a sport with a risk of injury to any of these areas (e.g., wrestlers who are at risk for auricular hematoma or blunt eye injuries), the physician should expand the physical to include a more comprehensive exam of the HEENT. Similarly, the rest of the physical examination depicted in Figure 2 should follow this screening format, using the medical history to focus the exam as indicate.

To follow the recommendation that a complete entry-level PPE be performed with subsequent annual limited reevaluations, the history and physical exam form has been organized accordingly. The athlete should complete the medical history annually, with special attention to question 13, "Have you had a medical problem or injury since your last evaluation?" and the physician's examination may be limited to that section labeled "Limited." Certainly an affirmative answer to question 13 should be pursued with more detailed history and pertinent physical examination.

A detailed discussion of each of the medical history questions as well as the recommended physi-

***TABLE 2.* Example of Station-Screening PPE Format**

Required Stations	Personnel
Sign-in height/weight, vital signs, vision screening	Ancillary staff (e.g., coach, nurse, booster club volunteers)
Medical history review, complete physical exam, assessment and clearance	Physician
Optional Stations	**Personnel**
Orthopedic-specific exam	Physician
Flexibility	Therapist or athletic trainer
Body composition	Exercise physiologist
Performance testing (i.e., strength, speed, agility, power, balance, endurance)	Therapist, athletic trainer, coach, exercise physiologist

Adapted from *Preparticipation Physical Evaluation* monograph, AAFP, AAP, AMSSM, AOSSM, AOASM, p. 11, 1992, with permission.

Preparticipation Physical Evaluation

History

Date ____________

Name ______________________ Sex ______ Age ______ Date of birth ____________

Grade ________ Sport ____________ ____________ ____________

Personal physician ____________ ____________ (Address) ____________ (Physician's phone)

Explain "Yes" answers below:

	Yes	No
1. Have you ever been hospitalized?	☐	☐
Have you ever had surgery?	☐	☐
2. Are you presently taking any medications or pills?	☐	☐
3. Do you have any allergies (medicine, bees or other stinging insects)?	☐	☐
4. Have you ever passed out during or after exercise?	☐	☐
Have you ever been dizzy during or after exercise?	☐	☐
Have you ever had chest pain during or after exercise?	☐	☐
Do you tire more quickly than your friends during exercise?	☐	☐
Have you ever had high blood pressure?	☐	☐
Have you ever been told that you have a heart murmur?	☐	☐
Have you ever had racing of your heart or skipped heartbeats?	☐	☐
Has anyone in your family died of heart problems or a sudden death before age 50?	☐	☐
5. Do you have any skin problems (itching, rashes, acne)?	☐	☐
6. Have you ever had a head injury?	☐	☐
Have you ever been knocked out or unconscious?	☐	☐
Have you ever had a seizure?	☐	☐
Have you ever had a stinger, burner or pinched nerve?	☐	☐
7. Have you ever had heat or muscle cramps?	☐	☐
Have you ever been dizzy or passed out in the heat?	☐	☐
8. Do you have trouble breathing or do you cough during or after activity?	☐	☐
9. Do you use any special equipment (pads, braces, neck rolls, mouth guard, eye guards, etc.)?	☐	☐
10. Have you had any problems with your eyes or vision?	☐	☐
Do you wear glasses or contacts or protective eye wear?	☐	☐
11. Have you ever sprained/strained, dislocated, fractured, broken or had repeated swelling or other injuries of any bones or joints?	☐	☐
☐ Head ☐ Shoulder ☐ Thigh ☐ Neck ☐ Elbow ☐ Knee ☐ Chest ☐ Forearm ☐ Shin/calf ☐ Back ☐ Wrist ☐ Ankle ☐ Hip ☐ Hand ☐ Foot		
12. Have you had any other medical problems (infectious mononucleosis, diabetes, etc.)?	☐	☐
13. Have you had a medical problem or injury since your last evaluation?	☐	☐

14. When was your last tetanus shot? ____________

When was your last measles immunization? ____________

15. When was your first menstrual period? ____________

When was your last menstrual period? ____________

What was the longest time between your periods last year? ____________

Explain "Yes" answers:

____
____
____
____
____
____

I hereby state that, to the best of my knowledge, my answers to the above questions are correct.

Date ____________

Signature of athlete ____________

Signature of parent/guardian ____________

From *Preparticipation Physical Evaluation* monograph, AAFP, AAP, AMSSM, AOSSM, AOASM, 1992, with permission.

FIGURE 1

cal exam has been reviewed elsewhere[17,25] and is beyond the scope of this chapter; therefore the following discussion is limited to the two areas requiring particular attention: the cardiovascular and musculoskeletal systems.

Cardiovascular Assessment

The primary goal of cardiovascular screening in the PPE is to identify cardiovascular conditions that may limit athletic participation or increase the risk

Preparticipation Physical Evaluation *continued*

Physical Examination

Date ______

Name ______ Age ______ Date of birth ______

Height ______ Weight ______ BP ______ / ______ Pulse ______

Vision R 20/____ L 20/____ Corrected: Y N Pupils ______

COMPLETE	LIMITED		Normal	Abnormal findings	Initials
		Cardiopulmonary			
		Pulses			
		Heart			
		Lungs			
		Tanner stage	1	2 3 4 5	
		Skin			
		Abdominal			
		Genitalia			
		Musculoskeletal			
		Neck			
		Shoulder			
		Elbow			
		Wrist			
		Hand			
		Back			
		Knee			
		Ankle			
		Foot			
		Other			

Clearance:

A. Cleared

B. Cleared after completing evaluation/rehabilitation for: ______

C. Not cleared for: ☐ Collision

☐ Contact

☐ Noncontact ____ Strenuous ____ Moderately strenuous ____ Nonstrenuous

Due to: ______

Recommendation: ______

______

______

Name of physician ______ Date ______

Address ______ Phone ______

Signature of physician ______

(Developed by the American Academy of Family Physicians, American Academy of Pediatrics, American Medical Society for Sports Medicine, American Orthopaedic Society for Sports Medicine and American Osteopathic Academy of Sports Medicine. Copyright © 1992.)

FIGURE 2

TABLE 3. Cardiovascular Causes of Sudden Death in Athletes

Common	Uncommon
Hypertrophic cardiomyopathy*	Aortic stenosis*
Anomalous coronary artery	Mitral valve prolapse*
Atherosclerotic heart disease	Myocarditis
Marfan's syndrome (aortic rupture)*	Right ventricular dysplasia
Idiopathic concentric left ventricular hypertrophy	Conduction system abnormalities
	Amyloidosis
	Sarcoidosis
	Cardiac tumors

*Screenable by history and physical exam.

of sudden death. More than 95% of sudden deaths in young athletes involve the cardiovascular system,[30] with the potential causes listed in Table 3. Although hypertension is not a cause of sudden death, it has been shown to be the most common reason why athletes are excluded from or allowed only limited sports participation.[18] Therefore, careful attention to the cardiovascular history is absolutely necessary.

The series of eight questions noted within question 4 on the recommended history form (Fig. 1) were designed to screen for the majority of cardiovascular problems. It is highly recommended that each of these questions be reviewed with the athlete to ensure that the athlete fully understood the questions and answered truthfully. A positive response to any of these questions may require more extensive questioning and should raise a red flag to direct the cardiovascular exam and possible further diagnostic testing. Exertional syncope may be indicative of hypertrophic cardiomyopathy, arrhythmias or conduction system abnormalities, or valvular pathology such as aortic stenosis. Although rare in athletes under the age of 30 in the absence of familial hyperlipidemia, atherosclerotic heart disease may be revealed by exertional chest pain. Chest pain may also indicate anomalous coronary arteries or mitral valve prolapse and frequently is the presenting symptom for exercise-induced asthma. Dizziness or palpitations may signify arrhythmias or conduction system abnormalities such as Wolff-Parkinson-White syndrome. Most frequently, the question regarding dizziness elicits an affirmative response in athletes with heat-related disorders. A history of previous high blood pressure or heart murmur is generally self-explanatory but may direct the physician to ask further questions about family history or any previous diagnostic evaluation. And finally, a family history of sudden cardiac death is pertinent, as several of the causes of sudden death (e.g., hypertrophic cardiomyopathy, Marfan's syndrome, and prolonged QT syndrome) have a familial component.

The cardiovascular portion of the physical examination should include blood pressure measurement—with the appropriate cuff size—and repeat measurements if the initial measurement is elevated. Recall that hypertension was the most common reason for restricting an athlete's participation in sports, and therefore, accurate blood pressure readings must be obtained, using caution both to prevent the hypertensive athlete from being overlooked and to prevent the normotensive athlete from being labeled hypertensive. Classification of hypertension by age has been outlined,[22,29] but a simple rule of thumb is that blood pressure greater than 125/75 in those younger than 10 years and greater than 135/85 in those older than 10 years requires further evaluation by the athlete's physician prior to clearance for participation.[17] The vital signs should include palpation of the radial pulse, but it is also highly recommended that the physician simultaneously check the femoral pulse as a simple screen for coarctation of the aorta.

Auscultation of the heart should be performed in two positions, preferably supine and standing, to increase the sensitivity of differentiating benign functional murmurs from pathologic murmurs such as hypertrophic cardiomyopathy and aortic stenosis. A careful assessment of heart sounds and the timing of any murmurs relative to those heart sounds also is important. Furthermore, various maneuvers such as Valsalva, deep inspiration, and squat-to-stand may assist the physician in differentiating murmurs.[14] Although benign functional murmurs are common in adolescents, it is of paramount importance to be certain that a murmur is indeed functional. If any question remains, then referral to a cardiologist is necessary prior to clearance for participation in sports. And finally, arrhythmias noted on auscultation require electrocardiographic evaluation to identify the arrhythmia and exclude structural heart disease even though disappearance of ectopic beats with exercise usually indicates a benign condition.

Musculoskeletal Assessment

The primary goal of musculoskeletal screening in the PPE is to identify orthopedic or rheumatologic disorders that may limit athletic participation or predispose the athlete to further injury or complications. It is rare for a musculoskeletal problem to preclude an athlete's participation but fairly common to identify a problem that may need rehabilitation or further evaluation.[18] Question 11 on the history form (Fig. 1) should be reviewed specifically with the athlete, and it is recommended that physicians follow the question with "Do you currently have any pain or swelling of any joints?" It is the author's opinion that that follow-up question may identify a nontraumatic orthopedic condition (e.g., an overuse syndrome such as chondromalacia patella or rotator cuff tendinitis) or rheumatologic condition (e.g., juvenile rheumatoid arthritis), which the athlete may have ignored because it was not severe enough to limit activity but which may require further evaluation or rehabilitation.

Any affirmative answers to the aforementioned musculoskeletal history questions necessitate a complete exam of that particular joint or area in addition to the general musculoskeletal screening exam outlined in Table 4. This screening exam was designed to identify musculoskeletal conditions that may limit athletic participation, predispose the athlete to injury, or require further evaluation or rehabilitation prior to clearance, but it certainly may be expanded to be more sport specific if the physician chooses.[13] For example, for athletes involved in a throwing or "overhead" sport, an exam of the shoulder for range of motion, joint laxity, and rotator cuff and scapular stabilizer strength could be performed. If any anatomic abnormalities or functional limitations are noted on the musculoskeletal screening exam despite a negative history, then a more detailed exam is essential.

A final thought regarding the musculoskeletal screening exam: an athlete's ability to complete these screening tests assumes an intact neurologic system. Should there be any findings referable to the neurologic system (e.g., radiculopathy with waist flexion or inability to stand on toes or heels), however, then a more complete neurologic assessment is necessary.

***TABLE 4.* Musculoskeletal Screening Examination**

Position/Functional Motion	Observation
1. Patient facing examiner	Symmetry of upper and lower extremities and trunk
2. Neck flexion, extension, right and left lateral flexion and rotation	Cervical spine range of motion
3. Resisted shoulder shrug	Trapezius strength
4. Resisted shoulder abduction	Deltoid strength
5. Shoulder internal and external rotation with arms 90 degrees abducted	Glenohumeral range of motion
6. Elbow flexion and extension	Elbow range of motion
7. Elbow and wrist pronation and supination with arms adducted at side and elbows 90 degrees flexed	Elbow and wrist range of motion
8. Making a fist, then spreading fingers	Hand and finger range of motion
9. Patient facing away from examiner	Symmetry of upper and lower extremities and trunk
10. Back flexion with knees straight	Thoracic and lumbosacral vertebral spine motion/curvature and hamstring flexibility
11. Lower extremity examination with patient facing examiner, then contraction of quadriceps simultaneously	Alignment of lower extremities and symmetry of muscle tone
12. Squat and "duck walk" 4 steps	Hip, knee, and ankle motion and general lower extremity strength and balance
13. Patient standing on toes (facing away from examiner) and then heels (facing examiner)	Calf muscle symmetry, leg strength, and balance

Adapted from *Preparticipation Physical Evaluation* monograph, AAFP, AAP, AMSSM, AOSSM, AOASM, pp. 21–29, 1992, with permission.

ROUTINE SCREENING TESTS

The use of screening laboratory, radiographic, and cardiovascular tests in the PPE has been the subject of much discussion and controversy. Currently, the use of routine laboratory tests for the screening of young athletes in the PPE is not recommended,[6,17] because the value of such proposed tests as urinalysis, complete blood count, chemistry profile, lipid assay, and ferritin level is unproven.[8,17,23,27,31] Likewise, extensive cardiovascular testing for routine screening in the PPE is not recommended,[1,17] as this also is unproven.[9,15,17,19]

If the medical history or physical examination warrants further evaluation by laboratory, radiographic, or other diagnostic testing, then such should certainly be performed. The athlete with poor eating habits, fatigue, performance decline, or excessive menstrual bleeding requires a complete blood count and possibly a ferritin level to exclude anemia or nonanemic hypoferritinemia. With a family history of premature atherosclerotic heart disease, an athlete should be screened for familial hyperlipidemia with a lipid profile. An example of when urinalysis is warranted would be the athlete with a family history of polycystic kidney disease with or without symptoms of flank pain, recurrent urinary tract infections, or hematuria. Cervical spine radiographs are indicated in athletes with recurrent burners/stingers (i.e., cervical nerve root or brachial plexus neurapraxia) to exclude cervical spinal stenosis. And a final example of the use of further tests warranted by findings in the history or physical exam is the athlete with exertional syncope, who would require an electrocardiogram, echocardiogram, and exercise stress test to exclude hypertrophic cardiomyopathy, arrhythmias, and conduction system abnormalities such as Wolff-Parkinson-White syndrome.

Although an answer is beyond the scope of this chapter, one other question is frequently asked in discussion of the use of screening tests in the PPE, and that is whether to routinely screen athletes for human immunovirus (HIV) and illegal drug use. Because this question elicits a multifaceted response involving medical, legal, ethical, and confidentiality issues, an answer acceptable to all involved (i.e., athletes, coaches, school administrators, health care providers) is not possible. However, it is this author's opinion that these two tests should not be performed as routine screening tools unless the medical history or physical exam indicates their necessity. If HIV or drug screening tests are performed, the physician should have a definite plan for utilizing the information with a view toward initiation of a treatment plan while ensuring confidentiality.

CLEARANCE FOR PARTICIPATION

After assimilating the information gathered from the medical history, the physical examination, and any diagnostic tests, the physician must determine an athlete's clearance status for sports participation. Physicians involved in clearance determinations should first be familiar with the demands of the sport the athlete anticipates participating in. These have been categorized in Table 5 based on the amount of contact as well as on intensity of exercise. If a particular sport is not listed in the table, then the physician should determine the category in which the sport may fall by comparing its physical demands and injury potential with similar sports.

Keeping in mind that the PPE is not meant to exclude athletes from participation but rather to enable them to compete safely, the physician should ask several questions when considering clearance for an identified problem:

1. Will this problem increase the athlete's risk of morbidity or mortality?
2. Will other participants be at increased risk of morbidity if this athlete is allowed to participate?
3. Will further evaluation, treatment, and/or rehabilitation allow full participation, and, while these are initiated, can the athlete participate in limited activities?
4. If the problem precludes full, unrestricted participation, can the athlete be cleared for participation in limited activities?

Because it is impossible to set rigid guidelines for clearance determinations, the physician must assess each situation individually. However, specific guidelines regarding cardiovascular abnormalities may be found in "16th Bethesda Conference: Cardiovascular Abnormalities in the Athlete: Recommendations Regarding Eligibility for Competition."[21] Furthermore, the general guidelines shown in Table 6 have been established by the American Academy of Pediatrics Committee on Sports Medicine's "Recommendations for Participation in Competitive Sports"[2] and may assist the physician in determining clearance for sports.

As noted on the bottom of the physical exam form (Fig. 2), clearance determinations can be categorized as follows: 1. unresticted clearance, 2. clearance after completion of specific evaluation and/or rehabilitation, 3. no clearance for the categories of sports noted.

Communication about any restrictions from participation and/or recommendations for further evaluation, treatment, or rehabilitation to the athlete and parent is of utmost importance. With the athlete's permission, this information may also be communicated to the coach. The use of a written record of the

***TABLE 5.* Classification of Sports**

Contact		**Noncontact**		
Contact/collisionous	*Limited contact/impact*	*Strenuous*	*Moderately strenuous*	*Nonstrenu-*
Boxing Field hockey Football Ice hockey Lacrosse Martial arts Rodeo Soccer Wrestling	Baseball Basketball Bicycling Diving Field (high jump, pole vault) Gymnastics Horseback riding Skating (ice, roller) Skiing (cross-country), downhill, water) Softball Squash/handball Volleyball	Aerobic dance Crew Fencing Field (discus, javelin, shot put) Running/track Swimming Tennis Weight lifting	Badminton Curling Table tennis	Archery Golf Riflery

From American Academy of Pediatrics, Committee on Sports Medicine: Recommendations for participation in competitive sports. Pediatrics 81:737–739, 1988, with permission.

TABLE 6. Recommendations for Participation in Competitive Sports

	Contact/ Collision	Limited Contact/ Impact	Noncontact		
			Strenuous	Moderately Strenuous	Nonstrenuous
Acute illnesses * Needs individual assessment, e.g., contagiousness to others, risk of worsening illness	*	*	*	*	*
Atlantoaxial instability * Swimming; no butterfly, breast stroke, or diving starts	No	No	Yes*	Yes	Yes
Cardiovascular					
Carditis	No	No	No	No	No
Hypertension					
Mild	Yes	Yes	Yes	Yes	Yes
Moderate	*	*	*	*	*
Severe	*	*	*	*	*
Congenital heart disease * Needs individual assessment † Patients with mild forms can be allowed a full range of physical activities; patients with moderate or severe forms, or who are postoperative should be evaluated by a cardiologist before athletic participation.	†	†	†	†	†
Eyes					
Absence or loss of function of one eye	*	*	*	*	*
Detached retina * Availability of American Society for Testing and Materials (ASTM)-approved eye guards may allow competitor to participate in most sports, but this must be judged on an individual basis. † Consult ophthalmologist	†	†	†	†	†
Inguinal hernia	Yes	Yes	Yes	Yes	Yes
Kidney: Absence of one	No	Yes	Yes	Yes	Yes
Liver: Enlarged	No	No	Yes	Yes	Yes
Musculoskeletal disorders * Needs individual assessment	*	*	*	*	*
Neurologic					
History of serious head or spine trauma, repeated concussions, or craniotomy	*	*	Yes	Yes	Yes
Convulsive disorder					
Well controlled	Yes	Yes	Yes	Yes	Yes
Poorly controlled * Needs individual assessment † No swimming or weight lifting ‡ No archery or riflery	No	No	Yes†	Yes	Yes‡
Ovary: Absence of one	Yes	Yes	Yes	Yes	Yes
Respiratory					
Pulmonary insufficiency	*	*	*	*	Yes
Asthma * May be allowed to compete if oxygenation remains satisfactory during a graded stress test	Yes	Yes	Yes	Yes	Yes
Sickle cell trait	Yes	Yes	Yes	Yes	Yes
Skin: Boils, herpes, impetigo, scabies * No gymnastics with mats, martial arts, wrestling or contact sports until not contagious	*	*	Yes	Yes	Yes
Spleen: Enlarged	No	No	No	Yes	Yes
Testicle: Absence or undescended * Certain sports may require protective cup.	Yes*	Yes*	Yes	Yes	Yes

From American Academy of Pediatrics, Committee on Sports Medicine: Pediatrics 81:737–739, 1988, with permission.

communication, such as a separate form similar to the one at the bottom of the physical exam form, is highly recommended. Medical documentation in the PPE is just as important as any other medical record keeping is, and therefore the physician should ensure accuracy and confidentiality. For this reason, if the school requires a copy of the medical history, physical exam, and clearance form, the physician should keep the original in the patient's medical chart, send copies to the school, and ask the school to keep the information in a confidential file (e.g., in the school nurse's office).

An additional medicolegal consideration beyond accurate and confidential medical record keeping is the effect that the federal Rehabilitation Act and Americans with Disabilities Act may have on team physicians and/or schools that restrict athletes from participation in competitive sports due to a medical condition. Recent interpretations of these federal acts state that individuals have the legal right to participate in any activity they choose regardless of their medical condition. For this reason, physicians are not permitted to exclude an athlete from participation but rather are allowed only to recommend the athlete not participate due to a medical condition that may increase risk of further injury and/or death as a result of participation.[11] In these situations, the use of an exculpatory waiver, though controversial, may become more common. An exculpatory waiver is based on assumption of risk and is a release executed by the "patient" (athlete) or parent that releases a physician from liability for negligence.[11] Physicians involved in PPEs of adolescent athletes must be aware that an exculpatory waiver is a form of contract, and therefore minors may not execute such an instrument independent of their parent.

Because a thorough discussion of frequently encountered medical conditions, musculoskeletal disorders, and clearance recommendations is beyond the scope of this chapter and has been detailed in the educational monograph *Preparticipation Physical Evaluation*,[17] cited earlier, it is highly recommended that physicians involved in performing PPEs on a regular basis who have further interest and/or questions refer to that monograph for assistance in determining an individual's clearance for athletic participation.

SUMMARY

Physicians involved in the care of young athletes have a certain responsibility that frequently begins with the PPE. A thorough, yet sport-specific, evaluation will help maintain the health and safety of athletes by determining their readiness to participate in training and competition. It also offers the chance to identify medical conditions that may limit competition or predispose to injury or illness. It is an opportunity both to evaluate health-risk behaviors and to counsel on health-related issues. It certainly must meet legal and insurance requirements and may go as far as determining fitness and performance levels.

The PPE should be done at least six weeks before the competitive season to allow adequate time to fully evaluate, treat, and/or rehabilitate any medical conditions or injuries that are identified. Depending on the setting in which physicians practice, the PPE may be performed in the office or in an organized, mass screening station format, as there are advantages and disadvantages to each. A complete entry-level evaluation with subsequent annual, limited reevaluations is suggested and is most effective if the athlete returns to the same physician for the reevaluation or if the initial complete evaluation record is available. The reevaluation should focus on a complete review of the medical history with attention to the cardiovascular system and any interim medical illnesses or injuries.

Routine screening laboratory, radiographic, and cardiovascular tests are not recommended, but certainly, if the medical history or physical examination indicates a need for specific screening or diagnostic testing, such should be performed prior to clearing the athlete for participation.

After assimilating the information elicited from the history, the physical examination, and any necessary screening or diagnostic tests, the physician must determine the athlete's clearance status for sports. It is not possible to adhere to a rigid set of guidelines, but rather, the physician must understand the demands of the sport and use established recommendations along with astute clinical judgment in each individual case to determine clearance status. If restrictions on an athlete's participation are imposed, the physician should not only allow but also encourage participation in alternative activities with less inherent risk of injury or illness.

In conclusion, the PPE should be more than a routine annual formality viewed by the athlete as a potential obstacle to participation in sports. Rather, it should be a positive experience in which the physician enables the athlete to participate safely in sports, thus opening the door for a trusting relationship and enhancing the medical care of young athletes.

REFERENCES

1. Ades PA: Preventing sudden death: Cardiovascular screening of young athletes. Physician Sportsmed 20(9):75–89, 1992.
2. American Academy of Pediatrics Committee on Sports Medicine: Recommendations for participation in competitive sports. Pediatrics 81:737–739, 1988.
3. American Medical Association: Evaluation of the Athlete: A Guide. Chicago, AMA, 1976.
4. Beasley A: Building better athletes: when even the fittest die (Sept. 4, pg. A1, A8, A9); Examining physicals: standards are absent (Sept. 5, pg. A1, A6, A7); They die because of ignorance (Sept. 6, pg. A1, A6, A7), Orlando Sentinel, Orlando, FL, 1988.
5. Commission on Public Health and Scientific Affairs, American Academy of Family Physicians: Athletic Competition Health Screening Form. Kansas City, MO, AAFP, 1984.

6. Committee on Sports Medicine and Fitness, American Academy of Pediatrics: Sports preparticipation exam. In Dyment PG (ed): Sports Medicine: Health Care for Young Athletes, 2nd ed. Elk Grove Village, IL, American Academy of Pediatrics, 1991.
7. Council on Scientific Affairs, American Medical Association: Ensuring the health of the adolescent athlete. Arch Fam Med 2:446–448, 1993.
8. Dodge WF, et al. Proteinuria and hematuria in schoolchildren: Epidemiology and early natural history. J Pediatr 88:327–347, 1976.
9. Epstein SE, Maron BJ. Sudden death and the competitive athlete: perspectives on preparticipation screening studies. J Am Coll Cardiol 7:220–230, 1986.
10. Feinstein RA, et al: A national survey of preparticipation physical examination requirements. Physician Sportsmed 16(5):51–59, 1988.
11. Gallup EM: Sports Medicine and the Law. A presentation to the Kansas City Sportsmedicine Roundtable, Kansas City, MO, March 4, 1993.
12. Goldberg B, et al: Preparticipation sports assessment: An objective evaluation. Pediatrics 66:736–745, 1980.
13. Kibler WB: The Sport Preparticipation Fitness Examination. Champaign, IL, Human Kinetics Publishers, 1990.
14. Lembo NJ, et al: Bedside diagnosis of systolic murmurs. N Engl J Med 318:1572–1578, 1988.
15. Lewis JF, et al: Preparticipation echocardiographic screening for cardiovascular disease in a large, predominantly black population of collegiate athletes. Am J Cardiol 64:1029–1933, 1989.
16. Lombardo JA: The preparticipation physical examination. Primary Care 11:3–21, 1984.
17. Lombardo JA, Robinson JB, Smith DM: Preparticipation Physical Evaluation. Kansas City, MO, American Academy of Family Physicians, American Academy of Pediatrics, American Medical Society for Sports Medicine, American Orthopaedic Society for Sports Medicine, American Osteopathic Academy of Sports Medicine, 1992.
18. Magnes SA, et al: What conditions limit sports participation? Physician Sportsmed 20(5):143–160, 1992.
19. Maron BJ, et al: Results of screening a large group of intercollegiate competitive athletes for cardiovascular disease. J Am Coll Cardiol 10:1214–1221, 1987.
20. McKeag DB: Preseason physical examination for the prevention of sports injuries. Sports Med 2:413–431, 1985.
21. Mitchell JH, Maron BJ, Epstein SE: Sixteenth Bethesda Conference: cardiovascular abnormalities in the athlete: recommendations regarding eligibility for competition. J Am Coll Cardiol 6:1186–1232, 1985.
22. National Heart, Lung, and Blood Institute: Report of the Second Task Force on Blood Pressure Control in Children—1987. Pediatrics 79:1–25, 1987.
23. Peggs JF, et al: Proteinuria in adolescent sports physical examinations. J Fam Pract 22:80–81, 1986.
24. Risser WL: Frequency of preparticipation sports examinations in secondary school athletes: Are the University Interscholastic League guidelines appropriate? Texas Med 81:35–39, 1985.
25. Smith DM, et al: The preparticipation evaluation. Primary Care 18:777–807, 1991.
26. Task Force on the Preparticipation Evaluation, American Medical Society for Sports Medicine, Middleton, Wisconsin: Personal communication.
27. Taylor WC, Lombardo JA: Preparticipation screening of college athletes: value of the complete blood count. Physician Sportsmed 18(6):106–118, 1990.
28. Tennant FS, et al: Benefits of preparticipation sports examinations. J Fam Pract 13:287–288, 1981.
29. The Fifth Report of the Joint National Committee on Detection, Evaluation, and Treatment of High Blood Pressure. National High Blood Pressure Education Program, National Heart, Lung, and Blood Institute, National Institutes of Health, October 30, 1992.
30. Van Camp SP: Sudden death in athletes. In Grana WA, Lombardo JA (eds): Advances in Sports Medicine and Fitness. Chicago, Year Book, 1988, pp 122–142.
31. Vehaskari VM, Rapola J: Isolated proteinuria: Analysis of a school-age population. J Pediatr 101:661–668, 1982.

2

Exercise Prescription and Cardiovascular Fitness Screening

Frank G. Yanowitz, M.D.

Public and professional interest in exercise training, physical fitness, wellness, and prevention has accelerated since the 1960s, creating an immense sports medicine industry with far-reaching economic and health-care implications. In 1980 the U.S. Department of Health and Human Services recommended that by 1990 all adults should participate in "exercise which involves large muscle groups in dynamic movement for periods of 20 minutes or longer, 3 or more days per week, and which is performed at an intensity of 60 percent or greater of and individual's cardiorespiratory capacity."[13] However, in spite of this increased interest and the wealth of data documenting the health benefits of exercise, fewer than 10% of the adult American population are exercising at this level.[19] Furthermore, fewer than 50 percent of adults exercise with intensity for more than 20 minutes a day, 3 or more days per week.[19]

The scientific evidence for the role of exercise and physical fitness in health maintenance and disease prevention continues to accumulate. The data are especially compelling for the prevention and management of coronary heart disease (CHD), the leading cause of death and disability in the United States.[9] Although studies of exercise in the primary prevention of coronary heart disease have been observational in design, a rigorous meta-analysis of 27 previously published cohort studies revealed a CHD risk reduction of 35–55% in physically active as compared to sedentary individuals.[3] In view of these data and taking into account the high costs and complexities of conducting randomized, placebo controlled exercise intervention studies, it is unlikely that more definitive scientific evidence on exercise training will be forthcoming. In addition to preventing the onset and progression of CHD, there are many other well documented health and physiologic benefits of exercise training (Table 1).[16] Together, these provide a strong argument for encouraging a life-long program of regular exercise.

The medical profession is beginning to recognize the important role of health promotion and disease prevention in controlling our nation's staggering health care costs. Nowhere is the saying "an ounce of prevention is worth a pound of cure" more applicable than in today's costly medical environment. Exercise is often considered to be the foundation of a program of "total" prevention. Thus, it is important that health care professionals working in prevention be knowledgable in exercise physiology and skilled in exercise prescription. This chapter discusses the principles of exercise prescription and screening for exercise programs. Current recommendations and guidelines published by the American College of Sports Medicine (ACSM) and other national organizations are considered, with an emphasis on practical applications of these guidelines for office practitioners.

EXERCISE PHYSIOLOGY

Although there are many components to total fitness (Table 2), this chapter is primarily concerned with the prescription of physical activity to improve **cardiorespiratory endurance,** the one fitness component likely to have an impact on cardiovascular health.[9] During dynamic isotonic exercise, oxygen is taken in by the lungs and transported by the cardiovascular system in increasing amounts to the exercising skeletal muscles. The oxygen is taken up by the muscle mitochondria and used to generate molecules of adenosine triphosphate (ATP) needed to energize the muscle contractile apparatus.[2] This *aerobic* process, called *oxidative phosphorylation,* provides the major source of chemical energy needed for sustained exercise activities. The carbon dioxide produced during aero-

TABLE 1. Health Benefits of Exercise Training

Physiologic Benefits
1. Increase in cardiorespiratory functional capacity
2. Reduced heart rate and blood pressure for given work load
3. Improved efficiency of myocardial work
4. Improved myocardial vascularization
5. Increased capillary density in skeletal muscles
6. Increased aerobic enzyme activity in skeletal muscles
7. Increased muscle strength
8. Improved structure and function of ligaments, tendons, and joints

Psychological Benefits
1. Increased sense of well-being
2. Improved mood, self-esteem, and work behavior
3. Reduced risk of developing depression
4. Reduction of depression and improved adaptations to stress

Disease-Related Benefits
1. Prevention and/or treatment of atherosclerosis
2. Prevention and/or treatment of hypertension
3. Reduction in obesity
4. Improved glucose tolerance (reduced insulin resistance) in diabetes mellitus
5. Improvement in blood lipid abnormalities (HDL/LDL ratios)
6. Reduced bone loss in osteoporosis
7. Antiarrhythmic effect due to reduced catecholamine levels
8. Antithrombotic effects due to enhanced fibrinolysis

TABLE 2. Components of Total Fitness

Health Related	Skill Related
1. Cardiorespiratory Endurance	1. Agility
2. Muscular Endurance	2. Balance
3. Muscle Strength	3. Coordination
4. Body Composition	4. Speed
5. Flexibility	5. Power
	6. Reaction Time

bic metabolism is transported in the reverse direction and eliminated by the lungs. The Fick equation represents the relationship of parameters in this sequence of events. At rest, the Fick equation for oxygen can be expressed as follows:

$$\dot{V}O_2 = \dot{Q} \times (CaO_2 - C\bar{v}O_2)$$

or

$$\dot{V}O_2 = (SV \times HR) \times (CaO_2 - C\bar{v}O_2)$$

where $\dot{V}O_2$ is the oxygen uptake (ml O_2/min), $\dot{Q}$ is the cardiac output (L/min), SV is the stroke volume (L), HR is the heart rate (bpm), CaO_2 is the arterial O_2 content (ml O_2 per L of blood) and $C\dot{\bar{v}}O_2$ is the mixed venous O_2 content. The term "$\dot{Q} \times CaO_2$" represents the quantity of oxygen transported to the tissues per minute. The term "$CaO_2 - C\bar{v}O_2$" is also called the a-$\bar{v}$ O_2 content difference and represents the amount of oxygen used by the tissues each minute. Oxygen uptake is often normalized for body weight and expressed in ml O_2/kg/min. One *metabolic equivalent,* or 1 MET, is the body's resting oxygen requirement in the sitting position and equals 3.5 ml O_2/kg/min.

Figure 1 illustrates the parameters of the Fick equation at rest, during several submaximal workloads, and at maximal exercise in a normal subject before and after an exercise training program.[11] Several important observations can be made from these relationships: (1) the $\dot{V}O_2$ response to exercise is linear until maximal $\dot{V}O_2$ is achieved; in many individuals there is a plateau near maximal exercise beyond which the $\dot{V}O_2$ does not change; (2) the SV response is curvilinear, increasing early in exercise with little change thereafter; (3) the heart rate response is linear up to a maximal heart rate which is approximately equal to "220 - age"; and (4) the a-$\bar{v}$ O_2 content difference widens during exercise as

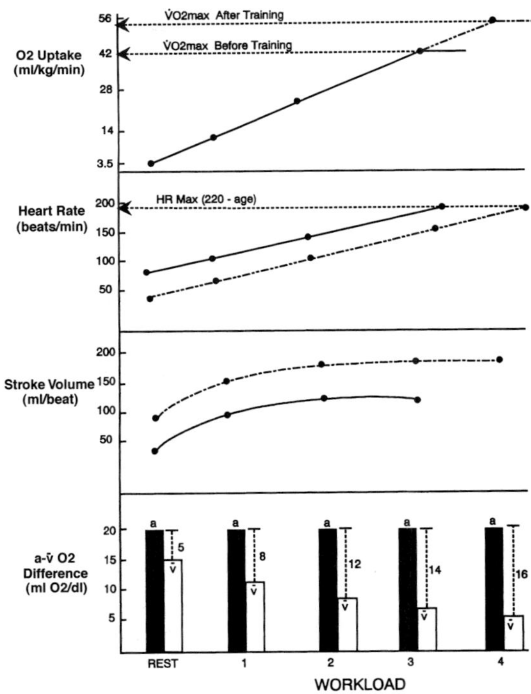

FIGURE 1. Hemodynamic response to incremental work exercise testing before and after an exercise training program. Solid lines indicate VO_2, heart rate, and stroke volume responses to progressive stages of exercise before training. Dashed lines represent the after-training responses. The a-v O_2 difference is represented by the difference in heights of the vertical bars. Workload 3 represents the maximal workload achieved before training; workload 4 is the maximal workload after training.

the mixed venous O_2 content decreases; arterial O_2 content does not change in normal subjects. The adaptive changes resulting from exercise training are also illustrated in Figure 1 and are further discussed below.

During an incremental exercise activity an increasing percentage of the oxygen uptake is redistributed to the exercising muscles until maximal exercise is reached. The Fick equation at maximal exercise,

$$\dot{V}O_{2max} = (SV_{max} \times HR_{max}) \times (CaO_{2max} - C\bar{v}O_{2min}),$$

reflects the maximal ability of the body to *take in, transport,* and *use* oxygen; this defines a person's *functional aerobic capacity*. $\dot{V}O_{2max}$ has become the "gold standard" laboratory measure of cardiorespiratory fitness. It is usually measured or estimated during treadmill or cycle ergometer exercise testing. Estimations of $\dot{V}O_{2max}$ are made from the maximal workload achieved during exercise testing and are reasonably accurate for routine assessments of functional capacity. Values of $\dot{V}O_{2max}$ normalized for body weight (ml O_2/kg/min) can be used to classify cardiorespiratory fitness in men and women based on age (Table 3).[12]

Exercise training results in several important adaptations in the Fick parameters that improve the body's efficiency during work. As seen in Figure 1, at every level of submaximal exercise (and cardiac output) the trained person is able to perform that work with a lower heart rate and greater stroke volume than before training. The lower heart rate response to submaximal exercise is also associated with a lower systolic blood pressure. Since the *double product* or *rate-pressure product* (HR × systolic BP) during exercise is a major determinant of myocardial oxygen needs,[15] this adaptation to exercise training improves the efficiency of cardiac work. In healthy individuals, increases in stroke volume during exercise are due to several factors: (1) increased ventricular diastolic size (preload); (2) decreased peripheral vascular resistance (afterload); and (3) improved contractility, which results in a greater ejection fraction. These adaptive changes in cardiac structure and function are called the *central adaptations* to exercise training.

There are also *peripheral adaptations* to exercise training which are reflected by an increased a-$\bar{v}$ O_2 content difference at maximal exercise (Fig. 1). Oxygen extraction by skeletal muscle fibers depends on a number of factors including exercise intensity, capillary density, maximal arteriolar vasodilatory capacity, and aerobic enzyme activity within the muscle mitochondria.[14] Exercise training results in increased density of capillaries within the muscle fibers, thus improving oxygen delivery per unit of muscle fibers. In addition, important increments in mitochondrial enzymes and mitochondrial size enable greater oxidative capacity of trained skeletal muscles. Approximately 50 percent of the increase $\dot{V}O_{2max}$ with training is accounted for by these peripheral adaptations.[4] In cardiac patients, moreover, peripheral adaptations often account for a greater percentage of aerobic benefits since the central adaptations are often limited by the compromised heart function.

Figure 2 summarizes the various factors that have both positive and negative effects on the Fick equation parameters that determine $\dot{V}O_{2max}$. In particular, functional aerobic impairment, or an abnormally low $\dot{V}O_{2max}$, can result from any factor or combination of factors that reduces maximal heart rate, maximal stroke volume, maximal arterial O_2 content, or maximal a-$\bar{v}$ O_2 content difference. Diseases of the lungs and skeletal muscles as well as hematologic disorders often have a profound effect on $\dot{V}O_{2max}$. An understanding of these various interactions is an important prerequisite to unraveling the many causes of exercise intolerance and differentiating various disease factors from those related to deconditioning and sedentary lifestyles.

To illustrate further the parameters of the Fick equation at rest and during exercise, Table 4 contrasts four hypothetical 30-year-old subjects: a world class athlete, a trained normal, a sedentary normal, and a post-MI patient with mild congestive heart failure (CHF).[21] These four subjects are compared at rest, during submaximal exercise, and at maximal exercise. The data illustrate important differences between sedentary and trained persons as

TABLE 3. **Physical Fitness Standards for Men and Women[12]**

	$\dot{V}O_{2max}$ (ml O_2/kg/min)*				
Age (yrs)	**Low**	**Fair**	**Average**	**Good**	**High**
MEN					
20–29	33.8	38.5	42.4	45.7	51.1
30–39	32.3	37.4	41.0	45.3	49.6
40–49	29.4	35.2	38.7	42.9	49.6
50–59	25.1	31.6	35.2	38.1	45.3
60–69	22.4	28.0	31.1	35.2	41.0
70–79	19.3	23.9	28.0	32.3	38.1
WOMEN					
20–29	28.0	31.6	35.2	39.5	44.3
30–39	25.1	30.2	33.8	36.7	41.0
40–49	23.7	28.0	30.9	33.8	38.5
50–59	22.2	25.1	28.0	30.9	35.2
60–69	19.5	23.7	25.8	28.2	32.3
70–79	19.3	22.2	25.3	29.4	32.5

*Data from Cooper Clinic Coronary Risk Factor Profile Charts,[12] Poor = 10th Percentile; Fair = 30th Percentile; Average = 50th Percentile; Good = 70th Percentile; High = 90th Percentile.

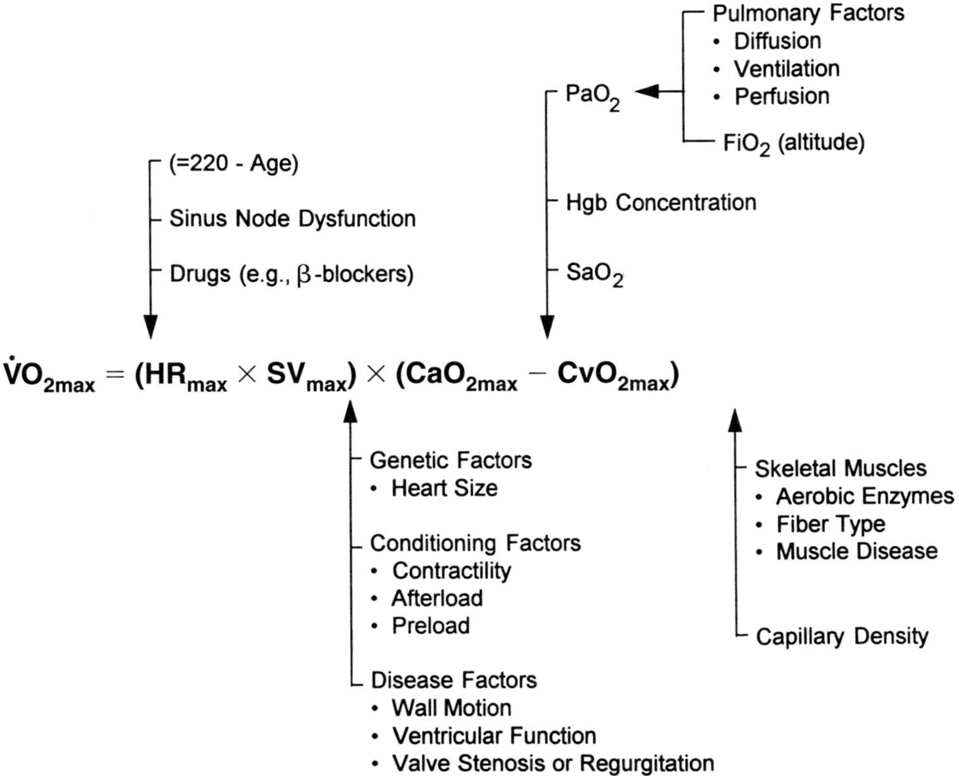

FIGURE 2. Determinants of $\dot{V}O_{2max}$ based on factors that influence the parameters of the Fick equation.

well as the more serious functional consequences of congestive heart failure.

At rest all four subjects have the same $\dot{V}O_2$ (normalized for body weight), the same cardiac output, and the same a-$\bar{v}$ O_2 content difference and oxygen utilization. Major differences, however, are seen in the two components that determine cardiac output. The world class athlete has the greatest stroke volume and slowest heart rate, while the other three subjects have progressively smaller stroke volumes and faster heart rates. End-diastolic volumes (EDV), end-systolic volumes (ESV), and ejection fractions (EF) also reflect these differences. The physiologic interpretation of these *central adaptations* to exercise training is that the resting cardiac output in trained individuals is more a function of a large stroke volume and is less dependent on heart rate. This implies an improved efficiency of cardiac work, since heart rate is a greater determinant of myocardial oxygen requirements than stroke volume. In sedentary individuals and in heart failure patients the lower stroke volumes necessitate higher heart rates and myocardial O_2 utilization to maintain the resting cardiac output. During submaximal exercise (e.g., 5 METS), the similarities and differences in Fick parameters measured in the four subjects are maintained (Table 4).

At maximal exercise significant differences are seen in all parameters of the Fick equation (Table 4). The wide range in $\dot{V}O_{2max}$ values reflects differences in cardiorespiratory endurance and the different maximal workloads achieved by each subject. Although heart rates are similar for the three normal subjects ($HR_{max} \approx 220$ - age in years), the patient with CHF has a lower maximal heart rate for reasons that are not entirely clear. The stroke volumes are also significantly different at maximal exercise as are the maximal cardiac outputs and ejection fractions. Unlike the resting and submaximal exercise data, however, the maximal a-$\bar{v}$ O_2 content difference is greatest in the athlete and is progressively smaller in the other three subjects. These differences among normal subjects reflect the *peripheral adaptations* to exercise training. Increases in the number and size of skeletal muscle mitochondria as well as in their aerobic enzyme content are well known training effects.[2] In addition, exercise training results in a greater density of blood capillaries per unit mass of skeletal muscle. These changes enable aerobically trained individuals to extract and use more oxygen during exercise in order to achieve higher maximal workloads.

The post-MI patient with heart failure has an additional handicap during exercise which limits oxy-

TABLE 4. **Four Hypothetical Cases: All Age 30 Years**

	VO_2 (ml/kg/min)	Heart Rate (BPM)	EDV (ml)	ESV (ml)	SV (ml)	Q (l/min)	C_aO_2 (mlO_2/L)	C_vO_2 (mlO_2/L)	a-v O_2D (mlO_2/L)	Q x CaO_2 (mlO_2/min)	O_2 extract (%)
Resting Data											
World Class	3.5	45	190	54	136	6.1	200	160	40	1220	20
Trained Normal	3.5	55	160	50	110	6.1	200	160	40	1220	20
Sedentary Normal	3.5	70	150	63	87	6.1	200	160	40	1220	20
Heart Failure	3.5	90	160	92	68	6.1	200	160	40	1220	20
Submaximal Exercise @ 5 METS											
World Class	17.5	70	200	24	176	12.3	200	100	100	2460	50
Trained Normal	17.5	90	170	33	137	12.3	200	100	100	2460	50
Sedentary Normal	17.5	120	150	47	103	12.3	200	100	100	2460	50
Heart Failure	17.5	160	160	83	77	12.3	200	100	100	2460	50
Maximal Exercise											
World Class	80	190	200	16	184	35	200	40	160	7000	80
Trained Normal	56	190	170	33	137	26.1	200	50	150	5220	75
Sedentary Normal	35	190	150	57	93	17.7	200	60	140	3500	70
Heart Failure	21	175	170	93	77	13.5	200	90	110	2680	60

EDV = end-diastolic volume; ESV = end-systolic volume; SV = stroke volume; Q = cardiac output; CaO_2 = arterial O_2 content; CvO_2 = mixed venous O_2 content; a-v O_2D = arterial-venous O_2 content difference gen extraction by the muscle fibers and maximal widening of the a-$\bar{v}$ O_2 difference. Patients with heart failure appear to have an impaired ability to maximally vasodilate during exercise, presumably because edema in the arteriolar wall limits the response to vasodilatory stimuli.[10] As a result, oxygen extraction and utilization is further compromised.

The preceding discussion is a brief introduction to cardiovascular exercise physiology to illustrate the beneficial adaptations of exercise training. Readers interested in the more in-depth reviews of exercise physiology will find an abundant literature on this subject.[2,4,12,14] The next section considers more practical aspects of screening for aerobic exercise training programs.

CARDIOVASCULAR FITNESS SCREENING

There are two main purposes in screening for cardiovascular fitness programs. The first is to evaluate health status to assess the safety of exercise and identify those at high risk for exercise-related complications. The second is to determine a fitness profile that can be used to develop an individualized exercise prescription. Although preexercise screening is usually done by primary care physicians and their professional staff, some patients may require additional studies by cardiovascular specialists.

Evaluation of Health Status

The American College of Sports Medicine (ACSM) continues to publish revised guidelines for exercise testing and prescription which provide extremely valuable information to health professionals who are evaluating individuals for exercise programs.[1] Exercise guidelines have also been published by the American Heart Association.[6] These guidelines offer explicit recommendations for assessing health status prior to initiating *vigorous* exercises activities. It is believed that most healthy adults can begin a gentle, slowly progressive exercise program, such as walking, without a formal medical examination or an exercise test[1].

Individuals who plan to begin an exercise program more vigorous than walking should have a current (within 2 years) medical evaluation including a medical history, physical examination, and laboratory tests.[1] Preexercise screening is primarily focused on detecting early coronary heart disease and other cardiopulmonary or metabolic abnormalities that might preclude vigorous unsupervised exercise. The evaluation is specifically designed to classify individuals into one of three risk categories:

***TABLE 5.* Major Coronary Risk Factors[1]**

1. Hypertension: Systolic BP ≥140 or diastolic BP ≥90 mm Hg on at least two occasions, or on antihypertensive medication.
2. Serum cholesterol ≥200 mg/dl
3. Cigarette smoking
4. Insulin dependent diabetes mellitus (≥ age 30, or for > 15 yrs duration) *or* noninsulin-dependent diabetes mellitus (≥ age 35)
5. Family history of premature coronary or other atherosclerotic disease (parents or siblings prior to age 55)

1. *Apparently healthy:* asymptomatic and apparently healthy persons with no more than one major coronary risk factor (Table 5)
2. *Higher risk:* individuals who have symptoms or signs suggestive of cardiopulmonary or metabolic diseases (Table 6) *or* those with two or more major coronary risk factors (Table 5).
3. *Disease:* individuals with known cardiac, pulmonary, or metabolic disease.

Apparently healthy individuals *at any age* can begin an exercise program of *moderate* intensity, such as walking, without the need for extensive medical screening or exercise testing as long as the program starts slowly, progresses gradually, and the person is taught to recognize unusual signs or symptoms (Table 6). The exercise activities should be well within the person's current capacity and remain within a comfortable range of intensities (i.e., 40 to 60% $\dot{V}O_{2max}$). If a person in this low-risk category is interested in participating in more vigorous exercise activities such as jogging, the ACSM guidelines recommend a more complete medical examination and a physician-supervised *maximal* exercise testing for men > age 40 and women > age 50. Submaximal exercise testing up to 75% of age-predicted maximal heart (i.e., 0.75 × "220-age") may be performed without physician supervision by appropriately trained personnel, although the use of such testing for the purpose of risk stratification and diagnosis of myocardial ischemia is questionable.

***TABLE 6.* Major Symptoms or Signs Suggestive of Cardiopulmonary or Metabolic Disease[1]**

1. Chest pain or discomfort suggestive of myocardial ischemia
2. Unusual dyspnea at rest or during mild exercise
3. Orthopnea or paroxysmal nocturnal dyspnea
4. Palpitations (irregular heart rhythms or tachycardias)
5. Dizziness or syncope
6. Ankle edema
7. Intermittent claudication
8. History of heart murmur or other cardiovascular diseases

Higher risk, symptomatic individuals and those with known cardiac, pulmonary, or metabolic disease should be strongly encouraged to undergo physician-supervised maximal exercise testing before starting a *vigorous* exercise program. Metabolic diseases include diabetes mellitus, thyroid disease, and liver and renal diseases. For those without symptoms or known disease, exercise testing is not necessary before starting a *moderate* exercise program as defined previously. Table 7 summarizes these ACSM guidelines for the different risk categories.[1]

Preexercise screening for sports participation and other vigorous exercise activities should rule out conditions associated with an increased incidence of sudden cardiac death. In individuals <35 years of age, hypertrophic cardiomyopathy and congenital heart lesions such as anomalous origin of a coronary artery are the most frequent causes of exercise-related sudden death.[8,18] These conditions often require careful auscultation of the heart and echocardiographic studies for definitive diagnosis. Hypertrophic cardiomyopathy is recognized clinically by a prominent apical impulse and a characteristic systolic ejection murmur which accentuates during the Valsalva maneuver and upon standing. The diagnosis is confirmed by echocardiography.

In older adults ischemic heart disease usually secondary to coronary atherosclerosis is the most common cause of exercise-related sudden cardiac death.[16] Minimal screening should include lifestyle and risk factor assessment, a careful review of symptoms paying particular attention to exercise-induced chest discomfort, dyspnea, palpitations or syncope, blood pressure and cardiovascular examination, and laboratory studies of glucose and blood lipids. Health professionals should be aware of the most recent recommendations of the National Cholesterol Education Program's Second Report on the Detection, Evaluation and Treatment of High Blood Cholesterol[5] and the Fifth Joint National Committee Report on the Detection, Evaluation, and Treatment of High Blood Pressure.[7] These valuable guidelines offer the most complete information on the management of individuals who are at high risk for CHD and its complications. Exercise testing, as discussed previously, should also be included for men ≥ aged 40 and women ≥ age 50.

Prescreening for elderly patients over age 65 should also focus on the peripheral circulation to identify patients with intermittent claudication, carotid bruits, and abdominal aortic aneurysms. Because coronary heart disease, and in particular silent myocardial ischemia, is common in elderly men and women, exercise testing is recommended for sedentary older people who wish to engage in vigorous physical activities. It is important for those testing the elderly to be aware of safety precautions and the various abnormalities that may occur during exercise in this population.[20] Guidelines for exercise testing laboratories and personnel have been published by the American Heart Association.[17] Patients should be given an opportunity to become familiar with the treadmill or bicycle ergometer activity at low workloads prior to the actual exercise test. Exercise testing protocols should be carefully tailored to the patient's usual level of physical activities.

TABLE 7. ACSM Recommendations for Maximal Exercise Testing Prior to Exercise Program[1]

Category	Maximal Test Needed?
Apparently Healthy	
Younger (Men ≤40; Women ≤50)	No
Older (moderate exercise)	No
Older (vigorous exercise)	Yes
Higher Risk (asymptomatic)	
Moderate exercise	No
Vigorous exercise	Yes
Higher Risk (symptomatic)	Yes
With Disease	Yes

THE EXERCISE PRESCRIPTION

The term *prescription* implies that a particular dosage is required to achieve specific therapeutic goals. If the dose is too small there will be an inadequate therapeutic response; if the prescribed dose is exceeded there is increased risk of toxic side effects. Exercise training is clearly a therapeutic intervention that requires careful dosing for some individuals, particularly those at high risk for cardiovascular complications. Even in the healthy population, excessive exercise training may lead to a variety of injuries which, although not life-threatening, can have a significant negative impact on continued exercise training.

There are five desirable features to incorporate in a well-designed exercise program: (1) the prescription should be *individualized* according to each person's needs and capabilities; (2) the exercise program should be structured to *improve or maintain functional capacity;* (3) the exercise activities should be *enjoyable* to ensure long-term compliance; (4) the program should promote health by reducing risk factors associated with the onset or progression of disease; and (5) the program should be designed to ensure the safety of the participant during the exercise activities. The individualized exercise prescription must be structured according to the interests of the participant, taking into consideration the person's overall health status and abilities.

Programs designed to reduce disease risk may be less intense than those structured to enhance cardiorespiratory functional capacity. For many individuals who are not interested in vigorous exercise, recommendations to increase their leisure time activities are often sufficient to attain many health-related benefits.

The five specific components to be addressed in the design of a structured exercise program are (1) type of exercise, (2) intensity, (3) duration, (4) frequency, and (5) mode of progression. The ACSM has developed explicit recommendations for each of the components that are applicable to all exercise prescriptions designed to enhance cardiorespiratory endurance.[1]

Type of Activity

The major requirements in selecting *aerobic* exercise activities are that they involve large muscle groups such as the legs in rhythmic and dynamic movements for a sustained period of time. Popular forms of outdoor exercise training include brisk walking, running or jogging, hiking, cycling, swimming, cross-country skiing, and skating. Indoor aerobic activities include aerobic dancing, rope skipping, swimming, and using treadmills, cycle ergometers, stair climbers, rowing machines, and cross-country ski devices. Beginners should choose an activity that can be easily sustained without variations in intensity and that does not require a great deal of skill. After 8–12 weeks and the development of conditioning, other more enjoyable activities may be substituted provided they meet the requirements of the prescription.

Intensity of Exercise

For cardiovascular conditioning to take place the intensity should exceed approximately 45–50% of a person's functional aerobic capacity (i.e., $\dot{V}O_{2max}$) and, for safety and comfort, not exceed 75–85%.[1] This usually translates to a heart rate training range of 55–90% of maximal heart rate.

Maximal heart rate can be estimated as "220-age" for apparently healthy men under age 40 and women under age 50. For older individuals and those with significant risk factors, symptoms, or disease manifestations (Table 5 and 6) a maximal exercise ECG test is recommended to screen for disease and determine the maximal heart rate for that person. This is especially important for those with known coronary heart disease and those taking heart-rate–lowering drugs (beta-blockers, some calcium channel blockers).

If an exercise test is performed, the recommended heart rate training range can be determined by plotting the linear relationship between exercise heart rate and exercise intensity measured in METs or $\dot{V}O_{2max}$ units. From this, the heart rates associated with a certain percentage of maximal exercise intensity, usually 45–85%, can be determined. Another common method for determining the heart rate training range is to use 70–85% of the measured or estimated maximal heart rate, which translates to approximately 60–80% of functional capacity. A third method is to take a percentage of the difference between resting and maximal heart rates and add that to the resting heart rate. For example, consider a resting heart rate of 60 bpm and a maximal heart rate of 180 bpm. Sixty percent of the difference in heart rates is 0.60×120 bpm, or 72 bpm; add this to 60 bpm to get 132 bpm, the lower heart rate limit for training. This corresponds to approximately 60% of that person's functional capacity. Eighty percent of the difference in heart rates is 96 bpm, which when added to resting heart rate is 156 bpm, the upper heart rate range and approximately 80% of functional capacity.

Regardless of which heart rate method is chosen, it is important to remember that the calculated training range is only a general guideline for exercise training. It also should be noted that this intensity range is quite broad, which allows for considerable flexibility in choice of exercise activities. Sedentary individuals, especially older adults and those with disease, should always begin at the lower end of the range in order to insure comfort, safety, and compliance to the exercise program. If the exercise is perceived as too strenuous or uncomfortable at the beginning of a program, it is unlikely that the program will be maintained for any length of time.

Exercise heart rates should be checked frequently during a beginning exercise program. This requires some practice in taking one's pulse, usually in the radial or carotid artery locations. Since it is often difficult to palpate the pulse during exercise, the pulse should be clocked for a period of ten seconds immediately after stopping the exercise activity, counting the first beat as "zero." Multiplying the 10-second count times 6 will estimate the minute heart rate. If this rate is below the prescribed training range, the intensity of exercise can be gradually increased; if the rate is above the range, the intensity should be reduced.

After the exercise program has become well established, frequent pulse checks are no longer necessary. The exerciser should be able to associate a certain perceived sense of exertion in the skeletal muscles and respirations with the prescribed training range. That perception becomes a substitute indicator of the intensity of effort. Most trained individuals know when they are below, within, or above the training heart rate range from their perception of how hard they are working. Once this relative perceived exertion has been learned the need for pulse checks is reduced, although it is recommended that occasional checks be obtained especially when exercising in unusual environmental conditions.

Duration of Exercise

To some extent the duration of an exercise session is inversely related to the intensity of effort for an equivalent training gain. If exercise activities are performed at the upper end of the prescribed heart rate range, the duration can be somewhat shorter. Beginning exercisers, however, should start out with a longer duration and lower intensity in order to maintain a level of comfort needed for enjoyment. The adage, "*train, don't strain*" is particularly important to emphasize in the early weeks of an exercise program.

There are several exercise duration strategies that can be prescribed for beginners. For someone who is quite limited because of age or disease, multiple short bouts of exercise (5–10 min) several times a day may be appropriate. Alternatively, 20–30 minutes of moderate-intensity exercise (i.e., 40–50% of functional capacity), exclusive of warm-up and cool-down, are recommended for most asymptomatic sedentary participants. The goal during the first months of an exercise training program is develop the exercise habit with a minimal risk for injury. Once physiologic adaptations take place, the duration and intensity can be increased appropriately based on the individual's personal goals and health status. Durations longer than 60 minutes per session are not necessary for developing or maintaining cardiorespiratory fitness. If symptoms of fatigue persist for one hour or longer after an exercise session, either the intensity, the duration, or both were excessive, and the subsequent sessions need to be adjusted accordingly.

Early in an exercise program it is a good idea to keep a log of exercise training sessions including time of day, heart rate responses, duration, distance, activities, and any unusual symptoms that occurred during or after exercising. Such a diary not only provides a psychological incentive to continuing an exercise program but also facilitates adjustments in training if necessary to improve the overall quality of the experience.

Frequency of Exercise

For most healthy adults exercising 3–5 days per week is sufficient. Beginning exercisers may prefer to workout every other day to allow for adequate rest needed to relieve muscle soreness that often accompanies weight-bearing exercises. For those who can sustain an exercise activity for only 5–10 minutes, exercising several times a day is recommended. In general, the more days a week a person exercises, the longer the duration of each session, and the higher the intensity, the more likely the development of unpleasant side effects that make it difficult to maintain compliance to the program.

Mode of Progression

A new exercise program involves three distinct phases: initial, improvement, and maintenance.[1] The rate of progression through these phases depends on functional capacity, age, health status, and particular needs or goals.

Most sedentary individuals require an initial phase lasting 4–6 weeks. During this period it is important to structure the exercise prescription to minimize discomfort. This is often a critical period for beginners, since a bad experience at the onset of a program may be detrimental to long-term adherence. As stated previously, a major goal during the transition from a sedentary to an active lifestyle is to develop a new and positively addicting exercise habit. This implies not only learning the various exercise activities but also restructuring daily routines to incorporate the exercise sessions. Activities during these initial weeks should include light calisthenics, gentle stretching exercises, and low intensity (40–50% $\dot{V}O_{2max}$) aerobic exercise. Duration should begin at 15–20 minutes per session, keeping the intensity on the low side of the target range by frequent heart rate checks.

During the improvement phase (4–6 months) the major physiologic adaptations to exercise training begin. The duration should be increased by about 3–5 minutes per session every few weeks until a total duration is reached which is compatible with the person's overall training goals. Increases in exercise intensity, measured by heart rate or perceived exertion, should occur when the duration of exercise can be sustained for at least 20 minutes, as long as the heart rate remains within the prescribed training range. Again, it is important to emphasize the need to progress slowly, especially for older and higher risk participants.

At the conclusion of the improvement phase the participant should have reached a level of cardiorespiratory fitness associated with long-term health benefits and optimal function. The final phase of the exercise program is designed to maintain these physiologic and other health benefits. It is during this phase that individuals may want to redefine their goals, incorporate more enjoyable activities or recreational games into their programs, and participate in competitive events. Also, by this time, the exercise program has become a routine with a high likelihood of long-term adherence. For maintenance of fitness it may not be necessary to exercise as long, frequently, or intensely as during the earlier phases of the program, although a minimum of three days per week, 30 minutes per session at the prescribed intensity, is recommended.

The Exercise Session

Regardless of which phase of exercise training, a typical exercise session should be structured to include warm-up, aerobic activities, and cool-down. Some individuals may also incorporate a strength training component if that is of particular interest. The exercise prescription for strength training, however, is not discussed in this chapter.

Warm-up should include light calisthenics, stretching, and activities similar to but lower in intensity than the aerobic exercises that have been selected in the exercise prescription. For example, if running is the desired aerobic activity, individuals should walk briskly for 5–10 minutes before beginning to run. Similarly, stationary cyclists should free-wheel for several minutes before increasing the workload on the cycle ergometer. The warm-up increases flexibility, which may minimize risk for musculoskeletal complications, and gradually increases the heart rate to the training range. Cool-down activities should follow the reverse sequence. This minimizes venous pooling in the lower extremities and enhances the overall sense of well-being associated with successful completion of the exercise session.

SUMMARY

This chapter has reviewed the principles of exercise prescription and screening for exercise programs. If exercise training is to have favorable outcomes in terms of cost-benefit effects on cardiovascular health and functional well-being, careful attention must be given by physicians and other health professionals to developing the most appropriate exercise prescription for each individual. This is particularly important in the sedentary, middle-aged and older segments of our population. There is an unfortunate tendency in our society to enthusiastically rush into new programs without careful preparation or knowledge of the skills required to safely carry out the activities of the program. With the increasing emphasis on wellness, health promotion, and disease prevention, health care professionals are becoming more involved in providing preventive services to their patients. There is now a great opportunity for promoting quality exercise programs that optimize the benefits and minimize the risks.

REFERENCES

1. American College of Sports Medicine: Guidelines For Exercise Testing and Prescription, 5th ed, Baltimore, Williams & Wilkins, 1995.
2. Astrand P, Rodahl K: Textbook of Work Physiology, 2nd ed. New York, McGraw-Hill, 1977.
3. Berlin JA, Colditz GA: A meta-analysis of physical activity in the prevention of coronary heart disease. Am J Epidemiol 132:612–28, 1990.
4. Clausen JP: Circulatory adjustments to dynamic exercise and effects of physical training in normal subjects and patients with coronary artery disease. Prog Cardiovasc Dis 18:459–95, 1976.
5. Expert Panel on Detection, Evaluation, and Treatment of High Blood Cholesterol in Adults: Summary of the second report of the National Cholesterol Education Program (NCEP) Expert Panel on Detection, Evaluation, and Treatment of High Blood Cholesterol in Adults. JAMA 269:3015–23, 1993.
6. Fletcher GF, Balady G, Froelicher VF, et al: Exercise standards. A statement for health professionals from the American Heart Association. Circulation 91:580–615, 1995.
7. Joint National Committee on Detection, Evaluation, and Treatment of High Blood Pressure: The fifth report of the Joint National Committee on Detection, Evaluation, and Treatment of High Blood Pressure (JNC V). Arch Intern Med 153:154–83, 1993.
8. Luckstead EF: Sudden death in sports. Pediatr Clin North Am 29:1355–62, 1982.
9. Manson JE, Tosteson H, Ridker PM, et al: The primary prevention of myocardial infarction. N Engl J Med 326:1406–16, 1992.
10. Mason DT, Zelis R, Longhurst J, Lee G: Cardiocirculatory responses to muscular exercise in congestive heart failure. Prog Cardiovasc Dis 19:475–489, 1976.
11. Mitchell JH, Blomqvist G: Maximal oxygen uptake. N Engl J Med 284:1018–1023, 1971.
12. Pollock ML, Wilmore JH: Exercise in Health and Disease, 2nd ed. Philadelphia, W.B. Saunders, 1990, pp 660–671.
13. Public Health Service: Promoting Health/Preventing Disease: Objectives for the Nation. Washington, DC, US Department of Health and Human Services, 1980.
14. Saltin B, Rowell LB: Functional adaptations to physical activity and inactivity. Fed Proc 39:1506–13; 1980.
15. Schlant RD, Sonneblick EH: Normal physiology of the cardiovascular system. In Hurst JW, et al: The Heart 7th ed, New York, McGraw-Hill, 1990, ch 3.
16. Simon HB: Exercise, health, and sports medicine. In Rubenstein E, Federmann DD (eds): Scientific American Medicine, New York, Scientific American, Inc., 1992.
17. Subcommittee on Rehabilitation Target Activity Group, American Heart Association: Standards for adult exercise testing laboratories. Circulation 59:421A–427A; 1979.
18. Tsung SH, Huang TY, Chang HH: Sudden death in young athletes. Arch Pathol Lab Med 106:168–78, 1982.
19. U.S. Preventive Services Task Force: Guide to Clinical Preventive Services: An Assessment of the Effectiveness of 169 Interventions. Baltimore, Williams & Wilkins, 1989.
20. Williams MA: Exercise Testing and Training in the Elderly Cardiac Patient. Human Kinetics Publishers, Champaign, IL, 1994, p 12.
21. Yanowitz FG: Functional exercise testing in chronic congestive heart failure. CARDIO April 1993.

3

Sports Nutrition

Kristin J. Reimers, M.S., R.D.
Jaime S. Ruud, M.S., R.D.
Ann C. Grandjean, Ed.D.

The role of the "team doc" grew into the discipline of sports medicine, the "pregame meal" into sports nutrition, and "focusing" into sports psychology. Sports science continues to change from an entity reliant on common sense, shared secrets, and trial and error to a field based on exercise physiology and biomechanics. The entire discipline of sports medicine continues to experience metamorphosis. Research and standards of practice have replaced conventional wisdom.

Like all aspects of sports medicine, sports nutrition continues to change. The "state" of sports nutrition currently lies somewhere between "tradition" and "prescription." Nutrition is scientifically grounded in biochemistry and physiology. Translation of nutrition principles into recommendations is strongly affected by psychological, physical, social, and environmental factors. As a result, nutrition for athletes will never be as straightforward as "take this pill" or "eat this bar."

Athletes need information on which to base food decisions. But just as important, they need the daily living skills necessary to keep food available despite erratic, hectic training schedules, school, work, and social life. Achieving a balanced nutrition program is difficult for the 8 to 5 office workers; it is often twice as difficult for the athlete.

Physicians are often in the position to provide answers to some of the sports nutrition questions frequently asked by athletes. "How much weight can I cut?" "Will iron supplements help my performance?" "Do I need to eat more protein to gain muscle?"

The focus of this chapter is on the fundamental components of an athlete's diet. To be meaningful, these components must be integrated into the life experiences, preferences, and schedule of the individual athlete.

ENERGY REQUIREMENTS OF ATHLETES

The energy requirement of an individual is defined as "the level of energy intake from food that will balance energy expenditure when the individual has a body size and composition, and level of physical activity, consistent with long-term good health; and that will allow for the maintenance of economically necessary and socially desirable physical activity".[149]

It is often assumed that athletes, by virtue of increased physical activity, have higher energy needs than their nonathlete counterparts. This may not be true in all cases, however.

Caloric requirements of athletes depend on body size, demands of the sport, training conditions, age, and nontraining activity level, with body size being the primary determinant. Energy demands vary greatly among sports, but almost any moderate sport can become one of high energy expenditure if it is continued in intensity for long enough. Energy expended for the same sport will vary; for example, energy expended riding a bicycle depends on the weight of the cyclist, the speed of the pace, and whether the bicycle is going uphill, downhill, or on level ground. The athlete's age, gender, and stage of maturation influence energy requirements. Adolescent males experiencing a growth spurt may double their energy requirements for a time. Although often not considered, the non-training activity of athletes also influences total calorie requirements.

As expected, surveys of male and female athletes participating in different sports show a wide range of energy intakes both between and within sport groups. In a review by Grandjean and Ruud, cyclists, triathletes, and basketball players reportedly had among the highest average daily energy intakes, ranging from 3533 to 5900 calories per day, and female gymnasts, dancers, and figure skaters had among the lowest energy intakes, ranging from 1174 to 1989 calories per day.[56]

Without sophisticated equipment, it is difficult, if not impossible, to determine the caloric requirement of an individual athlete, as two athletes of equal body size, body composition and age, involved in the same sport, and with similar training routines, may have caloric needs that differ significantly.

Our experience suggests that the most practical and perhaps most accurate means of determining total energy needs is by concurrently monitoring body weight and caloric intake. Energy balance is verified by a stable body weight, and thus consumption of calories equals requirement. If the athlete is consuming more calories than required, body weight will increase. A decrease in weight or an increase in height without a concurrent increase in weight signals a negative calorie balance.

WEIGHT LOSS

Rapid Weight Loss

Rapid weight loss, or "making weight," is a common practice in sports with weight classifications such as wrestling, judo, boxing, and weightlifting. The practice of making weight is an emotional and potentially divisive topic among parents, coaches, athletes, physicians, and other sports medicine professionals. Most physicians discourage the practice, warning young athletes about the potential health hazards.

The practice continues, however. It does appear that the practice of making weight is motivated by more than one purpose. One reason for propagation of the practices may be the belief among athletes and coaches that training at a heavier weight, then dropping weight right before competition, gives the athlete an edge. When asked "Why do you cut weight?", one All-American wrestler replied, "Because everybody does it. If one person does it, everybody else has to do it, too." Another reason may come purely from necessity. The weight classifications of wrestlers, for example, do not match the normal size distribution of young men. Thus, weight loss is one way for wrestlers to seize to spot on the varsity team.

Indeed, the practice is less of a peripheral artifact of certain sports; instead, it is an integral ritual of the sport. Does it create a psychological "high"? Does peer pressure start the cascade? The questions are many; the solution remains elusive.

Research examining the phenomenon of rapid weight loss on performance is equivocal. Some studies show reduced performance,[15,20,67,68,77,138,141] whereas others show no negative effect on performance.[2,47,73,122,126,130,139,143] The reason for the discrepancy probably lies in the duration and type of performance studied. The conclusion about the impact of making weight on performance appears to be that if weight loss does not exceed 5% total body weight and the parameter being measured is strength, rapid weight loss does not impair performance.

Statements, however, are frequently made regarding the effect of rapid weight loss on various parameters other than performance: development of eating disorders, growth delays, illness, and injury. Direct cause and effect of making weight on these variables has not been scientifically proved, however.

In an attempt to curtail the practice of making weight, it is sometimes suggested to these athletes that they achieve a gradual weight loss by moderately reducing caloric intake. While this method is ideal to achieve fat loss, many competitive athletes who make weight do not carry excess body fat, and the end result would not be fat loss, but lean tissue loss.

Gradual Weight Loss

If an athlete's goal is to maximize body fat loss while preserving lean body mass, gradual loss is recommended. This is achieved by creating a negative energy balance via increased energy expenditure with or without decreased caloric intake. Further increases in caloric expenditure may not be reasonable or desirable for the athlete already training several hours per day. On the other hand, if athletes are involved primarily in power or skill sports that may not require significant energy expenditure, increased aerobic activity may become necessary to achieve a negative energy balance. Reduced calorie intake is equally as critical, but must not be extended to the situation whereby energy is inadequate to support training. The appropriate calorie level will be determined primarily by the size and activity level of the athlete. The correctness of calorie intake is verified by weight loss of at least 0.5 lb, but usually no more than 2 lb per week, except in larger athletes.

Two types of athletes generally embark on weight loss. One type is obviously overly fat and needs to reduce fat for quickness and agility. Another is the athlete who is not really obese by conventional standards, but desires to lose body fat for aesthetic or performance purposes. Reducing body fat is known to improve performance for those required to move body mass through space, e.g., runners or jumpers. A very lean somatotype is expected and therefore often influences scoring in sports such as gymnastics and figure skating.

Athletes or their coaches may request from the physician a goal for body weight or body fat percentage. It is, however, challenging to provide such a number. For example, standard weight charts may not be applicable for athletes because of their above average lean body mass. Although assessing body fat percentage circumvents the above dilemma, no "ideal" body fat level for individuals in each sport exists. Somatotype, genetic predisposition, sport, position, expectations, and training requirements are critical factors in determining an optimal body fat level for an individual. A combination of factors may be used to determine the best weight or body composition for an individual athlete: performance, energy level, personal perception, and in females, menstrual status.

WEIGHT GAIN

The goal in gaining weight is to increase muscle mass, not fat. Muscle mass increases only after a sufficient period of progressive weight training. It cannot be increased by simply eating more food or more protein. Monitoring weight gain by using skinfold measurements along with scale weight will indicate the type of body weight being added. The rate of gain and location of added muscle mass, however will depend on the training program, gender, and somatotype of the athlete, as well as other genetic factors.

Whereas diet alone will not result in the desired gains, athletes engaged in an appropriate weight training program must also consume a diet that meets nutrient needs and provides the increased calories needed for growth. For some athletes, increasing calorie intake is difficult because increasing the size of meals may cause discomfort, especially if training takes place soon after eating. Additionally, the schedule of school, work, and training activities may make adding snacks or meals difficult. For most athletes the preferred solution is to increase intake at meals slightly and to include two to four snacks a day.

It is impossible to determine the exact number of calories needed by any one individual to increase muscle. Therefore, the first step is to increase food intake slightly and to monitor gains with routine weighings and skinfold measurements. An increase in weight, as measured on the scales, with a maintenance or decrease in fat-fold measurements will indicate a gain in muscle, whereas an increase in weight with an increase in fat-fold measurements indicates a gain in fat. Beware, however, that skinfold measurements taken during or immediately after a weightlifting session may be inaccurate due to blood engorgement and edema of the muscle.

PROTEIN

For centuries, athletes have believed in the power of protein to enhance athletic performance. Athletes in ancient Greece ate the meat of strong, swift animals they sought to emulate, and protein was once hypothesized to be the primary energy source for muscle. In more recent times, the pendulum has swung to a more conservative view of protein and performance. Many athletes' inquiries and dietary practices continue to focus on protein, however.

Questions remain regarding the role of protein in athletic performance, and research does suggest that some athletes require more protein than their sedentary counterparts. Two athlete populations that have been examined in terms of protein needs are endurance athletes and strength athletes.

Research shows that changes in protein metabolism occur with exercise. Prolonged exercise increases the oxidation of branched-chain amino acids (leucine, isoleucine, and valine), and under certain conditions, such as decreased muscle glycogen, total oxidation may become significant.[82,83,111]

Whereas data are not definitive on dietary protein requirements of endurance athletes, studies do indicate that these athletes need more than the Recommended Dietary Allowance (RDA) of 0.8 g/kg bw/d depending on the type, intensity and duration of exercise. Using nitrogen balance to estimate dietary protein requirements at three different protein intakes (0.6, 0.9, and 1.2 g/kg bw/d), Meredith et al.[91] reported that endurance exercise was associated with protein needs greater than 0.9 g/kg/d and that the minimum protein requirement to maintain positive nitrogen balance was 0.94 ± 0.5 g/kg/d, 17% higher than the RDA. Friedman and Lemon[51] found protein requirements to be 42 to 74% higher than the RDA (1.14 to 1.39 g/kg/d) for five well-trained endurance runners.

Strength athletes have historically made, and continue to make, efforts to consume high protein diets purportedly to support and promote muscle growth. Whether strength athletes require protein in excess of the RDA was the subject of a series of nitrogen balance and leucine turnover studies by Tarnopolsky et al[134,135,136]. This group concluded that protein requirements for trained strength athletes exceed those of sedentary controls by 98%; 1.76 vs. 0.89 g/kg/d, respectively. The balance of research to date suggests that protein requirements of strength athletes will vary depending on whether the athlete is conditioned or a novice, but most will meet protein requirements by consuming 1.5 to 2.0 g protein per/kg/bw.[81]

Perhaps more than any other factor, caloric intake has an impact on protein requirements, because a reciprocal relationship exists between protein and calories such that protein needs increase as calories decrease. The protein-sparing effect of calories, primarily in carbohydrate form, should be emphasized to athletes.

Physicians should encourage all athletes to eat sufficient carbohydrate, especially during periods of heavy training, not only to provide a protein-sparing effect but to also maintain hepatic and muscle glycogen stores.

CARBOHYDRATE

Athletes, coaches, and trainers are most aware of carbohydrate's role as an energy substrate for muscle tissue. More than fatty acids or amino acids, glucose is the most efficient energy source for humans. The essentiality of carbohydrate for athletic performance lies in the fact that glycogen is the primary source of energy for moderate to intense exercise.[24,80] Unlike fat or protein, carbohydrate stores within the body are severely limited. Approximately 400 g of carbohydrate are present in human muscle tissue and 70 g of carbohydrate are stored in liver tissue.[129] These carbohydrate stores of energy could be depleted during a marathon, triathlon, or other endurance activity. In comparison, only about 1% of the body's fat stores would potentially be depleted during such an activity.

Although the body stores of carbohydrate as muscle and liver glycogen are limited, the stores can be expanded through training and diet. For example, a trained athlete consuming a high carbohydrate diet may have twice as much glycogen as an untrained individual with equal muscle mass.[144] Training provides the adaptation allowing greater carbohydrate storage and dietary carbohydrate provides the only substrate for glycogenesis; both components are necessary to achieve increased glycogen availability.

Carbohydrate is second only to water in prolonging endurance exercise, thus, endurance athletes need to consume adequate dietary carbohydrate daily to replenish glycogen stores and to prevent diminished endurance capacity. It has been known for several decades that glycogen stores are a limiting factor in endurance exercise and that manipulation of glycogen stores can delay exhaustion in well trained athletes.[13,17,66,70] Studies have documented that cyclists or runners who consume carbohydrate and water are able to exercise for a longer period before exhaustion than those consuming only water.[32,34]

The ergogenic nature of carbohydrate is that of increasing capacity, not power nor intensity. A high carbohydrate diet will not make the athlete sprint faster, but may enable the athlete to run at a higher intensity for a longer period.[76,129,133,148]

Carbohydrate Requirements of Endurance Athletes

Training

For the endurance athlete, the athlete performing aerobically for more than 90 minutes per day, research suggests a daily consumption of approximately 10 g carbohydrate/kg bw/d will restore depleted glycogen within 24 hours.[1,79] For runners or cyclists who are training for shorter periods, e.g., 60 min/d, performance capabilities may be maintained at half that amount (5 g carbohydrate/kg bw/d) even though glycogen stores will be lower.[128]

Before Competition

The impact of manipulating timing and amount of carbohydrate consumption before and after endurance activity has received considerable attention by both scientists and athletes. Carbohydrate loading, the process of maximizing glycogen stores in the muscle by changing diet and exercise, was studied first in 1939.[24] Since then, a more conservative, safer and more effective method has been widely adapted. This method prescribes a diet high in carbohydrate in combination with tapering training to the point of complete rest the day before competition. For the athlete normally consuming 8 to 10 g carbohydrate/kg bw/d, diet does not need to change; training decreases will facilitate glycogen supercompensation.

Carbohydrate loading will only benefit athletes participating in sports that involve relatively high-intensity activity lasting longer than 60 to 90 minutes, such as distance runners, cross-country skiers, road cyclists, and some long distance swimmers. It is not recommended for athletes participating in short-term events, such as sprints, or for sports in which the activity may last for a long period of time, but in which the physical effort is characterized by brief periods of high-energy activity with alternate rest periods, such as football, baseball, and wrestling.

The degree of benefit derived from carbohydrate loading, even among endurance athletes, is individual; and therefore, athletes should determine prior to major competition the value of this regimen.

Although this week-long method of carbohydrate loading has proven effective in maximizing endurance, the impact on performance of carbohydrate intake immediately before competition has been less clear. Historically, ingesting simple sugars 1 to 2 hours before activity was not recommended due to incidence of hyperglycemia, hyperinsulinemia, subsequent hypoglycemia, and suppression of free fatty acids.[33,50] More recent data on this issue, however, show that the ingestion of carbohydrate shortly before performance does not enhance glycogen breakdown, nor adversely affect endurance time to exhaustion.[45,58,84] Thus, there are not consistently reported negative side effects of carbohydrate ingestion 30 to 60 minutes before exercise. A study of cyclists consuming 312 g sugar 4 hours before exercising should that blood glucose levels increased during exercise, and that increased carbohydrate oxidation prolonged performance.[127] Based on this study and others, endurance athletes may choose to consume an extra dose of carbohydrate prior to an event as a means of maximizing glucose oxidation during the activity. If the pre-exercise carbohydrate is consumed approximately 4 hours before exercise, the athlete may benefit from up to 4.5 g carbohydrate/kg bw. Closer to the event, less carbohydrate is advised; for example, one g carbohydrate/kg bw if consumption occurs 1 hour before activity.

After Competition

Timing and amount of carbohydrate intake after an endurance event may be critical for athletes requiring maximum glycogen stores day after day. It can also be argued that nonendurance athletes who practice two or three times each day are at risk of depleting glycogen stores and may benefit from methods to maximize rate of glycogen synthesis between and after training bouts. Because glycogen is synthesized most rapidly in the first few hours after activity, delaying carbohydrate consumption for even 2 hours can reduce the rate of glycogen repletion. A study by Ivy and colleagues[72] suggests that athletes who desire maximum glycogenesis should consume 1.5 g carbohydrate/kg bw immediately after exercise and again 2 hours later. Glucose or sucrose result in greater muscle glycogen replenishment than complex carbohydrate in the first 6 hours after exercise, but no difference remains 24 hours later.[110] To enhance intake and palatability, a combination of simple and complex, liquid and solid, carbohydrates may be consumed.

Carbohydrate Requirements of Nonendurance Athletes

The majority of research on carbohydrate requirements, as reviewed above, has been conducted on endurance athletes. The majority of athletes do not compete in marathons or road races, however, but in sports such as football, basketball, track, wrestling, volleyball, and other nonendurance sports. Such sports involve brief periods of high-energy activity with alternate rest periods, and may not reduce muscle glycogen to the same extent as continuous exercise for the same period of time.

Although exact recommendations for carbohydrate cannot be given, it is possible that nonendurance athletes who train daily and consume low-carbohydrate diets are at risk for a reduction in muscle glycogen levels that could negatively affect training and performance. For this reason, nonendurance athletes should consume sufficient carbohydrate to support training and workouts. Maintaining adequate dietary carbohydrate is especially important for non-endurance athletes who incorporate aerobic exercise into their training regimen. One 7-day study indicates that athletes who train aerobically for at least 60 minutes and incorporate sprint work into their training can maintain that training load when consuming 5 g carbohydrate/kg bw/d.[128]

Athletes differ in carbohydrate requirements based on body size, sport, and training routine. Whereas maximum requirements may differ, it is recommended that all athletes, regardless of sport or body size, consume a minimum of 200 g carbohydrate/d to replenish liver glycogen stores.

PRECOMPETITION NUTRITION

Few aspects of precompetition nutrition have been documented as having a significant effect on performance for the majority of athletes. Many guidelines appear in sports nutrition literature, and even more are recommended by coaches, parents and athletes themselves; but in practice, no one specific or combination of foods will be the right precompetition regimen for all athletes. The primary goal of precompetition nutrition is to provide fluid and energy to support the athlete during competition.[65] Pragmatically, the most important consideration is that the meal or snack not interfere with the physical demands of the upcoming activity; however, the psychological impact of foods eaten before competition may be of equal or even greater importance. Overall, the precompetition meal should consist of foods and beverages the athlete likes, foods that are well tolerated and foods the athlete generally eats. Having to eat foods one dislikes or is not accustomed to at a time when nervous tension is high will likely cause gastrointestinal (GI) distress.

More than other groups, runners tend to report GI symptoms such as increased GI motility during activity.[18,113,114] For those runners experiencing difficulty, altering pre-exercise foods may help alleviate symptoms. For example, some runners find it advantageous to consume a low-fiber, low-residue diet 1 to 3 days before competition.

Athletes in all areas occasionally experience nausea or vomiting when stress is high. A full stomach before competition will exacerbate the problem. Reducing fat in the precompetition meal will hasten stomach emptying, as will consuming a liquid meal instead of a solid one. An empty stomach will provide the nauseated athlete some relief.

Diaries can help athletes determine their best precompetition eating plan. Recording the types and amounts of foods consumed, when they were eaten in relation to competition (e.g., 2 hours before), and how the athlete felt during the event can serve as a learning tool, in analyzing the diary.

VITAMIN AND MINERAL SUPPLEMENTS

All vitamins needed by the human body can be obtained in adequate amounts by consuming a nutrient-dense, varied diet providing 1200 to 1500 calories. Nevertheless, sales of vitamin and mineral supplements generate a multimillion dollar business, and athletes are probably one of the biggest groups of consumers.[145] Surveys of athletes demonstrate that 54 to 84% use supplements.[6,54]

There are many factors that influence this practice in athletes. One is the attitude that nutrients are "good" and are therefore harmless; the other is the notion that if a little is good, a lot will be better. It is common for an athlete consuming five or six different supplements a day to be unaware of the nutrients provided by those supplements. Another factor that contributes to excessive use of supplements is the misperception that the RDA are minimum requirements rather than levels estimated to exceed the requirements of healthy individuals. Additionally, dangerously high levels of nutrients are consumed by people who are unaware of the fact that certain nutrients can be toxic or problematic.

Because many athletes have energy intakes above 4000 calories, the levels of nutrients consumed from food alone are often 200 to 300% of the RDA. With the addition of supplements, the combined food and supplement intake can result in megadoses. Toxicity and adverse effects resulting from high doses have been well documented for several nutrients.[52,92]

That physical performance will deteriorate during prolonged vitamin deficiency is well documented. Various studies on human subjects fed diets deficient in one or more of the water-soluble vitamins have shown deterioration in work performance, decrease in work output, increased fatigue, and increased muscle tenderness. Although the ability to do work is markedly diminished during states of severe vitamin deficiency, once vitamin requirements are met, there appears to be no value in consuming additional amounts. Numerous investigations have studied the effects of supplementing nutritionally adequate diets. Supplementation above an adequate diet did not improve work output, muscle strength, resistance to fatigue, recovery, cardiovascular function, endurance capacity, or oxygen consumption. (See Haymes' review[60] for more information in this area.) Scientific evidence supports the fact that supplementation of the diet with either single- or multi-nutrient preparations does not improve physical performance in athletes consuming a nutritionally adequate diet. The psychotherapeutic aspects of supplements cannot be ignored, however.

TABLE 1. Levels of Antioxidant Vitamin Supplementation Considered Safe, and Examples of Equivalent Food Sources

Vitamin	Food Source Equivalents
Vitamin E 100–400 IU	2–8 cups whole almonds 20–80 tbsp. corn oil 10–40 tbsp. mayonnaise 67–267 tbsp. peanut butter
Vitamin C 250–1000 mg	10½–40 tomatoes 2–8 cups fresh orange juice 2–8 cups boiled broccoli 3–12 kiwi fruit
Beta-carotene 3–20 mg (5000–33, 340 IU)	¼–1½ medium carrots 1–6 cups red pepper, sweet 1–6 cups cantaloupe cubes ⅓–2 cups spinach, boiled

One recent focus in the study of vitamin supplementation is the role of the antioxidants, vitamins C, E, and beta-carotene. A review of studies to date shows that supplementation of an adequate diet with antioxidants will not enhance performance, but evidence does suggest that antioxidant vitamins may help prevent oxidative damage induced by exercise.[147] If athletes desire to supplement their diets with antioxidants, Table 1 lists safe and appropriate levels. As demonstrated by the examples of foods necessary to achieve the supplemental levels, it is quite common for diets to provide vitamins A and C in relatively high levels, whereas it is less common for diets to contain high levels of vitamin E.

A nutrient by nutrient review of the literature is not practical here, but two nutrients demand further attention. Iron warrants individual attention because of the interest in this mineral shown by many coaches and athletes (especially endurance athletes). Calcium deserves brief mention because of the incidence of amenorrhea in female athletes and the role played by calcium in bone density and therefore in stress fractures and healing.

IRON

Iron is present in all cells of the body and plays a key role in many biochemical reactions, such as the transport of oxygen (hemoglobin, myoglobin), the activation of oxygen (oxidases and oxygenases), and electron transport (cytochromes). Thus, iron deficiency anemia is related to diminished work capacity, decreased endurance, diminished oxygen delivery, and increased lactic acid production.[3,36,53,105,108,123] Understandably, coaches, trainers, and athletes themselves seek optimal iron levels.

Iron Status and Physical Performance

Three questions arise when examining the relationship among athletes, iron and physical performance. (1) Does the iron status of athletes vary from the status of nonathletes? (2) What are the mechanisms influencing iron status among athletes? (3) What effect does iron status have on athletic performance?

The answer to the first seems straightforward, but is not. Difficulty is posed because varying standards have been used to define iron status. For example, most use ferritin <12 μg/L as the cutoff for iron depletion, but some use <20 μg/L. For clarification, Haymes[59] has defined three stages of negative iron status: Stage 1 is iron depletion defined as ferritin <12 μ/L. Stage 2 is iron-deficient erythropoiesis defined as ferritin μ12 μg/L and free-erythrocyte protoporphyrin exceeding 100 μg/dl RBC. Stage 3 is anemia defined as Hgb <12 g/dl for women and <13 g/dl for men.

Regardless of standards used, the majority of studies evaluating iron status in athletes indicates that distance runners, more so than sedentary controls, have some reduction in iron stores, but iron deficient erythropoiesis or anemia are uncommon. Low ferritin concentrations have been documented in male and female runners[5,19,27,39,43,62,99,104,146] as well as female athletes from other sports: field hockey, cross-country skiing, crew, basketball, and softball.[25,40,61,103,117,119] Considering current evidence, the physician should assume the incidence of decreased iron stores may be slightly higher in athletes than nonathletes, but that iron deficiency anemia is not more prevalent among athletes. The target group with the highest frequency of negative iron status is that of adolescent athletes. Limited data on female adolescent athletes suggest serum ferritin <12 to 20 μg/L exists in as many as 61% of this subpopulation, and anemia in as many as 11% of the female adolescent athlete population.[100,107,117,118]

Theories abound as to the causative mechanisms influencing iron status in athletes. These include hemodilution, decreased intestinal absorption, shunting of stores from the reticuloendothelial system to hepatocytes, increased urinary excretion due to hemolysis, losses via sweat and menses, and others.[5,44,107] Cook[29] contends that the primary variables influencing iron status of distance runners are blood loss from the GI tract, hemodilution, and a shift of iron from stores to an expanding red blood cell (RBC) compartment. He likens the changes in iron metabolism seen with endurance training to the changes during pregnancy: dilutional anemia with an expansion of RBC mass, decrease in iron stores that may progress to iron-deficient erythropoiesis, and a prompt reversal of negative iron balance after delivery or cessation of training.

One factor affecting status that cannot be overlooked, and is perhaps the most significant factor (other than menstrual loss) for many female athletes, is dietary iron intake. The amount of iron absorbed from the diet depends largely on the type of dietary iron. Heme iron, found in animal tissue including meat, liver, poultry, and fish, is absorbed in amounts directly correlated to status and is minimally influenced by other inhibiting or enhancing dietary factors. Nonheme iron, found in both animal and vegetable sources, is poorly absorbed, regardless of intraluminal factors. Historically, studies using single meals suggested that ingestion of ascorbic acid or meat appreciably enhanced absorption of nonheme iron by aiding conversion from the ferric to ferrous state. Conversely, ingestion of certain inhibiting factors such as the tannin in tea, polyphenols in coffee and spinach, oxalates in chocolate, and phytates in bran, were shown to significantly reduce nonheme iron absorption from a single meal. More recent studies, however, suggest that inhibition or enhancement of non-heme iron within the context of a diet is less significant than once thought.[30,71] Cook[30] concluded that "in the context of a varied Western diet, nonheme iron bioavailability is less important [to iron status] than absorption studies with single meals would suggest." Thus, meat consumption is a key dietary determinant of iron status.[28] Vegetarian diets are a significant risk factor for iron deficiency in endurance athletes.[125,131,142]

In addition to type of dietary iron, inadequate dietary intake of iron is often related to the low calorie diets of small athletes such as gymnasts, dancers, and figure skaters.[10,11,38,86,93,112] For example, for iron needs to be met, a female athlete consuming 1500 calories per day would need to ingest approximately 12.6 mg Fe/1000 kcal.[57] One study of runners by Manore[88] documented iron intakes ranged from 4.3 to 8.8 mg/1000 kcal.

And finally, a response to the third question—what is the impact of iron status on physical performance? Iron deficiency undoubtedly impairs performance. But does iron depletion in the absence of anemia impair performance? The argument that it does stems from findings of Finch and colleagues[46] showing that tissue depletion of iron in the presence of normal hemoglobin levels (transfused blood) negatively affected exercise capacity in rats. The majority of studies on humans fail to show a negative effect of iron depletion on performance, or more specifically, fail to show a positive effect of iron supplementation on performance in athletes who are not anemic.[48,98,117,123] Some, however, do suggest slight improvement.[87,119] Study in this area is convoluted due to failure to use standard identification of depletion and failure to correct for dilutional effect.

Supplementation

Regardless of the weak (and perhaps nonexistent) scientific link between benefits of iron supplementation in the absence of iron deficiency anemia, the mind set of many athletes is "the higher the ferritin the better." Thus supplementation among athletes, especially female endurance athletes, is prevalent.[7,39] Widespread prophylactic iron supplementation is not indicated in the absence of anemia. Contraindications include the recent evidence, though inconclusive, suggesting that excess iron stores may increase risk of cancer, stroke, and coronary heart disease.[121,132,137] Excess iron intake is also detrimental to the population with the autosomal recessive disease hemochromatosis, many of whom may not be aware of their condition.

Screening

The preparticipation examination provides a convenient setting to screen athletes for iron depletion and anemia. Those athletes found to be iron-deplete or deficient should receive diet counseling, and when indicated, supplemental iron.

CALCIUM

Calcium and Bone Health

The average human body contains 1.5 kg of calcium, all derived from dietary sources except that contributed by the mother during pregnancy. This observation alone suggests a vital link between dietary calcium and bone mineral content. Because of difficulties integral to the examination of the calcium-bone health relationship, however, the influence on bone density exerted by calcium has not been widely recognized by most experts until the past few decades.[4,8,89,102] Several well-controlled, double-blind, longitudinal studies substantiate calcium's potential to increase bone mass.[21,22,23,37,74,85,115]

A connection between bone mineral density (BMD) and injury continues to be explored. For example, Myburgh and colleagues[95] found that among 25 athletes (19 of them women) with similar training habits, bone density was significantly lower in athletes with fractures than in control athletes. Other factors associated with stress fractures were lower dietary calcium intake, current menstrual irregularity, and lower oral contraceptive use.

Because of calcium's important role in determining BMD, the question arises whether calcium supplementation prevents bone stress injuries.[90] To answer this question, it would be necessary to supplement an experimental group for a long period, i.e., several years, and subsequently compare to controls. One study[124] examined short-term supplementation and observed no results, as would be expected. Because no well-designed study exists which examines the effect of long-term calcium supplementation on injury in healthy women or women with documented low BMD, this question remains unanswered.

Other Factors in Bone Health

It is impossible to review, independent of other factors, the role of calcium as it relates to short-term (stress fracture) and long-term (osteoporosis) bone health. Many factors influence bone quality, many of which are not related to bone density, but may include the structure and architecture of the bone. Certainly calcium does not affect fatigue damage or trabecular connections that contribute to bone frailty. Calcium influences BMD, and as such, the connection of calcium intake to fracture risk is only as strong as the connection between BMD and fracture risk. Additionally, many factors besides calcium influence peak BMD. The three most influential, besides genetics, are calcium, gonadal hormone status, and mechanical loading, with hormone status exerting the greatest influence.[69]

In a four-year longitudinal study of women aged 19 to 30,[109] dietary calcium intake, as well as physical activity, exerted a positive effect on bone gain. Use of oral contraceptives exerted a further independent positive effect. Another notable finding was that the gain in bone mass in these healthy young women continued in the third decade of life. Heretofore, it had not been known whether appreciable gain in bone density could be achieved after late adolescence.

In studies of secondary amenorrhea in early post-menopausal women, neither exercise nor calcium intake compensated for decreased estrogen levels.[9,42,116,120,140] In fact, several studies indicate menstrual history and status is a primary determinant of bone density in athletes.[41,94,97] Of concern is the observation[41] that extended periods of oligomenorrhea and amenorrhea may have a residual effect on lumbar bone density.

Given a normal estrogenic state, exercise (more specifically, mechanical loading) appears to have an impact on bone mineral content,[75] but this fact is perhaps less significant than previously thought. Furthermore, the effects of exercise may be transient if it is discontinued.[35] For a comprehensive review of the role of exercise in bone mass, see Forwood's study.[49]

When a physician initially sees an athlete with amenorrhea, and co-morbidity (including eating disorders) has been ruled out, the physician should make recommendations to facilitate resumption of a normal estrogenic state, i.e., gradually decreased training and with increased food intake. If this treatment is not effective, oral contraceptives should be considered.

Intake

Calcium intake among female athletes has been documented to range from 60 to 120% of the RDA.[12,26,93,106] Lower than optimal intakes of calcium are common among female athletes, especially those restricting food to maintain thinness. In the 110 female athletes studied by Grandjean et al.,[55] 55% of those 18 years or younger consumed <70% of the RDA.

Calcium intake is, of course, not the only variable determining calcium balance. Several nutritional elements also play a role: vitamin D, protein, phosphorus, fiber, and sodium. Vitamin D is essential to increase the efficiency of calcium absorption. Protein, caffeine, and sodium increase urinary calcium loss (although the effect of caffeine is usually insignificant), whereas phosphorus decreases urinary calcium excretion.[64,78,96] Wheat fiber tends to decrease the availability of calcium in the gut. In the context of the daily diet, these factors become significant primarily when calcium intake is low and inhibiting factors high.

Requirements

The evolving data about calcium and bone health has generated debate regarding calcium requirements. The current RDSs tend to be lower than the levels some experts believe is necessary to meet absorptive thresholds.[63] An NIH expert panel[101] during a consensus development conference recommended 1200 to 1500 mg for 11 to 24 years olds, whereas the current RDA is 1200. Table 2 offers additional comparisons.

Supplements

Calcium supplements are used widely by female athletes. In 1985, $130 million was spent on calcium supplements in the United States.[140] As has been suggested, bone health depends on a multitude of environmental, genetic, and nutritional factors, so a single item, such as calcium supplements, is certainly only one piece in the puzzle. In light of the low-calcium intakes prevalent in young female athletes, however, supplements may be indicated for those athletes unwilling or unable to increase calcium intake by dietary modification.

***TABLE 2.* Comparison of NIH Expert Panel Recommendation to the Recommended Dietary Allowance of Calcium**

Ages	NIH Expert Panel	RDA
11–24 years	1,200–1,500 mg	1,200 mg
Women:		
25–49 years	1,000 mg	800 mg
50–65 years (taking estrogen)	1,000 mg	800 mg
50–65 years (not taking estrogen)	1,500 mg	800 mg
65+ years	1,500 mg	800 mg
Men:		
25–64 years	1,000 mg	800 mg
65+ years	1,500 mg	800 mg

Of the supplements available, calcium carbonate and calcium citrate both provide bioavailable forms of supplemental calcium. Calcium carbonate is often used in antacid preparations. Calcium citrate malate is used to fortify beverages such as orange juice.

As with iron supplements, calcium supplementation is not without risk and should not be advocated indiscriminately. For example, Bourgoin et al[16] have found significant levels of aluminum and lead in oyster shell supplements. Of equal importance is the antagonistic relationship of calcium and iron. Calcium ingestion of 300 to 600 mg may decrease iron absorption by 50 to 60%.[57] As noted by Cook,[30] taking calcium supplements with meals makes it more difficult for women to meet their daily iron requirements. Co-ingestion of food with the calcium supplement increases calcium absorption, however. A reasonable regimen for female athletes supplementing both iron and calcium is then to take the iron supplement with a meal, and the calcium supplement between meals with a light snack.

WATER

Water is of primary importance to the athlete. It gives structure and form to the body and provides the aqueous medium in which the functions of the body take place, and is also very important in the regulation of body temperature. During physical exercise great amounts of water may be lost through sweat as the body attempts to maintain normal temperature. Water replacement is of utmost importance to the athlete for optimal performance. This issue is discussed in greater detail in Chapter 6, "Fluids and Electrolytes for Exercise in the Heat."

SUMMARY

The term athlete is often used generically, but those who have experience with "athletes" know that no two are alike. As the discipline of sports nutrition evolves, this fundamental concept must be remembered: just as each athlete is different, so the nutrition goals for each athlete may vary.

Physicians should be cognizant of the fundamental components within sports nutrition—energy requirements, weight loss, weight gain, carbohydrate, protein, vitamins, minerals, and fluid—and recognize that slight changes will ensue as study continues within each area. A basic knowledge, however, of the principles presented will aid the physician in recognizing problems and making appropriate referrals and recommendations.

REFERENCES

1. Ahlborg B, Bergstrom J, Brohult et al: Human muscle glycogen content and capacity for prolonged exercise after different diets. Foersvarsmedicin 3:58–99, 1967.
2. Ahlman K, Karvonen MJ: Weight reduction by sweating in wrestlers, and its effects on physical fitness. J Sports Med 1:58–62, 1961.
3. Anderson H, Burkve H: Iron deficiency and muscular work performance. Scand J Clin Lab Invest 25(Suppl 114):9–37, 1970.
4. Arnaud CD, Sanchez SD: The role of calcium in osteoporosis. Annu Rev Nutr 10:397–414, 1990.
5. Balaban EP, Cox JV, Snell P, et al: The frequency of anemia and iron deficiency in the runner. Med Sci Sport Exerc 21:643, 1989.
6. Barnett DW, Conlee RK: The effects of a commercial dietary supplement on human performance. Am J Clin Nutr 40:586–590, 1984.
7. Barr SI: Nutrition knowledge of female varsity athletes and university students. J Am Diet Assoc 87:1660–1664, 1987.
8. Barrett-Connor E: The RDA for calcium in the elderly: too little, too late (editorial). Calcif Tissue Int 44:303–7, 1989.
9. Bauer DC, Browner WS, Cauley JA, et al: Factors associated with appendicular bone mass in older women. Ann Intern Med 118:657–665, 1993.
10. Benardot D, Schwarz M, Heller DW: Nutrient intake in young, highly competitive gymnasts. J Am Diet Assoc 89:401–403, 1989.
11. Benson JE, Alleman Y, Theintz GE, Howard H: Eating problems and calorie intake levels in Swiss adolescent athletes. Int J Sports Med 11:249–252, 1990.
12. Benson JE, Geiger CJ, Eiserman PA, Wardlaw GM: Relationship between nutrient intake body mass index, menstrual function, and ballet injury. J Am Diet Assoc 89: 58–63, 1989.
13. Bergstrom J, Hermansen L, Hultman E, Saltin B: Diet, muscle glycogen and physical performance. Acta Physiol Scand 71:140–150, 1967.
14. Bergstrom J, Hultman E, Roch-Norlund AE: Muscle glycogen synthase in normal subjects: Basal values, effects of glycogen depletion by exercise and of a carbohydrate-rich diet following exercise. Scand J Clin Lab Invest 29:231–6, 1972.
15. Bosco JS, Terjung RL, Greenleaf JE: Effects of progressive hypohydration on maximal isometric muscular strength. J Sports Med Phys Fitness 8:81–86, 1968.
16. Bourgoin BP, Evans DR, Cornett JR, et al: Lead content in 70 brands of dietary calcium supplements. Am J Public Health 83:1115–1160, 1993.
17. Brook JD: Variations in available carbohydrate and physical work ability with repeated prolonged severe exercise. Proc Nutr Soc 32:11A–12A, 1973.
18. Brouns F, Saris WHM, Rehrer NJ: Abdominal complaints and gastrointestinal function during long-lasting exercise. Int J Sports Med 8:175–189, 1987.
19. Brown RT, McIntosh SM, Seabolt VR, Daniel WA: Iron status of adolescent female athletes. J Adolesc Health 6:349, 1985.
20. Burge CM, Carey MF, Payne WR: Rowing performance, fluid balance, and metabolic function following dehydration and rehydration. Med Sci Sports Exerc 25:1358–1364, 1993.
21. Chan GM: Dietary calcium and bone mineral status of children and adolescents. Am J Dis Child 145:631–34, 1991.
22. Chan GM, Hess M, Hollis J, Book LS: Bone mineral status in childhood accidental fractures. Am J Dis Child 138: 569–79, 1984.
23. Chan GM, McMurry M, Westover K, et al: Effects of increased dietary calcium intake upon the calcium and bone mineral status of lactating adolescent and adult women. Am J Clin Nutr 46:319–23, 1987.
24. Christensen EH, Hansen O: Arbeitsfähigkeit und Ernährung. Skand Arch Physiol 81:160–171, 1939.
25. Clement DB, Lloyd-Smith DR, MacIntyre JG, et al: Iron status in winter Olympic sports. J Sports Sci 5:261, 1987.
26. Cohen JL, Potosnak L, Frank O, Baker H: A nutritional and hematologic assessment of elite ballet dancers. Physician Sportsmed 13:43–54, 1985.
27. Colt E, Heyman B: Low ferritin in runners. J Sports Med Phys Fitness 24:13, 1989.
28. Cook, JD: Adaptation in iron metabolism. Am J Clin Nutr 51:301–308, 1990.
29. Cook JD: The effect of endurance training on iron metabolism. Semin Hematol 31(2):1–3, 1994.
30. Cook JD, Dassenko SA, Lynch SR: Assessment of the role of nonheme-iron availability in iron balance. Am J Clin Nutr 54:717–722, 1991.
31. Cook JD, Dassenko SA, Whittaker P: Calcium supplementation: effect on iron absorption. Am J Clin Nutr 53:106–111, 1991.
32. Costill DL: Muscular exhaustion during distance running. Phys Sportsmed 2(10):36–41, 1974.
33. Costill DL, Coyle E, Dalsky G, et al: Effects of elevated plasma FFA and insulin on muscle glycogen usage during exercise. J Appl Physiol 43:695–99, 1977.
34. Coyle EF, Hagberg JM, Hurley BF, et al: Carbohydrate feeding during prolonged strenuous exercise can delay fatigue. J Appl Physiol 55:230–35, 1983.
35. Dalsky GP, Stocke KS, Ehsanii AA, et al: Weight-bearing exercise training and lumbar bone mineral content in postmenopausal women. Ann Intern Med 108:824–828, 1988.
36. Davies, KA, Maguire JJ, Brooks GA, et al: Muscle mitochondrial bioenergetics, oxygen supply, and work capacity during dietary iron deficiency and repletion. Am J Physiol 242:E418–E427, 1982.
37. Dawson-Hughes B, Dallal GE, Krall EA, et al: A controlled trial of the effect of calcium supplementation on bone density in post-menopausal women. N Engl J Med 323: 878–83, 1990.
38. Delistraty DA, Reisman EJ, Snipes M: A physiological and nutritional profile of young female figure skaters. J Sports Med Phys Fitness 32:149–155, 1992.
39. Deuster PA, Kyle SB, Moser PB, et al: Nutritional survey of highly trained women runners. Am J Clin Nutr 44:954–962, 1986.
40. Diehl DM, Lohman TG, Smith SC, Kertzer R: Effects of physical training and competition on the iron status of female field hockey players. Int J Sports Med 7:264, 1986.
41. Drinkwater BL, Bruemner MS, Chestnut CH: Menstrual history as a determinant of current bone density in young athletes. JAMA 263(4):545–548, 1990.

42. Drinkwater BL, Nilson K, Chesnut CH, et al: Bone mineral content of amenorrheic and eumenorrheic athletes. N Engl J Med 311:277, 1984.
43. Ehn L, Carlmark B, Hoglund S: Iron status in athletes involved in intense physical activity. Med Sci Sports Exerc 12(1):61–64, 1980.
44. Eichner ER: Runner's macrocytosis: A clue to footstrike hemolysis. Am J Med 78:321–325, 1985.
45. Fielding RA, Costill DL, Fink WJ, et al: Effects of pre-exercise carbohydrate feedings on muscle glycogen use during exercise in well-trained runners. Eur J Appl Physiol 56:225–229, 1987.
46. Finch CA, Miller LR, Inamdar AR, et al: Iron deficiency in the rat. Physiological and biochemical studies of muscle dysfunction. J Clin Invest 58:447–453, 1976.
47. Fogelholm GM, Koskinen R, Laakso J, et al: Gradual and rapid weight loss: Effects on nutrition and performance in male athletes. Med Sci Sports Exerc 25:371–377, 1993.
48. Fogelholm M, Jaakkola L, Lampisjarvi T: Effects of iron supplementation in female athletes with low serum ferritin concentration. Int J Sports Med 13:158–162, 1992.
49. Forwood MR, Burr DB: Physical activity and bone mass: Exercises in futility? Bone Miner 21:89–112, 1993.
50. Foster C, Costill DL, Fink WJ: Effects of pre-exercise feedings on endurance performance. Med Sci Sports Exerc 11:1–5, 1979.
51. Friedman JE, Lemon PWR: Effect of chronic endurance exercise on retention of dietary protein. Int J Sports Med 10:118–123, 1989.
52. Fumich RM, Essig GW: Hypervitaminosis A: Case report in an adolescent soccer player. Am J Sports Med 11:34, 1983.
53. Gardner GW, Edgerton VR, Senewiratne B, et al: Physical work capacity and metabolic stress in subjects with iron deficiency anemia. Am J Clin Nutr 30:910–917, 1977.
54. Grandjean AC: Vitamins, diet and the athlete. Clin Sports Med 2:105–114, 1983.
55. Grandjean AC: unpublished data, 1991.
56. Grandjean AC, Ruud JS: Energy intake of athletes. In Harries M, Williams, C, Stanish WD, Micheli LJ (eds): Oxford Textbook of Sports Medicine. New York, Oxford University Press, 1994, pp 53–65.
57. Hallberg L, Rossander-Hultin L: Iron requirements in menstruating women. Am J Clin Nutr 54:1047–1058, 1991.
58. Hargreaves M, Costill DL, Fink WJ, et al: Effect of pre-exercise carbohydrate feedings on endurance cycling performance. Med Sci Sports Exer 19:33–36, 1987.
59. Haymes EM, Trace minerals and exercise. In Wolinsky I, Hickson JF (eds.): Nutrition in Exercise and Sport, 2nd ed. Boca Raton, CRC Press, 1994, pp 223–230.
60. Haymes EM: Vitamin and mineral supplementation to athletes. Int J Sport Nutr 1:146–169, 1991.
61. Haymes EM, Puhl JL, Temples TE: Training for cross-country skiing and iron status. Med Sci Sports Exerc 18: 162–167, 1986.
62. Haymes EM, Spillman DM: Iron status of women distance runners, sprinters, and control women. Int J Sports Med 10(6):430–433, 1989.
63. Heaney RP: Nutritional factors in osteoporosis. Annu Rev Nutr 13:187–316, 1993.
64. Heaney RP: Protein intake and the calcium economy. J Am Diet Assoc 93:1256–60, 1993.
65. Hecker AL: Nutritional conditioning and athletic performance. Primary Care 9:545, 1982.
66. Hermansen L, Hultman E, Saltin B: Muscle glycogen during prolonged severe exercise. Acta Physiol Scand 71: 129–139, 1967.
67. Horswill CA, Hickner RC, Scott JR, et al: Weight loss, dietary carbohydrate modifications, and high-intensity physical performance. Med Sci Sports Exerc 22:470–76, 1990.
68. Houston ME, Marrin DA, Green HJ, Thompson JA: The effect of rapid weight loss on physiological functions in wrestlers. Physician Sportsmed 9:73–78, 1981.
69. Howat PM, Carbo ML, Mills GQ, Wozniak P: The influence of diet, body fat, menstrual cycling, and activity upon the bone density of females. J Am Diet Assoc 89:1305–1307, 1989.
70. Hultman E, Bergstrom J: Local energy-supplying substrates as limiting factors in different types of leg muscle work in normal man. In Keul J (ed): Limiting Factors of Physical Performance. Stuttgart, Thieme, 1973.
71. Hunt JR, Gallagher SK, Johnson LK: Effect of ascorbic acid on apparent iron absorption by women with low iron stores. Am J Clin Nutr 59:1381–5, 1994.
72. Ivy JL, Katz AL, Cutler CL, et al: Muscle glycogen synthesis after exercise: Effect of time of carbohydrate ingestion. J Appl Physiol 64:1480–1485, 1988.
73. Jacobs I: The effects of thermal dehydration on performance of the Wingate anaerobic test. Int J Sports Med 1:21–24, 1980.
74. Johnston CC, Miller JZ, Slemenda CW, et al: Calcium supplementation and increases in bone mineral density in children. N Engl J Med 327:82–87, 1992.
75. Kanders B, Dempster DW, Lindsay R: Interaction of calcium nutrition and physical activity on bone mass in young women. J Bone Miner Res 3:145–149, 1988.
76. Karlsson J, Saltin B: Diet, muscle glycogen and endurance performance. J Appl Physiol 31:203–206, 1971.
77. Klinzing JE, Karpowicz W: The effects of rapid weight loss and rehydration on a wrestling performance test. J Sports Med 26:149–156, 1986.
78. Knox TA, Zohrab K, Dawson-Hughes B, et al: Calcium absorption in elderly subjects on high- and low-fiber diets: Effect of gastric acidity. Am J Clin Nutr 53:1480–6, 1991.
79. Kochan RG, Lamb DR, Lutz SA, et al: Glycogen synthase activation in human skeletal muscle, effects of diet and exercise. Am J Physiol 236:E660–E666, 1979.
80. Krogh A, Lindhard J: The relative value of fat and carbohydrate as sources of muscular energy. Biochem J 14: 290–363, 1920.
81. Lemon PWR: Protein and amino acid needs of the strength athlete. Int J Sports Nutr 1:127–145, 1991.
82. Lemon PWR, Nagel FJ: Effects of exercise on protein and amino acid metabolism. Med Sci Sports Exerc 13(3): 141–149, 1981.
83. Lemon PWR; Yarosheski KE, Dolny DG: The importance of protein for athletes. Sports Med 1:474, 1984.
84. Levine L, Evans WJ, Cadarette BS, et al: Fructose and glucose ingestion and muscle glycogen use during submaximal exercise. J Appl Physiol 55:1767–1771, 1983.
85. Lloyd T, Andon MB, Rollings N, et al: Calcium supplementation and bone mineral density in adolescent girls. JAMA 270:841–844, 1993.
86. Loosli AR, Benson J, Gillien DM, Bourdet K: Nutrition habits and knowledge in competitive adolescent female gymnasts. Physician Sportsmed 14:118–130, 1986.
87. Magazanik A, Weinstein Y, Abarbancl J, et al: Effect of an iron supplement on body iron status and aerobic capacity of young training women. Eur J Appl Physiol 62:317–323, 1991.
88. Manore MM, Besenfelder PD, Wells CL, et al: Nutrient intakes and iron status in female long-distance runners during training. J Am Diet Assoc 89:257–259, 1989.
89. Marcus R: Calcium intake and skeletal integrity: Is there a critical relationship? J Nutr 117:631–35, 1987.
90. Matkovic V, Kostial K, Simonovic I, et al: Bone status and fracture rates in two regions of Yugoslavia. Am J Clin Nutr 32:540–49, 1979.
91. Meredith CN, Zackin MJ, Frontera WR, Evans WJ: Dietary protein requirements and body protein metabolism in endurance-trained men. Am J Physiol 66:2850–2856, 1989.

92. Miller DR, Hayes KC: Vitamin excess and toxicity. In Hathcock JH (eds): Nutritional Toxicity, Vol. I, New York, Academic Press, 1982.
93. Moffatt RJ: Dietary status of elite female high school gymnasts: Inadequacy of vitamin and mineral intake. J Am Diet Assoc 84:1361–1363, 1984.
94. Myburgh KH, Bachrach LK, Lewis B, et al: Low bone mineral density at axial and appendicular sites in amenorrheic athletes. Med Sci Sports Exerc 25:1997–1202, 1993.
95. Myburgh KH, Hutchins J, Fataar AB, et al: Low bone density in an etiologic factor for stress fractures in athletes. Ann Intern Med 113:754–59, 1990.
96. Need AG, Morris HA, Cleghorn DB, et al: Effect of salt restriction on urine hydroxyproline excretion in postmenopausal women. Arch Intern Med 151:757–759, 1991.
97. Nelson ME, Fisher EC, Catsos PD, et al: Diet and bone status in amenorrheic runners. Am J Clin Nutr 43:910–916, 1986.
98. Newhouse IJ, Clement DB, Taunton JE, McKenzie DC: The effects of prelatent/latent iron deficiency on physical work capacity. Med Sci Sports Exerc 21:263–268, 1989.
99. Nickerson HJ, Holubets MC, Weiler BR, et al: Causes of iron deficiency in adolescent athletes. J Pediatr 114: 658–663, 1989.
100. Nickerson HJ, Tripp AD: Iron deficiency in adolescent cross-country runners. Phys Sports Med 11(6):60–66, 1983.
101. NIH Consensus Development Conference: Optimal Calcium Intake. Washington, DC, June 6–8, 1994.
102. Nordin BEC, Heaney RP: Calcium supplementation of the diet: justified by present evidence. BMJ 300:1056–60, 1990.
103. Parr RB, Bachman LA, Moss RA: Iron deficiency in female athletes. Physician Sportsmed 12(4):81, 1984.
104. Pate RR, Dover V, Goodyear L, et al: Iron storage in female distance runners. In Katch FI (ed): Sport, Health, and Nutrition. Champaign, IL, Human Kinetics, 1986.
105. Pate RR, Maguire M, Wyuk JV: Dietary iron supplementation in women athletes. Physician Sportsmed 7:81, 1979.
106. Perron M, Endres J: Knowledge, attitudes, and dietary practices of female athletes. J Am Diet Assoc 85:573–576, 1985.
107. Raunikar RA, Sabio H: Anemia in the adolescent athlete. Am J Dis Child 146:1201–1205, 1992.
108. Read MH, McGuffin SL: The effect of B-complex supplementation on endurance performance. J Sports Med Phys Fitness 23:178–184, 1983.
109. Recker RR, Davies KM, Hinders SM, et al: Bone gain in young adult women. JAMA 268:2403–2408, 1992.
110. Reed MJ, Brozinick JT, Lee MC, Ivy JL: Muscle glycogen storage postexercise: effect of mode of carbohydrate administration. J Appl Physiol 66(2):720–726, 1989.
111. Refsum HE, Gjessing LR, Stromme SB: Changes in plasma amino distribution and urine amino acid excretion during prolonged heavy exercise. Scand J Clin Lab Invest 39:407–413, 1979.
112. Reggiani E, Arras GN, Trabacca S, et al: Nutritional status and body composition of adolescent female gymnasts. J Sports Med Phys Fitness 29:285–288, 1989.
113. Rehrer NJ, Brouns F, Beckers EFJ, et al: Physiological changes and gastrointestinal symptoms as a result of ultra-endurance running. Eur J Appl Physiol 64:1–8, 1992.
114. Rehrer NJ, Janssen GME, Brouns F, Saris WHM: Fluid intake and gastrointestinal problems in runners competing in a 25-km race and a marathon. Int J Sports Med 10(Suppl 1):S22–S25, 1989.
115. Reid IR, Ames RW, Evans MC, et al: Effect of calcium supplementation on bone loss in postmenopausal women. N Engl J Med 328:460–464, 1993.
116. Riggs BL, Meton LJ: The prevention and treatment of osteoporosis. N Engl J Med 327(9):620–627, 1993.
117. Risser WL, Lee EJ, Poindexter HBW, et al: Iron deficiency in female athletes: Its prevalence and impact on performance. Med Sci Sports Exerc 20(2):116–121, 1988.
118. Rowland TW, Deisroth MB, Green GM, et al: The effect of iron therapy on the exercise capacity of nonanemic iron-deficient adolescent runners. Am J Dis Child 142: 165–169, 1988.
119. Rowland TW, Kelleher JF: Iron deficiency in athletes: Insights from high school swimmers. Am J Dis Child 142:197, 1989.
120. Rus B, Thomsen K, Christiansen C: Does calcium supplementation prevent post-menopausal bone loss? N Engl J Med 316:173–77, 1987.
121. Salonen JT, Hyyssonen K, Korpela H, et al: High stored iron levels are associated with excess risk of myocardial infarction in Eastern Finnish men. Circulation 86:803–811, 1992.
122. Saltin B: Aerobic and anaerobic work capacity after dehydration. J Appl Physiol 19:1114–1118, 1964.
123. Schoene RB, Escourrou P, Robertson HT, et al: Iron repletion decreases maximal exercise lactate concentrations in female athletes with minimal iron-deficiency anemia. J Lab Clin Med 102:306–312, 1983.
124. Schwellnus MP, Jordaan G: Does calcium supplementation prevent bone stress injuries? A clinical trial. Int J Sport Nutr 2:165–74, 1992.
125. Seiler D, Nagel D, Franz H, et al: Effects of long-distance runners on iron metabolism and hematological parameters. Int J Sports Med 10:357–362, 1989.
126. Serfass RC, Stull GA, Alexander JF, Ewing JL: The effects of rapid weight loss and attempted rehydration on strength and endurance of the handgripping muscle in college wrestlers. Res Q Exerc Sport 55:46–52, 1984.
127. Sherman W, Brodozica G, Wright DA, et al: Effects of 4 h preexercise carbohydrate feedings on cycling performance. Med Sci Sports Exerc 21:598–604, 1989.
128. Sherman WM, Doyle JA, Lamb DR, Strauss RH: Dietary carbohydrate, muscle glycogen, and exercise performance during 7 d of training. Am J Clin Nutr 57:27–31, 1993.
129. Sherman WM, Wimer GS: Insufficient dietary carbohydrate during training: does it impair athletic performance? Int J Sport Nutr 1:28–44, 1991.
130. Singer RN, Weiss SA: Effects of weight reduction on selected anthropometric, physical, and performance measures of wrestlers. Res Q 39:361–369, 1968.
131. Snyder AC, Dvorak LL, Roepke JB: Influence of dietary iron source on measures of iron status among female runners. Med Sci Sports Exerc 21:7–10, 1989.
132. Stevens RG, Jones Dy, Micozzi MS, et al: Body iron stores and the risk of cancer. N Engl J Med 319:1047–1052, 1988.
133. Symons JD, Jacobs I: High intensity performance is not impaired by low intramuscular glycogen. Med Sci Sport Exerc 21:550–557, 1989.
134. Tarnopolsky MA, MacDougall JD, Atkinson SA: Influence of protein intake and training status on nitrogen balance and lean body mass. J Appl Physiol 64:187–93, 1988.
135. Tarnopolsky MA, Atkinson SA, MacDougall JD, et al: Whole body leucine metabolism during and after resistance exercise in fed humans. Med Sci Sport Exerc 23: 326–331, 1991.
136. Tarnopolsky MA, Atkinson SA, MacDougall JD, et al: Evaluation of protein requirements for trained strength athletes. J Appl Physiol 73(5):1986–1995, 1992.
137. Terada LS, Willingham IR, Repine JE: Iron and stroke. In Lauffer RB (ed): Iron and Human Disease. Boca Raton, FL, CRC, 1992, 313.

138. Torranin C, Smith DP, Byrd RJ: The effect of acute thermal dehydration and rapid rehydration on isometric and isotonic endurance. J Sports Med Phys Fitness 19:1–9, 1979.
139. Tuttle WW: The effect of weight loss by dehydration and the withholding of food on the physiologic responses of wrestlers. Res Q Exerc Sport 14:158–166, 1943.
140. Walden O: The relationship of dietary and supplemental calcium intake to bone loss and osteoporosis. J Am Diet Assoc 89:397–400, 1989.
141. Webster S, Rutt R, Weltman A: Physiological effects of a weight loss regimen practiced by college wrestlers. Med Sci Sports Exerc 22:229–234, 1990.
142. Weight LM, Jacobs P, Noakes TD: Dietary iron deficiency and sports anaemia. Br J Nutr 68:253–260, 1992.
143. Widerman PM, Hagan RD: Body weight loss in a wrestler preparing for competition: a case report. Med Sci Sports Exerc 14:413–418, 1982.
144. Williams C: Carbohydrate needs of elite athletes. In Simopoulos AP, Ravlou KN (eds): Nutrition and Fitness for Athletes. Basel, Karger, 1993, Vol. 71, 34–60.
145. Williams MG: Nutritional aspects of human physical and athletic performance. Springfield, IL, Charles C Thomas, 1985.
146. Wishnitzer R, Vorst E, Berrebi A: Bone marrow iron depression in competitive distance runners. Int J Sports Med 4:27, 1983.
147. Witt EH, Reznick AZ, Viguie CA, et al: Exercise, oxidative damage and effects of antioxidant manipulation. J Nutr 122:766–773, 1992.
148. Wooden SA, Williams C: Influence of carbohydrate status on performance during maximal exercise. Int J Sports Med 5(Suppl):126–127, 1984.
149. World Health Organization, Energy and Protein Requirements. Report of Joint FAO/WHO/UNU Expert Consultation. Technical Report Series 724, Geneva, World Health Organization, 1985.

4

Drugs and Doping in Athletes

James C. Puffer, M.D., FAAFP, FACSM

Drug use and abuse has become a national concern; we are bombarded daily with media reports of drug-related deaths, drug arrests, and prominent personalities entering drug rehabilitation programs. Athletes have not been immune from problems associated with drugs. Indeed, the pressures of participating in a highly visible environment, the desire to gain the competitive edge, and the drive to excel have frequently placed athletes in situations where they have felt compelled to use drugs in order to succeed. The deaths of Maryland basketball player Len Bias and Cleveland Browns football player Don Rogers, as well as the revelation that Canadian sprinter Ben Johnson had been found to be using anabolic steroids at the 1988 Summer Olympic Games, have underscored these issues and have led many to reexamine the value systems that underlie competitive sport. Yet, while these events have dramatized the extent to which drugs have pervaded the world of athletics today, this problem is not new; in fact, it has existed for hundreds of years.

HISTORICAL PERSPECTIVE

Doping has become a common term in international athletic circles in the past 5 years. This term actually originated in Southeast Africa where Kaffirs used a local liquor called "dop" as a stimulant. The first use of drugs in athletic competition appears to have predated the birth of Christ. Homer documented ingestion of mushrooms by Greek athletes in the third century B.C. to enhance performance.[49] In the nineteenth century there were reports of widespread use of caffeine, alcohol, nitroglycerin, ethyl ether, and opium by European athletes in efforts to enhance their athletic prowess.

It was not until the unfortunate death of Danish cyclist Kurt Enemar Jensen at the 1960 Summer Olympic Games in Rome that considerable attention was focused on this mounting problem. Jensen and two of his teammates had taken amphetamines and Roniacol to improve their performance in the 100-kilometer team trials. Jensen died, and his two teammates were taken to an Italian hospital in critical condition and subsequently survived. This unfortunate incident led to a convention of European sports governing bodies in January 1963 to address the problem of drugs in sport. From this meeting came a definition of doping that was later adopted by the International Doping Conference of the Federation Internationale de Medicine Sportive in Tokyo in October 1964 and the International Olympic Committee:[7] "Doping is the administration to, or the use by, a competing athlete of any substance foreign to the body or any physiological substance taken in abnormal quantity or by an abnormal route of entry into the body, with the sole intention of increasing in an artificial and unfair manner his performance in competition."

The International Olympic Committee subsequently developed drug testing procedures which were initiated for the 1968 Winter and Summer Olympic Games. Although these procedures have been refined, they have remained in place for every subsequent Olympiad. More recently, drug testing has been adopted by the NCAA and the National Football League, and drug policies have been developed by the National Basketball Association and professional baseball.

PREVALENCE

The prevalence of drug use by athletes has been documented in numerous surveys. The Big Ten Conference conducted a study comparing drug use by male athletes to that of the general student body in 1981.[26] This study found that there was basically little difference in the use of alcohol and marijuana between the two groups (approximately 80% and 20% for each drug respectively); however, 2% of the athletes reported using anabolic steroids, while none of the general student body did so. A Canadian

TABLE 1. Drug Use by Intercollegiate Athletes*

Drug	Percentage of Athletes Using
Alcohol	88%
Amphetamines	8%
Anabolic steroids	6.5%
Anti-inflammatories	31%
Caffeine	68%
Cocaine	17%
Marijuana	36%

*Adapted from Anderson WA, McKeag DB: The substance use and abuse habits of college student athletes. National Collegiate Athletic Association, June 1985.

study by Clement, investigating drug use among 1,687 Olympic athletes in Canada, revealed that 5% used anabolic steroids, 21% were contemplating the use of anabolic steroids, 10% used psychomotor stimulants, 57% used alcohol, 23% used marijuana and 4% used cocaine.[19] A more recent study, completed in 1985 by Anderson and McKeag for the NCAA, investigated drug use by intercollegiate athletes throughout the United States.[5] A summary of this study is found in Table 1. A replication study recently completed for the NCAA by the same authors found strikingly similar results.

From this data, it is apparent that four major categories of drugs are used frequently by athletes. These include anabolic steroids, stimulants, nonsteroidal anti-inflammatory drugs, and recreational drugs. Each of these categories will be reviewed in detail. The use of human growth hormone, blood doping, the use of recombinant erythropoietin, and phosphate/bicarbonate loading, four doping procedures that have recently gained considerable attention, will also be discussed.

ANABOLIC STEROIDS

The use of testosterone or testosterone-like synthetic drugs results in both anabolic and androgenic activity in those using these substances. In other words, they increase protein synthesis, resulting in an increase in muscular bulk, and they also enhance the development of secondary sexual characteristics in the male. In the female, these drugs have masculinizing effects. Anabolic steroids first became available for experimental and therapeutic use in the 1930's and were used extensively during World War II to help restore positive nitrogen balance in victims of starvation.[42] Although these substances have been used for the treatment of refractory anemia, as replacement therapy in hypogonadal males, and in the management of burn victims, there is limited application of these substances for therapeutic purposes at present. Nevertheless, they continue to be used by increasing numbers of athletes to enhance muscular strength and power. When used by athletes, they are frequently taken in amounts 10 to 40 times greater than therapeutic doses, and are usually used in combination ("stacked") or cycled in a pyramid fashion with other erogenic substances.[14] A survey by Buckley in 1988 found that 6.6% of a national sample of high school students used anabolic steroids, with 38% of these students beginning before the age of 15.[12] It is estimated that more than one million people use or have used anabolic steroids in this country. This has generated a 2 million dollar a year black market industry in trafficking these substances.

At the cellular level, the anabolic steroids are bound by cytoplasmic proteins and are subsequently transported to the nucleus, where they then activate DNA-dependent RNA polymerase. This results in the production of messenger RNA, which forms the template for subsequent protein synthesis. Numerous studies have been published supporting both improvement in strength,[6,8,35,59,64] as well as no significant improvement in strength in male athletes.[34,38,42,60] Although there has been considerable confusion in the literature with regard to the benefits of these substances, a review by the American College of Sports Medicine on the use of these agents resulted in the following conclusions:[4] (1) Anabolic steroids in the presence of an adequate diet can contribute to increases in body weight and lean mass; (2) the gains in muscular strength achieved through high-intensity exercise and proper diet can occur by increased use of anabolic steroids in some individuals; (3) anabolic steroids do not increase aerobic power.

Although, after careful review of the literature, this group of experts concluded that the use of these substances may result in the enhancement of muscular strength, it should be noted that the use of these substances has been associated with numerous adverse effects;[43] these are outlined in Table 2. Most of these side effects are well known, but the least appreciated are those that are attributable to the powerful psychoactive properties of these agents.

The work of Pope and Katz first highlighted the potential psychiatric problems with long term anabolic steroid use in 41 body builders and football players who met DSM III-R criteria for significant psychopathology.[48] This included the demonstration of a full affective syndrome in 22% and psychotic symptoms in 12% of the athletes. More importantly, a dependence pattern has been reported with the use of these drugs with features similar to opioid addiction.[10] The treatment of athletes demonstrating such dependence patterns may be particularly challenging for the clinician.

TABLE 2. Reported Adverse Effects of the Anabolic Steroids

Cardiovascular	Psychiatric
increase in total and LDL cholesterol	aggressive behavior
decrease in HDL cholesterol	mood disorders including depression
hypertension	changes in libido
myocardial infarction	dependence disorder
cerebrovascular accident	psychosis
Gynecologic	Male Reproductive
oligo/amenorrhea	oligo/azospermia
male pattern alopecia	decreased testicular size
hirsutism	gynecomastia
clitoromegaly	prostatic hypertrophy
deepening of the voice	adenocarcinoma of the prostate
Gastrointestinal	Miscellaneous
hepatocellular dysfunction	premature closure of the epiphyses in youth
peliosis hepatis	acne
adenocarcinoma of the liver	spontaneous tendon rupture
	blood-borne infection from needle sharing, including AIDS

HUMAN GROWTH HORMONE

Human growth hormone is a polypeptide hormone consisting of 191 amino acids. Normally, 5–10 mg are stored in the pituitary, and adults produce this hormone at a rate of approximately 0.4–1.0 mg/day. With the significant improvement in detection methods for anabolic steroids, many athletes have turned to the use of human growth hormone as an anabolic agent; this substance cannot be detected by current drug testing procedures. While the true prevalence is difficult to estimate, it is widely believed that this preparation is used by football players, weightlifters, and track and field athletes.[44]

It is well known that human growth hormone promotes positive nitrogen balance and stimulates skeletal and soft tissue growth in hormone-deficient children,[62] and it increases the rate of growth in some short-statured children who are not deficient in growth hormone.[57,63] Little evidence exists that this agent has anabolic properties in athletes. However, a report of decreased body fat and increased fat-free weight in highly conditioned adults who were given growth hormone has been shown in a prospective double-blind, randomized trial that used an intense training regimen.[22]

While 25 years of experience have indicated that therapeutic replacement of growth hormone is safe for growth-hormone–deficient children, considerable concern has been expressed over the use of this potent metabolic agent in those who are not growth hormone–deficient.[2,62] While most existing data has been obtained from cohorts in which growth hormone has been used as replacement therapy rather than a pharmacologic agent, several important clinical observations should be noted. Formation of antibodies to growth hormone has been common, and hypothyroidism has occurred. Insulin resistance, hyperinsulinism, and impaired glucose tolerance are likely to occur in those using this substance, as may frank diabetes mellitus and hypertension.

Acromegaly is a potential serious side effect in those abusing this substance. It has been estimated that acromegalic patients with growth hormone concentrations in the range of 5–30 ng/ml have production rates of 1.5 to 9 mg/day.[2] At commonly used doses, a 50-kg person would receive 1 mg/day. Therefore, as little as a twofold increase in dose might result in levels which could cause some of the clinical or biochemical changes noted in acromegaly. Such data should not be taken lightly given that many athletes acquire drugs illegally and self administer them in doses which commonly exceed pharmacologic ranges.

Finally, reports of iatrogenic Creutzfeldt-Jakob disease associated with human growth hormone therapy have added an additional concern.[40] While the production of genetically engineered growth hormone obviates this problem as it replaces cadaver preparations, strict regulations placed on the use of the synthetic preparation will result in many athletes continuing to use nonsynthetic sources, thereby increasing their potential risk for acquiring this catastrophic neurologic disorder.

STIMULANTS

Historically, these drugs have been well known for their potential use as ergogenic aids. At present, three drugs in this category are most frequently used to enhance performance: amphetamine, cocaine, and caffeine.

Amphetamine

Amphetamines are perhaps the drugs best known by the public to be abused by athletes. Considerable publicity concerning the use of these drugs by professional athletes and the well-publicized suspension of Dr. Arnold Mandell's medical license in conjunction with his role in prescribing amphetamines to addicted players while serving as consulting team physician for the San Diego Chargers have brought these issues to the forefront.

There is considerable literature describing the effects of amphetamines on human performance, dating back to the 1950's. Smith and Beecher demonstrated the enhancement of timed trials in selected swimming events.[55] A subsequent study by the same authors demonstrated that athletes using these substances experienced increased feelings of being "revved up" before athletic events as well as feeling more vigorous, energetic, and alert.[56] A report by Chandler demonstrated no substantial improvement in athletic performance with use of amphetamines when selected physiologic components were evaluated.[18] The differences in these two studies most likely can be attributed to the activities that were assessed. Tasks that were sufficiently simple and repetitive so as to permit sustained attention and habituation could be predicted to result in evidence of enhanced performance while using the amphetamines, whereas more complicated maneuvers would not. The dose-related relationship of these phenomena are well described by Mandell in his now classic description of the "Sunday syndrome" in professional football players using these substances.[45]

The amphetamines exert a number of physiologic responses, including increases in blood pressure and heart rate, mild bronchodilation, increased metabolic rate, and increases in plasma-free fatty acids. They are known to disrupt thermoregulatory mechanisms and predispose athletes to heat illness. Large doses and long-term use lead to toxic effects and psychological addiction; these effects include restlessness, tremor, dizziness, anxiety, insomnia, provocation of angina pectoris, arrhythmias, convulsions, coma, and cerebral hemorrhage.

Cocaine

Cocaine has gained much exposure recently, not only for its use in professional sports, but also as a commonly used recreational drug. This drug acts as a central nervous system stimulant, and for this reason has been used by many athletes in an effort to enhance performance. This drug increases the release and blocks the reuptake of norepinephrine from neurons in the nervous system; this results in more available epinephrine to bind to receptor sites, causing euphoria, increased speed of peripheral reflexes, and increased blood pressure and heart rate. In the inexperienced user, peripheral reflexes are frequently dyssynchronous, resulting in marked diminishment of performance. This substance has a half-life of approximately 2 to 6 hours, and can be detected in the urine 24 to 36 hours after being taken.

As noted previously, the use of cocaine by athletes is increasing, and the tragic deaths of Maryland basketball star Len Bias and Don Rogers of the Cleveland Browns have underscored precisely how lethal the use of this drug can be. Increased catecholamine levels associated with cocaine used intranasally, intravenously, or by smoking can directly induce ventricular dysrthymias, coronary vasospasm, vasospasm with thrombosis, and myocardial infarction.[21,37] Any of these events, alone or in combination, can obviously lead to sudden death. A report by Isnek and colleagues has documented that acute cardiac events and sudden death can occur in the absence of underlying cardiac disease and with doses of the drug that are not massive.[37] Cerebrovascular accidents and rupture of the aorta have also been reported in those using cocaine.[21]

Because this drug is frequently taken by sniffing the substance through the nasal passages, it can result in swelling and congestion of the nasal mucosa, as well as ulceration of the nasal septum. Rhinitis, sinusitis, and bronchitis are common side effects in frequent users. Frequent nosebleeds with nasal septum necrosis and ulceration can also be seen in chronic users. It has been hypothesized that sprint-trained athletes may be at greater risk for severe lactic acidosis and subsequent cocaine induced seizures due to the higher percentage of glycolytic muscle fibers frequently found in these athletes.[31] Toxic psychosis, agitation, insomnia, depression, paranoia and rapid addiction may occur in those who use this drug.[21]

Caffeine

Caffeine is a powerful stimulant of the central nervous system and has been used extensively by athletes. It appears abundantly in tea, coffee, and cola drinks and is used frequently by athletes as a stimulant prior to athletic events. Laurin and Letorneau found significant amounts of caffeine in large numbers of urine samples collected from athletes competing in the 1976 Olympic Games in Montreal.[41] Work by Ivy and colleagues has demonstrated that caffeine results in increased work output, most likely secondary to increased mobilization of free fatty acids and increased rates of lipid metabolism.[36] More recent work by independent investigators, however, has cast some doubt on the ability of caffeine to enhance or prolong work output.[15,17] If caffeine does have a benefit in improving athletic performance, it is probably limited to endurance activities and most likely is a result of increased mobilization of free fatty acids, increased rate of lipid metabolism and direct effects on muscle contraction secondary to increases in calcium permeability of the sarcoplasmic reticulum.[65]

Because of the potential for abuse of this substance, the IOC developed quantitative standards for the detection of this substance in urine for the 1984 Olympic Games. Any athlete who was found to have greater than 15 μg/ml in his or her urine was subject to disqualification. Recently, the IOC has lowered this standard to 12 μg/ml. Concern is always raised by athletes as to how much coffee, tea, or cola they can drink without risking subsequent disqualification. Approximately 4–8 cups of coffee would need to be consumed to reach disqualifying levels, depending upon the strength of the coffee, the size of the athlete, and the rate of metabolism. Table 3 provides additional information concerning caffeine levels.

Sympathomimetic Amines

The sympathetic amines are synthetic congeners of naturally occurring catecholamines. One of the powerful sympathomimetic amines, amphetamine, has already been discussed separately. However, several weaker sympathomimetic amines have the potential to be abused by athletes as well; these include drugs such as phenylpropanolamine, phenylephrine and pseudoephedrine, which are frequently found in many over-the-counter medications. The sympathomimetic amines are also commonly found in most asthma preparations. Perhaps no category of drugs has created more confusion and furor in international competition than the sympathomimetic amines. The most celebrated case involved the disqualification of swimmer Rick De Mont at the 1972 Summer Olympic Games for the use of a commonly prescribed asthma preparation.

The question of whether these substances enhance athletic performance has been controversial. Several studies have demonstrated no significant increases in performance with the use of these substances.[24,52] However, a recent study demonstrated an ergogenic effect of inhaled albuterol, a commonly used asthma preparation, on short-term power output in healthy nonasthmatic patients.[53]

***TABLE 3.* Caffeine Content of Commonly Used Substances**

Substance	Caffeine Concentration (mg/100 ml)	Caffeine Level* (μg/ml)
Coffee	55–85	1.5–3 (one cup)
Tea	55–85	1.5–3 (one cup)
Cola	10–15	.75–1.5 (one cup)
Medication	(mg/tablet)	
Cafergot	100	3–6
NoDoz	100	3–6
Anacin	32	2–3
Midol	32	2–3

*Level depends on size of athlete and rate of metabolism. These figures represent general estimates based on average size and rate of metabolism.

NONSTEROIDAL ANTI-INFLAMMATORY DRUGS

The nonsteroidal anti-inflammatory drugs (NSAIDs) have become an important tool in the physician's treatment of common musculoskeletal disorders in athletes. They are frequently prescribed to assist in the management of tendinitis, sprains, strains, and other soft-tissue derangements. Although NSAIDs are extremely effective in the amelioration of soft-tissue inflammation, they do have known side effects, including dyspepsia, gastrointestinal bleeding, decreased platelet aggregation, and sedation. The antiprostaglandin activity of these drugs can result in reduced renal perfusion, and it is well known that the kidney can retain salt and water in response to the use of these medications. However, NSAIDs also uncouple oxidative phosphorylation in skeletal muscle, which can have an effect on oxygen consumption; they directly stimulate ventilation as well as promote sweating and dehydration.[23] Given this information, it is obvious that these drugs interfere with thermoregulatory mechanisms and may predispose athletes to heat illness. These facts should be considered by physicians prescribing these medications for common soft-tissue injuries. NSAIDs have analgesic properties and are frequently used in international competition for the management of pain because they do not appear on the IOC's banned list.

RECREATIONAL DRUGS

Numerous recreational drugs are used on a regular basis by many athletes. These include alcohol, marijuana, and cocaine. As mentioned previously, cocaine does have a stimulatory effect on the central nervous system, and for this reason appears on the IOC's banned list. This drug has previously been discussed in detail along with other psychomotor stimulants.

Alcohol

Alcohol is perhaps the drug most frequently used by intercollegiate and elite athletes.[19,26] Social acceptance of this drug has been high, and it has not been until recently that abuse of this substance has been recognized as a significant problem. The physiologic effects of alcohol are well known and will not be reviewed here. What does deserve mention is the manner in which alcohol may affect performance. Much interest has been generated in this area because of the recent ingestion of alcoholic beverages by marathon runners as a carbohydrate source and a fluid and electrolyte replacement.

A position statement by the American College of Sports Medicine has addressed the use of alcohol by athletes and made several key statements that are substantiated by a thorough review of the literature:[3]

1. The acute ingestion of alcohol has a deleterious effect on many psychomotor skills, including reaction time, hand-eye coordination, accuracy, balance, and complex coordination.

2. Alcohol consumption does not substantially influence physiologic functions crucial to physical performance (VO_{2max}, respiratory dynamics, cardiac function).

3. Alcohol ingestion will not improve muscular work capacity and may decrease performance levels.

4. Alcohol may impair temperature regulation during prolonged exercise in a cold environment.

Some have contended that alcohol may serve as a supplemental energy substrate. Animal studies, however, have demonstrated that ethanol ingestion results in depressed mitochondrial function in skeletal muscle.[29] Although mitochondrial respiration and cytochrome content were significantly depressed in sedentary animals given ethanol, these effects could be offset by exercise, as demonstrated by the normal levels present in trained animals given ethanol. Although there has been some interest in the possibility that alcohol dehydrogenase induction could supplement normal glucogenic pathways in the liver and boost endurance performance, no findings to date would tend to support this conclusion.[54] It would appear that there are no advantages to using alcohol during or prior to athletic competition, and that the known effects of fine motor skill retardation and discoordination would speak against the use of this substance.

Marijuana

Marijuana is a recreational drug also used frequently by athletes. Its active ingredient, Δ-9 tetrahydrocannabinol (THC), results in the impairment of coordination, perception, and vigilance. It has been demonstrated that motor coordination is impaired by doses commonly taken in social settings by both naive and long-term users of this drug. Impairment of short-term memory and alteration of time sense also have been noted. An amotivational syndrome has been described that is characterized by apathy, difficulty in concentrating, loss of ambition, and decline in work performance.[9] Reduction in plasma testosterone levels, oligospermia, and gynecomastia are also well-recognized side effects in those using marijuana chronically.

With regard to exercise performances, work by Renaud and Cormier has demonstrated a reduction of maximal exercise performance with premature achievement of maximal oxygen uptake after smoking marijuana.[40] No effect was noted on tidal volume, arterial blood pressure, or carboxyhemoglobin levels when compared with the control group.

While marijuana is not banned by the IOC, it has been banned by the NCAA. Retention of this substance by adipose tissue results in the ability of sophisticated testing procedures to detect the drug as long as 2–4 weeks after it has been used. Depending upon the sensitivity of the testing procedures used, passive inhalation of secondary smoke theoretically could result in a positive test.

BLOOD DOPING AND EPO

A discussion of doping would not be complete without a discussion of blood doping. This procedure, which also has been known as blood boosting or blood packing, results in the induction of erythrocythemia by removing blood from an individual and storing it in a frozen state while allowing the individual's red cell mass to reequilibrate. At some later time after this equilibration, the red blood cells that have been donated previously are reinfused, resulting in a marked increase in red blood cell mass. The earliest report of this procedure appeared in the literature in 1947 and described the infusion of 2000 ml of freshly transfused blood from matched donors to armed forces personnel.[46] The infusion of fresh, matched blood resulted in a 26% increase in hematocrit over that of controls as well as a 34% increase in endurance capacity. Subsequent studies using refrigerated blood failed to show increases as dramatic as those of this original study performed in 1947. However, in these instances the blood had been refrigerated, and one could expect that 30–40% of the red cells had been lost secondary to processing and normal cell aging during the storage period. Subsequent studies that have used blood frozen at minus 80°C have shown much more impressive results. Buick and colleagues studied the effect of blood doping on aerobic power in elite runners.[13] They demonstrated significant improvements in both maximal oxygen consumption and total exercise time, in addition to significant increases in hemoglobin concentration when compared with controls. Additional work has confirmed these results and demonstrated that the reinfused blood does not significantly compromise the cardiovascular system.[32,58,66] Although transfused blood does not represent a drug per se, it is a physiologic substance that is introduced into the body in a foreign manner with the explicit intent of improving performance, and therefore blood doping obviously is in violation of the definition of doping mentioned previously.

The IOC, after reports of blood doping by American cyclists at the 1984 Summer Olympic Games, has officially banned the practice of blood doping. From a practical standpoint, however, techniques are not available for detecting the presence of transfused autologous or donor blood. Enforcement of this policy, therefore, will be extremely cumbersome, and effective deterrence of this practice by those athletes who wish to employ it difficult to accomplish.

Obviously considerable risks attend the transfusion of blood or blood products. The use of improperly matched donor blood may result in potentially fatal transfusion reactions and also carries the risk of transmission of infectious disease. The use of blood products by athletes for enhancing performance contravene the ethics of both sport and good medicine, and therefore, this practice should be deplored by physicians and athletes alike.

The practice of blood doping, however, may well have become outdated by the recent development of human recombinant erythropoietin (EPO). This synthetically produced substance has been used extensively to treat the anemia of chronic renal failure as well as refractory anemias. The use of this substance results in a predictable increase in red blood cell mass in a typical dose-response relationship.[27] Abuse of this agent, however, can result in marked polycythemia and the potential for subsequent thromboembolism, stroke, and myocardial infarction. The deaths of of 18 Belgian and Dutch racing cyclists over a 4-year period from 1987 to 1991 have been attributed in the lay press to the use of EPO, although this cannot be confirmed with hard medical evidence.

BICARBONATE/PHOSPHATE LOADING

The latest developments in doping have centered around ingestion of significant amounts of either bicarbonate or phosphate in an effort to favorably alter physiologic parameters that influence maximum performance. While neither of these substances is banned by the IOC, their ingestion solely for the purpose of artificially increasing performance violates the definition of doping defined earlier.

Bicarbonate Loading

During steady state exercise, sufficient oxygen is supplied to and used by working muscle. Under these conditions lactic acid homeostasis is maintained. If exercise intensity increases and aerobic metabolism is insufficient to meet energy demands, however, anaerobic glycolysis contributes to energy requirements and lactic acid is formed. Almost all of the lactic acid generated during anaerobic metabolism is buffered by bicarbonate. However, regulation of pH becomes progressively more difficult during strenuous exercise secondary to an increase in hydrogen ion concentration from both carbon dioxide and lactic acid formation. Eventually intramuscular pH rises as a result of lactate accumulation, and this not only restricts glycolysis but also decreases lipolysis. This results in diminished energy production and decreased muscular work.

Since extracellular bicarbonate enhances diffusion of hydrogen and lactate ions from the intracellular to the extracellular space, it would seem logical that increasing the concentration of bicarbonate available for these purposes would forestall fatigue and improve performance. In fact, this has been demonstrated.[20,39] Pate and coworkers have studied the effect of orally administered bicarbonate on performance of high-intensity exercise by highly trained endurance athletes.[47] They demonstrated that with a 0.3 g/kg oral dose blood pH was significantly increased immediately before, immediately after, and three minutes after exhaustive treadmill exercise as compared with placebo in a controlled, double-blind protocol. Additionally, run time to exhaustion was significantly increased (578 vs. 564 seconds) after athletes ingested bicarbonate rather than placebo.

Phosphate Loading

It is well known that increasing serum phosphate results in an increase in red blood cell 2,3 diphosphoglycerate (2,3DPG) levels. Since increased 2,3DPG levels shift the oxygen-hemoglobin dissociation curve to the right and thereby enhance oxygen delivery to tissues, it might seem logical that increasing serum phosphate would improve maximum oxygen consumption. Cade and colleagues at the University of Florida studied the effect of 1 gm of sodium phosphate taken four times daily for three consecutive days compared with placebo in 10 highly trained athletes who served as their own controls.[16] They found that after oral phosphate loading there was a significant increase in serum phosphate and red blood cell 2,3DPG. Maximum oxygen consumption increased and correlated with the rise in 2,3DPG.

DRUG TESTING

Drug testing has been used to deter the use of performance-enhancing substances by athletes and guarantee a drug-free environment in which athletes can compete fairly. The employment of drug testing, however, has not been without considerable expense. Three million dollars were spent to equip the drug testing laboratory used in Montreal during the Summer Olympic Games in 1976, and in 1984 the Olympic Organizing Committee in Los Angeles spent approximately 1.8 million dollars to establish the UCLA Olympic Analytic Laboratory. The NCAA spends over one million dollars annually to run its drug testing program. Despite the expense, drug testing is at present the only effective way to attempt to enforce drug policy and deter the use of performance enhancing drugs.

Three types of testing procedure are used that have varying degrees of sensitivity, specificity, and cost. Thin layer chromatography is the least expensive screening test but has low specificity and cannot provide unequivocal identification of a banned substance. The Centers for Disease Control reviewed 13 laboratories using thin layer chromatography techniques and found that these laboratories were often unable to detect drug concentrations called for by their contracts.[33] Radioimmunoassay (RIA) and enzyme-multiplied immunoassay (EMIT) are two of the most commonly used screening methods. The manufacturers of these tests claim that they are 97–99% accurate; however, such is usually not the case. This creates the need for a second, highly specific test to confirm the presence of a banned substance and to avoid false-positive results. Gas chromatography and mass spectroscopy (GC/MS) serves as the "gold standard" test because it provides a precise fingerprint of the substance under question and thus provides exact identification.

Because of the extreme accuracy of GC/MS technology, athletes have attempted to employ several techniques to avoid detection. The first of these methods was the substitution of exogenous testosterone for the synthetic anabolic steroids. Prior to 1984, the qualitative tests used to detect banned substances could not distinguish exogenous testosterone from naturally occurring testosterone. For these reasons, many athletes avoided detection of anabolic steroids by stopping these substances well before the projected time of known drug testing and then switched to injectable testosterone preparations until the time of competition. At the 1980 Summer Olympic Games in Moscow, Donike and colleagues independently tested urine specimens that were submitted by randomly selected athletes for anabolic steroid testing for the presence of abnormal quantities of testosterone.[25] As many as two thirds of these samples had quantities of testosterone that were nonphysiologic. Subsequently, a method was developed for detecting exogenous testosterone using the known one-to-one relationship of testosterone to its isomer epitestosterone. When exogenous testosterone is administered, serum testosterone is elevated out of proportion to epitestosterone. A positive test was defined as a ratio which exceeded six to one.

This analytic method was introduced into the 1984 Olympic Games and has been widely used since then. However, recent caution has been used in interpreting these results, as it has been found on several occasions that athletes who have not used exogenous testosterone have levels that exceed or are very close to the six-to-one ratio. Furthermore, a recent Swedish study has found that the ingestion of ethanol may increase this ratio as well.[28]

A number of novel methods have been used by athletes to avoid the detection of banned substances in the urine. This includes the use of diuretics and the use of blocking agents, such as probenecid, as well as the substitution of "clean" urine by means of self-catheterization or the development of "innovative" delivery systems. These problems have been obviated by banning the aforementioned substances and attempts at manipulating the urine specimen.

Drug testing occurs at all levels. As previously mentioned, the International Olympic Committee instituted routine drug testing at the Olympic Games beginning in 1968. Restricted and banned substances and methods that are used by this international governing body can be found in Table 4. The NCAA began drug testing in 1986 at postseason football games and championship events. This program has been broadened to include random, unannounced testing as well. A number of member institutions have instituted their own drug programs. A 1986 survey of 257 NCAA affiliate schools found that 28 percent had a drug screening program for athletes and that 52 percent of those schools without such a program were considering

***TABLE 4.* Restricted and Banned Substances and Methods: International Olympic Committee**

DOPING CLASSES
- Stimulants
  - psychomotor stimulants
  - sympathomimetic amines
  - miscellaneous CNS stimulants (including caffeine—urinary concentration > 12 μg/ml)
- Narcotics
- Anabolic Steroids
- Beta-Blockers
- Diuretics
- Growth Hormone
- human Chorionic Gonadotropin
- EPO

DOPING METHODS
- Blood Doping
- Pharmacologic, Chemical, and Physical Manipulation of the Urine

CLASSES OF DRUGS SUBJECT TO CERTAIN RESTRICTIONS
- Alcohol (levels may be requested by specific international federations)
- Local Anesthetics (permitted when medically indicated and documented in writing to the IOC Medical Commission)
- Corticosteroids (banned, except when used topically, locally, intra-articularly, or via inhalation and documented in writing to the IOC Medical Commission)
- Beta-2 Agonists (permitted in the aerosol or inhalant form for the treatment of asthma)

TABLE 5. Restricted and banned substances and procedures: National Collegiate Athletic Association

BANNED DRUG CLASSES
- Psychomotor and Central Nervous System Stimulants
  - Including Caffeine (urinary concentration > 15 mcg/ml)
- Anabolic Steroids Including Testosterone
  - (testosterone to epitestosterone ratio greater than 6)
- Substance Banned for Specific Sports
  - Alcohol (rifle)
  - beta-blockers
- Diuretics
- Street Drugs
  - heroin
  - marijuana and THC (urinary concentration greater than 25 ng/ml)

DRUGS AND PROCEDURES SUBJECT TO RESTRICTION
- Blood Doping
- Growth Hormone
- Urine Manipulation
- Local Anesthetics (procaine, carbocaine, xylocaine without vasoconstrictor may be used locally or topically when medically justified and submitted in writing to the NCAA crew chief in charge of testing; cocaine is not permitted)

developing one.[61] It is important to note that the NCAA drug testing policy and list of banned substances differ significantly from that of the International Olympic Committee, and this is listed in Table 5 for purposes of comparison.

The organizations that oversee professional sports have varying drug policies. Major league baseball conducts random tests for cocaine, marijuana, heroin, and morphine among players with specified drug testing clauses in their contracts as well as among owners, mangers, executives, and umpires. The National Basketball Association can test with "reasonable cause" individual players for cocaine and heroin without prior notice. The National Football League currently conducts an extensive testing program throughout the NFL season for street drugs, anabolic steroids, and amphetamines.

Given the cost of drug testing, the effectiveness of these programs in preventing drug use has been questioned. A 1987 NCAA survey of 407 football players from Division One schools revealed that 63 percent believed drug testing was a deterrent to drug use.[1] While drug testing certainly is not perfect, it provides, along with a sound educational program, the only means of deterring the use of performance-enhancing substances by athletes.

SUMMARY

The use of drugs to enhance athletic performance poses tremendous potential risk to sport and athletes. The incidence of drug usage by athletes is increasing, and many athletes are turning to new drugs or alternative doping methods in an effort to avoid detection. Future success in eradicating drug usage by athletes will result only from increased efforts directed at enhancement of athlete education, development of strict policies dealing with athletes who use banned substances, refinement of drug testing procedures, and a shift in public attitude from "winning at all costs" to one that fosters the basic values sports were intended to promote.

REFERENCES

1. Abdenour TE, Miner MJ, Weir N: Attitudes of intercollegiate football players toward drug testing. Athl Train 22: 199–201, 1987.
2. Ad Hoc Committee on Growth Hormone Usage, the Lawson Wilkins Pediatric Endocrine Society, and the Committee on Drugs: Growth hormone in the treatment of children with short stature. Pediatrics 72:891–894, 1983.
3. American College of Sports Medicine: Position statement on the use of alcohol in sports. Med Sci Sports Exerc 14:ix–x, 1982.
4. American College of Sports Medicine: Stand on the use of Anabolic-androgenic steroids in sports. American College of Sports Medicine, 1984.
5. Anderson WA, and McKeag DB: The substance use and abuse habits of college student athletes. National Collegiate Athletic Association, June 1985.
6. Ariel G: The effect of anabolic steroid upon skeletal muscle contractile force. J Sports Med Phys Fitness, 13:187–190, 1973.
7. Barnes L: Olympic drug testing: Improvements without progress. Phys Sportsmed 8:21–24, 1980.
8. Berg A, and Keul J: Der Einfluss von anabolen Substanzen auf das Verhalten der freien Serumaminosauren von Normalperson und Scwerathleten in Rule and bei Korperarbeit. Oester Z Sportsmed 4:11–18, 1974.
9. Biron S, and Wells J: Marijuana and its effect on the athlete. Athletic Training 18:295–303, 1983.
10. Brower KJ, et al: Anabolic-androgenic steroid dependence. J Clin Psychiatry 50:31–33, 1989.
11. Brown P, Gajdusek DC, Gibbs CJ, et al: Potential epidemic of Creutzfeldt-Jakob disease from human growth hormone therapy. NJ Med 313:728–731, 1985.
12. Buckley WE, et al: Estimated prevalence of anabolic steroid use among male high school seniors. JAMA 260:3441–3445, 1988.
13. Buick FJ, Gledhill N, Froese AB, et al: Effect of induced erythrocythemia on aerobic work capacity. J Appl Physiol 48:636–642, 1980.
14. Burkett LN, and Falduto MT: Steroid use by athletes in a metropolitan area. Phys Sports Med 12:69–74, 1984.
15. Butts NK, Crowell D: Effect of caffeine ingestion on cardio-respiratory endurance in men and women. Res Q Exerc Sport 56:301–305, 1985.
16. Cade R, Conte M, Zauner C, et al: Effects of phosphate loading on 2, 3 diphosphoglycerate and maximal oxygen uptake. Med Sci Sports Exerc 16:263–268, 1984.
17. Casal DC, Leon AS: Failure of caffeine to affect substrate utilization during prolonged running. Med Sci Sports Exerc 17:174–179, 1985.
18. Chandler JV, Blair SN: The effects of amphetamines on selected physiological components related to athletic success. Med Sci Sports Exerc 12:65–69, 1980.
19. Clement DB: Drug use survey: Results and conclusions. Physician Sportsmed 11:64–67, 1983.

20. Costill DL, Verstappen F, Kuipers H, et al: Acid-base balance during repeated bouts of exercise with HCO_3. Med Sci Sports Exerc 15:115, 1983.
21. Cregler LL, Mark H: Medical complications of cocaine abuse. N Engl J Med 315:1495–1500, 1986.
22. Crist DM, Peake GT, Egan PA, Water DL: Body composition response to exogenous GH during training in highly conditioned adults. J Appl Physiol 65:579–584, 1988.
23. Day RO: Effects of exercise performance on drugs used in musculo-skeletal disorders. Med Sci Sports Exerc 13: 272–275, 1981.
24. DeMeersman R, Getty D, Schaefer DC: Sympathomimetics and exercise enhancement: All in the mind? Pharmacol Biochem Behav 28:361–365, 1987.
25. Donike, M: Personal communication, 1983.
26. Duda, M: Drug testing challenges: College and pro athletes. Phys Sportsmed 11:64–67, 1983.
27. Ersler AJ: Erythropoietin. N Engl J Med 324:1339–1344, 1991.
28. Falk O, Palonek E, Bjorkhem I: Effect of ethanol on the ratio between testosterone and epitestosterone in urine. Clin Chem 34(7):1482–1484, 1988;15:225–32, 1979.
29. Farrar RP, Martin TP, Abraham LD, et al: The interaction of endurance running and ethanol on skeletal muscle mitochondria. Life Sci 30:67–75, 1982.
30. Frasier SD: Human pituitary growth hormone (hGH) therapy in growth hormone deficiency. Endocr Rev 4:155–170, 1983.
31. Giammarco RA: The athlete, cocaine, and lactic acidosis: A hypothesis. Am J Med Sci 294:412–414, 1987.
32. Goforth HW Jr, Campbell NL, Hodgdon JA, et al: Hematologic parameters of trained distance runners following induced erythrocythemia. Med Sci Sports Exerc 14:174, 1982.
33. Hansen HJ, et al: Crisis in drug testing: Results of CDC blind study. JAMA 253(16):2382–7, 1985.
34. Hervey GR: Are athletes wrong about anabolic steroids? Br J Sports Med 9:74–77, 1975.
35. Hervey GR, Knibbs AV, Burkinshaw L, et al: Effects of methandienone on the performance and body composition of men undergoing athletic training. Clin Sci 60:457–461, 1981.
36. Ivy JL, Costill DL, Fink WJ, et al: Role of caffeine and glucose ingestion on metabolism during exercise. Med Sci Sports Exerc 10:66, 1978.
37. Isnek JM, Estes NAM, Thompson PD, et al: Acute cardiac events temporally related to cocaine abuse. N Engl J Med 315:1438–1443, 1986.
38. Johnson LD, Roundy ES, Allsen PE, et al: Effect of anabolic steroid treatment on endurance. Med Sci Sports, 7:287–289, 1975.
39. Jones NL, Sutton JR, Taylor R, et al: Effect on pH on cardiorespiratory and metabolic responses to exercise. J Appl Physiol 43:959–964, 1977.
40. Koch TK, Berg BO, De Armand SJ, et al: Creutzfeldt-Jakob disease in a young adult with idiopathic hypopituitarism: Possible relation to the administration of cadaveric human growth hormone. N Engl J Med 313:731–733, 1985.
41. Laurin CA, Letorneau G: Medical report on the Montreal olympic games. Am J Sports Med 6:54–61, 1978.
42. Loughton SV, Ruhline RO: Human strength and endurance responses to anabolic steroids and training. J Sports Med Phys Fitness 17:285–296, 1977.
43. MacDougall D: Anabolic steroids. Phys Sports Med 11: 95–99, 1983.
44. Macintyre JG: Growth hormone and athletes. Sports Med 4:129–42, 1987.
45. Mandell AJ, Stewart KD, Russo PV: The Sunday syndrome: From kinetics to altered consciousness. Fed Proc 40:2693–2698, 1981.
46. Pace N, Lozner EL, Consolazio WV, et al: The increase in hypoxia tolerance of normal men accompanying the polycythemia induced by transfusion of erythrocytes. Am J Physiol 148:152–163, 1947.
47. Pate RR, Smith PE, Lambert MI et al: Effect of orally administered sodium bicarbonate on performance of high intensity exercise. Med Sci Sports Exerc 17:200–201, 1985.
48. Pope HG, Katz DL: Affective and psychotic symptoms associated with anabolic steroid use. Am J Psychiatry, 145:487–90, 1988.
49. Puffer JC: The use of drugs in swimming. Clin Sports Med 5(1):77–89, 1986.
50. Renaud AM, Cormier Y: Acute effects of marijuana smoking on maximal exercise performance. Med Sci Sports Exerc 18:685–689, 1986.
51. Ryan AJ: Anabolic steroids are fool's gold. Fed Proc 40:2682–2688, 1981.
52. Sidney KH, Lefcoe NM: The effects of Tedral upon athletic performance: A double blind cross-over study. Quebec City International Congress of Physical Activity Sciences, 1976.
53. Signorile JF, Kaplan JA, Applegate B, Perry AC: Effects of acute inhalation of the bronchodilator, albuterol, on power output. Med Sci Sports Exerc 24:638–42, 1992.
54. Shepard RJ: 1982 Yearbook of Sports Medicine. Chicago, Year Book, 1982, p 140.
55. Smith GM, Beecher HK: Amphetamine sulphate and athletic performance. I. Objective effects. JAMA 170:542–547, 1959.
56. Smith GM, Beecher HK: Amphetamine, secobarbital and athletic performance. II. Subjective evaluation of performances, mood states, and physical states. JAMA 172: 1502–1514, 1960.
57. Spiliotis BE, August GP, Hung W, et al: Growth hormone neurosecretory dysfunction: A treatable cause of short stature. JAMA 251:2223–2330, 1984.
58. Spriett LL, Gledhill N, Forese AB, et al: The effect of induced erythrocythemia on central circulation and oxygen transport during maximal exercise. Med Sci Sports Exerc, 12:122, 1980.
59. Stamford BA, Moffatt R: Anabolic steroid: Effectiveness as an ergogenic aid to experienced weight trainers. J Sports Med Phys Fitness 14:191–197, 1974.
60. Stromme SB, Meen HD, Aakvaag A: Effects of an androgenic anabolic steroid on strength development and plasma testosterone levels in normal males. Med Sci Sports 6:203–208, 1974.
61. Summary Report of Drug Screening Questionnaire. The National Collegiate Athletic Association, December 1986.
62. Underwood LE: Report of the conference on uses and possible abuses of biosynthetic human growth hormone. N Engl J Med, 311:606–608, 1984.
63. VanVliet G, Styne DM, Kaplan SL, et al: Growth hormone treatment for short stature. N Engl J Med 309:1016–1022, 1983.
64. Ward P: The effect of an anabolic steroid on strength and lean body mass. Med Sci Sports 5:277–282, 1973.
65. Welch JM, Aubier M, Jardin M, et al: Effect of caffeine on skeletal muscle function before and after fatigue. J Appl Physiol 54:1303–1305, 1983.
66. Williams MH, Wesseldine S, Somma T, et al: The effects of induced erythrocythemia upon 5-mile treadmill run time. Med Sci Sports Exerc 13:169–175, 1981.

5

Thermoregulation, Heat Illness, and Safe Exercise in the Heat

Morris B. Mellion, M.D.
Guy L. Shelton, M.A., P.T., A.T.C.

TEMPERATURE REGULATION

The human body is well adapted to exercise in the heat. Our muscles can generate 20 times as much energy during exercise as they do at rest. At maximal exercise intensity the human body's work efficiency is approximately 25%. Therefore, about 75% of the muscle energy consumption is converted to heat rather than work.[85] Conditioned endurance athletes can generate 1033 Kcal/hr of heat safely for up to three hours.[28] We have a highly efficient thermoregulatory system that allows us to dissipate this heat load into our environment. Otherwise, within 10 to 15 minutes of beginning intense exercise, our body temperature could rise to life-threatening levels.[23]

Heat Transfer and Heat Dissipation

Most of the heat generated by exercise is transported by the cardiovascular system from the working muscles back to the body core. Only a small amount is conducted passively from muscle through overlying tissue to skin for dissipation. Additionally, a small amount of heat is lost from superficial veins to the adjacent skin as the warmed blood travels to the heart.

The blood from the working muscles mixes in the heart with the venous return from the rest of the body to form the cardiac output. Early in exercise heat production exceeds heat loss, producing an increase in body core temperature. The rise in core temperature is sensed by thermodetectors in the hypothalamus, spinal cord, and limb muscles and provides a sympathetically mediated stimulus to increase the skin blood flow and initiate sweating.[28] Additional thermodetectors indicate skin temperature increases to the hypothalamus. High ambient temperature or severe radiant heat from the sun can trigger the heat-dissipating mechanisms even before exercise is begun.[23]

The warm blood from the body's core carries much of its heat load into the dilated vessels of the skin. When the ambient temperature is less than 68°F (20°C), most of the heat loss to the environment is by convection and radiation from the skin. When the environment itself is warm, these mechanisms are inefficient; and above 68°F most of the heat is lost through evaporative cooling. At 95°F (35°C) convection and radiation no longer contribute to heat loss.[28] Since the evaporative heat loss of a single liter of water at 30°C is 580 Kcal,[93] and the hypothetical 70-kg individual sweats 1 to 2 liters per hour during intense exercise in the heat, this is an extremely efficient way to dissipate heat.[23]

After the heat-dissipating mechanisms are brought into play, the core temperature reaches a plateau, where it remains until the exercise demand is finished.[73] In elite endurance athletes this level may be over 104°F (40°C) without compromising performance. Body temperatures in athletes may even exceed so called "survival" limits (40–42°C) transiently without injury.[39] If the heat-dissipating mechanisms fail, or if there is an overwhelming heat stress, the core temperature may continue to rise, even to dangerous levels.[39]

Distribution of Cardiac Output

There are competing demands for cardiac output and blood volume in the exercising human.[39,46,60] During the first 10 to 20 minutes of exercise, approximately 15% of the intravascular fluid volume is shunted to the working muscles. Increases of skin blood flow for cooling and the gravitational displacement of blood volume to the lower extremities during upright exercise shunt additional blood from the central circulation and lower central plasma volume. Additionally, sweating can easily cause losses of 1 to 2 liters/hour (more in larger athletes), and further diminish plasma volume.

As central blood flow decreases, reflex vasoconstriction in the renal and splanchnic circulation helps maintain adequate intravascular volume.[46] However, with continued sweat loss there is less blood returning to the heart to be pumped. Consequently, stroke volume decreases, and the body attempts to compensate by increasing heart rate in order to maintain cardiac output. Finally, a point is reached at which a higher heart rate cannot be maintained. If adjustments are not made to this process, the system will collapse.[28,33,39,60]

The body does respond. In some individuals, the vasomotor center, triggered by baroreceptor signals indicating hypovolemia and by osmolarity measures of hypertonic plasma, transmits efferent messages that lower skin blood-flow and reduce sweat rate.[23,46,61,77,79] The obvious problem is that, if the cooling mechanisms are reduced significantly without a concurrent drop in the exercise level, and therefore in the heat load, core temperature may rise dangerously. The athlete can change this process favorably by reducing the exercise load (slowing down) or by building the plasma volume through hypotonic fluid (water) consumption, or preferably both.

In other athletes, the reduced cardiac return causes decreased blood pressure with a concomitant fall in metabolic activity without decreased skin blood flow. These individuals may collapse with their sweating mechanism still functioning with a normal or slightly elevated core temperature.[39]

Dehydration reduces the heat dissipation process, causing greater heat storage and a reduced physical performance.[77] Severe dehydration during exercise in the heat is a major factor in heat illness. Figure 1 characterizes typical effects of dehydration on physical performance. Some athletes may be more susceptible than indicated in this figure, but some elite, highly trained, acclimated athletes may tolerate severely reduced hydration without significant consequences.

Metabolic Considerations

Although dehydration is a critical factor in most cases of exertional heat stroke, the fact that heat stroke can occur in the absence of clinically significant dehydration has focused attention on the effects of increased heat load on metabolism. There is good evidence that submaximal heart rate and rectal temperature changes during an exercise challenge in a temperate environment correlate well with the same individual's response to exercise in the heat.[83] Furthermore, a study of 30 marathoners revealed that their post-race rectal temperature correlated with their metabolic rates during the race, but not with their percent of fluid loss (dehydration).[67] These findings point to the importance of metabolic efficiency during exercise in the heat.

The importance of metabolic pathophysiology in the development of heat injury has led Hubbard to hypothesize that thermally driven metabolic events could actually drain an individual's energy supply, even in a state of euhydration. His Energy Depletion Model has three major components. First, elevated skeletal muscle temperature increases the

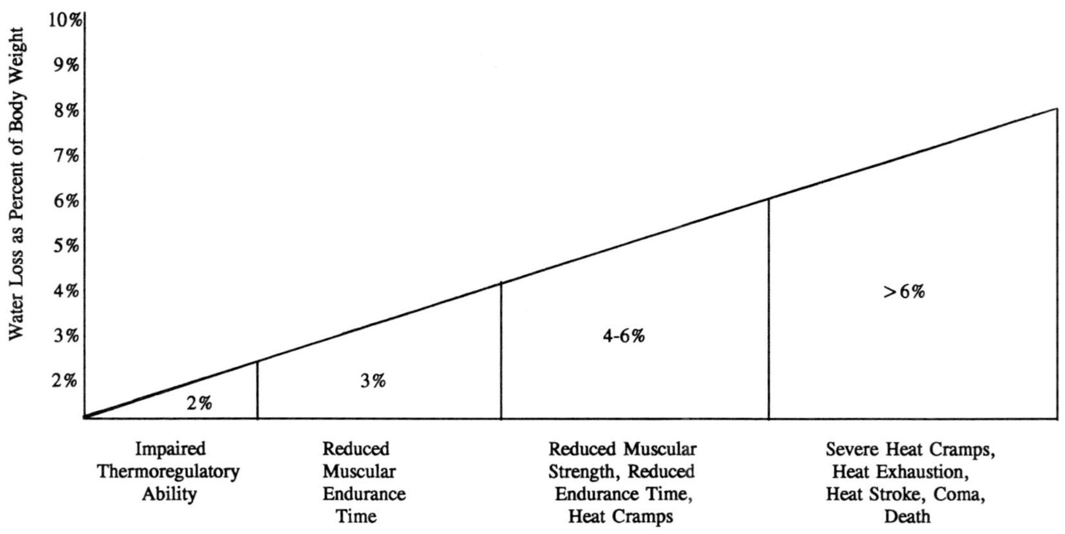

FIGURE 1. Effect of dehydration on physical performance. (From Wheeler KB: Effect of hypohydration on performance—fluid and electrolyte requirements. NSCA Journal 10(5):46–48, 1988, with permission.)

muscle metabolic rate and magnifies the energy cost of force development. Second, elevated temperature causes increased cell membrane permeability with leakage of sodium and potassium ions. The compensatory transmembrane ion pumping necessary to restore homeostasis causes a large energy drain. Evidence for the increased membrane permeability comes from elevations of serum creatine kinase and lactate dehydrogenase. Third, intracellular lactic acidosis develops, promoting fatigue and cell swelling. This model demonstrates a "fundamental problem with energy availability." The heat load increases the metabolic rate and decreases metabolic efficiency. Muscle weakness and fatigue occur with extreme energy deficiency, and muscles fail to relax and remain contracted. Muscle weakness, tightness, and fatigue are common symptoms of heat illness.[38]

Effect of Upright Posture

When humans exercise in an upright position, 70% of their total blood volume is below the level of the heart, much of it in distensible, dependent veins. With exercise, muscle contraction pumps the column of blood in the veins up to the heart as venous return. During moderate exercise in a cool environment, this muscle pump works efficiently. Cutaneous vasoconstriction stimulated by the upright position limits the rate of venous refilling and inhibits peripheral venous pooling. During exercise in the heat, however, cutaneous vasodilation diverts more blood flow to the skin, thereby increasing peripheral venous volume. In this setting the muscle pump is less efficient.[39,46,76] Consequently, upright exercise in the heat places an extra stress on the maintenance of adequate cardiac output.

Thermoregulation in Women

Research on the influence of gender difference in thermoregulation is in its early stages. There is evidence that thermoregulatory responses, plasma volume and serum electrolytes are better maintained in female than in male runners during prolonged running in a hot, humid environment.[55] Young adult and post-pubescent females exercising in the heat also demonstrated significantly lower loss of sweat electrolytes.[53] In reproductive-age women exercising during the post-ovulatory (luteal) phase of the menstrual cycle, heat dissipation may be reduced because of an increased temperature set point during this phase and perhaps because of smaller plasma volume.[37,72,89] Postmenopausal women have the same thermoregulatory sweating response to core temperature elevation during heat exposure as do premenopausal women; estrogen replacement therapy generally lowers their resting core temperature and the threshold for onset of sweating and cutaneous vasodilation during exercise.[89]

Acclimation and Training Effect

Both acclimation to exercise in the heat and physical conditioning improve the individual's ability to tolerate heat stress, and the results are to some extent additive. Acclimation consists to 4 to 7 episodes of exercise in the heat for 1 to 4 hours each, with gradually increasing intensity over approximately 7 to 10 days for adults and slightly longer for children.[8] Fifty percent of acclimation is lost between 10 to 15 days without continued exposure to exercise in the heat.[75] Table 1 demonstrates the physiologic effects of acclimation and physical conditioning that enable the athlete to tolerate a high level of exercise heat stress. One particular aspect of acclimation deserve special attention. Table 2 demonstrates that the acclimatized athlete has a significantly increased ability to control temperature loss by sweating. Total sweat capacity is also increased in the acclimated athlete. Even though the sweat sodium concentration is reduced, the increased sweat capacity may result in an increased maximum sodium loss.[3] In long exercise sessions and competitions, the total sodium loss may be quite significant.

Fever, Exercise, and Antipyretics

Stimulated by endotoxin, microbes or immune system components, mononuclear phagocytes release the pyrogen interleukin-1, which, in turn, triggers the hypothalamus to raise the body's core temperature set point. The result is the form of

***TABLE 1.* Physiologic Effects of Acclimation to Exercise in the Heat Combined with Physical Conditioning**

Heat Dissipation
Earlier initiation of sweating[3,8,23,28,49,60]
Increased rate of sweating[3,8,15,23,60]
Increased maximum sweating capacity[3]
Lower sweat sodium concentration[3,8,49]
Cardiovascular Effects
Increased basal plasma volume[3,12,33,39,60]
Decreased heart rate at given work load and heat stress[3,8,10,39,49]
Metabolic Effects
Increased aldosterone production[3]
Reduced urinary sodium excretion[3]
Increased skeletal muscle mitochondrial density[3]
Increased skeletal muscle myoglobin[3]
Increased skeletal muscle glycogen[3]
Thermal Effects
Increased exercise capacity in the heat[3]
Lower core and skin temperature at given work load and heat stress[3,8,10,49]
Reduced perceived intensity of exercise[8]
Increased thermal comfort[8]

***TABLE 2.* Sweat Rate and Sweat (NA+) Concentration in Man**

	Maximal Sweating Rate	(Na+) Concentration	Maximum (Na+) Loss/hr
Unacclimatized	1.5 L/hr	100 mEq/L	150 mEq/hr
Acclimatized	2.5 L/hr	75 mEq/L	175 mEq/hr

*Reprinted from Anderson RJ, Reed G, Knochel J: Heatstroke. Adv Int Med 28:115–141, 1983, with permission.

temperature elevation known as fever. Core temperature rises caused by fever are additive to those caused by exercise. Temperature rises caused by fever may be reduced by antipyretics such as aspirin and acetaminophen, whereas those caused by exercising will not respond to these medications.[28,43,84]

EXERTIONAL HEAT ILLNESSES

There are at least six common syndromes of exercise-induced heat illness. Heat edema is a transitory reaction of peripheral swelling when an unacclimated individual is exposed to the heat. Heat syncope is a transient hypovolemic syncopal episode. Heat cramps, heat exhaustion, and heat stroke form a spectrum of increasingly severe heat illnesses due to dehydration, electrolyte losses, and failure of the body's heat-dissipating mechanisms. Hyponatremic collapse is a recently described syndrome that occurs predominantly in ultraendurance athletes, but which has been reported in marathoners.

Heat Edema

When an unacclimated individual is exposed to even mild exercise in a hot environment, a marked peripheral vasodilatation and sweating may cause a decreased plasma volume and a resultant marked increase in aldosterone production. The aldosterone-mediated sodium and water retention may result in a transitory dependent edema, usually most noticeable in the hands and feet. Generally, the healthy body will respond over the first few days of exposure to heat with a more thorough adaptive response and the edema will appear to resolve spontaneously.[3]

Heat Syncope

If an athlete who is maximally vasodilated and somewhat dehydrated after a workout or competition in the heat stops exercising abruptly and stands still, as some do at the end of a race, he or she may feel lightheaded and faint. Much of the athlete's central blood volume "pools" in the vessels of the lower extremities, and there is too little venous return for the heart to pump an adequate blood flow to the brain. Once recognized, this is a relatively trivial problem. Treatment consists of having the athlete lie down with legs slightly elevated in a cool or shaded place, drink cold water, and rest. Complications and sequelae are rare. This syndrome can be prevented by maintaining adequate hydration before and during exercise, acclimatizing properly to exercise in the heat, and ending exercise sessions with proper cool-down.

Heat Cramps

Heat cramps are a form of muscle tightening and spasm occurring during or after intense, prolonged exercise in heat. They may be exquisitely painful, and they rarely respond to muscle kneading or massage. Typically, the gastrocnemius and thigh muscles are affected, but abdominal and intercostal muscles can be involved as well.

Hyponatremia has been implicated as the underlying cause of heat cramps. Typically, this syndrome occurs after prolonged sodium depletion with inadequate dietary replacement between exercise sessions. The already hyponatremic athlete exercises in the heat, loses more sodium in sweat, and then drinks large amounts of water during a break or after exercise. The further dilutional drop in serum sodium triggers the cramps. This problem is common in poorly acclimatized athletes, but it is also seen in well-acclimatized, highly conditioned athletes who lose large amounts of sodium relatively slowly over long bouts of exercise in the heat.[3] It also occurs in athletes on diuretics, particularly during the first few weeks of medication.

Treatment consists of rest and cooling down, gentle stretching, and oral hypotonic salt solutions (1 teaspoon salt/1 quart water). Occasionally, contracting the antagonistic muscle group against firm resistance relieves the spasm. A liter of intravenous normal saline usually provides dramatic relief if these other measures fail. If sodium replenishment fails to remedy heat cramps, evaluation of potassium, calcium, and magnesium levels may provide an answer.

The athlete should always be reminded that heat cramps may be a warning of impending heat exhaustion.

Heat Exhaustion

Heat exhaustion is a serious acute heat injury caused by sodium depletion, dehydration, or both.

Commonly, marked deficiencies of both sodium and water characterize the problem. **Sodium depletion heat exhaustion** occurs most commonly in unacclimated athletes who replace sweat losses with water but do not maintain adequate dietary compensation for sodium losses. Athletes limiting their sodium intake as part of a so-called healthy diet are at particular risk for this problem. The sodium depletion generally occurs over several days, but the actual symptom onset is acute. The syndrome is characterized by fatigue, profound weakness, lightheadedness, sweating, and muscle cramps. Temperature elevations, if present, are moderate; and the patient usually exhibits a tachycardia and occasionally hypotension. A variety of "flu-like" symptoms may be present, including headache, myalgias, nausea, vomiting, or diarrhea. Mental status is generally normal or mildly impaired. Loss of consciousness is rare.[3]

Water depletion heat exhaustion occurs in individuals exercising in a hot environment with inadequate water intake. This syndrome includes intense thirst, headache, and mild anxiety, agitation, and confusion. Muscle weakness, generalized fatigue, and neuromuscular incoordination often occur. Individuals with this pattern of heat exhaustion are generally febrile with skin turgor changes typical of dehydration. Tachycardia and hypotension are particularly marked in more severe episodes. These patients generally are still able to sweat, but as the serum sodium concentration and osmolarity increase in response to dehydration, sweating may be reduced.[3]

Pure sodium depletion or water depletion forms of heat exhaustion are rare in athletes. Generally, there is some element of each mechanism. Treatment consists of rest, rapid cooling, and fluid and electrolyte replacement. Traditionally, hypotonic fluids have been given orally or intravenously. If cooling and oral fluids fail to induce clinical improvement, it has been considered safe to administer a liter of D5/½ normal saline intravenously over 30–60 minutes while obtaining serum electrolyte levels. When the serum sodium is markedly elevated, it is wise to continue hydration cautiously in order to avoid an iatrogenic cerebral edema.[3]

Heat Stroke

Traditionally, exertional heat stroke has been defined as an acute medical emergency with three major manifestations: profound dysfunction of the central nervous system; a hot, dry skin; and a rectal temperature exceeding 40.6°C (105°F).[47] This symptom complex, represented a failure of the body's thermoregulatory mechanism. The keys to the diagnosis were the extreme temperature elevations of at least 105°F and often as high as 107°F or 108°F. The hot, dry skin indicated the failure of the body's sweating mechanism.

TABLE 3. Common Electrolyte and Metabolic Abnormalities in Exertional Heat Stroke

Hyperkalemia or hypokalemia
Hypernatremia or hyponatremia
Hypocalcemia
Hypophosphatemia
Hypoglycemia
Lactic acidosis
Uremia

It is now well known that although rectal temperature may be high when measured at the time of collapse from heat stroke, delayed measurements may be considerably lower, even in the normal range.[14,82] It is also now well established that in most cases of heat stroke the sweating mechanism is still functioning.[14,82] The central nervous system impairment varies from moderate confusion, disorientation, and agitation in milder cases to hysterical behavior, delirium, and coma in the more severe situations.

The central nervous system characteristics of heat stroke differentiate it from heat exhaustion.[14] Heat stroke is a more severe problem which is not spontaneously reversible. Without prompt intervention it progresses inexorably to cardiovascular and central nervous system collapse. At this point, it involves a myriad of electrolyte and metabolic problems that require careful monitoring and therapy (Table 3) and causes severe complications to virtually every organ system (Table 4).

TABLE 4. Severe Complications of Heat Stroke

Cardiovascular	Arrhythmias
	Myocardial infarction
	Pulmonary edema
	Shock
Central Nervous System	Confusion
	Coma
	Seizures
	Cerebral or spinal infarction
Gastrointestinal	Diarrhea and vomiting
	Hepatocellular necrosis
	Upper gastrointestinal bleeding
Hematologic	Fibrinolysis
	Thrombocytopenia
	Disseminated intravascular coagulation
Musculoskeletal	Rhabdomyolysis
	Myoglobinemia
Pulmonary	Hyperventilation
	Respiratory alkalosis
	Adult respiratory distress syndrome
	Pulmonary infarction
Renal	Acute renal failure

In a study comparing 13 Marine Corps recruits with exertional heat stroke sustained during basic training with 14 recruits suffering from severe heat exhaustion, the majority of the heat stroke patients were not acclimated. By comparison, all but one of the severe heat exhaustion patients had been in training over three weeks in the heat and were acclimated.[14]

Rhabdomyolysis, a problem which may occur both as a comorbidity and as a complication of heat stroke, deserves special mention. Muscle membrane injury is a predictable consequence of extreme exertion. The risk is compounded if an untrained individual performs eccentric exercise in a hot environment.[56] When the muscle cell membrane integrity is lost, much of the intracellular content leaks out and is absorbed into the blood stream. Myoglobinuria results. Ferrihaemate, a myoglobin breakdown product, is toxic to the renal tubules. The resulting tubular injury, combined with a decreased glomerular filtration rate due to dehydration and lactic acidosis, may lead to acute renal failure.[56,91] Hypokalemia may predispose to rhabdomyolysis. It may occur in athletes exercising in a hot climate because of cumulative potassium loss in the sweat with concurrent high urinary potassium excretion due to increased aldosterone production.[47,48]

Heat Stroke Treatment

For the hypothermic heat stroke patient the cornerstone of management is external cooling because the patient's own thermal control system has failed. Rectal temperature should be determined immediately in all exercise-induced collapse patients. In moderate to cool ambient temperatures, the collapse is often due to hypothermia, with or without accompanying dehydration.[74] Obviously, hyperthermic casualties should be cooled; and hypothermic victims should be warmed.

Treatment in the field or in an ambulance may involve packing the victim with ice bags, wrapped in wet towels and applied to the major areas of heat loss: the neck, axillae, and groin.[74] After transportation to a more controlled setting, such as a hospital emergency room, thermal management may be achieved by either ice bath immersion or evaporative techniques. Ice bath immersion consists of placing the heat stroke victim in a tub of ice and water and massaging the extremities vigorously to facilitate heat exchange from the skin to the core. This process usually takes 10 to 40 minutes and may be discontinued when the core temperature falls to 102°F (38.9°C).[3,13,14] Another excellent option is to wet the patient down with a tepid or cool spray and use a large fan to speed evaporative cooling.[3,7,32]

An intravenous line should be placed at the earliest possible time as a safety measure in heat stroke patients, but massive fluid administration to correct hypotension before cooling should be avoided.[3] Vasoconstriction during the cooling process often increases venous return and cardiac output. If the patient remains hypotensive after cooling, 250–500 ml boluses of normal saline may be given by rapid infusion and monitored with blood pressure measurement. If hypotension persists, appropriate pressor agents may be used judiciously.[3]

Heat stroke patients manifest incipient, if not actual, cardiac, respiratory, and metabolic collapse. Vigorous management, preferably in the modern hospital emergency room or intensive care unit, is necessary. Heat stroke patients frequently require airway management, oxygenation, careful fluid and electrolyte administration, circulatory support, and cardiac, metabolic, and laboratory monitoring.

Similarities between some cases of heat stroke and the malignant hyperthermia syndrome seen in patients undergoing general anesthesia have been noted,[41,42,51] and although some authors have suggested treating subsets of heat stroke patients with dantrolene, the drug's efficacy has not been firmly established in this disease.[42,51,54] Its greatest promise appears to be in heat stroke patients taking neuroleptic medications which predispose them to heat injury.[51,54,69]

Hyponatremia

Early reports of clinically significant hyponatremia occurring in ultraendurance athletes were published in 1985. Noakes et al reported four cases of athletes in ultramarathons who ran from 7–10 hours and were hospitalized with major complications of hyponatremia. Using a hypothetical analysis of fluid and electrolyte balance, they concluded that the athletes developed hyponatremia as a result of water intoxication by drinking too much hypotonic fluid during the races. Only in one case was there substantial evidence of a weight gain (4.5 kg) to support this theory.[66] Another group reported two cases of hyponatremic collapse in ultramarathon runners the following year and adhered to the water intoxication theory.[25] Subsequently, a case of hyponatremic collapse was reported in a runner competing in a standard-length marathon.[62]

Hiller et al measured serum electrolytes in 53 men and 11 women competing in the Hawaiian Ironman Triathlon. Nineteen (29%) had post-race hyponatremia. Nine of the 64 subjects were treated for dehydration or heat injury and six of them had low sodium, chloride, or glucose levels. Thus, most of the hyponatremic competitors tolerated their electrolyte abnormality without collapse. The authors believed that the treated competitors manifested a sodium depletion form of heat exhaustion in which the salt depletion occurred in a single hot, extremely demanding day, rather than cumulatively over several days.[35,36]

There is general agreement that hyponatremia is often found in ultraendurance athletes. Recent work suggests that the incidence of decreased serum sodium in this setting is 9–29%.[36,68] The etiology is not yet determined. Water intoxication, sodium depletion, heat exhaustion, atrial natriuretic peptide, and anti-diuretic hormone excess have all been postulated as causes.[2,25,35,36,50,62,66]

Controversy developed when Noakes et al. suggested that the recommended fluid intake for prolonged exercise in mild environmental conditions be 1/2 liter per hour[63,64] and that intravenous fluid therapy not be used routinely for treatment of collapsed runners.[65] Their pronouncements stimulated a vociferous response because they generalized some of their recommendations to all athletes with heat exhaustion and heat stroke from the small percent of collapsed runners who participate in ultraendurance events.[9,16] Clearly, for individuals exercising either for prolonged periods of time or at high intensity, or both, in the heat, the real threat is dehydration and not water intoxication.[16]

Perhaps the best recommendation to ultraendurance runners is to determine their own fluid replacement levels by keeping accurate records of pre- and post-exercise body weight and of individual fluid consumption at different ambient temperatures during long runs in training. Projecting race needs from this data is a simple, practical way to prevent dehydration as well as overhydration. As for treatment of ultraendurance athletes with exercise-associated collapse, the recommendations in the "Heat Stroke Treatment" section above antedate the controversy but are, nevertheless, still safe and reasonable.

TABLE 5. Populations at Increased Risk for Exertional Heat Stroke

Healthy Individuals
Poorly acclimatized
Poorly conditioned
Inexperienced competitor
Salt or water depletion
Large and/or obese
Age extremes: children, elderly
Previous heat injury
Sleep-deprived
Acute Illnesses
Febrile illnesses
Gastrointestinal illnesses
Chronic Illnesses
Alcoholism and substance abuse
Cardiac disease
Cystic fibrosis
Diabetes, uncontrolled
Eating disorders
Hypertension, uncontrolled
Skin problems with impaired sweating
Thyrotoxicosis
Medications
Anticholinergics
Antidepressants: tricyclics, MAO inhibitors
Antihistamines
Beta blockers
Diuretics
Neuroleptics

POPULATIONS AT INCREASED RISK

Healthy Individuals

Certain populations are at increased risk for exertional heat injury. Those commonly encountered are listed in Table 5, and many deserve discussion. As already noted, inadequate acclimatization and conditioning create vulnerability. Athletes with lack of experience either in the sport or in exercising in the heat tend to have poorer judgment about heat risk. If the participant has become gradually water- or salt-depleted over several days, susceptibility is increased.

Large athletes, even when well-conditioned, generate more heat to perform the same activity than smaller athletes; moreover, they dissipate the heat less efficiently due to a smaller body surface to mass ratio.[18,45,90] In addition to these factors, obese individuals have higher tissue temperature elevations for the same heat load because adipose tissue has a lower specific heat then lean tissue.[45] They also have fewer heat-activated sweat glands in areas overlying adipose tissue.[45,86]

Children are less efficient in heat than adults. They sweat less, and they require a greater increase in core temperature to trigger perspiration.[19,20] They acclimate to heat more slowly, and they are less efficient in the heat. Since they have a lower cardiac output at a given metabolic rate, they are more likely to lack sufficient blood flow to maintain their activity level in the heat while providing adequate cooling flow to the skin. Children have a high surface area to body mass ratio, which works well for them in a temperate environment, but when the sun is strong or temperature is high, they absorb relatively more heat from their environment than do adults.[8,88] The transition to an adult thermoregulatory response occurs after puberty.[20]

At high levels of heat stress, the elderly are more prone to heat injury. This may be partly related to reduced fitness levels, but there also appears to be an age-related limitation on full heat acclimatization.[45] The vasodilatory response to exercise in the heat is decreased in the elderly, with first changes seen as early as age 50. This decrease is probably due to structural changes in the vascular bed of aging skin.[46] There is also a reduced thirst response after water deprivation in the elderly which may predispose to dehydration in the heat.[71]

Victims of previous heat injury may have increased susceptibility to thermal heat stress.[6,26,47,81] This susceptibility may be related to decreased work efficiency in the heat,[18] or to the entire group of predisposing factors for heat injury.[47] It is often unclear whether the susceptibility was entirely premorbid, but there is evidence that the heat intolerance persists in a small percentage of prior heat stroke patients.[6,18,47] It has been suggested that heat tolerance of heat stroke patients should be formally tested 8–12 weeks post-episode to detect possible residual decrements of thermoregulation capacity.[47] This approach is important when heat stroke victims anticipate continued heat exposure because the time course of recovery is highly variable and sequelae may persist up to a year in severe cases.[45] The increased susceptibility to recurrent heat stroke may also be due to an underlying malignant hyperthermia syndrome.[41,42] This effect may be idiosyncratic, as with the malignant hyperthermia syndrome.[42]

Reproductive age women may have reduced heat tolerance during the luteal phase of their menstrual cycle.[37,72,89]

Sleep deprivation lowers both the sweat rate and skin blood-flow responses to exercise heat load.[78]

Acute Illnesses

Febrile illnesses reduce exercise heat tolerance by reducing the heart's ability to maintain cardiac output while, at the same time, increasing the metabolic demand for blood flow throughout the body. Gastrointestinal illnesses compromise heat tolerance by increasing blood flow to the gastrointestinal tract in competition with skin flow and by causing dehydration and electrolyte disturbances in anorexia, vomiting, and diarrhea.

Chronic Illnesses

Alcohol and substance abuse predispose individuals to heat illness.[45] Until recently it was not clear whether the susceptibility was related to the substances themselves or only to the related behaviors, but recent research demonstrates a residual effect of alcohol consumption reducing thermoregulation in heat-acclimated males.[30] Because many patients with cardiac diseases have reduced cardiac output, they manifest decreased heat-dissipating capacity. Cystic fibrosis patients are at increased risk due to marked sweat sodium losses. Uncontrolled diabetics are at increased risk owing to their potassium and water balance problems, but well-controlled insulin-dependent diabetics without microangiopathy or neuropathy exhibit normal heat tolerance.[22] Diabetics may develop decrements in sweating capacity due to peripheral neuropathy.[21] Anorexics and bulimics are prone to exercise-induced heat disorders, both because of their characteristic behaviors, which lead to dehydration and electrolytic disturbances, and because of the frequent obsessive patterns of over-exercise that they exhibit. Unmedicated or inadequately treated essential hypertensives exhibit reductions in heat transfer capacity and skin blood-flow when exercising in the heat.[44,45]

Medications

Many medications influence the body's capacity for exercise in the heat. This discussion is limited to those commonly demonstrating major effects in exertional heat illness. Anticholinergics, and, to a lesser extent, antihistamines, may reduce the body's sweating capacity. Beta blockers reduce the cardiac output and peripheral circulation necessary for heat dissipation.[31,45,70,80] Diuretics have been shown to reduce athletic performance.[5,11] They contract fluid volume and may reduce cardiac output and provide less plasma volume for sweating. They also induce frequent electrolyte abnormalities, which may be more significant in heat stress. Neuroleptic agents predispose to, and may trigger, malignant hyperthermia. Many sunscreens may reduce heat tolerance by impeding sweat evaporation.[92]

PREVENTION OF HEAT ILLNESS

Heat-related injuries in athletics are best treated through prevention. The adage that "an ounce of prevention is worth a pound of cure" is more than true in cases of heat illness. Several factors must be considered when advising athletes about how to prevent these injuries.

Medical History, Medical Evaluation, Level of Fitness, and Level of Acclimatization

Athletes who are susceptible to heat stress and those with conditions that would predispose them to heat stress should be identified and counselled. The preparticipation athletic evaluation should include screening for the heat stress risk factors listed in Table 5. Further work-up, correction of the risk factor, education of the athlete, and restriction of athletic activity should be instituted where appropriate.

Atmospheric Conditions

High levels of heat and humidity severely limit the exercising body's ability to dissipate heat. Athletes, coaches, athletic trainers, and team physicians need an increased level of awareness of the

TABLE 6. Heat Stress* (Apparent Temperatures in ° F.)

		AIR TEMPERATURE (°F)										
		70	**75**	**80**	**85**	**90**	**95**	**100**	**105**	**110**	**115**	**120**
Relative Humidity (%)	0%	64	69	73	78	83	87	**91**	**95**	**99**	**103**	**107**
	10%	65	70	75	80	85	**90**	**95**	**100**	**105**	**111**	**116**
	20%	66	72	77	82	87	**93**	**99**	**105**	**112**	**120**	**130**
	30%	67	73	78	84	**90**	**96**	**104**	**113**	**123**	**135**	**148**
	40%	68	74	79	86	**93**	**101**	**110**	**123**	**137**	**151**	
	50%	69	75	81	88	**96**	**107**	**120**	**135**	**150**		
	60%	70	76	82	**90**	**100**	**114**	**132**	**144**			
	70%	70	77	85	**93**	**106**	**124**	**144**				
	80%	71	78	86	**97**	**113**	**136**					
	90%	71	79	88	**102**	**122**						
	100%	72	80	**91**	**108**							

DANGER ZONE = +90°F. (temperatures in bold-faced type, above)
*Source: National Weather Service

prevailing atmospheric conditions during practice, competition, or workout. The exercising athlete cannot depend only on "how hot or humid it feels" to judge the situational heat stress from the environment. More objective measurements of temperature and humidity can be compared with published guidelines to give suggested adjustments in exercise intensity, duration, and precautions.

Weather reports from the United States Weather Service or local radio and television stations can provide approximate temperature and humidity readings. Using Table 6 or Figure 2, relative degrees of heat stress can be determined. This is the most simple and convenient method for athletes involved in fitness, recreational, or individual sports activities. However, these remote temperature and humidity readings do not allow for variances due to local geography or distance between the weather reporting site and the workout area.

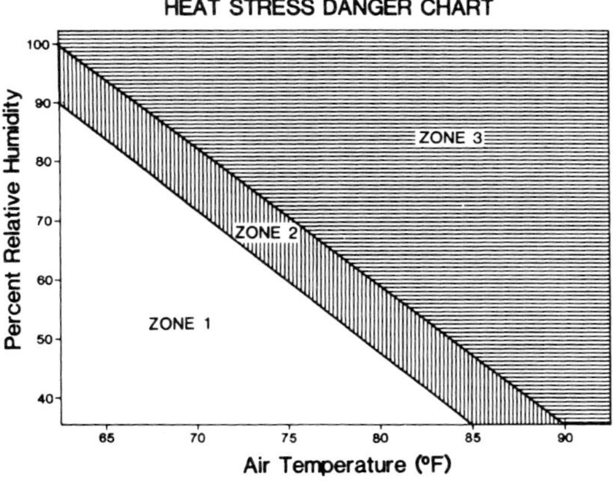

FIGURE 2. Heat Stress Danger Chart. Environmental conditions in **Zone 1** are fairly safe for participation. Normal heat stress precautions should be taken. In **Zone 2,** moderate heat stress precautions should be taken. Workouts should be less intense, shorter, and with more frequent fluid breaks, with more careful observation of individuals at increased risk. In **Zone 3,** heat stress danger is at its greatest. Workouts should be rescheduled to a cooler part of the day. Workouts should be relatively easy. Light clothing and a minimum of equipment should be worn. Extra fluids for everyone and close observation for early heat injury symptoms are essential. (Adapted from Fox EL, Mathews DK: The Physiological Basis of Physical Education and Athletics, 3rd Ed. Philadelphia, Saunders College Publishing, 1981.)

A **sling psychrometer** (Fig. 3) is used to measure dry bulb (DB) and wet bulb (WB) temperature at the activity site. The relative humidity can then be determined from a chart supplied with the instrument. Table 6 or Figure 2 can be consulted to determine the degree of environment heat stress for the given workout time.

An alternative method of estimating heat stress is to average the dry bulb and wet bulb temperatures. Using the centrigrade scale, 22–24 signifies a light heat load, 24–28 indicates a moderate heat load, and over 28 specifies a severe heat load.[82] The sling psychrometer is readily available (School Health Supply, Addison, Illinois), reasonably inexpensive, accurate, portable, and easy to learn to use.

The **heat index thermometer** is a more complex and expensive system used to measure DB, WB, and black bulb (BB) temperatures. The BB thermometer is enclosed in a black globe. First used in the military,[57] it provides for a measure of the radiant heat gained in the heat stress index. Figure 4 shows a homemade heat index thermometer system. The Wet Bulb Global Temperature (WBGT) index is then calculated, using the following formula:

$$\text{WBGT} = 0.7\ (\text{WB}) + 0.1\ (\text{DB}) + 0.2\ (\text{BB})$$

The WBGT index can also be determined using a commercially available heat index thermometer (Reuter-Strokes, Cambridge, Ontario).

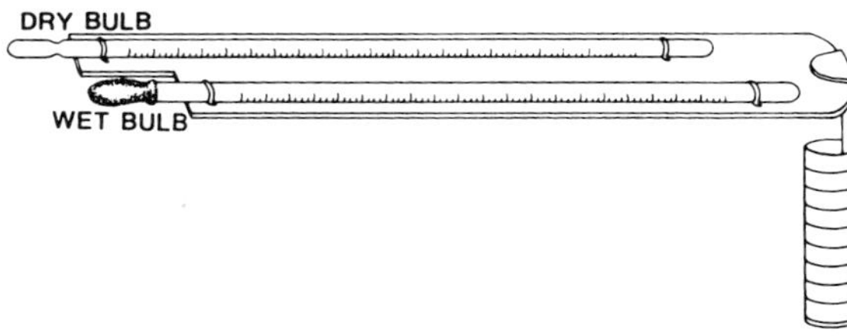

FIGURE 3. Sling Psychrometer. Wick on wet bulb is moistened with distilled water and the unit is rotated overhead. Evaporative cooling causes the wet bulb temperature to decrease. The dry bulb and wet bulb readings are used to determine percent of relative humidity.

The WBGT index is compared with published guidelines that indicate relative levels of heat-stress risk and provide suggestions for activity modifications. Such guidelines have been outlined for football[4,15,27] and distance running[1,40] and can be adapted for other activities.

Workout Schedule

Identifying stressful environmental conditions has absolutely no benefit unless appropriate steps are taken to adjust the practice or competition schedule. Several authors have suggested various levels of modification in the football practice schedule in the presence of different levels of heat stress.[4,15,27] The American College of Sports Medicine[1] has proposed a system of flags to advise race participants of heat stress conditions during races. Each flag color suggests certain adjustments in running intensity.

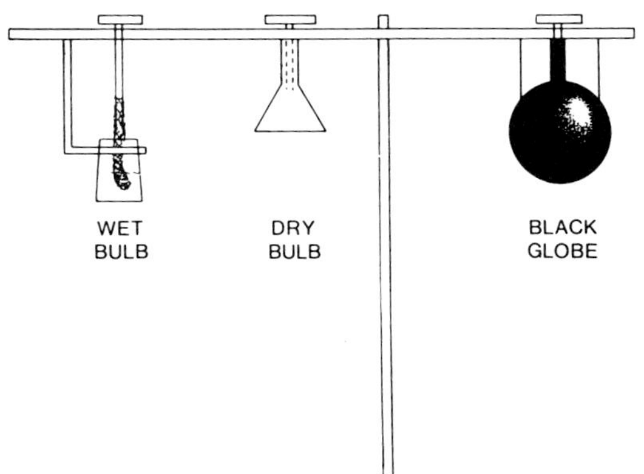

FIGURE 4. Heat Index Thermometers. Homemade unit consists of three thermometers mounted on a board. The bulb of the wet thermometer is enclosed in a moistened wick. The bulb of the dry thermometer is in an inverted funnel to shield it from direct sunlight. The bulb of the black globe thermometer is enclosed in a black copper globe to absorb radiant energy.

During times of the year when environmental stress is likely to be the greatest, competition and workouts should be scheduled away from the middle of the day. Other extra precautions should also be taken (Fig. 2). These general suggestions should also be applied to athletes who participate in sports and activities other than football or running.

Clothing

As ambient temperatures increase, evaporation becomes the primary means for the body to dissipate heat. Restrictive clothing can severely limit evaporative cooling. Core temperature, heart rate, and weight loss are significantly increased during exercise in football gear compared to exercise in shorts, even in mild environmental conditions.[52] Excessive protective equipment limits the skin-surface area available for evaporative cooling.[4]

Air trapped next to the skin and in the clothing itself creates an insulating layer, limiting convective air currents from assisting evaporation. Rectal temperatures in exercising subjects wearing vapor-impermeable garments are increased significantly compared with those in exercising subjects dressed in vapor-permeable garments.[29] The use of rubberized workout suits creates a super-saturated environment around the skin and limits evaporative cooling. It has been suggested that certain sunscreens containing an oil or gel base allow sweat to run off before evaporative cooling takes place.[92]

Several authors have suggested the use of short-sleeved, short-midriff shirts under football shoulder pads and loose-fitting, openweave "fishnet" jerseys to facilitate evaporative cooling.[4,27,59,87] Light-colored uniforms[4,27] help reflect radiant energy. Sweat-soaked clothing should be changed to decrease the humidity directly adjacent to the skin.[58] In males, wearing no shirt further facilitates evaporative cooling but may allow some radiant heat gain.[1]

Body Weight

Acute weight loss of as little as 2% can impair thermoregulatory ability.[34] Greater than 3% weight loss causes deterioration of performance parameters. Dehydration is evidenced by acute weight loss. Therefore, ongoing monitoring of the athletes' weight is a reasonably accurate method of assessing their state of hydration. Several authors have suggested weighing the athlete before and after workouts.[4,27,58] These recorded weights should be checked daily by the athletic trainer, coach, or other responsible person. Caution should be exercised with individuals showing a practice weight loss of 3–5%. Particular caution should be conveyed to athletes who have not regained the previous day's weight loss by practice time the next day. This residual weight loss is due to dehydration. Athletes with large or persistent acute weight loss should be restricted from activity until rehydrated.

Observation

Careful observation of athletes identified as being at risk is essential to preventing heat illness. Particular attention should be paid to those athletes who are out of shape or overweight. Athletes who give 100% may not recognize the early signs of heat illness.[87] In extreme environmental heat stress and before acclimation, all athletes should be watched more carefully for signs of heat illness. Those with excessive practice weight loss and/or failure to rehydrate should be closely monitored, even once their weight is regained.

Education

All people involved with athletics and fitness should have a basic understanding of heat illness, its causes, treatment, and prevention. Medical personnel should be able to provide sound advice on the prevention, recognition, and treatment of various types of heat illness. Good communication with the coaches and athletes is essential.

Coaches must set aside all of the myths that can contribute to additional heat stress.[47] They must be trained to recognize early signs of heat illness and apply appropriate first aid measures. The coach also serves as the coordinator of the prevention program in the absence of an athletic trainer.

The athlete must be taught to recognize the early signs and symptoms of heat illness and the appropriate initial steps to take in treating it. The athlete should have a working knowledge of heat illness prevention principles. Emphasis should be placed on environmental factors, fluid replacement, acclimatization, and clothing. Further, the athlete should be versed in how to adjust his or her training program to accommodate to the heat.

REFERENCES

1. American College of Sports Medicine: Position stand on prevention of thermal injuries during distance running. Med Sci Sports Exerc 19:529–533, 1987.
2. Anderson JV, Bloom SR, Somers VK, et al: Hyponatremia and ultramarathons (letter) JAMA 256:213–214, 1986.
3. Anderson RJ, Reed G, Knochel J: Heatstroke. Adv Intern Med 28:115–141, 1983.
4. Andrews JR, Massey M, Mullins L, et al: Heat illness in athletes. J Med Assoc State Alabama 45(2):29–32, 1975.
5. Armstrong LE, Costill DL, Fink WJ: Influence of diuretic-induced dehydration on competitive running performance. Med Sci Sports Exerc 17:456–461, 1985.
6. Armstrong LE, DeLuca JP, Hubbard RW: Time course of recovery and hat acclimation ability of prior exertional heatstroke patients. Med Sci Sports Exerc 22:36–48, 1990.
7. Barner HB, Masar M, Wettach GE, Wright DW: Field evaluation of a new simplified method for cooling heat casualties in desert. Milit Med 149:95–97, 1984.
8. Bar-Or O: Climate and the exercising child. In Baro-Or O: Pediatric Sports Medicine for the Practitioner: From Physiologic Principles to Clinical Applications. New York, Springer-Verlag, 1983, pp 260–299.
9. Barr SI, Costil DL, Fink WJ: Response to clinical commentary. Med Sci Sports Exerc 24:626, 1992.
10. Cadarette BS, Sawka MN, Toner MM, Pandolf KB: Aerobic fitness and the hypohydration response to exercise-heat stress. Aviat Space Environ Med 55:507–512, 1984.
11. Caldwell JE, Ahonen E, Nousiainen U: Diuretic therapy, physical performance, and neuromuscular function. Phys Sportsmed 12(6):73–85, 1984.
12. Convertino VA: Blood volume: Its adaptation to endurance training. Med Sci Sports Exerc 23:1338–1348, 1991.
13. Costrini A: Emergency treatment of exertional heatstroke and comparison of whole body cooling techniques. Med Sci Sports Exerc 22:15–18, 1990.
14. Costrini AM, Pitt HA, Gustafson AB, Uddin DE: Cardiovascular and metabolic manifestations of heat stroke and severe heat exhaustion. Am J Med 66:296–302, 1979.
15. Davidson M: Heat illness in athletics. Athletic Training 20(2):96–101, 1985.
16. Eichner ER: Sacred cows and straw men (editorial). Phys Sportsmed 19(7):24, 1991.
17. Epstein Y: Heat intolerance: Predisposing factor or residual injury? Med Sci Sports Exerc 22:29–35, 1990.
18. Epstein Y, Shapiro Y, Brill S: Role of surface area-to-mass ratio and work efficiency in heat intolerance. J Appl Physiol 54:831–836, 1983.
19. Falk B, Baro-Or O, Calvert R, MacDougall JD: Sweat gland response to exercise in the heat among pre, mid-, and late-pubertal boys. Med Sci Sports Exerc 24:313–319, 1992.
20. Falk B, Baro-Or O, MacDougall JD: Thermoregulatory responses of pre-, mid-, and late-pubertal boys to exercise in dry heat. Med Sci Sports Exerc 24:688–694, 1992.
21. Fealey RD, Phillip AL, Thomas JE: Thermoregulatory sweating abnormalities in diabetes mellitus. Mayo Clin Proc 64:617–628, 1989.
22. Fortney SM, Koivisto VA, Felig F, Nadel ER: Circulatory and temperature regulatory responses to exercise in a warm environment in insulin-dependent diabetics. Yale J Biol Med 54:101–109, 1981.
23. Fortney SM, Vroman NB: Exercise, performance and temperature control: Temperature regulation during exercise and implications for sports performance and training. Sports Med 2:8–20, 1985.
24. Fox EL, Mathews DK: The Physiological Basis of Physical Education and Athletics, 3rd ed, Philadelphia, Saunders College Publishing, 1981, pp 454–485.
25. Frizzell RT, Lang GH, Lowance DC, Lathan SR: Hyponatremia and ultramarathon running. JAMA 255:772–774, 1986.
26. Gerstein SM: Risk factors for collapse of runners. Phys Sportsmed 18(12):72–85, 1990.
27. Gieck J: Heat and activity. Athletic Training 9:78–81, 1974.
28. Gisolfi CV, Wenger CB: Temperature regulation during exercise: Old concepts, new ideas. Exerc Sports Sci Rev 12: 339–72.
29. Gonzalez RR, Cena K: Evaluation of vapor permeation through garments during exercise. J Appl Physiol 58: 928–935, 1985.
30. Goodpaster BH, Sinning WE, Roemmich J, et al: The residual effects of alcohol consumption on thermoregulation in heat acclimated males. Med Sci Sports Exerc 25(5 Suppl):S28, 1993.
31. Gordon NF, Myburgh DP, Schwellnus MP, et al: Effect of β-blockade on exercise core temperature in coronary artery disease in patients. Med Sci Sports Exerc 19: 591–596, 1987.

32. Graham BS, Lichtenstein MJ, Hinson JM, Theil GB: Nonexertional heatstroke: Physiologic management and cooling in 14 patients. Arch Intern Med 146:87–90, 1986.
33. Harrison MH: Heat and exercise: Effects on blood volume. Sports Med 3:214–223, 1986.
34. Hecker AL, Wheeler KB: Impact of hydration and energy intake on performance. Athletic Training 19:260–264, 311, 1984.
35. Hiller WDB: Dehydration and hyponatremia during triathlons. Med Sci Sports Exerc 21(5 Suppl):S219–S221, 1989.
36. Hiller WDB, O'Toole ML, Massimino F: Plasma electrolyte and glucose changes during the hawaiian ironman triathlon. Med Sci Sports Exerc 17:219, 1985.
37. Hirata K, Nagasaka T, Hirai A, et al: Effects of human menstrual cycle on thermoregulatory vasodilation during exercise. Eur J Appl Physiol 54:559–565, 1986.
38. Hubbard RW: Heatstroke pathophysiology: The energy depletion model. Med Sci Sports Exerc 22:19–28, 1989.
39. Hubbard RW, Armstrong LE: An introduction: The role of exercise in the etiology of exertional heatstroke. Med Sci Sports Exerc 22:2–5, 1989.
40. Hughson RL, Staudt LA, Mackie JM: Monitoring road racing in the heat. Phys Sports Med 11(5):94–105, 1983.
41. Hunter SL, Rosenberg H, Tuttle GH, et al: Malignant hyperthermia in a college football player. Phys Sportsmed 15(12):77–84, 1987.
42. Jardon OM: Heat stroke, stress, and malignant hyperthermia. Neb Med J 70:195–199, 1985.
43. Johnson SC, Ruhling RO: Aspirin in exercise-induced hyperthermia: Evidence for and against its role. Sports Med 2:1–7, 1985.
44. Kenney WL: Decreased core-to-skin heat transfer in mild essential hypertensives exercising in the heat. Clin Exp Hypertens A7:1165–1172, 1985.
45. Kenney WL: Physiologic correlates of heat intolerance. Sports Med 2:279–286, 1985.
46. Kenney WL, Johnson JM: Control of skin blood flow during exercise. Med Sci Sports Exerc 24:303–312, 1992.
47. Knochel JP: Dog days and siriasis: How to kill a football player. JAMA 233:513–515, 1975.
48. Knochel JP, Dotin LN, Hamburger RJ: Pathophysiology of intense physical conditioning in a hot climate: I. Mechanisms of potassium depletion. J Clin Invest 51:242–255, 1972.
49. Kobayashi Y, Ando Y, Takeuchi S, et al: Effects of heat acclimatization of distance runners in a moderately hot environment. Eur J Appl Physiol 45:189–198, 1980.
50. Lathan SR, Lowance DC, Frizzell RT: Hyponatremia and ultramarathons (letter). JAMA 256:214, 1986.
51. Lydiatt JS, Hill GE: Treatment of heat stroke with dantrolene. JAMA 246:41–42, 1981.
52. Mathews DK, Fox EL, Tanzi D: Physiological responses during exercise and recovery in a football uniform. J Appl Physiol 26:611–615, 1969.
53. Meyer F, Bar-Or O, MacDougall JD, et al: Electrolyte loss in sweat and urine during exercise in the heat: effects of gender and maturation. Med Sci Sports Exerc 23(4 Suppl):S68, 1991.
54. Meyers EF, Meyers RW: Thermic stress syndrome. JAMA 247:2098–2099, 1982.
55. Millard M, Sparling PB, Rosskopf LB, et al: Gender differences in fluid requirements during prolonged running in the heat? Med Sci Sports Exerc 24(5 Suppl):S63, 1992.
56. Milne CJ: Rhabdomyolysis, myoglobinuria and exercise. Sports Med 6:93–106, 1988.
57. Minard D, O'Brien RL: Heat casualties in the Navy and Marine Corps, 1959–1962, with appendices on the field use of the wet globe thermometer index. U.S. Navy Medical Research Institute Report 7:1, 1964.
58. Murphy RJ: Heat illness. J Sports Med 1(4):26–29, 1973.
59. Murphy RJ: Heat illness in the athlete. Am J Sports Med 12:258–261, 1984.
60. Nadel ER: Recent advances in temperature regulation during exercise in humans. Fed Proc 44:2286–92, 1985.
61. Nadel ER, Fortney SM, Wenger CB: Effect of hydration state on circulatory and thermal regulations. J Appl Physiol 49:715–721, 1980.
62. Nelson PB, Robinson AG, Kapoor W, Rinaldo J: Hyponatremia in a marathoner. Phys Sportsmed 16(10):78–88, 1988.
63. Noakes TD: Hyponatremia during endurance running: A physiological and clinical interpretation. Med Sci Sports Exerc 24:403–405, 1992.
64. Noakes TD, Adams BA, Myburgh KH, et al: The danger of an inadequate water intake during prolonged exercise. Eur J Appl Physiol 57:210–219, 1988.
65. Noakes TD, Berlinski N, Solomon E, Weight L: Collapsed runners: Blood biochemical changes after IV fluid therapy. Phys Sportsmed 19(7):70–82, 1991.
66. Noakes TD, Goodwin N, Rayner BL, et al: Water intoxication: A possible complication during endurance exercise. Med Sci Sports Exerc 17:370–375, 1985.
67. Noakes TD, Myburgh KH, Du Plessis J: Metabolic rate, not percent dehydration, predicts rectal temperature in marathon runners. Med Sci Sports Exerc 23:443–449, 1990.
68. Noakes TD, Norman RJ, Buck RH, et al: The incidence of hyponatremia during prolonged ultraendurance exercise. Med Sci Sports Exerc 22:165–170, 1990.
69. Paasuke RT: Drugs, heat stroke, and dantrolene. Can Med Assoc J 130:341–343, 1984.
70. Pescatello LS, Mack GW, Leach CN, et al: Thermoregulation in mildly hypertensive men during beta-adrenergic blockade. Med Sci Sports Exerc 20(2 Suppl):S63, 1988.
71. Phillips PA, Rolls BJ, Ledingham JGG, et al: Reduced thirst after water deprivation in healthy elderly men. N Engl J Med 311:753–759, 1984.
72. Pivarnik JM, Mariachal CJ, Spillman HT, et al: Menstrual cycle phase affects temperature regulation during endurance exercise. Med Sci Sports Exerc 22(2 Suppl): S119, 1990.
73. Pugh LGE, Corbett JL, Johnson RH: Rectal temperatures, weight losses, and sweat rates in marathon running. J Appl Physiol 23:347–352, 1967.
74. Roberts WO: Exercise-associated collapse in endurance events: A classification system. Phys Sportsmed 17(5): 49–56, 1989.
75. Rogers GG: Loss of acclimatization to heat in man during periods of no heat exposure. South African Med J 52: 412, 1977.
76. Rowell LB: Cardiovascular aspects of human thermoregulation. Circ Res 52:367–379, 1983.
77. Sawka MN, Francesconi RP, Young AJ, Pandolf KB: Influence of hydration level and body fluids on exercise performance in the heat. JAMA 252:1165–1169, 1984.
78. Sawka MN, Gonzalez RR, Pandolf KB: Effects of sleep deprivation on thermoregulation during exercise. Am J Physiol 246 (1 Pt 2):R72–R77, 1984.
79. Sawka MN, Young AJ, Francesconi RP, et al: Thermoregulatory and blood responses during exercise at graded hypohydration levels. J Appl Physiol 59:1394–1401, 1985.
80. Shannon LM, Mack G, Leach CN, et al: The effect of nonselective beta-blockade on thermoregulation during exercise. Med Sci Sports Exerc 18(2 Suppl):S50, 1986.
81. Shapiro Y, Magazanik A, Udassin R, et al: Heat intolerance in former heatstroke patients. Ann Intern Med 90:913–916, 1979.
82. Shapiro Y, Seidman DS: Field and clinical observations of exertional heat stroke patients. Med Sci Sports Exerc 22:6–14, 1990.

83. Shvartz E, Meroz A, Magazanik A, Shapiro Y. Prediction of heat tolerance and VO_2 max from heart rate and rectal temperature. In Landry F, Orban WAR (eds): Exercise Physiology: Fitness and performance capacity studies. Miami, Symposia Specialists, Inc., 1978, pp 521–528.
84. Simon HB: Extreme hyperpyrexia. Hosp Pract 21(5A):123–129, 1986.
85. Simon HB: Hyperthermia. N Engl J Med 329:483–487, 1993.
86. Smith NJ: Weight control and heat disorders in youth sports. J Adolescent Health Care 3:231–236, 1983.
87. Spickard A: Heat stroke in college football and suggestions for prevention. South Med J 61:791–796, 1968.
88. Squire DL: Heat illness. Pediatr Clin North Am 37:1085–1109, 1990.
89. Stephenson LA, Kolka MA: Thermoregulation in women. Exerc Sports Sci Rev 21:231–62, 1993.
90. Wailgum TD, Paolone AM: Heat tolerance of college football linemen and backs. Phys Sportsmed 12(5):81–86, 1984.
91. Ward MM: Factors predictive of acute renal failure in rhabdomyolysis. Arch Intern Med 148:1553–1557, 1988.
92. Wells TD, Jessup GT, Langlotz KS: Effects of sunscreen use during exercise in the heat. Phys Sportsmed 12(6): 132–144, 1984.
93. Wenger CB: Heat of evaporation of sweat: Thermodynamic considerations. J Appl Physiol 32:456–9, 1972.
94. Wheeler KB: Effect of hypohydration on performance-fluid and electrolyte requirements. NSCA Journal 10(5):46–48, 1988.

6

Fluids and Electrolytes for Exercise in the Heat

Jaime S. Ruud, M.S., R.D.
Kristin J. Reimers, M.S., R.D.
Ann C. Grandjean, Ed.D.

Fluid and electrolyte balance is important in all of medicine, and sports medicine is certainly no exception. Water, more than electrolytes, has a crucial role in athletic endeavors. Hypohydration not only may affect performance but also may cause serious physical disorders, even death, if not managed properly.

Water has many functions in the body. An extremely important one for athletes is thermoregulation. At rest, body heat is dissipated by convection and radiation, but when large amounts of metabolic heat are produced, such as during exercise, these systems are not sufficient and sweating becomes the primary cooling system.

The rate of sweating depends on several factors and is increased in proportion to the intensity and duration of exercise, fitness of the individual, environmental temperature, and humidity. In athletes, the highest sweat rates occur during prolonged strenuous exercise in the heat.[43] Athletes who are exposed to high temperature, high humidity, and sunlight can experience sizeable fluid losses, up to 1.5 to 2.0 liters of sweat per hour.[5] Unreplaced sweat loss can cause reduction in strength, power, endurance, and aerobic capacity in some athletes.[44] Fluid loss equal to 1% of body weight impairs thermoregulation; at 3% to 5% the body's ability to efficiently utilize oxygen is impaired; and at 7% loss collapse is likely (Fig. 1). These adverse effects of dehydration are assumed to result from a decreased blood volume (hypovolemia) and increased plasma osmolality.[45] Thus, adequate fluid intake during exercise in the heat is critical to the athlete's health and performance.

DEHYDRATION AND EXERCISE

Involuntary Dehydration

Unlike some mammals, humans will not maintain euhydration during periods of stress when fluid is consumed ad libitum. As Pitts[40] demonstrated, thirst alone is an inadequate stimulus to prevent dehydration. This phenomenon of involuntary dehydration appears in situations of heat or cold stress, altitude, water immersion, and exercise. Greenleaf[20] proposed several mechanisms responsible for involuntary dehydration, including social customs controlling what is offered to drink, capacity and rate of fluid absorption from the GI system, level of cellular hydration, upright posture, and hypovolemic angiotensin II stimuli.

Psychological, physiologic and environmental factors influence water consumption. One factor known to influence water consumption in man is water temperature. Boulze et al.[4] found that during induced dehydration, subjects maximized drinking when water temperature was 15 degrees centrigrade (59°F) and drank less when warmer or colder water was offered. Likewise, Hubbard et al.[23] found that cooling and flavoring water were additive in increasing water intake in a group of

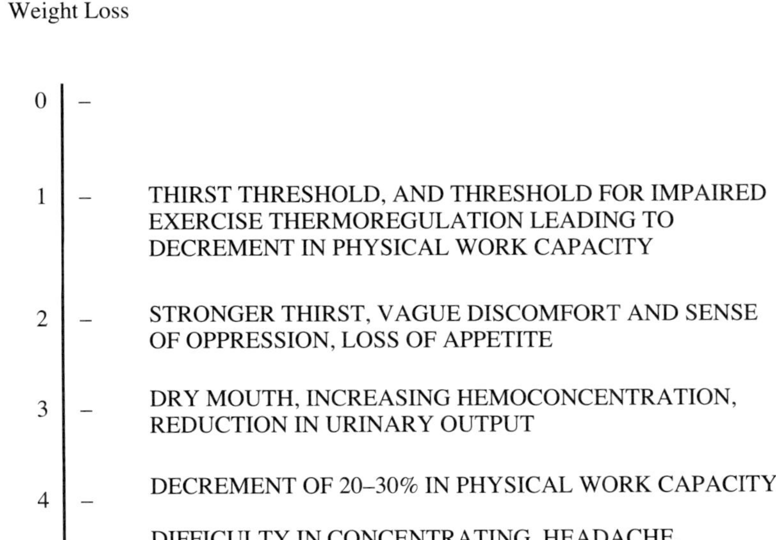

FIGURE 1. Adverse Effects of Dehydration. (Adapted from Greenleaf JE, Harrison MH: Water and electrolytes. In Layman DK (ed): Nutrition and Aerobic Exercise, Washington, DC, American Chemical Society, 1986, p 107–124.)

dehydrated subjects. Food consumption will also increase fluid intake and reduce the degree of involuntary dehydration.[49]

During exercise, involuntary dehydration can occur rapidly during competition or practice (acute), or over a period of several days (chronic). An example of acute dehydration resulting in heat exhaustion was witnessed by millions on television when Swiss runner Gabriela Andersen-Schiess entered Olympic Stadium and nearly collapsed during the women's marathon at the 1984 Olympic Summer Games. Usually, acute dehydration is prevented when fluids are consumed before, during, and after physical activity. Chronic dehydration is less visible and usually occurs when athletes practice or train in hot environments without consuming adequate fluids to completely rehydrate on a daily basis. Chronic dehydration is not uncommon in football players during fall practice. Monitoring daily weights of such athletes enables coaches and trainers to identify athletes experiencing chronic dehydration. Typically, the athlete should not be allowed to practice until baseline weight (± 1%) is achieved.

Deliberate Dehydration

Although most athletes attempt to avoid dehydration, some athletes, such as wrestlers, boxers, weightlifters, and light-weight rowers, purposely dehydrate themselves in order to reach a desired weight class before competition. Rapid dehydration methods may include fluid restriction, exercise, rubberized sweat suit, saunas, diuretics, and laxatives.[48]

Despite physiologic dangers posed by dehydration, high-power performance lasting 30 seconds or less may not be affected if weight loss through dehydration is <5% of body weight.[1,24,42,46,47,51,53] A study by Fogelholm et al.[18] also documented no change in performance tests (vertical jump, 30-m sprint, and Wingate anaerobic test) before and after rapid weight loss of 6% followed by a 5-hour "loading" period.

However, some degree of performance impairment may occur at higher levels of dehydration and/or longer periods of exercise. In a study by Webster et al.[52] college wrestlers achieved a 5% decrease in body weight by exercising and not consuming food or fluid 12 hours before testing. The tests revealed decreases in upper body strength, anaerobic power output, anaerobic capacity, the lactate threshold, and aerobic power. A study by Burge et al.[7] examined the effect of rapid dehydration and partial rehydration on performance and physiologic function during an approximate 7-minute high-intensity rowing bout by elite lightweight rowers. Body weight was reduced using exercise together with food and fluid restriction over 24 hours and was followed by consumption of 1.5 liters of water over 2 hours. The results showed that the dehydration/rehydration protocol increased rowing time by 22 seconds compared with the euhydrated trial.

FLUID REPLACEMENT

The amount of ingested fluid that enters the circulating blood depends on two factors: gastric emptying and intestinal absorption. Table 1 displays those factors known to effect gastric emptying. Gastric emptying increases in proportion to the volume of fluid consumed with a maximal rate of emptying attained at a volume of 600 mL.[16]

Fluid Volume

How much and which beverage an athlete needs is a question frequently asked by both coaches and athletes. The ideal fluid replacement regimen will depend on the duration and intensity of exercise, the environmental temperature, and the athlete. There is great variation between individuals, and the optimal type and amount of fluid consumed can be determined only by experience.[31] The most accurate method of determining fluid replacement needs is for athletes to weigh themselves, nude, before and after practice sessions or competitions. For every pound lost, the athlete should consume 2 cups (16 oz) of water. When athletes have determined their sweat loss patterns and are able to match fluid consumption with variable environmental and training conditions, weighing may no longer be necessary. Experienced athletes will be able to accurately predict fluid needs based on the weather and type of training planned.

TABLE 1. Factors Affecting the Rate of Gastric Emptying

Volume	pH
Caloric density	Intensity of exercise
Electrolyte content	Mode of exercise
Osmolality	Hydration status
Temperature	Individual variation

*Adapted from: Costill DL: Gastric emptying of fluids during exercise. In Gisolfi CV, Lamb DK (eds): Perspectives in Exercise Science and Sports Medicine. Vol 3: Fluid Homeostasis During Exercise. Indianapolis, Benchmark Press, 1990, pp 97–121.

It is important that athletes and their coaches understand the principles of fluid replacement. In a study by Bedgood and Tuck[3] 77% of the high school coaches surveyed did not know that thirst is not an adequate indicator of the need for water, a fact that was recognized more than 50 years ago.[40] One study found that 3 hours of ad libitum drinking was inadequate to achieve complete rehydration after exercise.[8] Athletes must be encouraged to drink fluids before they become thirsty.

Several pitfalls impede optimal fluid replacement practice for athletes. These include absence of a scale to determine fluid losses, impracticality of weighing nude, lack of drink breaks during practice or training, inexperience with sport drinks, drinking only in response to thirst, and others. Successful athletes overcome these problems through trial and error, ultimately devising a practical fluid replacement regimen suitable to their preferences and training demands.

Fluid Type

Water replacement is the major concern; however, research shows that endurance athletes (those athletes exercising aerobically for more than 60–90 minutes) may benefit from use of carbohydrate-containing beverages, i.e., sport drink. The addition of carbohydrate and electrolytes to water can enhance fluid intake and absorption, and can delay fatigue during endurance exercise.[6,25]

Millard-Stafford et al.[33] evaluated the effects of a 7% carbohydrate beverage on physiologic responses, hydration status, and exercise performance in male distance runners during a 40-km road race under warm, humid conditions. Using a double-blind procedure, subjects consumed 400 mL of either a carbohydrate-electrolyte drink or a placebo 30 minutes prior to exercise and 250 mL at 5 km intervals throughout the race. Mean performance time during the last km of the run was significantly faster ($p<0.03$) when subjects consumed the carbohydrate drink (21.9 ± 1.0 min) compared with the placebo (24.4 ± 1.5 min). This finding is in agreement with previous studies showing improved performance with a carbohydrate solution.[17,34]

Studies show that sport beverages containing 6% to 8% carbohydrate in the form of glucose, glucose polymers, or sucrose are all absorbed quickly and help maintain blood glucose levels during exercise.[17,33,34] However, when carbohydrate concentration exceeds 12%, data show that the absorption of fluid is impaired and exercise performance decreases.[17] For a more complete discussion on sport drinks, see Puhl and Buskirk.[41]

Glycerol

Athletes participating in endurance events in the heat may experience significant dehydration despite efforts to replace fluids.[11] Consuming fluids with glycerol before exercise in the heat may improve hydration status. Glycerol, or glycerin, is a clear, colorless, viscous liquid obtained from the hydrolysis of fats and oils. It is found naturally in many foods and is also used as a food additive.

Montner and co-workers[35] compared the effects of prehydration with equal volumes of water and a glycerol and water solution (1 g/kg body weight) on endurance time, rectal temperature, hydration status, and heart rate during cycling. Compared with water, glycerol was associated with significantly longer endurance times (94 minutes vs. 77 $p < 0.05$). Those who drank the glycerol and water had lower body temperature and lower heart rate. The researchers concluded that the increase in performance time was due to enhanced expansion of plasma volume.

Although glycerol appears to be a promising method of hyperhydrating, more research is needed. Currently, it is recommended that glycerol intake not exceed 1 g/kg body weight every 6 hours. High doses of glycerol have been associated with symptoms of lightheadedness, bloating, and nausea in some athletes. For this reason, athletes should experiment with glycerol solutions during training rather than actual competition.

ELECTROLYTES

Sweat is composed primarily of water, but it does contain a number of nutrients. Three of these nutrients are the electrolytes sodium, chloride, and potassium, which are often added to sport drinks. Electrolytes play a fundamental role in regulation of body water distribution between various fluid compartments; sodium, in particular, has a major influence on fluid regulation. Changes in the extracellular concentration of sodium will stimulate adjustments in thermal regulation, water and ion excretion, and drinking behavior. Electrolytes are essential to muscle and nerve excitation, electromechanical coupling in muscle contraction, and enzymatic control of cellular reactions.

Theoretically, any great disturbance in the balance of electrolytes in body fluids could interfere with performance. Electrolyte supplementation during heavy physical work with profuse sweating is based on the concept that large quantities of electrolytes are lost in sweat and need to be replaced. Table 2 compares the concentrations of electrolytes in sweat to those in other body fluids. Compared with other body fluids, sweat is hypotonic. The ionic concentration of sweat varies among individuals, however, and is influenced by the rate of sweat, the athlete's state of heat acclimatization, and the dietary intake of electrolytes.[15] Excessive sweating during prolonged heavy physical activity can produce large losses that can potentially disturb fluid and electrolyte balance.

TABLE 2.* Electrolyte Concentrations and Osmolality in Sweat, Muscle, and Plasma

	Electrolytes (mmol/L)				Osmolarity
	Na	Cl	K	MG	(mOsmol/L)
Sweat	40–60	30–50	4–5	1.5–5	80–185
Plasma	140	101	4	1.5	302
Muscle	9	9	162	31	302

*From Costill DL, Miller JM: Nutrition for endurance sport: carbohydrate and fluid balance. Int J Sports Med 1:2–14, 1980, with permission.

Sodium

Sodium is the electrolyte most affected by physical exercise. Under extreme conditions, athletes who sweat profusely, who are not acclimated to the heat, or who have relatively low sodium intakes (less than 2–4 g/day) may experience heat cramps or exhaustion due to sodium imbalance. Thus, in some situations, increased sodium consumption at meals and/or sodium replacement during activity may be warranted.

Research shows that rehydration during and after exercise in hot weather will occur more quickly when sodium accompanies fluids. Nose et al.[39] studied how the sodium content of ingested fluids affects drinking and restoration of body fluids following thermal dehydration in humans. Six subjects underwent two exposures to a heat and exercise program that caused a relatively mild dehydration (2.3% decrease in body weight). Each subject then rehydrated at his own pace with water and capsules containing either sodium or a placebo. The subjects rehydrating with water alone restored 68% of the lost fluid after three hours. The subjects rehydrating with water and sodium over the three hours replaced 82% of their lost fluids. Similar results were reported by Carter and Gisolfi,[8] who found that a carbohydrate-electrolyte drink containing sodium consumed after exercise resulted in greater fluid intake and increase in plasma volume than when water alone was consumed.

Hyponatremia

Several isolated cases of hyponatremia (serum sodium concentrations <130 $mmol.l^{-1}$) were reported during the 1980s in athletes competing in ultraendurance events. Some researchers attributed the occurrence to excess consumption of plain water and thus recommended that athletes curtail their fluid intake during such events. Others argued that the etiology of the condition is primarily salt depletion from massive sweat loss associated with net dehydration and thus recommended increased sodium intake.

Research on hyponatremia is limited. Barr and colleagues[2] conducted a study under laboratory conditions to assess the need to replace sodium during moderate endurance exercise of up to 6 hours duration. Noakes and colleagues[38] have conducted studies designed to determine the incidence of hyponatremia during ultraendurance events and provide insight into the mechanisms involved.

Barr et al.[2] confirmed the deleterious effects of fluid restriction and concluded that saline intake versus water did not prevent a decrease in plasma sodium. They also found that no subject in their study had to terminate exercise because of plasma sodium falling to ≤ 130 mmol.1^{-1}. It can thus be concluded that adequate fluid intake during moderate endurance exercise is important, and, provided that plasma sodium concentrations are normal at the start of exercise, sodium replacement does not appear necessary during events of moderate intensity of less than 6 hours duration.

Results of Noakes' study indicate that even when most of the foods and fluid ingested during the races contained little or no sodium chloride, hyponatremia occurs in less than 0.3% of all competitors during prolonged exercise. However, of those athletes who collapsed, it was found to occur in 9%.

Based on the limited research, it is impossible to determine the exact mechanism whereby hyponatremia develops in select individuals. Factors indicated, however, include overhydration and chronic consumption of a diet low in sodium.[2,38] Additionally, it appears that slower runners may be more likely to develop hyponatremia.[37]

Although the incidence of hyponatremia is extremely low in runners and triathletes, physicians should be aware that a significant proportion of collapsed ultraendurance athletes may be hyponatremic.

Potassium

Potassium plays an essential role in muscular contraction and nerve conduction, and helps in the transport of glucose across cell membranes and in the storage of glycogen, thus it is of interest to coaches and athletes. More than 90% of ingested potassium is absorbed from the gastrointestinal tract, but due to the kidneys' regulatory role in potassium balance, higher and lower intakes are not reflected in fluctuations in plasma potassium. Potassium is lost from the body in the urine and, to a lesser extent, in gastrointestinal secretions. Although potassium is a component of sweat, only minimal amounts are excreted, although losses can increase under profuse sweating.

Although early studies caution that significant potassium depletion may occur in young men training in the heat, with potassium losses via sweat being the probable primary cause,[27,28] more recent studies have not substantiated the need for caution.[13] The most frequent cause of potassium deficiency is excess loss, usually through the alimentary tract or the kidneys. Such loss may accompany prolonged vomiting, chronic diarrhea, or laxative abuse. The use of diuretics is the most common cause of excessive renal loss. This is a common concern in the treatment of hypertension; however, it may be of limited concern for the athlete.

There is widespread perception in the world of sport that mineral supplements may be advantageous to individuals engaged in strenuous exercise. There is no doubt that during profuse sweating, which is defined as greater than 5 liters per day, mineral losses can be substantial. The most extensive body of research on fluid and electrolyte requirements in extreme conditions has been collected by the U.S. Army Research Institute of Environmental Medicine.[10] Based on the available research, the Military Recommended Dietary Allowances (MRDA) for potassium are 1875–5625 mg (50–150 mEq). It was the conclusion of the Committee on Military Nutrition Research that current data do not indicate requirements above this level, even under extreme conditions of heat for prolonged periods of time. The National Research Council's Recommended Dietary Allowance (RDA)[36] for potassium is 1600–2000 mg (40–50 mEq) per day, significantly lower than the MRDA.

Potassium is widely distributed in food, with the richest dietary sources being unprocessed food, especially fruits, nuts, many vegetables, fresh meats, and dairy products (Table 3). Potassium intakes of Americans vary considerably, with people who consume large amounts of fruits and vegetables consuming as much as 8000–11,000 mg (205–282 mEq) per day.[36] Urban whites eat about 2500 mg/d (64 mEq),[26] while intakes as low as 1000 mg/d (26 mEq) have been reported in blacks.[22,29]

For most athletes, even those performing prolonged exercise in the heat on repeated days, potassium replacement is not a major concern because losses are minimal compared with normal intake. However, athletes who have recently suffered severe vomiting or diarrhea or possess conditions predisposing them to excessive potassium losses may be at increased risk of hypokalemia. Ingestion of potassium in supplement form should be discouraged because of the possibility of gastric distress, sharp elevation of plasma potassium, and risk of cardiac toxicity.

***TABLE 3.* Foods that Provide 5.0 mEq (200 mg) or More of Potassium per Average Serving**

Cereals	All Bran	Bran Buds
	100% Bran	Bran Chex
Meat	Beef	Turkey
	Lamb	Veal
	Pork (except bacon)	
Fish	Bass	Perch
	Carp	Pike
	Catfish	Pollack
	Cod	Red snapper
	Flounder	Salmon
	Haddock	Sole
	Halibut	Tuna
	Herring	
Dairy	Milk	Cottage cheese (2% fat)
	Buttermilk	Yogurt
Vegetables	Broccoli, boiled	Potato
	Brussels Sprouts	Pumpkin
	Carrots, raw	Spinach
	Celery, boiled	Squash, winter
	Lentils and legumes	Tomato
	Kale, boiled	Zucchini, boiled
	Parsnips	
	Kale, boiled	
Fruits	Apricots, raw	Pear, fresh
	Avocado	Pineapple
	Banana	Prunes
	Cantaloupe	Raisins
	Honeydew melon	Rhubarb
	Kiwi	Strawberries
	Mango	Tangelos
	Orange	Peach
Nuts/Seeds	Almonds	Pistachios
	Chestnuts	Soybean nuts
	Peanut butter	Sunflower seeds

Magnesium

Magnesium is the second most concentrated cation within the cell. Magnesium is pertinent to physical performance because it is cofactor in carbohydrate metabolism and plays a role in glucose transport across cell membrane. During endurance exercise, serum magnesium levels decline approximately 10% due to sweat losses and shunting to erythrocytes, adipocytes, and muscle cells.[9,14,19,30,32] The significance of this decline is not certain; however, the phenomenon has raised several questions: Do endurance athletes require more magnesium than the general population? Do endurance athletes require magnesium supplementation? Would increased magnesium intake improve performance?

In an attempt to answer these questions, Terblanche et al.[50] studied marathon runners. The runners did not routinely ingest magnesium supplements. They were split into two groups: one received placebo, and the other a magnesium supplement. Pre- and post-marathon tests revealed no differences between the groups in all parameters measured: skeletal muscle magnesium concentration, serum magnesium concentration, serum creatine kinase activity, urinary hydroxyproline/creatine ratio, maximum voluntary contraction of quadriceps or muscle soreness. Thus, these athletes did not demonstrate a deficient state that improved with supplementation, nor did they demonstrate performance improvement with higher magnesium intake.

The RDA for magnesium is 350 mg/day for men and 280 mg/day for women.[36] Foods that are good sources of magnesium include nuts, whole-grain products, legumes, and green vegetables. It appears that athletes consuming a normal, varied diet probably do not require nor benefit from magnesium supplementation.

SUMMARY

Consuming enough water to replace fluids lost in sweat is the top hydration priority for athletes. While plain water meets this goal for most athletes, endurance athletes may benefit from carbohydrate added to water. Replacement of electrolytes during exercise is not necessary in most cases, as a typical diet should provide adequate sodium, chloride, potassium, magnesium, and other nutrients to replace sweat losses.

REFERENCES

1. Ahlman K, Karvonen MJ: Weight reduction by sweating in wrestlers, and its effects on physical fitness. J Sports Med 1:58–62, 1961.
2. Barr SI, Costill DL, Fink WJ: Fluid replacement during exercise: Effects of water, saline, or no fluid. Med Sci Sports Exerc 23:811–817, 1991.
3. Bedgood BL, Tuck MB: Nutrition knowledge of high school athletic coaches in Texas. J Am Diet Assoc 83: 672, 1983.
4. Boulze D, Montastruc P: Water intake, pleasure and water temperature in humans. Physiol Behav 30(1):97–102, 1983.
5. Brouns F: Heat–sweat–dehydration–rehydration: A praxis oriented approach. J Sports Sci 9:143–152, 1991.
6. Brouns F, Saris W, Schneider H: Rationale for upper limits of electrolyte replacement during exercise. Int J Sports Nutr 2:229–238, 1992.
7. Burge CM, Carey MF, Payne WR: Rowing performance, fluid balance, and metabolic function following dehydration and rehydration. Med Sci Sports Exerc 25:1358–1364, 1993.
8. Carter JE, Gisolfi CV: Fluid replacement during and after exercise in the heat. Med Sci Sports Exerc 21(5):532–539, 1989.
9. Casoni I, Guglielmini C, Graziono L, et al: Changes of magnesium concentrations in endurance athletes. Int J Sports Med 11:234–237, 1990.
10. Committee on Military Nutrition Research: Nutritional Needs in Hot Environments. Washington D.C., National Academy Press, 1993.
11. Costill DL: Sweating: Its composition and effects on body fluids. Ann NY Acad Sci 301:160–174, 1977.
12. Costill DL: Gastric emptying of fluids during exercise. In Gisolfi DV, Lamb DK (eds): Perspectives in Exercise Science and Sports Medicine, Vol. 3: Fluid Homeostasis

During Exercise. Indianapolis, Benchmark Press, 1990, pp 97–121.

13. Costill DL, Cote R, Fink W: Dietary potassium and heavy exercise: Effects on muscle water and electrolyte. Am J Clin Nutr 36:266–275, 1982.
14. Costill DL, Cote R, Fink W: Muscle and electrolytes following various levels of dehydration in man. J Appl Physiol 40:60–71, 1976.
15. Costill DL, Miller JM: Nutrition for endurance sport: Carbohydrate and fluid balance. Int J Sports Med 1:2–14, 1980.
16. Costill DL, Saltin B: Factors limiting gastric emptying during rest and exercise. J Appl Physiol 37:679–683, 1974.
17. Davis JM, Burgess WA, Slentz CA, et al: Effects of ingesting 6% and 12% glucose/electrolyte beverages during prolonged intermittent cycling in the heat. Eur J Appl Physiol 57:563–569, 1988.
18. Fogelholm GM, Koskinen R, Laakso J, et al: Gradual and rapid weight loss: Effects on nutrition and performance in male athletes. Med Sci Sports Exerc 25:371–377, 1993.
19. Franz KB, Ruddel H, Todd GL, et al: Physiologic changes during a marathon, with special reference to magnesium. J Am Coll Nutr 4:187–194, 1985.
20. Greenleaf JE: Problem: Thirst, drinking behavior, and involuntary dehydration. Med Sci Sports Exerc 24(6):645–656, 1992.
21. Greenleaf JE, Harrison MH: Water and electrolytes. In Layman DK (ed): Nutrition and Aerobic Exercise. Washington DC, American Chemical Society, 1986, pp 107–124.
22. Grim CE, Luft FC, Miller JZ, et al: Racial differences in blood pressure in Evans County, Georgia: Relationship to sodium and potassium intake and plasma renin activity. J Chronic Dis 33:87–94, 1980.
23. Hubbard RW, Sandick BL, Matthew WT, et al: Voluntary dehydration and alliesthesia for water. J Appl Physiol 57(3):868–875, 1984.
24. Jacobs I: The effects of thermal dehydration on performance of the Wingate anaerobic test. Int J Sports Med 1:21–24, 1980.
25. Johnson HL, Nelson RA, Consolazio CF: Effects of electrolyte and nutrient solutions on performance and metabolic balance. Med Sci Sports Exerc 20:26–33, 1988.
26. Khaw KT, Barrett-Connor E: Dietary potassium and stroke-associated mortality: A 12-year prospective population study. N Engl J Med 316:235–240, 1987.
27. Knochel JP: Potassium deficiency during training in the heat. Ann Acad Sci 301:175–189, 1977.
28. Knochel JP, Vertel RM: Salt loading as a possible factor in the production of potassium depletion, rhabdomyolysis, and heat injury. Lancet 9:659–661, 1967.
29. Langford HG: Dietary potassium and hypertension. In Horan MJ, Blaustein M, Dunbar JB, et al (eds): NIH Workshop on Nutrition and Hypertension: Proceedings from a Symposium. New York, Biomedical Information Corp., 1985.
30. Lukaski HC, Bolonchuk WW, Klenay LM, et al: Maximal oxygen consumption as related to magnesium, copper and zinc nutriture. Am J Clin Nutr 37:407–415, 1983.
31. Maughan RJ: Fluid balance and exercise. Int J Sports Med 13(Suppl 1):S132–135, 1992.
32. McDonald R, Keen CL: Iron, zinc and magnesium nutrition and athletic performance. Sports Med 5:171–184, 1988.
33. Millard-Stafford ML, Sparling PB, Rosskopf LB, Dicarlo LJ: Carbohydrate-electrolyte replacement improves distance running performance in the heat. Med Sci Sports Exerc 24(8):934–940, 1992.
34. Mitchell JB, Costill DL, Houmard JA, et al: Effects of carbohydrate ingestion on gastric emptying and exercise performance. Med Sci Sports Exerc 20:110–115, 1988.
35. Montner P, Chick T, Reidesel M, et al: Glycerol hyperhydration and endurance exercise. Med Sci Sports Exerc 24:S157, 1992.
36. National Research Council: Recommended Dietary Allowances, 10th ed. Washington DC, National Academy Press, 1989.
37. Noakes TD, Goodwin N, Rayner BL, et al: Water intoxication: A possible complication during endurance exercise. Med Sci Sports Exerc 17(3):370–375, 1985.
38. Noakes TD, Norman RJ, Buck RH, et al: The incidence of hyponatremia during prolonged ultraendurance exercise. Med Sci Sports Exerc 22(2):165–170, 1990.
39. Nose H, Mack GW, Shi X, Nadel ER: Role of osmolality and plasma volume during rehydration in humans. J Appl Physiol 65(1):325–331, 1988.
40. Pitts GC, Johnson RE, Consolazio CF: Work in the heat as affected by intake of water, salt, and glucose. Am J Physiol 142:253, 1944.
41. Puhl SM, Buskirk ER: Nutrient beverages for exercise and sport. In Wolinsky I, Hickson JF (eds): Nutrition in Exercise and Sport, 2nd ed. Boca Raton, FL, CRC Press, Inc., 1994, pp 264–294.
42. Saltin B: Aerobic and anaerobic work capacity after dehydration. J Appl Physiol 19:1114–1118, 1964.
43. Sawka MN: Physiological consequences of hypohydration: Exercise performance and thermoregulation. Med Sci Sports Exerc 24(6):657–670, 1992.
44. Sawka MN, Francesconi RP, Young AJ, Pandolf KB: Influence of hydration level and body fluids on exercise performance in the heat. JAMA 252:1165–1169, 1984.
45. Sawka MN, Young AJ, Francesconi RP, et al: Thermoregulatory and blood responses during exercise at graded hypohydration levels. J Appl Physiol 59:1394–1401, 1985.
46. Serfass RC, Stull GA, Alexander JF, Ewing JL: The effects of rapid weight loss and attempted rehydration on strength and endurance of the handgripping muscle in college wrestlers. Res Q Exerc Sport 55:46–52, 1984.
47. Singer RN, Weiss SA: Effects of weight reduction on selected anthropometric, physical, and performance measures of wrestlers. Res Q 39:361–369, 1968.
48. Steen SN, Brownell KD: Patterns of weight loss and regain in wrestlers: Has the tradition changed? Med Sci Sports Exerc 22:762–768, 1990.
49. Szlyk PC, Sils IV, Francesconi RP, Hubbard RW: Patterns of human drinking: Effects of exercise, water temperature, and food consumption. Aviat Space Environ Med 61:43–48, 1990.
50. Terblanche S, Noakes TD, Dennis SC, et al: Failure of magnesium supplementation to influence marathon running performance or recovery in magnesium replete subjects. Int J Sport Nutr 2:154–164, 1992.
51. Tuttle WW: The effect of weight loss by dehydration and the withholding of food on the physiologic responses of wrestlers. Res Q 14:158–166, 1943.
52. Webster S, Rutt R, Weltman A: Physiological effects of a weight loss regimen practiced by college wrestlers. Med Sci Sports Exerc 22:229–234, 1990.
53. Widerman PM, Hagan RD: Body weight loss in a wrestler preparing for competition: A case report. Med Sci Sports Exerc 14:413–418, 1982.

7

Special Issues in Youth Sports

Morris B. Mellion, M.D.

One of the most difficult tasks facing the physician who treats children is to counsel them and their parents about a broad range of perplexing, often controversial, issues involving youth sports. Questions about organized sports programs, weight lifting, safety, motivation, and injuries often indicate both a desire for information and a need for family guidance in dealing with important matters. This chapter examines some of the more commonly encountered issues that transcend the boundaries of sports, medicine, psychology, and physiology.

ORGANIZED COMPETITIVE YOUTH SPORTS

"Should my child play competitive sports?" How many times does the practicing physician hear this simple question to which there is no simple answer? The increasing popularity of organized competitive youth sports has paralleled the growing recognition that physical fitness is a basic component of a healthy lifestyle for all ages. It is important to understand that children are not merely small adults, and their needs are not the same as those of their parents. Youth sports programs, properly organized and conducted, offer excellent opportunities for a positive growth experience for children. Unfortunately, not all youth sports programs live up to that potential.

Effective Coaching

The key to a successful youth sports program is the coach, particularly at the entry level. In the United States, approximately 20 million children are coached by 2.5 million adult volunteers participating in nonschool youth sports programs.[54] Many of these volunteer coaches have little or no formal training and tend to fall back on their past sports experience—usually at the high school or college level—for coaching young children. On the other hand, there exist specific training programs that teach the educational and motivational skills essential to good coaching.

In order to meet the training needs of prospective youth coaches, Rainer Martens, Ph.D., a leading sports psychologist, founded the American Coaches Effectiveness Program (ACEP). ACEP sponsors both coaching effectiveness clinics to prepare entry-level coaches and leadership clinics to train coaching effectiveness instructors around the country. YMCA, the Boys Clubs of America, 19 of the 37 National Governing Bodies of Olympic Sports, a long list of other national and state sports organizations, and many colleges and universities use the ACEP. Table 1 lists the addresses of ACEP and three other major organizations concerned with the training and competency of youth coaches.

Coaching Young Athletes, the textbook for ACEP level 1 courses, is also available to the public.[55] The authors start from the premise "Athletes First—Winning Second." By doing so, they confront the central issue. Youth sports have value only inasmuch as they contribute to a child's growth as a person and offer an opportunity for the child to have fun. We live in an extremely competitive society. The notion of "winning" in sports is carried to almost every home virtually every day by electromagnetic waves. Television sports are an entertainment area in which the focus on winning and the hype of stardom tend to be overemphasized. It is important that these exaggerations not be carried over to the sports experiences of youngsters.

Although we are rightly concerned with the threat to our children of an unbridled concentration on winning, there is legitimate merit to competition, which Martens defines as "a process of striving for a valued goal." Indeed, youth sports may provide an excellent setting in which to teach children about achieving a balance between competition and cooperation in their life.[53] "The intensity of competition should be low, increasing only as the children's skill level and interest increase."[56]

TABLE 1. Organizations Concerned with the Training and Competency of Youth Coaches

American Coaching Effectiveness Program
P.O. Box 5076
Champaign, IL 61820

Canadian National Certification Program
Coaching Association of Canada
333 River Road
Ottawa, ON K1L 8H9
Canada

Little League Baseball Incorporated
P.O. Box 3485
Williamsport, PA 17701

National Youth Sports Coaches Association
2611 Okeechobee Boulevard
West Palm Beach, FL 33409

TABLE 2. The 10 Most Important Reasons I Play My Best School Sport

1. To have fun
2. To improve my skills
3. To stay in shape
4. To do something I'm good at
5. For the excitement of competition
6. To get exercise
7. To play as part of a team
8. For the challenge of competition
9. To learn new skills
10. To win

Sample: 2,000 boys and 1,900 girls, grades 7–12, who identified a "best" school sport. Answers above were among 25 responses rated on a 5-point scale. (From Ewing ME, Seefeldt V: Participation and Attrition Patterns in American Agency-sponsored and Interscholastic Sports: An Executive Summary. East Lansing, MI; Youth Sports Institute, Michigan State University, 1989, with permission.)

Smoll and Smith have developed a four-part "philosophy of winning," which they believe should characterize youth sports. If the philosophy is properly applied, they believe, young athletes will have the greatest possibility of enjoying sport and benefiting from the experience: Winning isn't everything, nor is it the only thing. Failure is not the same thing as losing. Success is not synonymous with winning. Children should be taught that success is found in striving for victory (i.e., success is related to effort.)[91] "Youngsters should be taught that they are never losers if they give maximum effort. A major source of athletic stress is fear of failure; knowing that making a mistake or losing a game while giving maximum effort is acceptable to coaches and parents should remove important sources of pressure from the child."[91] A high level of self-esteem is essential for emotional health. Research has shown that children led by coaches with effectiveness training made significant gains in self-esteem when compared to a control group supervised by untrained coaches. Moreover, "it is the low-self-esteem child who probably is in the greatest need of a positive athletic experience and who appears to respond most favorably to . . . desirable coaching practices and most unfavorably to negative practices."[90] The coach makes the biggest impact on the most vulnerable children. And the well-trained coach can provide the most positive experience for the child who needs it the most.

Children worry about how their parents, coaches, and teammates view their performance. Young children have a great desire to please and a low tolerance for negative verbal and nonverbal criticism. Repeated challenges to their self-esteem may cause them to drop out of sports. Unrealistic expectations by parents and coaches may also damage a child's self-esteem. It may be too much to expect that a youngster be "the best," but it may be just right to suggest that the child "do his or her best."[37]

Why Play Sports?

Ewing and associates of the Youth Sports Institute of Michigan State University addressed the issues of why youngsters and adolescents play sports and why they drop out. They surveyed 10,000 seventh- to twelfth-grade students with the cooperation of school systems in 11 cities. Their studies reveal that both the desire to participate and actual participation in sports declined sharply and consistently between the ages of 10 and 18. At the age of 10, 45% of children indicated that they participated or intended to participate in nonschool team sports. By the age of 18, the response dropped to 26%. The decline was steady and included almost all forms of school and community-organized sports. "Having fun" was the primary reason for participating, and "lack of fun" was the number one reason for dropping out (Tables 2, 3, and 4).[26] When students who

TABLE 3. The 11 Most Important Reasons I Stopped Playing a Sport

1. I lost interest
2. I was not having fun
3. It took too much time
4. Coach was a poor teacher
5. Too much pressure (worry)
6. Wanted nonsport activity
7. I was tired of it
8. Needed more study time
9. Coach played favorites
10. Sport was boring
11. Overemphasis on winning

Sample: 2,700 boys and 3,100 girls who said they had recently stopped playing a school or nonschool sport. Answers above were among 30 responses rated on a 5-point scale. (From Ewing ME, Seefeldt V: Participation and Attrition Patterns in American Agency-sponsored and Interscholastic Sports: An Executive Summary. East Lansing, MI; Youth Sports Institute, Michigan State University, 1989, with permission.)

TABLE 4. The 12 Most Important Reasons I Play My Best School Sport

Boys	Girls
1. To have fun	1. To have fun
2. To improve skills	2. To stay in shape
3. For the excitement of competition	3. To get exercise
4. To do something I'm good at	4. To improve skills
5. To stay in shape	5. To do something I'm good at
6. For the challenge of competition	6. To be part of a team
7. To be part of a team	7. For the excitement of competition
8. To win	8. To learn new skills
9. To go to a higher level of competition	9. For the team spirit
10. To get exercise	10. For the challenge of competition
11. To learn new skills	11. To go to a higher level of competition
12. For the team spirit	12. To win

Sample: 2,000 boys and 1,900 girls, grades 7–12, who indicated they had a "best" school sport. They rated a total of 25 answers on a 5-point scale. (From Ewing ME, Seefeldt V: Participation and Attrition Patterns in American Agency-sponsored and Interscholstic Sports: An Executive Summary. East Lansing, MI; Youth Sports Institute, Michigan State University, 1989, with permission.)

TABLE 5. The 6 Most Important Changes I Would Make to Get Involved Again in a Sport I Dropped

"I would play again if . . ."

BOYS

1. Practices were more fun
2. I could play more
3. Coaches understood players better
4. There were no conflict with studies
5. Coaches were better teachers
6. There were no conflict with social life

GIRLS

1. Practices were more fun
2. There were no conflict with studies
3. Coaches understood players better
4. There were no conflict with social life
5. I could play more
6. Coaches were better teachers

Sample: 2,700 boys and 3,100 girls, grades 7–12, who said they had recently stopped playing a school or nonschool sport. They rated 21 different responses on a 5-point scale. (From Ewing ME, Seefeldt V: Participation and Attrition Patterns in American Agency-sponsored and Interscholastic Sports: An Executive Summary. East Lansing, MI; Youth Sports Institute, Michigan State University, 1989, with permission.)

had dropped out of a sport were asked under what condition would they play again, both boys' and girls' leading response was that they would play again if "practices were more fun" (Table 5).[26] Significantly, winning was not a strong motivator for participation. It was only the eighth most important reason boys play their best school sport and the twelfth most important reason girls play[26] (Table 4).

Whereas "winning" proved to be a relatively poor motivator for sports participation, self-improvement achieved a high rating among the students surveyed. Overall, improving skills was second only to having fun. The study demonstrated that both boys and girls were much more concerned about the experience of participating in sports than about the issue of winning. Ewing et al. have continued this research and expanded their database. The resulting material is the basis for a book they will be publishing in the near future.

Parents of Athletes

The other major influence determining the quality of a child's experience in organized sports is the role the parents play. The interactions between the athlete, the parents, and the coach are so important that the relationship is often called the "athletic triangle." Skillful parenting and coaching fills the triangle with fun and growth (Fig. 1), but when such skillfulness is lacking, the triangle may be hollow.

Parental involvement can produce a wide variety of responses ranging from pleasure and elation to anger and sadness in the young athlete. Parents who know how to encourage their children's efforts and praise their successes, no matter how small, enhance the sports experience greatly. Those who are overly critical about their children's performance may trigger an undesired response that endures long after the time spent on the playing field.

Here again, self-esteem is the issue. Children tend to view their worlds globally. Frequent criticism of their performance on the athletic field may lead children to think that they are a general disappointment to their parents. This reaction may diminish their self-esteem and reduce their motivation to perform well, not only in athletics but also in other aspects of their life as well.

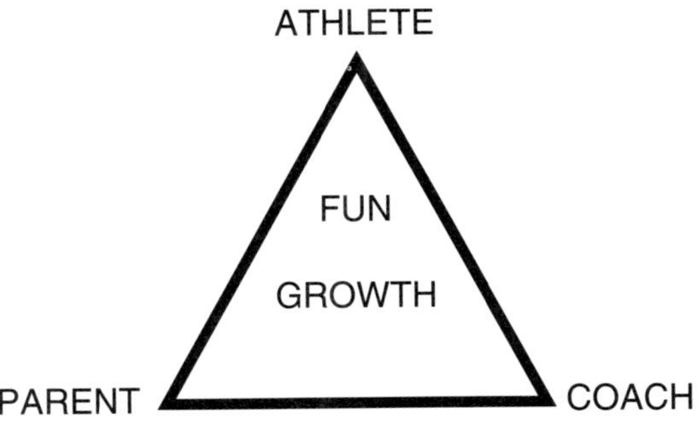

FIGURE 1. The athletic triangle.

There is a particularly difficult type of parent who may be appropriately called the "Vicarious Athlete." This parent pressures the child to excel in athletics so that the parent can experience the child's successes vicariously. The Vicarious Athlete generally recruits the spouse into an alliance in which they both provide an extremely confining, bizarre form of support and encouragement for the child. They may become overly involved in the administration and logistics of the youth sports program often to the point of manipulating the coach or other parents.

Such parents demonstrate a "conditional love."[62] They communicate a lifelong message to the child, both subtly and overtly: "Winning is what counts." In this setting, children realize they are not loved for who they are but for how they perform in the athletic arena. Their sense of worth becomes tied to athletic performance.

The Vicarious Athlete (and spouse) place the ever-increasing burden of expectations on their child-athlete. In response, the child must narrow his or her athletic participation to a single sport, which then becomes a year-round endeavor. The parents reward improving performance with a seemingly never-ending round of athletic camps and sports clinics in order to ensure their child's path to championship. The normal activities of childhood are set aside to allow more time for practice. If the child has the natural potential to become a truly elite athlete, this process may go on for many years.

Most children of Vicarious Athletes reach a point at which they can no longer achieve the ever-increasing expectations of their parents. The children have been trapped in this aberrant parent-child relationship for so many years that it is unthinkable to tell the parents that it is time to stop. Instead, they may develop injuries typical of their sport. Gymnasts get back pain, skiers get knee pain, and swimmers get shoulder pain. When these children arrive in the physician's office, they present a major diagnostic challenge. Are they elite athletes with overuse injuries, as their parents contend, or are they burned-out child-athletes? Is their pain a psychosomatic attempt to escape what they subconsciously, or perhaps consciously, recognize is a trap their parents have set? The solution to the physician's dilemma is rarely obvious at the first encounter. Over time, however, the patient has the opportunity to either heal or reveal the underlying problem. In the latter case, the physician's task is to help the family establish a new basis for communication that replaces the child's athletic career as the only tie that binds them together. The child should be allowed a choice of continuing the intense athletic career or diversifying and participating in many of the activities of normal childhood previously set aside.

Fortunately, most parents do not fall into this pattern. They are able to let their children know that they are loved for what they are, not for how they perform either on the playing field or in the classroom. The important issue is that the child learns that his or her worth is as a person, not as a performer.

Parents as Coaches

"Should I coach my own child?" This question is asked often in youth sports. The answer usually is found in practical necessity. Since one coach is needed for roughly every eight children, and there are 20 million children participating in organized youth sports in the United States, many parents find that they have to coach in order to create an opportunity for their children to play.

It is a major challenge for parents to coach their own children, but one can be met with proper training and preparation. The first stop in meeting this challenge is to undergo ACEP or other coaching effectiveness training. If such training is not available through a community league or the local YMCA, assistance in finding or even establishing a coaching effectiveness program can usually be obtained by contacting the physical education department of any nearby college or state university.

The trained parent-coach will still have to walk the fine line between appearing too critical or too approving of his or her own child either at practice or during a competition. It is helpful to learn to focus approval or criticism to the specific effort made or skill demonstrated. Global criticism is never appropriate with children. Parent-coaches are generally well advised to praise their own children's efforts moderately on the field and more generously in the car on the way home.

Youth Sports Burnout

Hellstedt defines burnout in youth sports as "a loss of energy and enthusiasm for sports" and states that it is caused by anxiety and stress. "The child no longer has fun, becomes overwhelmed by the demands of competition and training, and seeks to escape in order to cope."[37] Hellstedt describes competitive stress as a persistent form of excessive anxiety, which develops in young athletes who "worry that they will fail the team or be negatively evaluated by others." Such athletes may show signs of agitation in the form of sleep disturbance, skin rashes, nausea, headaches, and muscle tightness, as well as signs of depression, including lack of energy, sadness, frequent illness, and loss of interest in the sport.[37]

For many, the competition to earn a place on the team may be the greatest source of stress. In research on stressors in junior high school-age students, Coddington determined that not qualifying for participation in an extracurricular activity such as an athletic team ranked in severity as a stressor between birth of a sibling and a parent's losing his or her job. It ranked higher on the stress scale than breaking up with a boyfriend or girlfriend or the death of a grandparent.[20]

Such excluded athletes may also develop lingering injuries as "an acceptable alternative to high-pressure competition."[62] Smoll and Smith indicate that an overemphasis on winning and a lack of fun while participating are two major predictors of postcompetition anxiety.[91] Pillemer and Micheli describe a group of young athletes with initially relatively minor injuries who, despite appropriate care and rehabilitation, continue "to complain of severe discomfort and inability to participate in normal routines, including athletic training."[70] They indicate that these children may have secondary gain from being "an injured athlete." The injured status is a "saving face," which they define as "a sociably acceptable manner of removing oneself from athletic competition."[70] They identify a number of potential secondary gains related to family concerns. Injury status is often a dysfunctional solution for an adjustment reaction to problems unrelated to sports.[70]

Not all athletic decline is due to burnout. Rowland emphasizes that before concluding that symptoms such as declining performance, chronic fatigue, and mental lassitude are the result of psychosocial factors or overtraining, the physician should undertake a thorough history and physical. He mentions anemia, nonanemic iron deficiency, exercise-induced bronchospasm, medication side effects, abnormal weight, insufficient athletic training, cardiovascular disease, and neuromuscular disorders as other potential etiologies of a patient's symptoms, which should be ruled out.[78]

ISSUES OF PARTICIPATION

Age Guidelines. Children vary in their rates of emotional and physical maturity; consequently, there is no specific age at which all children should begin to participate in organized or competitive sports. Generally, children will cue their parents in many subtle and not-so-subtle ways that they are ready to play. In 1980, Martens developed a set of age guidelines for beginning participation in competitive youth sports based on "available evidence and judgment of youth sports leaders" (Table 6).[54] In 1991, Nelson combined sports participation guidelines with the developmental characteristics of various age groups (Table 7).[65] He offers valuable information to be used when making a determination for an individual young athlete.

Maturity and Matching. One of the most difficult problems in organized youth sports is how to organize the programs into different levels of participation. The problem is most acute in the peripubertal years because the hormonal changes of puberty accelerate growth in size, strength, coordination, and endurance, as well as epiphyseal closure. The onset of puberty varies normally from 8.5 to 13.0 years in girls and 9.5 to 13.5 years in boys. Even more significantly, the period of most rapid growth, known as peak height velocity, varies greatly as well, averaging 12.1 years in girls and 14.1 years in boys.[51,52]

TABLE 6. Age Guidelines For Beginning Participation in Competitive Youth Sports

Age	Type of Sport	Examples
6	Noncontact	Swimming Tennis Track and field
8	Contact	Basketball Soccer Wrestling
10	Collision	Tackle football Ice hockey

Adapted from Martens R: The uniqueness of the young athlete: Psychological considerations. Am J Sports Med 8:382–385, 1980.

Traditionally, children have been matched by age or grade in school. This method results in frequent mismatches in size, strength, speed, and agility and weakens the quality of a sports program. A much preferred method is to match participants, especially in contact and collision sports, by level of sexual maturation using the generally accepted Tanner scales.[51,52] In pubertal girls, age at menarche is also extremely useful. Daniel and Slap have correlated the Tanner development stages with the clinical changes that take place during the maturation process.[22,89] Pratt has correlated maturity with strength and flexibility in adolescent males.[71] Duke et al. developed a self-assessment system for adolescents, which indicates their level of sexual maturation; he also demonstrated excellent agreement between the outcome of the adolescence rating and that of the physician.[24] Matching by sexual maturation requires a very tactful and sensitive approach. The greatest problem with this method is that it often cuts across school grades and other social patterns. In some girls' sports, such as gymnastics and swimming, physical immaturity may actually correlate with a higher level of performance.

Boys and Girls Together? Should boys and girls play organized sports together on the same teams? This question was rarely, if ever, seriously asked until the 1970s. As social assumptions have changed, however, physicians and physical educators have addressed the issue. There is now general consensus that prepubertal boys and girls can play together without concern for increased physical or emotional risk.[4]

After puberty, the situation is much more complicated. The differences in strength and size between pubertal and postpubertal boys and girls is

TABLE 7. Developmental Characteristics of and Sports Participation Guidelines for Various Age-Groups

	Infancy (0–2 yr)	Early Childhood (3–5 yr)	Childhood (6–9 yr)	Late Childhood (10–12 yr)
Motor skills	Skills primarily reflex; posture depends on visual input	Fundamental skills limited; balance skills limited	Fundamental skills improved; transitional skills begin; balance control becomes automatic	Transitional skills improved; balance control declines at puberty
Learning skills	Response to training minimal; benefits of training not long term	Attention span short; attention overexclusive; response to training limited	Attention span limited; attention overinclusive; cooperation improved	Attention selective: memory strategies used
Vision	Farsighted	Farsighted; eye movements imprecise; tracking of speed and direction of moving objects difficult	Tracking of speed and direction of moving objects improved, but still difficult	Patterns same as for adults
Guidelines for sports participation	Recognize that swimming programs and exercise programs offer no advantage; encourage free play; provide safe, unstructured play environment	Avoid competition; provide limited instruction verbally and by demonstration; emphasize fun play	Keep competition minimal; keep rules of sport flexible; emphasize fundamental skills; keep instruction time short	Minimize competition; emphasize fundamental and transition skills; decrease intensity of sports involvement at puberty
Recommended activities	Free play	Walking, running, swimming, tumbling, throwing, catching	Swimming, running, gymnastics, entry-level soccer and baseball; complex-skill sports such as football, hockey, basketball, and wrestling are difficult	Entry-level football, basketball, wresting, and other contact/collision sports

From Nelson MA: Developmental skills and children's sports. Physician Sportsmed 19(2):67–79, 1991, with permission.

often great enough to pose an increased risk for coeducational participation in contact or collision sports. This risk is only one factor, however, because in most situations when schools or sports leagues have resisted participation by girls in boys' sports programs, court rulings have allowed the girls to play.

The issue has a different meaning in parts of the country where field hockey has traditionally been a girls-only sport. Here, boys have asserted their right to play field hockey. By dint of the increased speed and strength of the boys, the team with the most boys will have a decided advantage. Thus, participation by boys actually threatens the quality of the sport. The theoretical solution to the problem would be to develop a boys' field hockey team. But that solution is not practical because of lack of adequate interest among boys at the present time to form such teams, limited financing, and the limited number of playing fields at most schools.[25]

Every Child Plays. If the main reason for developing youth sports programs is to provide a safe setting for children to develop athletically while also having fun, then all children have the right to play. It is grossly unfair to allow youngsters to commit large amounts of time and energy to learning and practicing a sport without the benefit of actually playing. Children agree. When surveyed, "more than 90% of the boys questioned would rather play on a losing team than sit on the bench of a winning team. In short, playing is more valued than winning."[54]

Dangerous Sports. Although there is inherent risk involved in most sports, two specific sports present extreme risks—boxing and trampoline.

Because of the high risk of head injury and chronic brain damage, the American Medical Association, the American Academy of Family Physicians, and the American Academy of Pediatrics have all opposed boxing. They contend it is difficult to find any benefits from boxing that cannot be obtained from other, safer, and more appropriate sports. Proponents of amateur boxing take issue with these medical organizations. They assert that with proper protective equipment, good coaching, and competent officiating, amateur boxing is a safe sport.

Because of growing public awareness that trampoline accidents produce a high incidence of head and neck injuries and because of the ensuing liability insurance problems, trampoline availability and use have dropped way off. There is a valid, limited role for the trampoline in youth sports, but it should be used only under the immediate supervision of highly trained instructors. It has no place in the home or recreational settings, and it should not be left unsecured in an open space when a qualified instructor is not present.[2] When used properly, it may be a valuable tool for teaching athletic skills, especially in gymnastics and diving.

Safety in Youth Sports. Several aspects of youth sports programs can help to reduce the risk of injury inherent in athletics. Preparticipation physical examination can identify children with limiting conditions and those with problems warranting treatment and rehabilitation. The five major medical organizations whose members care for most young athletes have agreed on a common protocol.[46] Proper supervision by well-trained coaches and officials is the cornerstone of a safe program. The rules of play should be designed to protect young athletes. Adequate physical conditioning reduces the frequency and severity of injuries, as does matching for maturity, already discussed. Properly fitting protective equipment, adequate footwear, and well-maintained practice and competition facilities are essential. The importance of all of these factors is demonstrated by the existence of the Bill of Rights for Young Athletes:

The Bill of Rights for Young Athletes

Right to participate in sports
Right to participate at a level commensurate with each child's maturity and ability
Right to have qualified adult leadership
Right to play as a child and not as an adult
Right of children to share in the leadership and decision-making of their sport participation
Right to participate in safe and healthy environments
Right to proper preparation for participation in sports
Right to an equal opportunity to strive for success
Right to be treated with dignity
Right to have fun in sports

Reprinted with permission of the American Alliance for Health, Physical Education, Recreation and Dance, 1900 Association Drive, Reston, VA 22091.

STRENGTH TRAINING AND WEIGHTLIFTING

Athletes are constantly searching for ways to enhance performance, and strength training is a well-documented technique for the physically mature athlete. The trend is that the training methods successfully employed by high-level competitors are being used by athletes at all levels and ages. Consequently, there has been increasing interest in strength training among prepubertal and pubertal athletes. At the same time, there has been concern over the value and safety of strength training at these levels of maturity.

What is strength? Webb defines it as "the ability to exert muscular force against resistance."[98] But, he notes, what many coaches are interested in developing is the "explosive strength" of a football running back or a powerful hitter in baseball. In this sense, the proper term is "power," which is "a function of both the amount of muscular force exerted and the rate of body or limb movement. Most strength athletes are in fact power athletes."[98]

In 1985, three major national organizations with interest in sports medicine and athletics published position papers on strength training and weightlifting in young athletes.[6,23,63] One, the National Strength and Conditioning Association, presented the following definitions, which have already received widespread acceptance:

Resistance training is any method or form used to resist, overcome, or bear force.

Weight training is the use of barbells, dumbbells, or machine-type apparatuses as resistance.

Weightlifting and **power lifting** are the competitive sports that contest maximum lifting ability in the Olympic snatch and clean and jerk, or squat, bench press and dead lift, respectively. (The military press or overhead lift has been discontinued as a dangerous lift, both within the United States and in Olympic competition since 1972.[39])

Strength training is the use of resistance methods to increase one's ability to exert to resist force. The training may utilize free weights, the individual's own body weight, machines, and/or other devices to attain this goal. In order to be measurably effective, the training sessions must include timely progressions in intensity that impose sufficient demand to stimulate strength gains that are greater than those associated with normal growth and development.[63]

With these definitions in mind, this discussion will address the following questions: (1) Can prepubertal and pubertal athletes gain significant strength through strength training? (2) Does strength training cause injuries to children at these levels of maturity? (3) Does strength training reduce the incidence of sports-related injuries at these levels of maturity? (4) If strength training is safe and useful, are there guidelines available for the young athlete's benefit? (5) Is there a role for weightlifting and power lifting before puberty has been completed?

Strength Gains

The traditional view in sports science has been that before the hormonal changes of puberty, children are unable to produce significant muscle response to strength training. This view was supported by the early work of Vrijens, whose study failed to demonstrate strength gain in prepubescent athletes.[97]

In retrospect, the lack of significant strength gain shown by Vrijens's work and other early research appears due to an inadequate training stimulus.[45,69] For many years it was believed that all apparent gains in strength were really the result of attaining new skills and improving coordination by repetition. Several recent studies of prepubertal and pubertal athletes challenge this conception by demonstrating significant strength gains.[19,30,67,69,72,73,82,85,86,88,99]

There is now general recognition that prepubescent and pubescent athletes can achieve strength gains through well-supervised weight training programs.[5,27,45,92,94,98] However, research on how they achieve the strength gains is limited. In a study measuring integrated electromyographic amplitude, Ozmun et al. concluded that early gains in muscle strength result from increased muscle activation rather than muscle hypertrophy.[67] Ramsay et al. used percutaneous electrical stimulation to evoke muscle contractual properties and achieved similar results.[72] Neither of these groups found significant increase in muscle size compared to controls.[67,72] Fukunaga et al. did find an increase in cross-sectional muscle area in a controlled study of 52 elementary school children participating in a 12-week strength-training program.[30] They noted that the strength-training effect on cross-sectional muscle area in strength for these prepubescent students was similar in direction but lower in magnitude and changes found in a similar study they had performed on adults some years before.[30] The conflicting insights provided by these studies signal a need for further research to determine the mechanism(s) of strength gain in prepubescent and pubescent athletes.

Safety of Strength Training

Many concerns are frequently expressed about the safety of strength training, with only a paucity of data to substantiate or refute them. A large, controlled, prospective study focusing on the safety of strength training is lacking in the sports medicine literature at this time. In several well-controlled studies demonstrating the efficacy of strength training in prepubertal and pubertal athletes, there was no evidence of an increase incidence of injuries, but these studies were small and relatively short term, even though well supervised.[36,69,73,85,86,99]

There are, however, both documented reports and an extensive mythology about injuries related to strength training, weightlifting, and power lifting. Because resistance training for sports conditioning has become common practice among so many junior high school and high school athletes,it is important that the practicing physician be able to offer credible advice to young athletes and their parents.

First, at least two types of injuries appear to be common in this population in the performance of unsupervised or poorly supervised overhead weight lifting: epiphyseal fractures of the wrists and damage to the pars interarticularis. Proponents of strength training maintain that epiphyseal wrist injuries are the product only of competitive-style overhead lifting, and the reports in the literature tend to support their analysis as far as they go.[11,34,81] Rians et al. performed a two-phase bone scan on 17 prepubescent subjects and 8 controls before and after a 14-week strength-training program and found no damage to bones or growth plates.[73] Moreover, there have been only rare reports of epiphyseal wrist injuries in the recent studies that have evaluated injuries during strength training.[13,36,73,85,86,99]

Pars interarticularis injuries are much more problematic. Low-back injuries constitute half or more of all injuries sustained by adolescent weight lifters.[10,11,74] There is little question that spondylolysis and spondylolisthesis occur more frequently than previously observed in young athletes performing strength training and Olympic-style weightlifting.[11,38,41–43,45,47,58,98] It is also clear that certain types of resistance-training equipment are more likely to cause low-back injury; such equipment requires competent supervision when and if it is used.[10] May of the young athletes using various forms of resistance training to develop strength are also stressing their backs by playing football or performing gymnastics at the same time.[40,101] It is not clear whether strength training even with proper equipment and competent on-site supervision increases the risk of pars damage in young athletes. Good prospective, controlled studies are needed.

Second, a group of overuse syndromes is seen in athletes performing resistance training. Most common among these are musculotendinous strains and patellofemoral syndrome. They are often related to attempting too much too fast and/or using improper technique. Generally speaking, these problems respond well to rehabilitation and thus are not as worrisome. They do, however, teach the importance of having a knowledgeable coach or teacher individualize and supervise strength training for young athletes.

Third is the accusation that strength training will reduce flexibility and make the young athlete muscle bound. In fact, there is evidence that just the opposite is true. Well-designed strength programs in which the exercises are performed throughout the full range of joint motion tend to increase flexibility,[12,86] The athlete who is extremely inflexible initially may be well advised to perform an intensive stretching program prior to or along with strength training.

Protective Aspect of Strength Training

One benefit of strength training is that it seems to confer on the athlete an element of protection against injury. Preseason conditioning has been shown to reduce the incidence and severity of knee injuries in high school football players.[12] It has also been associated with a dramatic reduction in the incidence of injuries in a cohort of strength-trained high school boys and girls participating in a variety of sports compared with an untrained controlled group. In addition, when injuries did occur, those in the strength-trained group experienced greatly reduced average recovery and rehabilitation times.[36] Certainly, more research about the potential protective role of strength training is needed.

Guidelines for Safe Strength Training

Whether physicians agree with the notion that strength training is valuable or not, they often find themselves faced with the reality that such programs already exist in their communities and wonder if there are guidelines designed to make strength training as safe as possible. In 1985, the American Orthopedic Society for Sports Medicine (AOSSM) convened a workshop including representatives of eight organizations involved in sports medicine in order to establish such a set of guidelines. Their recommendations were published the following year.[23] Also in 1985, the National Strength and Conditioning Association published its "Position Paper on Prepubescent Strength Training."[63]

Most major issues are treated with similar recommendations by the two documents. Following are the common guidelines suggested by both groups: (1) the need for preparticipation physical examination; (2) the requirement that the child have adequate emotional maturity to accept coaching; (3) supervision by competent coaches trained in strength training specifically for this age group; (4) strength training only as part of a broader program designed to increase other motor skills and fitness level; (5) adequate warm-up and cool-down; (6) all exercises performed through full joint range of motion; (7) no lifting to attain the individual's maximum single-repetition capacity; (8) initial training without resistance, so as to learn proper techniques; (9) 6–15 repetitions per set; (10) small load increments (maximum 3 pounds) when building up resistance level; and (11) 20- to 30-minute strength-training sessions up to three times per week.[23,63] The AOSSM recommendations also prohibit competition and call for emphasis on dynamic concentric contractions (exercises in which the major resistance occurs while the muscles are shortening and tightening rather than while lengthening and releasing).[23]

A commonly asked question is, How can a young athlete's strength be assessed using commonly acknowledged terminology without determining the athlete's maximum single-repetition capacity? Webb suggests that when a measurement of strength is deemed necessary, a one-repetition maximum equivalent may be calculated using a previously published formula:

$$\text{1 RM equivalent} = (\text{weight lifted} \times \text{number of repetitions} \times 0.03) + \text{weight lifted}$$ [98]

What should be included in a strength-training program for prepubescent and pubescent athletes? Leo Totten of the U.S. Weightlifting Federation provides some poignant insights:

> First, all aspects of physical and psychological development must be incorporated into the program. Strength is important, but it must not be emphasized to the point of neglecting flexibility, power, endurance, skill work, or psychological training. The chain is only as strong as its weakest link, so even if one aspect of growth and development is ignored, the athlete will suffer. . . .
>
> Fun must be a key ingredient of any program, strength or otherwise. Kids will perform amazing amounts of work for the ingenious coach or teacher who can make it seem like fun instead of drudgery.[94]

In Table 8, Rooks and Micheli give age-scaled guidelines for what should be included in a weight training program.[75]

Weightlifting and Power Lifting

As defined earlier, weightlifting and power lifting are competitive sports, whereas strength training is a type of physical conditioning. Because of concerns about the higher injury potential of these sports, AOSSM and the American Academy of Pediatrics (AAP) guidelines consider them inappropriate for prepubertal children.[6,23] In a 1990 policy

TABLE 8. **Recommendations for Developing a Weight-training Program**

Ages	9–11	12–14	15–16	17+
Exercises per body part	1	1	2	>2
Sets	2	3	3 or 4	4–6
Repetitions	12–15	10–12	7–11	6–10
Maximum weight (resistance)	Very light	Light	Moderate	Heavy

From Rooks DS, Micheli LJ: Musculoskeletal assessment and training: The young athlete. Clin Sports Med 7:641–677, 1988.

statement, the AAP Committee on Sports Medicine expanded its stand on weightlifting and power lifting to include body building and "the repetitive use of maximal amounts of weight in strength training programs." The committee recommends that children and adolescents not participate in these activities until they have reached the Tanner stage 5 level of developmental maturity.[5]

Extreme caution and close supervision are advised for young athletes participating in any form of overhead lifting.

Some Reservations

The evidence about safety of strength training is thin, and more research is necessary. The present guidelines represent valuable interim measures, because they offer the practicing physician a basis for counseling patients and parents, but they will require a great deal of refinement over the next few years as more data become available.

One reservation about weight training has been whether it can contribute to hypertension in children and adolescents. In a study on the effect of weight training in six adolescents with persistent essential hypertension, Hagberg et al. concluded that weight training "appears to maintain the reductions in blood pressure achieved by endurance training, and may even elicit further reductions in blood pressure."[35] Servedio et al. measured blood pressure during workload in prepubescent boys performing Olympic-style lifts.[85] They noted no change in systolic blood pressure but a decrease in diastolic blood pressure during workload. Echocardiogram revealed that left ventricular and diastolic dimension and volume during workload was increased compared to a control group. Thus, their data also indicated hemodynamic benefit.[85] Rians et al. found no change in resting blood pressure or heart rate in 18 prepubescent males participating in a 14-week strength-training program consisting of three 45-minute circuit training sessions using hydraulic resistance machines.[73] A note of caution is inserted by Fleck et al. who studied 12 junior elite Olympic weight lifters by way of cardiomagnetic resonance imaging and demonstrated increased left ventricular mass and smaller than normal systolic and diastolic diameters of their ventricles, indicating a pressure overload phenomenon similar to that previously shown in older resistance-trained athletes.[28,29]

Other concerns about strength training, weightlifting, and power training include the relationship between increased strength, speed, and upper body mass and the incidence of knee injuries—in sports that require frequent cutting and pivoting—and the clinical syndrome of syncope—during heavy weight lifting.

Endurance Training in Children

As more young children participate in running and other competitive sports, research on the aerobic response to endurance training in this age group has flourished. The research has often been characterized by significant methodological and design limitations and has produced mixed results. A critical review of this research indicates that with adequate training programs, prepubescent children can make significant gains in aerobic capacity (VO_{2max}) through endurance training.[8,76,96] Analyzing previous studies, Rowland noted that those children's training regimens that failed to demonstrate increased aerobic fitness also failed to comply with "adult" standards of duration (15–60 minutes), frequency (three to five times weekly), and intensity (heart rate 60–90% of maximum). Conversely, he noted that those programs that did meet these adult criteria often showed VO_{2max} increases similar to those observed in adults. Part of the research problem may stem from uncertainty about how to determine VO_{2max} in pubescent children.[77] Mahon and Vaccaro provided additional proof of the endurance-training effect by measuring ventilatory threshold, which is believed to be "the point where anaerobic metabolism begins to provide energy." They demonstrated that an 8-week stimulus of endurance training improved both ventilatory threshold and aerobic capacity in eight previously untrained male children with an average age of 12.4 years.[49]

Despite the substantial evidence that endurance training programs can improve aerobic power in children, several questions still remain: (1) What are the proper guidelines for endurance training in prepubescent and pubescent athletes? (2) Are there negative effects of high-level endurance training in these age groups? (3) What are the emotional benefits and concerns about high-intensity training in young athletes? These questions should be addressed by future research, with a view toward development of effective, safe training programs for serious young athletes.

Injuries

The risk of injury to children in sports is an important concern on the part of athletes, parents, coaches, and administrators. Not many years ago, organized medicine openly opposed contact sports for young children because it was feared that youngsters would be more susceptible to injury than high school or college athletes.[3] In fact, research has shown that such fears were unfounded: contact and even collision sports are now regularly played in some elementary and most middle level schools as well as in a myriad of community leagues.

TABLE 9. Injury Rate by Division

Division	Age (yr)	Weight (lb)	No. of Children	No. (%) of Injuries: Moderate (7–21 d)	Major (21 d)	Total
Jr Pee Wee	8–11	49.5–84.3	692	8 (1.2)	5 (0.7)	13 (1.9)
Pee Wee	9–12	64.5–99	1,610	29 (1.8)	15 (0.9)	44 (2.7)
Jr Midget	10–13	79.2–103.6	1,489	50 (3.4)	36 (2.4)	86 (5.8)
Midget	11–14	89.1–133.80	1,160	59 (5.1)	38 (3.3)	97 (8.4)
Bantam	12–15	108.9–148.5	177	11 (6.2)	6 (3.4)	17 (9.6)
Total			5,128	157 (3.1)	100 (2.0)	257 (5.0)

Modified from Goldberg B, Rosenthal PP, Robertson LS, Nicholas JA: Injuries in youth football. Pediatrics 81:255–261, 1988.

A community-wide study of a midwestern U.S. city of 100,000 by Zaricznyj et al. demonstrated that younger children had fewer injuries and that the rate of injury increased with age until high school age was attained: 3% of elementary school students, 7% of junior high school students, and 11% of high school students sustained injuries severe enough to be either treated by a physician, noted in official sports records, or reported to the school insurance carrier over the course of a year. There were approximately twice as many injuries in nonorganized sports and in physical education classes as there were in organized sports, but is it possible that these data merely reflect the numbers of children participating in these activities. Twenty percent of the injuries were considered serious, but only 1.2% caused permanent damage. The authors felt that 27% of the injuries "could have been avoided had nominal safety precautions been observed."[103] Other authors have suggested that 63% of youth sports injuries evaluated in a different setting could have been avoided.[33]

Goldberg et al. studied the injury experience of 5,128 boys representing 71 towns in six New England Pop Warner football leagues. They found that the injury rates were lowest in the youngest and lightest divisions and increased in proportion to the age and weight categories of the divisions (Table 9).[32]

Boys and girls have similar injury rates in sports played by both sexes.[31,95] However, the overall injury rate for boys is much higher due to greater participation in contact and collision sports.[31,87,103]

At the high school level, most athletes are postpubertal and therefore stronger, larger, and faster. Here, the injury rate rises precipitously in proportion to the intensity of contact involved in the sport. In addition, overuse injuries in the running sports begin to be frequent problems in this age group. Garrick and Requa provide data on injuries sustained by athletes in four large metropolitan high schools (Table 10).[31] McLain and Reynolds provide data on injuries sustained in a single large high school with 1,283 participating student athletes experiencing 280 injuries (Table 11). Their study included an analysis of the days lost per injury by girls and boys in each sport (Table 12).[48]

Epiphyseal Injuries

Injuries involving the bony growth plate deserve special attention in any discussion of youth sports medicine. Although a thorough analysis of the diagnosis and management of these problems would be more appropriate for an orthopedic text, a general understanding of some basic issues is essential for any physician treating young athletes.

In growing children, the physis, or bony growth plate, is considerably weaker than the surrounding ligamentous tissue. This difference in strength between the two types of tissue appears to be greatest at puberty, the time of peak bone growth.[14,44,60,68,100] Consequently, an injury that would likely result in a torn ligament in a postpubertal athlete is more likely to cause a disruption of the growth plate in the prepubertal or pubertal competitor.[7,14,44,59] The

TABLE 10. Injury Rate Per Season in Four Metropolitan High Schools

Sport	Boys (%)	Girls (%)
Badminton	–	6
Baseball	–	18
Basketball	31	25
Cross-country	29	35
Football	81	–
Gymnastics	28	40
Soccer	30	–
Softball	–	44
Swimming	9	1
Tennis	3	7
Track and field	35	33
Volleyball	–	10

Adapted from Garrick JG, Requa RK: Injuries in high school sports. Pediatrics 61:465–469, 1978.

TABLE 11. Athletes and Injuries in 24 Sports

Sport/Sex	No. of Athletes	No. of Athletes with Injuries	% of Athletes with Injuries
Football	179	109	61
Gymnastics			
Girls	24	11	46
Boys	20	8	40
Wrestling	65	26	40
Basketball			
Boys	57	21	37
Girls	45	14	31
Volleyball	64	11	17
Baseball	68	10	15
Cross-country			
Boys	54	7	13
Girls	40	3	7
Soccer			
Boys	99	13	13
Girls	72	12	17
Softball	54	7	13
Track			
Boys	70	7	10
Girls	65	12	18
Badminton	40	3	7
Field hockey	46	3	6
Water polo			
Boys	36	2	5
Girls	16	0	0
Tennis			
Girls	30	1	3
Boys	32	0	0
Golf	26	0	0
Swimming			
Boys	40	0	0
Girls	41	0	0
All	1,283	280	22

From McLain LG, Reynolds S: Sports injuries in a high school. Pediatrics 84:446–450, 1989, with permission.

physician, aware of this phenomenon, will often wisely obtain stress x-rays of joints that appear to be "sprained" but that actually have sustained growth plate fractures.

In addition to the increase in epiphyseal fractures at the time of puberty, there is a concomitant increase in fractures of all types. Blimkie et al. studied the relationship of fracture incidence to physical activity and growth velocity in adolescent Belgian boys. The peak fracture rate occurred during "mid-adolescence," which the authors defined as the age at peak height velocity +/– two standard deviations. In this population, they noted, fracture incidence occurred when the amount of time the boys spent in sports physical activity was low compared with later years. They attributed the high fracture rate predominantly to a lag in cortical bone thickness and mineralization relative to linear skeletal growth.[9]

Another factor in the high incidence of injuries at the time of puberty is the relative disparity between the growth of bones and musculotendinous units at the time of peak height velocity. Typically, the long bones grow faster than the muscles and tendons, resulting in decreased flexibility and increased stress to the bone and joints.[60,66,79]

With the increase in popularity of gymnastics, one particular kind of epiphyseal injury has become increasingly common. Young gymnasts often develop stress fractures at the distal radial growth plate. Symptomatically, these injuries are characterized by distal radial pain aggravated by forced dorsiflexion. In male gymnasts, the pain is most notable on the pommel horse. On examination, there is tenderness at the distal radius, most prominent at the radial styloid. Occasionally, there is a mild degree of dorsal swelling. Radiographs typically reveal widening of the physis with narrowing of the epiphysis and cystic changes of the distal metaphysis. Often these findings are accompanied by a haziness within the epiphyseal plate.[1,17,18,50,64,80,102] This process may lead to premature radial growth plate closure,[1] but in most cases the problem resolves without premature growth plate closure.[18,50,64,80,102] A gymnast with this

TABLE 12. Severity of Injuries

Sport/Sex	Days Lost per Injury
Track	
Girls	32.0
Boys	23.1
Basketball	
Girls	28.6
Boys	11.8
Cross-country	
Girls	26.7
Boys	4.1
Wrestling/boys	22.6
Baseball	21.5
Gymnastics	
Girls	19.0
Boys	10.1
Soccer	
Girls	9.8
Boys	10.6
Tennis	
Girls	10.0
Boys	0
Softball/girls	9.4
Volleyball	8.3
Football	6.7
Badminton	5.3
Water polo	
Girls	0
Boys	5.0
Field hockey	3.3
Swimming	
Girls	0
Boys	0
Golf	0

From McLain LG, Reynolds S: Sports injuries in a high school. Pediatrics 84:446–450, 1989, with permission.

problem often develops a length discrepancy between the radius and the ulna. Known as a positive ulnar variance, the problem may be due either to inhibited growth of the distal radius or to the ulna's adapting to recurrent stress with hypertrophy.[1,50,64]

Growth cartilage also occurs in bony prominences where major muscle tendons insert. These sites, called apophyses, are prone to two types of injury: avulsion and traction. Whereas the older athlete might sustain a muscle "pull," the peripubertal athlete is vulnerable to the avulsion of the tendinous insertion.[100] Such injuries, though not common, do occur at the origins of several major muscle groups on the pelvis. These include the anterior superior iliac spine, the anterior inferior iliac spine, the ischium, the iliac crest, and the adjacent lesser trochanter of the femur.[57] When a physician suspects a muscle strain at either end of the muscle in this age athlete, x-rays should be considered in order to rule out apophyseal avulsion.

Repetitive forceful contractions of large muscles may cause traction injuries of the apophysis, known variably as apophysitis and epiphysitis. The process appears to start as an inflammatory reaction to repeated stress a the tendinous insertion and is followed by reactive bone formation. There is growing acceptance of the theory that these lesions are "the result of tiny avulsion fractures and the body's resultant healing processes."[59] The most common traction apophysitis is Osgood-Schlatter's disease, which occurs at the insertion of the patella tendon and often produces painful bony hypertrophy of the tibial tubercle. Common apophyseal overuse injuries are listed in Table 13.

The popularity of endurance running and even marathon competition in recent years has spread to children, and many are involved in intensive training programs with extremely high mileage. The research literature does not give a clear understanding about whether such rigorous activity can be tolerated safely by the growth plates of the weight-bearing bones in the young athlete. Until better information is available, most authorities are recommending a cautious approach to extreme distance running until puberty is complete.[14]

For many years physicians were concerned that the epiphyses and apophyses were so prone to injury that children should avoid contact sports until completing puberty. Larson dispelled those concerns by demonstrating that only 933 (19%) of 4,854 athletic injuries evaluated in a group orthopedic practice had occurred in children 15 years old or younger. Of the 933, 84 (9%) had disruptive injuries, and 54 (6%) had other epiphyseal problems, mostly apophysitis.[44]

Concussion

Concussion is defined as "a clinical syndrome characterized by immediate and transient posttraumatic impairment of neural function, such as the alteration of consciousness, disturbance of vision,

TABLE 13. Common Sites of Apophyseal Overuse Injuries

Site	Apophyseal Injury
Elbow	Medial epicondylitis
Pelvis	Iliac crest apophysitis
	Anterior superior iliac spine (sartorius)
	Anterior inferior iliac spine (rectus femoris)
	Ischial tuberosity
Knee	Sinding-Larsen-Johansson syndrome (distal pole of patella)
	Osgood-Schlatter's disease (tibial tubercle)
Foot	Sever's disease (os calcis apophysitis)
	Accessory navicular syndrome

Modified from Micheli LJ: The traction apophysitises. Clin Sports Med 6:389–404, 1987.

equilibrium, etc., due to brainstem involvement."[21] Although on-the-field management of head injury is beyond the context of this book, the issue of when and if it is safe for the athlete who has sustained one or more concussions to return to collision sports is certainly germane.

The physician reading the current sports medicine literature regarding concussion is likely to be confused and frustrated by encountering the well over a half dozen classification and grading systems for concussion, each with a different set of guidelines for an athlete's return to play. There is a well-justified general trend, however, to be much more conservative in decision making.

In 1984, Saunders and Harbaugh as well as Cantu defined what has since become known as the second impact syndrome. They noted that "sequential minor impacts may occasionally lead to major cerebral pathological conditions." An initial minor head injury reduces compliance of the brain and, thereby, its ability to withstand the shock of a second relatively minor blow. The result may be severe intracranial injury and death.[16,83] Two cases of athletes' developing almost immediate cerebral edema and dying after having sustained prior concussions had been reported previously.[84] Similarly, athletes recovering from infectious mononucleosis with encephalitis have sustained major head injury from minor trauma.[93]

Our current understanding of the second impact syndrome makes it clear that there is no justification for an athlete with *any* persisting signs or symptoms related to a concussion or postconcussion state to return to play in a contact sport until long after the sequelae have resolved. The athlete with even brief loss of consciousness or posttraumatic amnesia should be kept out of contact play until symptom free for a week, and longer if it is a recurrent concussion in the same season.[15] The athlete with symptoms that persist several days after even mild concusion or with symptoms that progress at any time warrants computerized tomography or magnetic resonance imaging evaluation. Three mild concussions should lead to termination of the athlete's season.[15] At the high school level or lower, three concussions with flaccid unconsciousness should end participation in collision sports permanently.[4]

CONCLUSION

The issues discussed in this chapter are of vital concern to all those involved in youth sports. The responsibility for counseling athletes, their parents, and their coaches often falls on the shoulders of the physician. It is a responsibility that should always be treated with utmost care.

REFERENCES

1. Albanese SA, Palmer AK, Kerr DR, et al: Wrist pain and distal growth plate closure of the radius in gymnasts. J Pediatr Orthop 9:23–28, 1989.
2. American Academy of Pediatrics: Committee on Accident and Poison Prevention and Committee on Pediatric Aspects of Physical Fitness, Recreation, and Sports. Trampolines II. Pediatrics 67:438, 1981.
3. American Academy of Pediatrics, Committee on School Health: Competitive athletics: A statement of policy. Pediatrics 18:672–676, 1956.
4. American Academy of Pediatrics, Committee on Sports Medicine: Dyment PG (ed): Sports Medicine: Health Care for Young Athletes, 2nd edition. Elk Grove Village, IL, American Academy of Pediatrics, 1991.
5. American Academy of Pediatrics, Committee on Sports Medicine: Strength training, weight and power lifting, and body building by children and adolescents. Pediatrics 86:801–803, 1990.
6. American Academy of Pediatrics, Committee on Sports Medicine: Weight training and weightlifting: Information for the pediatrician. Physician Sportsmed 11(3): 157–161, 1983.
7. Bailey DA, Wedge JH, McCulloch RG, Martin AD, Bernhardson SC: Epidemiology of fractures of the distal end of the radius in children as associated with growth. J Bone Joint Surg 71-A:1225–1231, 1989.
8. Bar-Or O: Trainability of the prepubescent child. Physician Sportsmed 17(5):65–81, 1989.
9. Blimkie CJR, Lefevre J, Beunen GP, et al: Fractures, physical activity, and growth velocity in adolescent Belgian boys. Med Sci Sports Exerc 25:801–808, 1993.
10. Brady TA, Cahill BR, Bodnar LM: weight training-related injuries in the high school athlete. Am J Sports Med 10:1–4, 1982.
11. Brown EW, Kimball RG: Medical history associated with adolescent powerlifting. Pediatrics 72:636–644, 1983.
12. Cahill BR, Griffith EH: Effect of preseason conditioning on the incidence and severity of high school football knee injuries. Am J Sports Med 6:180–184, 1978.
13. Caine DJ: Growth plate injury and bone growth: an update. Pediatr Exerc Sci 2:209–229, 1990.
14. Caine DJ, Lindner KJ: Growth plate injury: A threat to young distance runners? Physician Sportsmed 12(4): 118–124, 1984.
15. Cantu RC: Guidelines for return to contact sports after a cerebral concussion. Physician Sportsmed 14(10):75–83, 1986.
16. Cantu RC: Second impact syndrome: immediate management. Physician Sportsmed 20(9):55–66, 1992.
17. Carek PJ, Fumich RM: Stress fractures of the distal radius: NOT just a risk for elite gymnasts. Physician Sportsmed 20(5):115–118, 1992.
18. Carter SR, Aldridge MJ: Stress injury of the disal radial growth plate. J Bone Joint Surg 70-B:834–6, 1988.
19. Claiborne JM, Donolli JD: Effects of resistance training on female prepubescent swimmers. Med Sci Sports Exerc 21(2 Suppl):S83, 1989.
20. Coddington, RD: The significance of life events as etiologic factors in the diseases of children I—a survey of professional workers. J Psychosom Res 16:7–18, 1972.
21. Congress of Neurologic Surgeons: Ad Hoc Committee to Study Head Injury Nomenclature. Glossary of head injury including some definitions of injury to the cervical spine. Clin Neurosurg 12:386–394, 1966.
22. Daniel WA Jr: Growth at adolescence: Clinical correlates. Semin Adol Med 1:15–24, 1985.
23. Duda M: Prepubescent strength training gains support. Physician Sportsmed 14(2):157–161, 1986.

24. Duke PM, Litt IF, Gross RT: Adolescents' self-assessment of sexual maturation. Pediatrics 66:918–920, 1980.
25. Dyment PG: Controversies in pediatric sports medicine. Physician Sportsmed 17(7):57–71, 1989.
26. Ewing ME, Seefeldt V: Participation and Attrition Patterns in American Agency-sponsored and Interscholastic Sports: An Executive Summary. East Lansing, MI; Youth Sports Institute, Michigan State University, 1989.
27. Faigenbaum AD: Strength training: A guide for teachers and coaches. Nat Strength Condit Assoc J 15(5):20–29, 1993.
28. Fleck SJ, Heinke C, Wilson W: Cardiac MRI of elite junior olympic weight lifters. Med Sci Sports Exerc 20(2 Suppl): S54, 1988.
29. Fleck SJ, Pattany PM, Stone MH, et al: Magnetic resonance imaging determination of left ventricular mass: junior Olympic weightlifters. Med Sci Sports Excerc 25: 522–527, 1993.
30. Fukunaga T, Funato K, Ikegawa S: The effects of resistance training on muscle area and strength in prepubescent age. Ann Physiol Anthropol 11:357–364, 1992.
31. Garrick JG, Requa RK: Injuries in high school sports. Pediatrics 61:465–469, 1978.
32. Goldberg B, Rosenthal PP, Robertson LS, Nicholas JA: Injuries in youth football. Pediatrics 81:255–261, 1988.
33. Goldberg B, Witman PA, Gleim GW, Nicholas JA: Children's sports injuries: Are they avoidable? Phys Sportsmed 7:93–101, 1979.
34. Gumbs VL, Segal D, Halligan JB, Lower G: Bilateral distal radius and ulnar fractures in adolescent weight lifters. Am J Sports Med 6:375–379, 1982.
35. Hagberg JM, Ehsani AA, Goldring D, et al: Effect of weight training on blood pressure and hemodynamics in hypertensive adolescents. J Pediatr 104:147–151, 1984.
36. Hejna WF, Rosenberg A, Buturusis DJ, Krieger A: The prevention of sports injuries in high school students through strength training. Nat Strength Condit Assoc J 4:28–31, 1982.
37. Hellstedt JC: Kids, parents and sports: Some questions and answers. Physician Sportsmed 16(4):59–71, 1988.
38. Hensinger RN: Spondylolysis and spondylolisthesis in children and adolescents. J Bone Joint Surg 71-A:1098–1107, 1989.
39. Herrick RT (letters to the editor): Am J Sports Med 11:369, 1983.
40. Jackson DW, Wiltse LL, Cirincoine RJ: Spondylolysis in the female gymnast. Clin Orthop 117:68–73, 1976.
41. Jackson DW, Wiltse LL, Dingeman RD, Hayes M: Stress reactions involving the pars interarticularis in young athletes. Am J Sports Med 9:304–312, 1981.
42. Jesse JP: Olympic lifting movements endanger adolescents. Physician Sportsmed 5(9):61–67, 1977.
43. Kotani PT, Ichikawa N, Wakabayashi W, et al: Studies of spondylolysis found among weightlifters. Br J Sports Med 6:4–8, 1971.
44. Larson RL: Epiphyseal injuries in the adolescent athlete. Orthop Clin North Am 4:839–851, 1973.
45. Lillegard WA: Strength training for the young athlete. J Back Musculoskel Rehabil 1(2):29–37, 1991.
46. Lombardo J, Robinson J, Smith D: Preparticipation physical evaluation, Kansas City, MO: American Academy of Family Physicians, American Academy of Pediatrics, American Medical Society for Sports Medicine, American Orthopaedic Society for Sports Medicine, American Osteopathic Academy of Sports Medicine, 1992.
47. McCarroll JR, Miller JM, Ritter MA: Lumbar spondylolysis and spondylolisthesis in college football players: A prospective study. Am J Sports Med 14:404–406, 1986.
48. McLain LG, Reynolds S: Sports injuries in a high school. Pediatrics 84:446–450, 1989.
49. Mahon AD, Vaccaro P: Ventilatory threshold and VO_{2max} changes in children following endurance training. Med Sci Sports Exerc 21:425–431, 1989.
50. Mandelbaum BR, Bartolozzi AR, Davis CA, et al: Wrist pain syndrome in the gymnast pathogenetic, diagnostic, and therapeutic considerations. Am J Sports Med 17: 305–317, 1989.
51. Marshall WA, Tanner JM: Variations in the pattern of pubertal changes in boys. Arch Dis Child 45:13–23, 1970.
52. Marshall WA, Tanner JM: Variations in the pattern of pubertal changes in girls. Arch Dis Child 44:291–303, 1969.
53. Martens R: Kids sports: a den of iniquity or a land of promise. In Magill RA, Ash MJ, Smoll FL (eds): Children in Sport: A Contemporary Anthology. Champaign, IL, Human Kinetics, 1978, 201–216.
54. Martens R: The uniqueness of the young athlete: Psychological considerations. Am J Sports Med 8:382–385, 1980.
55. Martens R, Christina RW, Harvey JS, Sharkey BJ: Coaching Young Athletes. Champaign, IL, Human Kinetics, 1981.
56. Martens R, Seefeldt V (eds): Guidelines for Children's Sports. Reston, VA, American Alliance for Health, Physical Education, Recreation and Dance, 1979.
57. Metzmaker JN, Pappas AM: Avulsion fractures of the pelvis. Am J Sports Med 13:349–358, 1985.
58. Micheli LJ: Back injuries in gymnastics. Clin Sports Med 6:85–93, 1985.
59. Micheli LJ: Overuse injuries in children's sports: The growth factor. Orthop Clin North Am 14:337–360, 1983.
60. Micheli LJ: Pediatric and adolescent sports injuries: Recent trends. Exerc Sports Sci Rev 14:359–74, 1986.
61. Micheli LJ: The traction apophysitises. Clini Sports Med 6:389–404, 1987.
62. Nash HL: Elite child-athletes: How much does victory cost? Physician Sportsmed 15(8):129–133, 1987.
63. National Strength and Conditioning Association: Position paper on prepubescent strength training. Nat Strength Condit Assoc J 7:27–31, 1985.
64. Nattiv A, Mandelbaum BR: Injuries and special concerns in female gymnasts detecting, treating, and preventing common problems. Physician Sportsmed 21(7):66–82, 1993.
65. Nelson MA: Developmental skills and children's sports. Physician Sportsmed 19(2):67–79, 1991.
66. O'Neill DB: Preventing injuries in young athletes. J Musculoskel Med 6(11):21–35, 1989.
67. Ozmun JC, Mikesky AE, Surburg PR: Neuromuscular adaptations during prepubescent strength training. Med Sci Sports Exerc 23(4 Suppl):S31, 1991.
68. Pappas AM: Epiphyseal injuries in sports. Phys Sportsmed 11(6):140–148, 1983.
69. Pfeiffer RD, Francis RS: Effects of strength training on muscle development in prepubescent, pubescent, and post-pubescent males. Physician Sportsmed 14(9):134–143, 1986.
70. Pillemer FG, Micheli LJ: Psychological considerations in youth sports. Clin Sports Med 7:679–689, 1988.
71. Pratt, M: Strength, flexibility, and maturity in adolescent athletes. Am J Dis Child 143:560–563, 1989.
72. Ramsay JA, Cameron JR, Blimkie R, et al: Strength training effects in prepubescent boys. Med Sci Sports Exerc 22:605–614, 1990.
73. Rians CB, Weltman A, Cahill BR, Janney CA, Tippett SR, Katch FI: Strength training for prepubescent males: Is it safe? Am J Sports Med 15:483–489, 1987.
74. Risser WL, Riser JMH, Preston D: Weight-training injuries in adolescents. Am J Dis Child 144:1015–1017, 1990.
75. Rooks DS, Micheli LJ: Musculoskeletal assessment and training: The young athlete. Clin Sports Med 7:641–677, 1988.

76. Rowland TW: Aerobic response to endurance training in prepubescent children: A critical analysis. Med Sci Sports Exerc 17:493–497, 1985.
77. Rowland TW: Does peak VO_2 reflect VO_{2max} in children?: Evidence from supramaximal testing. Med Sci Sports Exerc 25:689–693, 1993.
78. Rowland TW: Exercise fatigue in adolescents: Diagnosis of athlete burnout. Physician Sportsmed 14(9):69–77, 1986.
79. Rowland TW: Overtraining hazards in prepubertal athletes. J Musculoskel Med 7(2):52–60, 1990.
80. Roy S, Caine D, Singer KM: Stress changes of the distal radial epiphysis in young gymnasts: A report of twenty-one cases and a review of the literature. Am J Sports Med 13:301–308, 1985.
81. Ryan JR, Salciccioli GG: Fractures of the distal radial epiphysis in adolescent weightlifters. Am J Sports Med 4:26–27, 1976.
82. Sailors M, Berg K: Comparison of responses to weight training in pubescent boys and men. J Sports Med Phys Fit 27:30–37, 1987.
83. Saunders RL, Harbaugh RE: The second impact in catastrophic contact-sports head trauma. JAMA 252:538–539, 1984.
84. Schneider RC: Head and Neck Injuries in Football: Mechanisms, Treatment, and Prevention. Baltimore, Williams & Wilkins, 1973.
85. Servedio FJ, Bartels RL, Hamlin RL, et al: The effects of weight training, using Olympic-style lifts, on various physiological variables in prepubescent boys. Med Sci Sports Exerc 17:288; 1985.
86. Sewell L, Micheli LJ: Strength training for children. J Pediatr Orthop 6:143–146, 1986.
87. Shively RA, Grana WA, Ellis D: High school sports injuies. Phys Sportsmed 9(8):46–50, 1981.
88. Siegel JA, Camaione DN, Manfredi TG: Upper body strength training and prepubescent children. Med Sci Sports Exerc 20(2 Suppl):S53, 1988.
89. Slap GB: Normal physiological and psychosocial growth in the adolescent. J Adolesc Health Care 7:13S–23S, 1986.
90. Smith RE, Smoll FL, Curtis B: Coach effectiveness training: A cognitive-behavioral approach to enhancing relationship skills in youth sport coaches. J Sports Psychol 1:59–75, 1979.
91. Smoll FL, Smith RE: Psychology of the young athlete: stress-related maladies and remedial approaches. Pediatr Clin N Am 37:1021–1046, 1990.
92. Tanner SM: Weighing the risks: Strength training for children and adolescents. Physician Sportsmed 21(6):105–116, 1993.
93. Torg JS, Beer C, Bruno LA, Vegso J: Head trauma in football players with infectious mononucleosis. Phys Sportsmed 8:107–110, 1980.
94. Totten L: The prepubescent athlete: practical considerations in strengthening the prepubescent athlete. Nat Strength Condit Assoc J 8(2):38–40, 1986.
95. Tursz A, Crost M: Sport-related injuries in children: A study of their characteristics, frequency, and severity, with comparison to other types of accidental injuries. Am J Sports Med 14:294–299, 1986.
96. Vaccaro P, Mahon A: Cardiorespiratory responses to endurance training in children. Sports Med 4:352–363, 1987.
97. Vrijens: J. Muscle strength development in the pre- and post-pubescent age. Med Sport 11:152–158, 1978.
98. Webb DR: Strength training in children and adolescents. Pediatr Cliin N Am 37:1187–1210, 1990.
99. Weltman A, Janney C, Rians CB, et al: The effects of hydraulic resistance strength training in pre-pubertal males. Med Sci Sports Exerc 18:629–638, 1986.
100. Wilkins KE: The uniqueness of the young athlete: Musculoskeletal injuries. Am J Sports Med 8:377–382, 1980.
101. Wiltse LL, Widell EH, Jackson DW: Fatigue fracture: The basic lesion in isthmic spondylolisthesis. J Bone Joint Surg 57A:17–22, 1975.
102. Yong-Hing K, Wedge JH, Bowen CVA: Chronic injury to the distal ulnar and radial growth plates in an adolescent gymnast: A case report. J Bone Joint Surg 70A: 1087–1089, 1988.
103. Zaricznyj B, Shattuck LJM, Mast TA, et al: Sports-related injuries in school-aged children. Am J Sports Med 8: 318–324, 1980.

8

The Athletic Woman

Margot Putukian, M.D.

During the past several decades, girls and women in sports have enjoyed tremendously increased opportunities, and they have demonstrated their excellence in various athletic activities. At the same time, the field of sports medicine is also growing and expanding in exponential proportions. As the sports medicine literature rapidly grows, we begin to realize there is still much to learn, especially regarding the female athlete. We already have a good understanding of the physiological adaptations that occur with training and of the numerous injuries that are common to various sports, but most of that information has been gleaned from studies of men. As women move forward in their involvement in athletics, many medical concerns have been raised that are specific to the female athlete.

The benefits of competitive exercise, both physically and mentally, are numerous.[16,44,54,118] The long-term effects with regard to overall health and quality of life are also well-known.[117,136,160] Today, women along with men are at risk for cardiac disease, and coronary artery disease is the leading cause of heart disease in women, accounting for 28% of all fatalities. Exercise can play a positive role in decreasing the risk factors of coronary artery disease by having an effect on lipid profile, body mass index, and diabetes mellitus.[171] Participation in athletics can be an important part of an individual's growth in the area life skills, and it confers general health benefits as well.

There do not appear to be major differences between men and women in terms of response to strengthening and conditioning exercise. The types of muscle fibers utilized, the ability to metabolize fat,[46,175] and the physiologic responses to exercise in males and females are similar.[46,175] Although there are absolute differences in some of those physiologic variables (such as maximal oxygen uptake), the differences disappear when related to lean body weight.[10] What remains unclear are the effects of competitive athletics on the female reproductive, endocrinological and musculoskeletal systems. It is therefore important to address the medical issues relating specifically to the female athlete so that health providers can recognize problems early, provide education, and treat patients, with a view toward patients' continued athletic participation.

Osteoporosis, menstrual dysfunction, and eating disorders—what has been termed the female triad[179,180]—along with exercise during pregnancy are all entities that concern the athletic woman. There are also musculoskeletal and nutritional problems of the female athlete that may differ from those seen in their male counterparts.

Are there health concerns that accompany exercise training at the competitive level, and if so, are they irreversible, and/or can they be prevented? Is exercise beneficial for pregnant women, and are there any specific concerns with exercise during pregnancy? What effect does exogenous hormonal administration have on exercise and performance? What musculoskeletal problems are unique to the female athlete, and how can they be prevented? These are just some of the many questions to address, and exciting work in several areas is under way. This chapter outlines some of the special concerns of female athletes and how health care providers can identify them so that safe and enjoyable participation in sports can continue.

MENSTRUAL FUNCTION AND DYSFUNCTION

The menstrual cycle and the hormones that regulate it are commonly affected by exercise, although the exact mechanisms remain unclear. How the reproductive hormones affect exercise and performance is an issue that has been studied by many researchers. Menstrual dysfunction and amenorrhea occur more commonly in athletes than in the general population, and the mechanisms involved are becoming clearer. It is important that the health care provider be familiar with the normal menstrual cycle, the influence of the cycle on sports performance and potential injury, and the risks involved with menstrual dysfunction. It is also important to understand the potential risks and benefits of exogenous hormonal medications when prescribing them for the active woman.

Normal Menstrual Cycle

The normal menstrual cycle is regulated by hormones secreted from the hypothalamus, posterior pituitary, and ovary, and it depends on an intact female genital system. If there is normal anatomy, then function depends on the proper interplay of hormonal signals and feedback systems. Gonadotropin hormone–releasing hormone (GnRH) is released from the median eminence of the hypothalamus and acts on the anterior pituitary to produce follicle-stimulating hormone (FSH) and luteinizing hormone (LH). There are a follicular phase and a luteal phase in the menstrual cycle, demonstrated in Figure 1.

In the follicular phase, FSH stimulates the granulosa cells to produce estradiol, which in turn stimulates further growth of the follicle. A negative feedback eventually occurs at the level of the pituitary, and FSH production decreases. The dominant follicle is able to continue growing despite this, however, and a positive feedback system at the pituitary increases LH release during the mid to late follicular phase. Just before ovulation and during the late follicular phase, progesterone levels increase slightly, which in combination with estrogen causes an increase in the release of LH and FSH. Estradiol levels reach their peak (about 300 pg/ml), the LH surge occurs approximately 14 to 24 hours later, and ovulation occurs approximately 34 to 36 hours later.[43] Progesterone levels increase during the luteal phase and act on the granulaso cells producing the corpus luteum, which has a life span of approximately 14 days. The uterus prepares for potential implantation of a fertilized ovum, and if that does not take place, then endomentrial sloughing occurs, causing menstrual blood flow.

The normal cycle consists of 23 to 35 days, with 10 to 13 cycles per year; women with such a menstrual pattern are termed regular, or eumenorrheic. Oligomenorrhea means having 3 to 6 cycles per year at intervals of >36 days. "Amenorrhea is defined as

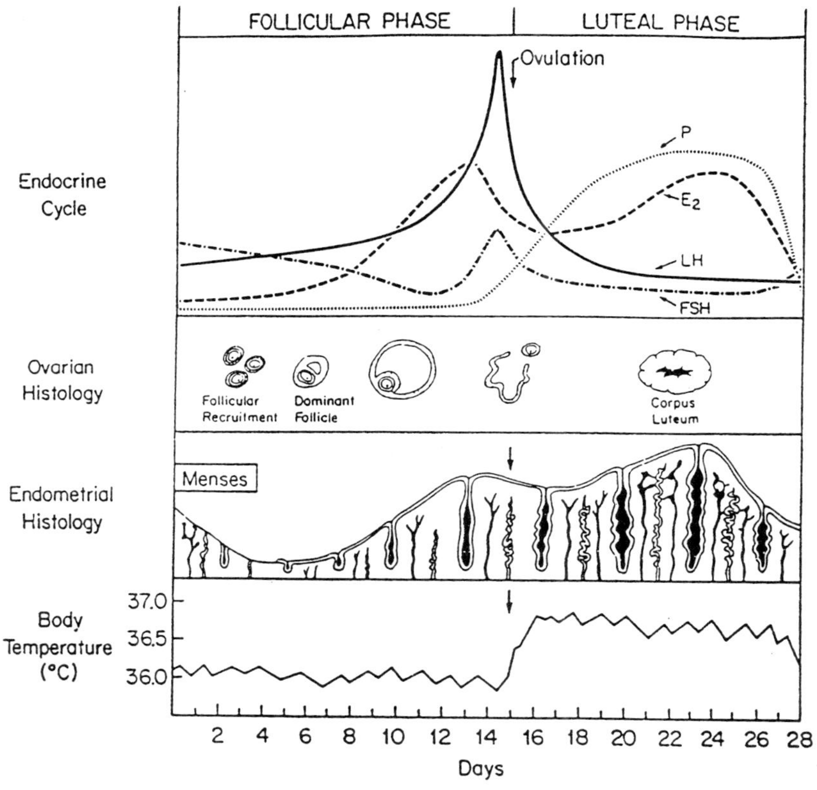

FIGURE 1. The hormonal, ovarian, endometrial, and basal body temperature changes and relationships throughout the normal menstrual cycle. (From Carr BR, Wilson JD: Disorders of the ovary and female reproductive tract. In Braunwald E, Isselbacher KJ, et al (eds): Harrison's Principles of Internal Medicine, 11th ed. New York, McGraw-Hill, 1987, pp 1818–1836, with permission.)

the absence or cessation of menstrual flow and is the clinical manifestation of a variety of disorders."[43] Primary amenorrhea is the absence of menarche by the age of 16; secondary amenorrhea is the absence of 3 to 12 consecutive menstrual periods after normal menarche has occurred. Physical training can cause many changes in the female athlete, including changes in body weight, body composition, energy utilization, and cardiovascular adaptations.

THE MENSTRUAL CYCLE AND ORAL CONTRACEPTIVES: EFFECT ON EXERCISE AND PERFORMANCE

There is much more to learn about the effects of the menstrual cycle on exercise and performance, as well as the effects of exercise on the reproductive and endocrinological systems. These areas are difficult to study and have only recently become more clearly elucidated.

In a recent review, Lebrun outlined the effects of the menstrual cycle on performance and the effects of oral contraceptives on performance.[92] In studies to date, no difference in performance was related to cycle phase in 37% to 63% of athletes, whereas an improvement was noted during menstruation in 13% to 29%. The worst performances were noted just prior to menses, and the best shortly afterward. Studies regarding individual physiologic responses during different phases of the cycle and regarding the effect of oral contraceptives have been somewhat conflicting. Briefly reviewing some of the information on the menstrual cycle's effects on various physiological parameters is helpful in understanding the effects on performance. Unfortunately, it is difficult to measure certain of the subjective changes noted during the menstrual cycle, and hormonal replacement, too, affect performance.

Performance

Some females believe their menses adversely affects performance,[8] but others feel that menses has no effect on performance.[54] Some studies have shown there may be a slight increase in performance during the luteal phase of the cycle, as measured by time to exhaustion[82,128] and increased VO_2 max.[143] Other studies have found no significant difference in performance variables.[38,42]

The effects of oral contraceptives on performance have not been conclusively researched, and it is difficult to compare studies because studies usually use different pill preparations and different caliber athletes from each other. No significant differences in performance were demonstrated with oral contraceptive use in some studies,[37,78] whereas more recent data suggest that low-dose oral contraceptive use may be associated with a decline in VO_2 max by as much as 5%-8%.[93,129] Women usually find that their molimenal symptoms such as cramps, bloating, nausea, vomiting, breast tenderness, and emotional lability are lessened when they are physically active compared to when they are inactive. In a recent prospective study of soccer players, those on oral contraceptives were found to have fewer injuries than those not on oral contraceptives.[118a] This was thought to be secondary to the decreased incidence of molimenal symptoms that oral contraceptives had on these women. Some of the effects of estrogen and progesterone are demonstrated in Table 1.

***TABLE 1.* Effects of Estrogen and Progesterone**

Estrogen	Progesterone
Promotes fat deposition in buttocks, breasts, thighs	Increases glandular elements in breast
Decreases cholesterol	Increases basal body temperature
Increases high-density lipoproteins	Increases exertional H_2O and Na loss from kidney
Increases capillary wall strength	Hyperventilation (luteal phase)
Increases glycogen storage in liver and muscle	Increases ventilatory drive
Glycogen sparing —> free fatty acid	

Adapted from LeBrun C: Effects of the phases of the menstrual cycle and oral contraceptives on athletic performance. Presented at Medical and Orthopedic Issues of Active and Athletic Women, April 30, 1993, Penn State University.

Cardiovascular System

The effects of the menstrual cycle on the cardiovascular system have been assessed by many authors. Several variables have been addressed, including hemoglobin, heart rate, free fatty acids, oxygen uptake (VO_2), ventilation, and respiratory exchange ratio. When the stage of the cycle has been documented by basal body temperature measurements or direct hormone levels, the data have been conflicting. One of the well-known reponses to endurance training is an increase in plasma volume, with a concomitant but lesser increase in red blood cell volume resulting in a pseudoanemia based on dilution. This may represent an adaptation that occurs in order to promote the movement of blood through the vasculature. Both hemoglobin and hematocrit levels were lower during the luteal phase in some studies,[42,167] whereas in others, no significant difference was noted.[94]

Some authors have noted an increase in heart rate during the luteal phase,[74,135] whereas others have, again, noted no significant difference.[38,77,94] The studies by DeSouza et al.,[38] Dombovy, et al.,[42] and Nicklas et al.[128] are also consistent in demonstrating no significant difference in the ratings of either perceived exertion or oxygen uptake during different phases of the menstrual cycle. DeSouza et al.,[38] Dombovy et al.,[42] Horvath and Drinkwater,[77] and Lebrun[94] did not show any significant difference in ventilation. Therefore, although the information is mixed regarding the cardiovascular reponses during the menstrual phase, there does not appear to be much effect on performance. Hoveath and Drinkwater did find an increase in the VO_2 during the luteal phase of the cycle at rest, but that difference disappeared with exercise.[77]

The data regarding the effects of menstrual function on cardiovascular response with oral contraceptive medications have been similarly equivocal. Although there is evidence that cardiac index, pulmonary distensibility, heart rate, and blood pressure do not vary in women taking an estrogen-progestin combined pill compared to a progestin-only pill or placebo, there does appear to be greater cardiac output with the combined pill compared to the progestin-only pill, and with both pill formulations compared to placebo.[99] Higher blood volume, stroke volume, and cardiac output were also demonstrated in women taking lynestrenol- and mestranol-containing contraceptives.[96] If an increase in cardiac output occurs, along with an increase in blood volume, then theoretically, one might see an improvement in performance. In addition, with oral contraceptive use there may be a decrease in menstrual flow and thus a decrease in the loss of iron, which together with increased cardiac output might increase performance.

Ventilatory Response

The ventilatory response changes that occur with the menstrual cycle and with oral contraceptive administration appear to be related to progesterone, although estrogen may have an enhancing effect. Progesterone appears to increase the ventilatory response seen during the luteal phase; the same response has been found in studies of men given medroxyprogesterone.[11,42,154] Increased sensitivity to both hypoxia and hypercarbia during the luteal phase has also been demonstrated.[42,154] Progesterone levels do not correlate with the changes seen and there appears to be no effect on performance variables. In recent studies of oral contraceptive use, there do not appear to be any changes in ventilation, despite a small decrement in VO_2 max.[94]

Strength Changes

There do not appear to be any strength gains during various phases of the menstrual cycle.[39,75,140] Some earlier studies have shown a decrease in strength during the luteal phase of the cycle.[132,176] A recent prospective study by Lebrun et al.[94] looking at isokinetic knee extension and flexion strength did not show any difference between the luteal and follicular phases. Although the data are limited, oral contraceptives do not seem to alter strength either.[93,132]

Thermoregulatory Changes

The relationship of thermoregulation and the menstrual cycle is another variable that has been addressed by several researchers, and again the result are conflicting. Some studies have shown no changes in heat stress response during different parts of the menstrual cycle.[22,135,170] Others have demonstrated core temperature increases both preexercise and postexercise during the luteal phase, as well as a decrease in exercise performance related to altered thermoregulation.[73,74] There have been few data about the effect of oral contraceptives on heat stress responses.

Metabolic Changes

Metabolic changes that occur during the menstrual cycle and with use of the oral contraceptive pill are somewhat clearer. Estradiol alters resting metabolism by increasing triglyceride (TG) synthesis and HDL_2 levels, by increasing lipolysis in fat and muscle tissue, and by inhibiting gluconeogenesis and glycogenolysis.[19] During exercise, estrogen again appears to spare glycogen and favor lipid metabolism.[68] Estradiol has also been studied during different phases of the menstrual cycle, and it appears that during the luteal phase, glycogen sparing occurs secondarily to lower lactate production.[82] Progesterone also acts to increase the uptake of glucose into both liver and muscle.[110,166] Oral contraceptives have a negative effect on both cholesterol and the blood lipid profile, but may have a positive effect on glucose utilization during high-intensity endurance exercise.[9]

THE FEMALE TRIAD

The number of females involved in competitive athletics has increased dramatically in the past 50 years, and with that expanded interest has come a broader understanding of the effects of training on the female athlete. Although exercise has had a profoundly positive effect on many exercising girls and women, certain medical concerns have surfaced. Eating disorders and menstrual dysfunction have been shown to occur with increased frequency in female athletes. Together with osteoporosis, they have become known as the female triad.[179,180] So much more needs to be researched in this area because of concerns that menstrual dysfunction and eating disorders can lead to hypoestrogenism and, concomitantly, to a decrease in bone mineral density that can engender increased risk for both stress fractures and osteoporosis. There is a great need for education at all levels of involvement so that those problems can be identified and treated early on. As our understanding of these complex areas grows, we shall become better able to offer treatment guidelines and recommendations that will ensure healthy and enjoyable sports participation by the female athlete

Osteoporosis

The first component of the female triad is osteoporosis, a major cause of morbidity and mortality in the United States. Bone is a dynamic tissue undergoing constant formation and remodeling and is essential to maintenance of calcium homeostasis. It is composed of both trabecular and cortical components, with varying amounts of each found in different sites throughout the body. Trabecular bone is found in the spine, the pelvis, and the ends of long bones and flat bones, and it is more metabolically active than cortical bone. Cortical bone is found in the shafts of long bones and composes two-thirds of the skeleton. There are different methods for measuring bone density, and these are compared in Table 2.

Osteoporosis consists of a decrease in bone mass and tensile strength that leads to microarchitectural deterioration and carries with it the increased risk of skeletal fragility and fracture. Osteoporosis causes more than 1.3 million fractures per year at an annual cost of $6 billion in the United States. In many individuals it represents the final straw that ends independent living, with 20% of those suffering a hip fracture dying within a year.[64] In postmenopausal women, 40% suffer at least one osteoporotic fracture, highlighting the concern for identification of risk factors.[34] Risk factors that have been identified are shown in Table 3.

Establishing adequate calcium intake—especially in childhood and young adulthood, when peak bone mass forms—is crucial, as is the maintenance of normal estrogen levels. Other risk factors include sedentary lifestyle and decreased bone mineral content. In a recent study of twins, tobacco use was demonstrated to lower bone density and thus would also be expected to increase the risk for osteoporosis.[76]

Exercise and estrogen therapy both have been shown to prevent bone loss in postmenopausal women.[15,16,21,24,52,163] Thus the primary prevention of osteoporosis consists in maximizing attainment of peak bone mass, which in turn is dependent on adequate Ca++ intake in childhood and early adulthood, as well as on exercise, although too much of the latter may be detrimental if it leads to amenorrhea or is associated with anorexia nervosa. Secondary prevention consists in estrogen therapy,[53] although other treatment protocols including calcium, calcitonin, and fluoride are currently under investigation.

Menstrual Dysfunction

Estrogen plays an important role in many different systems, some of which are listed in Table 4. Without the presence of estrogen, there may be increased risk for coronary artery disease, diabetes mellitus, hypertension, embolic disease, stroke, and cancer along with the aforementioned stress fractures and osteoporosis. It has been demonstrated that amenorrheic track runners have a higher low-density lipoprotein cholesterol (LDLC) than either regularly menstruating runners and regularly menstruating sedentary controls,[84] and therefore the absence of normal menstrual function may negate the positive effects of exercise on the lipid profile.

Understanding some of the acute and chronic responses to exercise can help health care providers appreciate how exercise can alter the menstrual cycle and lead to menstrual dysfunction. The mechanism of menstrual dysfunction often plays a crucial role in treatment decisions. Although the variables that lead to menstrual dysfunction are complex and often interactive, a look at each of them can be helpful in determining the best plan of action. The variables that have been identified include exercise-related changes in stress and sex hormones; nutrition; body composition; and energy drain.

In chronic exercise, many positive gains have been seen in body composition, cardiovascular fitness, strength, and modification of some of the risk factors leading to coronary artery disease, hypertension, and diabetes mellitus. However, there is also a concern that if increased exercise results in altered menstrual function, then there may be some negative effects as well that may have long-term health

TABLE 2. Comparison of Bone Density Measurement Methods

Technique	Site	Radiation Exposure	Cost
Single-photon absorptiometry (SPA)	Radius (integral bone)	10 rads	$60–$100
Dual-photon Absorptiometry (DPA)	Spine/hip (trabecular)	100 rads	$125–$150
Quantitative computed tomography scanning	Spine/hip(integral and trabecular)	1,000 rads	$250–$350
Dual-energy x-ray absorptiometry (DEXA)	Spine/hip/total BMD* (integral)	3 rads	$75–$100

*BMD=bone mineral density
Adapted from Pearl AJ (ed): The female athlete. Champaign, IL, Human Kinetics, 1993.

TABLE 3. Osteoporosis: Risk Factors

Female sex	Decreased bone mineral density
Asian or Caucasian race	Prolonged corticosteroid use
Age	Decreased calcium
Sedentary lifestyle	Estrogen deficiency
Thinness	
Tobacco use	

consequences. Although the exact mechanism is unclear, both delayed puberty[58,104,168] and estrogen-deficient states have been demonstrated in athletes.

Acute exercise causes increases in estradiol (follicular and luteal phases), progesterone (luteal phase), testosterone, prolactin, catecholamines, and cortisol.[14,41,106] There are also increases in B-endorphin and B-lipotropin levels.[19,70] With long-term exercise training other changes can occur. It has been demonstrated that athletes have a reduction in the frequency and amplitude of the LH surge[33] and that such decrease in the LH surge may represent the first abnormality of menstrual function that occurs.[157] Naloxone, an opiate antagonist, has been shown to restore the normal LH surge and amplitude in some amenorrheic athletes.[111] In another study, Veldhuis showed that there was a decrease of LH pulses in amenorrheic runners, which responded normally to exogenous GnRH stimulation.[166a] This would suggest that the dysfunction is at the level of the hypothalamus and not at the pituitary secretory level. Some researchers have felt that the changes in temperature that occur with exercise might affect GnRH release, thereby causing exercise-associated menstrual dysfunction.[67]

In 1974, the idea was proposed that a minimum body fat of 17% was necessary in order to initiate menarche and that below 22%, menarche could not be maintained.[60] Although body fat is a factor, it has since been shown that it is not the only factor. Normal menstrual flow has been seen in athletes with body fats as low as 4%.[108]

Diet and nutrition also play an important role in normal menstrual function. A higher risk for amenorrhea has been shown in diets low in protein, fat, or calories.[137,155] Marcus et al. found that in elite runners, 50% of amenorrheic versus 40% of normally cycling runners were getting less than two-thirds of the recommended daily allowance for Ca++.[108] Iron and protein consumption were also lower among the amenorrheic versus eumenorrheic runners.

TABLE 4. Effects of Estrogen on Various Body Systems

System	Effects
Endocrinological system	Alters glucose metabolism and adiopose metabolism
Hematological system	Alters fibrinolytic activity
Cholesterol metabolism	Increases triglycerides, HDL_2; enhances lipolysis in muscle and adipose tissues
Bone	Promotes osteoblastic activity
Reproductive system	Necessary for ovulation
Immune system	Modulates cell function

The age of menarche is delayed in athletes,[104,168] and Frisch et al. found that an average 2.3-year delay in menarche occurred in girls who were involved in vigorous activity, with each year of training causing a delay of 0.4 year.[58] What comes first in this situation is often difficult to determine: does delayed menarche offer an advantage to a young girl participating in gymnastics or endurance running, or do such activities in and of themselves cause a delay in menarche? Many factors interact, affecting the menstrual cycle, and with time the puzzles they present are being slowly put together.

The incidence of menstrual irregularity in athletes and in the general population has differed depending on the study. Most studies have shown that menstrual irregularities and amenorrhea are more common in athletic women compared to their sedentary counterparts. The incidence of amenorrhea in the general population has been reported as 2% to 5%[102] compared to 3.4% to 66% in athletic women.[13,103] Three main subsets of menstrual dysfunction are seen in response to training: luteal-phase deficiency, anovulation,[138] and exercise-associated amenorrhea.

Luteal-phase Deficiency. Luteal-phase deficiency consists in a shortening of the luteal phase, which is associated with decreased levels of progesterone. Studies on swimmers and runners have documented abnormal FSH:LH ratios consistent with luteal-phase shortening and progesterone deficiency.[12,59,155] Menstrual cycle length and pattern remain unchanged, and therefore these individuals may be unaware of any dysfunction. Luteal-phase deficiency has been related to decreased bone density[137] and infertility[158] and therefore has important clinical significance.

Anovulation. In anovulatory individuals, estrogen is present without progesterone, and cycles are irregular. Cycle length can be as short as 21 days or as long as 35 to 150 days between menstruations.[137] The main concern in this situation is unopposed estrogen, which can increase the risks for endomentrial hyperplasia, adenocarcinoma, and breast cancer.[65,172] Anovulation has many causes, and it prompts further evaluation and treatment.

Exercise-associated Amenorrhea. Exercise-associated amenorrhea (EAA) is a diagnosis of exclusion, but remains the most frequent cause of amenorrhea in athletes. Its causes are multifactorial, and it appears that an alteration at the hypothalamic-pituitary level is the common pathway leading to menstrual dysfunction. EAA is not limited to a specific sport, even though much of the information has been reported among ballet dancers. Factors that seem to play a role in the development of EAA include nutrition, changes in body composition, exercise-induced changes in hormones, stress, amount of training and training intensity, and reproductive immaturity (nulliparity, delayed menarche, and oligomenorrhea).[131,172]

Amenorrheic athletes have a lower bone mineral density than their eumenorrheic counterparts, and this is felt to be secondary to the low-to-absent levels of estrogen present in amenorrheics.[21,48,108] The low bone density seen in amenorrhea is a risk factor for premature osteoporosis and stress fractures. Other features of hypoestrogenic states include atrophic vaginitis and hot flashes. The absence or diminished levels of estrogen may lessen some of the protective effects estrogen confers and may increase the risk for other disorders. Lamon-Fava et al. demonstrated that amenorrheic runners lose the improvements in lipid profiles seen with exercise compared to their eumenorrheic counterparts.[90] Menstrual dysfunction also carries with it an increased risk for infertility.[159]

Bone formation is enhanced by exercise,[35,36,106,109,162] and weight-bearing exercise is better than non-weight-bearing exercise in this regard.[172] However, if amenorrhea results, then the benefits may be lost. In 1984, Cann et al. demonstrated a 22% to 29% decrease in spinal bone mineral density(BMD) in amenorrheic women compared to age-matched eumenorrheic controls.[21] The bone loss was greater in individuals who had been amenorrheic for longer than 2 years compared to those amenorrheic for less than 1 year. Low levels of estrogen were uniformly decreased in the amenorrheic women.

These findings were confirmed by Drinkwater et al. in runners, whose study found that vertebral BMD estradiol levels, and peak progesterone levels in amenorrheic runners were significantly lower than the levels seen in eumenorrheic runners.[48] There was no correlation between estradiol levels and BMD, and there was no difference between groups in terms of calcium intake, percentage of body fat, age at menarche, number of years of training, or frequency and duration of training. In a follow-up study, Drinkwater et al. retested 9 of the 14 amenorrheic runners, 7 of whom had spontaneously regained their menses.[49] The 7 who regained their menses had a significant, 6.2%, increase in BMD over 14.4 months. whereas the 2 who remained amenorrheic had a further decrease in BMD. The BMD of both groups still remained lower than that of the eumenorrheics. The women who regained their menses had increased their body weight by 1.9 kg and decreased their training levels by 10%; in addition, their estrogen levels had normalized.

In a later study by Drinkwater et al. menstrual patterns were compared to bone density, and a linear relationship was found, with the highest BMD being present in those individuals with currently normal and historically normal cycles and the lowest BMD seen in those with a history of amenorrhea who were currently amenorrheic.[47] Athletes who had occasional irregularities in their menstrual cycle had a bone density 6% less than normal cyclers (1.18 g/cm^2), and runners always irregular had a bone density of 17% lower (1.05 g/cm^2). Thus, both the current menstrual status and the past history of menstrual abnormalities are important in terms of decreased BMD.

Stress fractures have been shown to occur at an increased rate in individuals with menstrual dysfunction compared with normal menstrual function. Myburgh et al. found that "in athletes with similar training habits, those with stress fractures are more likely to have low bone density, lower dietary calcium intake, current menstrual irregularity, and lower oral contraceptive use."[123] These findings have been confirmed.[83,97] In 1984, Lindberg et al. showed that amenorrheic runners had significantly lower BMD (both trabecular and cortical) than other runners, with effects more evident in trabecular bone.[98] Forty-nine percent of the amenorrheic runners had a history of stress fracture during the previous year compared to no stress fracture in the eumenorrheic runners or the nonathletic controls.

These studies demonstrate that menstrual dysfunction, in particular, amenorrhea, is associated with decreased BMD, which may carry with it an increased risk for stress fractures and osteoporosis later in life. Since peak bone density is attained early in life, it is important to recognize amenorrhea early so that proper intervention can be initiated. The natural history of EAA is unknown. Although the study by Drinkwater et al. revealed an initial 6.2% increase in the bone density of amenorrheic runners who spontaneously regained their menses, the following year the increase in bone density dropped to 3% and remained unchanged for the 2 years following.[49] After 4 years, these individuals had a BMD that remained significantly lower than that of the eumenorrheic controls. Therefore, although some of the effects on bone marrow density are reversible, the extent and time frame of reversal remain unclear.

Evaluation of Amenorrhea. Evaluation of amenorrhea should include a complete physical examination, including pelvic examination; determination of FSH, LH, and prolactin levels, and thyroid function tests. Pregnancy is the most common cause of amenorrhea, and in sexually active women it is important to obtain a pregnancy test. Additional testing may include roentgenographic studies—to assess bone age—and chromosomal analysis—if

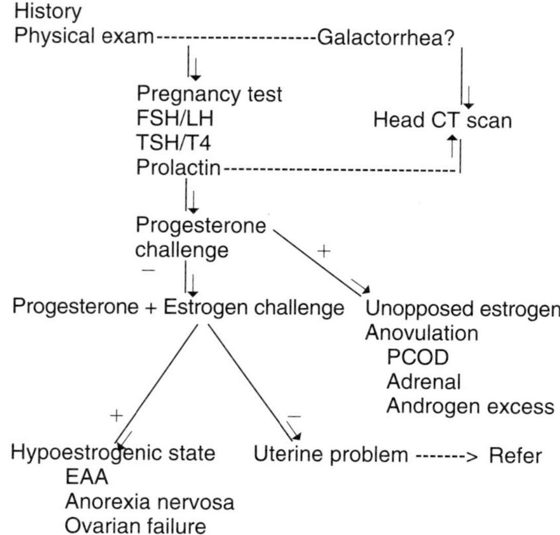

FIGURE 2. Algorithm for amenorrhea workup (+ = menstrual bleeding; − = no bleeding).

the possibility of Turner's syndrome is raised by history and/or physical examination. An algorithm for evaluation is presented in Figure 2. Although many different algorithms have been presented for evaluation of amenorrhea, it is important to individualize evaluation and treatment based on a patient's history and physical examination.

A progesterone challenge represents the next step in evaluation of amenorrhea and consists of medroxyprogesterone acetate given at a does of 5 to 10 mg per day for 7 to 10 days. If the uterus is under the influence of estrogen but lacks progesterone, then withdrawal bleeding will occur 3 to 4 days after completing this regimen. If no bleeding occurs, then both estrogen and progesterone are absent. This step is important to perform, because the risks of hypoestrogenism and the risks of unopposed estrogen are very different, and their treatments may be different.

If the progesterone challenge test produces bleeding, then only progesterone is lacking, and treatment consists of cyclical oral progesterone for 10 days at the end of the patient's cycle (or 10 days out of a month if the patient is amenorrheic). If the progesterone challenge test is negative, the practitioner can add 0.3 to 0.6 mg estrogen each day for 25 days—with progesterone added from day 14 to day 25—to learn whether functioning of the genital tract is intact. Different treatment options are available depending on whether contraception is an issue, whether the woman wants to become pregnant, and whether risk factors for hormonal treatment are present.

Treatment. Other disease processes need to be excluded before making the diagnosis of EAA. Once that diagnosis is made, treatment centers on trying to reestablish normal menses. Just as the etiology of EAA is multifactorial, so is the treatment plan. It includes decreasing the athlete's training intensity by roughly 10%; increasing the body weight or percentage of fat if it is low; ensuring adequate caloric intake, especially calcium, iron, and protein intake; and estrogen therapy.

This treatment plan is sometimes difficult for female athletes to accept. Few want to decrease their intensity of training, often considering amenorrhea as evidence that they are training adequately. Few want to gain weight. Even fewer are concerned about missing the monthly inconvenience and premenstrual symptoms that often accompany it. Therefore, trainers, coaches, parents, and athletes themselves must be educated so that they understand the health risks associated with menstrual dysfunction. Even if they cannot appreciate the long-term risks of osteoporosis that they may face prematurely, many are aware that stress fractures can cause the premature finish of an otherwise promising season.

The administration of estrogen makes sense from a theoretical standpoint, for there is no question that estrogen levels in menstrual dysfunction are diminished and that those low levels constitute the main risk for low bone density. What the optimal estrogen regimen is, however, remains unclear, but the absolute contraindications to systemic estrogen therapy are given in Table 5. Some investigators have preferred using cyclical estrogen for the first 25 days of the menstrual cycle along with progesterone added in the last 14 to 21 days; others recommend using oral contraceptives. Although the data conflict concerning estrogen replacement in individuals with hypoestrogenic states relative to bone density,[51,118] to date there has not been a good study examining the effect of estrogen replacement specifically with EAA.

Oral contraceptive pills (OCP) do not provide the same amount of estrogen as the amount used in a cycled regimen (that does not provide contraception), yet the ideal estrogen-progestin regimen that would allow optimal bone deposition remains unknown. From some of the studies in which OCP use appeared to be protective, one would infer that the estrogen

***TABLE 5.* Absolute Contraindications to Systemic Estrogen Therapy**

1. Unexplained vaginal bleeding	5. Breast cancer
2. Past history of cerebrovascular accident	6. Uterine cancer
3. Deep-vein thrombosis	7. Cervical cancer
4. Cardiac disease with right to left shunting	8. Active hepatic disease
	9. Pregnancy

Adapted from White CM, Hergenroeder AC: Amenorrhea, osteopenia, and the female athlete. Pediatr Clin North Am 37:1125–1141, 1990.

provided by OCP is adequate. Oral contraceptives allow for additional protection against pregnancy, which other regimens do not, and therefore may represent a reasonable regimen for the sexually active female. In addition, the side-effect profile and ease of administration usually make this regimen the one that athletes most easily and successfully adhere to. Although these issues still remain to be addressed, it seems prudent to offer some form of combined estrogen and progesterone therapy given the long-term risks of hypoestrogenism.

Eating Disorders

Eating disorders make up the third component of the female triad. Women account for 90% of those with eating disorders,[72] and therefore such disorders are a major concern for female athletes. As is the case with menstrual dysfunction, there is an increased risk for decreased bone mineral content in individuals with eating disorders, and therefore the concomitant increased risk for both stress fractures an osteoporosis. Eating disorders also carry with them a high morbidity and mortality.

Health care providers who work with the female population at large, and particularly those who deal with female athletes, need to be familiar with eating disorders. In addition, trainers, coaches, parents, and athletes themselves should be aware of the signs of disordered eating, methods to help identify and treat athletes, and the short- and long-term health consequences of these disorders.

Anorexia nervosa, bulimia nervosa, and eating disorders not otherwise specified make up the three subsets of eating disorders. These may be very different in their presentation, in the individual's willingness to receive treatment, and in their overall morbidity and mortality. The Diagnostic Statistical Manual IV Draft Criteria for these disorders are given in Table 6.

Individuals with eating disorders are often hard to separate from otherwise healthy athletes, and in fact the two groups may share some common features. Some of the features that athletes share with persons with eating disorders, and some of the features that can be used to help distinguish athletes from persons with eating disorders, are shown in Table 7.

Anorexia nervosa is a psychiatric syndrome consisting of severe weight loss by self-starvation due to distorted body image and the extreme desire to be thin. It is seen most commonly in the adolescent and young adult age groups. Anorectic individuals are very difficult to identify because of their denial and secretive behavior.

Those affected with bulimia nervosa share a similar desire for thinness, but their body weight is often at or above normal. Bulimia nervosa is characterized by recurrent bingeing eating episodes

TABLE 6. Criteria for Anorexia and Bulimia

Anorexia nervosa

A. Refusal to maintain normal body weight at or above a minimally normal weight for age and height (e.g., < 85% of that expected or failure to make expected weight loss leading to maintenance of body weight gain during period of growth, leading to body weight <85% of that expected).
B. Intense fear of gaining weight or becoming fat, even though underweight.
C. Disturbance about the way one's body weight or shape is experienced, undue influence of body weight or shape on self-evaluation, or denial of the seriousness of current, low body weight.
D. In postmenarchal females, amenorrhea, (i.e., the absence of at least three consecutive menstrual cycles). (A women is considered to have amenorrhea if her periods occur only following hormone [e.g., estrogen] administration.)

Specify type

Restricting type: During the espisode of anorexia nervosa, the individual does not regularly engage in binge-eating or purging behavior (i.e., self-induced vomiting or the misuse of laxatives or diuretics).
Binge-eating/purging type: During the episode of anorexia nervosa, the individual regulary engages in binge-eating or purging behavior (i.e., self-induced vomiting or the misuse of laxatives or diuretics).

Bulimia nervosa

A. Recurrent episodes of binge eating. An episode of binge eating is characterized by *both* of the following:
   1. Eating, in a discrete period of time (e.g., within any 2-hour period), an amount of food that is definitely larger than most people would eat during a similar period of time and under similar circumstances.
   2. A sense of lack of control over eating during the episode (i.e., a feeling that one can neither stop eating nor control what or how much one is eating).
B. Recurrent inappropriate compensatory behavior in order to prevent weight gain, such as self-induced vomiting; misuse of laxatives, diuretics, or other medications; fasting; and excessive exercise.
C. Binge-eating and inappropriate compensatory behaviors both occur, on average, at least twice a week for 3 months.
D. Self-evaluation is unduly influenced by body shape and weight.
E. The disturbance does not occur exclusively during periods of anorexia nervosa.

Specify type

Purging type: The individual regularly engages in self-induced vomiting or the misuse of laxatives or diuretics.
Nonpurging type: The individual uses other inappropriate compensatory behaviors, such as fasting or excessive exercise, but does not regularly engage in self-induced vomiting or the misuse of laxatives or diuretics.

Task Force on DSM-IV: DSM-IV Draft Criteria. Washington, DC, American Psychiatric Association, 1993, pp 1–2, with permission.

TABLE 7. Shared Features (Athlete and Anorectic)

Dietary faddism
Controlled caloric comsumption
Specific carbohydrate avoidance
Low body weight
Resting bradycardia and hypotension
Increased physical activity
Amenorrhea or oligomenorrhea
Anemia (may or may not be present)

Distinguishing features

Athlete

Purposeful training
Increased exercise tolerance
Good muscular development
Accurate body image
Body fat level within defined normal range
Increased plasma volume
Increased O_2 extraction from blood
Efficient energy metabolism
Increased HDL_2

Anorectic

Aimless physical activity
Poor or decreasing exercise performance
Poor muscular development
Flawed body image (believes oneself to be overweight)
Body fat below normal level
Electrolyte abnormalities if abusing laxatives and/or diurectics
Cold intolerance
Dry skin
Cardiac arrhythmias
Lanugo hair
Leukocyte Dysfunction

Adapted from McSherry JA: The diagnostic challange of anorexia nervosa. Am Fam Physican 29:144, 1984.

usually followed by purging behavior that includes self-induced vomiting, laxative use, or diuretic use. Weight fluctuations are very common, as is an awareness that one's eating behavior is abnormal. Bulimic individuals may be fearful of their inability to control their eating behaviors.

Eating disorders not otherwise specified (EDNOS) are characterized by individuals who are usually of average weight but who are preoccupied with body image, weight, and guilt surrounding eating. Individuals with EDNOS can be thought of as anorectic patients who are not amenorrheic and bulimic patients who do no binge.

The statistics for eating disorders are worrisome, especially in athletes, although the numbers reported in the general population may be underestimates. Anorexia occurs in 0.5% to 1.0%, bulimia in 2% to 5%,[71] and EDNOS in 3% to 5% of women aged 15–30. The rates among athletes are higher, ranging anywhere from 15% to 62% depending on the study.

Athletes are at increased risk for eating disorders, because many of the characteristics that describe the best athletes also describe those individuals at risk for eating disorders. Those characteristics include heightened body awareness, perfectionism, compulsiveness, and high achievement expectations. In addition, athletes are always trying to gain the extra edge in competition, and they will often go to extraordinary measures to reach the weights they feel will give them that performance advantage. Unfortunately, certain subtle messages given by parents, teammates, or even coaches can reinforce disordered eating behaviors.

Etiology of Eating Disorders. The origins of eating disorders are multifactorial and include social climate, family issues, biologic issues, response to victimization, identity issues, low self-esteem, and role conflicts. Certainly societal issues contribute to the development of disordered eating behaviors by normalizing many of these pathogenic behaviors and by prizing thinness. Persons with eating disorders often come from families whose members do not have good coping skills and in whom self-worth has been related to and centered on appearance.

Biological changes can occur as the result of severe dieting, and they may affect one's psychological and physiological cues for satiety. Approximately 20% to 35% of persons with eating disorders report a history of sexual abuse, and 67% of bulimics report being subjects of sexual and/or physical abuse. Unfortunately, many individuals with eating disorders do not feel good self-worth, and controlling their eating represents one of few areas in their lives that they believe they can feel good about. They may not be able to control how they are treated by others or what they accomplish in their lives, but they *can* control what they eat; therefore, for many of them, eating disorders are the desperate result of trying to gain control over some part of their lives.

Risks of Eating Disorders. The risks of eating disorders are numerous, and nutritional deficiencies are by far the rule. Deficient nutrition impairs both wound healing and the ability to fight infections. Long-term sequelae include infertility, electrolyte disturbances, gastrointestinal disease, psychiatric problems, decreased immune function, malnutrition, and decreased bone density. Fully 6% of anorexics will die from starvation, sepsis, cardiac arrhythmias, or suicide, with the latter accounting for most of the mortality.[72]

Identification. Identifying individuals with eating disorders can be very difficult and yet remains crucial to early institution of treatment. Because morbidity and mortality are significant, the earlier such individuals can be recognized, the more likely they are to recover successfully. Some of the features that can help identify athletes with eating disorders are given in Table 8. Although anorectic individuals are easy to spot because of their very low weights, they also have a strong amount of denial, which makes them difficult to approach. Bulimics,

TABLE 8. Signs of Disordered Eating

Repeatedly expressed concerns about feeling fat, even when weight is average or below average
Refusal to maintain the minimal normal weight consistent with height.
Preoccupation with food, calories, weight
Increasing self-criticism of one's weight
Consumption of huge amounts of food not consistent with weight
Secretly eating or stealing food
Eating large meals, then disappearing/make trips to the bathroom
Bloodshot eyes, especially after trips to the bathroom, swollen parotid glands at the jaw angle, giving chipmunklike appearance
Vomitus, or odor of vomitus, in sink, toilet, or shower
Foul breath, poor dental hygiene, frequent sore throats
Wide fluctuations of weight over short time spans
Excess use of diet pills, laxatives, diuretics
Periods of severe caloric restriction or repeated fasting
Relentless, excessive physical activity that is not part of the training regimen
Depressed mood and self-deprecating thoughts after eating
Avoidance of situations in which one may be observed while eating
Appearing preoccupied with the eating behavior of other people such as friends, relatives, and teammates
Mood swings, irritability, poor concentration, fatigue
Wearing baggy or layered clothing
Complaints of bloating or light-headedness that cannot be attributed to other medical causes

on the other hand, may be more willing to come forth with their problem, because they feel loss of control due to their bingeing and purging episodes and they reach out for help. Bulimic individuals, however, may not be suspected, because they are at or above their ideal body weight.

A trainer, coach, teammate, or parent who is concerned about an individual athlete should take the first step by discussing this openly with the athlete, in a nonconfrontational manner. Athletes should be assured that their position on the team is not threatened and that there exists genuine concern about their well-being and health. If the athlete has been identified by a teammate or roommate, such concern should be emphasized. Athletic participation can usually continue as long as the health of the athlete is not compromised and as long as there is no associated risk for significant injury with such continued participation.

Treatment. Once an eating-disordered individual has been identified, the treatment plan is multifaceted, tending to involve the physician, the psychology team, and the nutritionist. Although the nutritionist is often the first person consulted, this is probably where help is needed last. Eating is often *not* the problem but is a symptom of an underlying psychiatric problem. Treatment centers on psychotherapy, and although individuals may at first be wary of obtaining counseling, this step must be emphasized. Additional counseling with a sports psychologist or the physician can also be instrumental. Once the individual is starting to make progress, the nutritionist can be very helpful by further educating the athlete and helping to make good nutritional decision. Eating disorders remain difficult to treat, however, and are often very frustrating for the individual, the family, teammates, coaches, and anyone else involved. Treatment is lengthy, difficult, and, unfortunately, often unsuccessful, but because the consequences can be tragic, education and prevention are paramount.

The female triad is a new concept that is only recently starting to be written about.[139,180] There is exciting work currently under way and more that needs to be done to address the many questions that the triad's components raise. Is there a way to prevent the triad from occurring? What regimen should be universally applied to EAA to prevent bone loss? Is the bone loss seen in both amenorrhea and anorexia reversible? If so, is there a limited time frame to initiate therapy, as there seems to be in postmenopausal women? At what point in the diagnostic workup should bone densitometry be utilized?

EXERCISE AND PREGNANCY

Because more women have made exercise an important part of their everyday life, the issue of how exercise affects pregnancy has been readdressed. Pregnancy in the exercising female is a topic that has received both positive and negative attention. In 1985, the American College of Obstetricians and Gynecologists (ACOG) published guidelines for exercise during pregnancy,[1] but recent studies question whether the ACOG recommendations may be too conservative.[177] More recently, the recommendations by ACOG have been updated, and these are given in Table 9. For women who exercise regularly and, at times, at high levels, exercise recommendations during pregnancy may be very different from the ones given a sedentary woman who decides to start an exercise program after she becomes pregnant. This area of study is exciting, and thus far, the information appears to demonstrate that exercise during pregnancy is safe as well as beneficial to both the woman and the developing fetus as long as certain precautions are taken.

The risks and the benefits of exercise during pregnancy may well differ in women who are fit and who train at competitive levels prior to pregnancy compared to sedentary women, and therefore a complete history including an exercise history should be taken prior to pregnancy so as to better individualize rec-

TABLE 9. American College of Obstetricians and Gynecologists Guidelines for Exercise During Pregnancy and Postpartum

Exercise guidelines

There are no data on humans to indicate that pregnant women should limit exercise intensity and lower targeted heart rates because of potential adverse effects. For women who have no additional risk factors for adverse maternal or perinatal outcome, the following recommendations may be made.

1. During pregnancy, women can continue to exercise and derive health benefits even from mild-to-moderate exercise routines. Regular exercise (at least three times per week) is preferable to intermittent activity.
2. Women should avoid exercise in the supine position after the first trimester. Such a position is associated with decreased cardiac output in most pregnant women. Thus, because the remaining cardiac output will be preferentially distributed away from splanchnic beds (including away from the uterus) during vigorous exercise, such regimens are best avoided during pregnancy. Prolonged periods of motionless standing should also be avoided.
3. Women should be aware of the decreased oxygen available for aerobic exercise during pregnancy. They should also be encouraged to modify the intensity of their exercise according to maternal symptoms. Pregnant women should stop exercising once they are fatigued and should not exercise to exhaustion. Weight-bearing exercises may under some circumstances be continued throughout pregnancy at intensities similar to those prior to pregnancy. Non-weight-bearing exercises such as bicycling or swimming minimize the risk of injury and facilitate the continuation of exercise during pregnancy.
4. Morphologic changes in pregnancy should serve as a relative contraindication to types of exercise in which loss of balance could be detrimental to maternal or fetal well-being, especially in the third trimester. Further, any type of exercise involving the potential for even mild abdominal trauma should be avoided.
5. Pregnancy requires an additional 300 kcal per day in order to maintain metabolic homeostasis. Thus, women who exercise during pregnancy should be particularly careful to ensure an adequate diet.
6. Pregnant women who exercise in the first trimester should augment heat dissipation by attending to adequate hydration, wearing appropriate clothing, and ensuring optimal environmental surroundings during exercise.
7. Many of the physiologic and morphologic changes of pregnancy persist 4–6 weeks postpartum. Thus, prepregnancy exercise routines should be resumed gradually based on a woman's physical capability.

Contraindications to exercise

The foregoing recommendations are intended for women who have no additional risk factors for adverse maternal or perinatal outcome. A number of medical or obstetric conditions may lead the obstetrician to recommend modifications to those guidelines. The following conditions should be considered contraindications to exercise during pregnancy:

1. Pregnancy-induced hypertension
2. Preterm rupture of membranes
3. Preterm labor during the previous or current pregnancy or both
4. Incompetent cervix/cerclage
5. Persistant second- or third-trimester bleeding
6. Intrauterine growth retardation

In addition, women with certain other medical or obstetric conditions, including chronic hypertension or active thyroid, cardiac, vascular, or pulmonary disease, should be evaluated carefully in order to determine whether an exercise program is appropriate.

Adapted from ACOG Technical Bulletin, Exercise during pregnancy and the postpartum period. Number 189, February 1994.

ommendations. Most authors argue that a moderate amount of exercise can be beneficial during pregnancy, with few, if any, associated risks as long as precautions are observed. Certain situations in which exercise may place the woman or the fetus at unwarranted risk dictate that exercising should be limited. In considering a patient's exercise during pregnancy, the physician may find it helpful to assess both maternal risks and fetal risks, as well as potential benefits,[80,114,173] keeping in mind that such recommendations must always be individualized.

Changes with Pregnancy

Pregnancy causes increases in heart rate, stroke volume, and cardiac output. Pivarnik et al. demonstrated that women whose walking and running speeds are kept constant have a 10% increase in VO_2 during the course of pregnancy.[134] This increase may not be significant when body weight is taken into account. Pregnancy does not appear to affect maximal VO_2, although this may depend somewhat on the exercise modality. By neither cycle ergometry[149,150,151] or treadmill exercise[101] is VO_2 max affected, whereas in swimming ergometry,[112] VO_2 max decreases as pregnancy progresses.

Pregnancy causes a decrease in expiratory reserve volume and a decrease in functional reserve capacity. Vital capacity remains unchanged. Pregnancy increases tidal volume by 40% and oxygen consumption by 20%.[14] It affects the ventilatory response to exercise and has been examined at both submaximal and maximal exercise intensities. In both situations, pregnancy appears to increase the ventilatory response, possible due to a direct progesterone effect and an increased CO_2 sensitivity. The ventilation at maximal exercise is increased by 7% to 8% in both cycle ergometry and treadmill exercise.[101]

Pregnancy increases cardiac output due to an increase in both heart rate[101,113,121] and stroke volume,[133] with both of these variables increasing throughout the course of pregnancy. Stroke volume may play the greater role as pregnancy progresses, with an increase in plasma volume being the primary cause.

The stress response to exercise in the pregnant woman is not clearly understood, and research examining the effects of cortisol, catecholamines, prolactin, gulcagon, growth hormone, and insulin are under way.[114] The release of these substances in response to exercise may be altered during pregnancy, with a blunting of the overall stress response. Why and to what purpose these changes occur have not been fully elucidated.

Hyperthermia is a true concern for the exercising woman during pregnancy. Animal studies have demonstrated that an increase in core temperature can lead to an increase in fetal neural defects. The critical core temperature above which defects occur appears to 39°[87,153] Hydration, proper clothing, and adequate cooling mechanisms need to be addressed when exercising, and they are of prime importance during pregnancy.

Other changes that occur with pregnancy are related to anatomical alterations made to accommodate the fetus, and they include an increase in the lumbar lordosis, increased ligamentous laxity, and an increase in the anterior tilt of the pelvis.[144] The center of gravity moves upward and anteriorly, with the increase in lubar lordosis and rotation of the pelvis on the femur compensating for this. These changes often make exercise or other activities requiring balance more difficult. Neither is it uncommon for total body weight to increase by 15% to 25%,[4] which may increase the incidence of injury caused by the combined effect of increased load with altered biomechanics.

Swimming is an excellent form of exercise for the pregnant woman[86] and may also represent an exercise modality that is beneficial for keeping the core temperature from rising. There may be other benefits in that the supine position may allow for better blood flow to the fetus, and the woman does not experience the balance control problems of land exercise. In addition, the increase laxity that accompanies pregnancy may put the woman at more risk during land exercise compared to water exercise. Swimming may not be an available option for all women, but should be considered in the exercise prescription.

Risks of Exercise during Pregnancy

The fetal risks during pregnancy can be thought of as any increase in fetal stress, assessed by changes in fetal heart rate, amniotic fluid volume, fetal movements and breathing, and muscular tone. The most common and easiest screen for fetal distress is a change in fetal heart rate or biophysical profile. The range of normal fetal heart rates is approximately 120 to 160 beats per minute (bpm). Fetal tachycardia occurs if fetal heart rate is greater than 160 bpm for longer than 10 minutes, and fetal bradycardia occurs if fetal heart rate is less than 120 bpm for longer than 1 min.[115]

In a recent review by McMurray and VanDoorn,[115] the fetal heart rate increase in response to exercise averaged 10 to 30 bpm, with little alteration secondary to exercise intensity or length of gestation. Mild or moderate exercise caused an increase in fetal heart rate, which returned to normal within 15 minutes, whereas 30 minutes was required after strenuous exercise. Hauth et al. examined women by means of a nonstress test at 28 to 38 weeks of gestation who jogged 1.5 miles three time weekly prior to and during pregnancy. They found that there was no evidence of fetal distress with that regimen.[69] In another study of women swimming three times a week for 30 to 45 minutes, there was again no evidence of fetal distress produced by exercise.[44] These latter women were at 32 to 39 weeks of gestation, and although maternal heart rate reached 80% of their predicted maximum, increased fetal movement occurred but fetal heart rate averaged 149 beats per minute and no exercise-induced tachycardia or bradycardia was noted. These studies show that although maternal heart rate may increase with exercise, it may not unduly stress the fetus.

These is also concern that exercise may increase fetal risk by causing a relative hypoxemia. Exercise during the third trimester can cause a shunting of blood away from the uterus to increase blood flow to muscles, which in turn may lead to fetal hypoxemia.[2] There is some evidence that conditioning may blunt this response, which is felt to be due in part to an increase in catecholamine release.[122] Therefore, in a woman who is not conditioned, concern over hypoxia may be more valid than in a woman who is in good physical condition.

Concerns have also been raised about advocation of exercise during pregnancy in situation of different barometric pressures. Living at high altitude and activities such as mountain climbing or mountain skiing are examples of situations of decreased barometric pressure. At levels above 2,500 meters, an increase in the maternal ventilatory response to hypoxia occurs and may represent increased fetal risk.[119] It is important to consider other medical conditions that may alter a woman's ability to respond to environmental stresses. These include preeclampsia, anemia, and diabetes, and caution should be taken in consideration of exercise to be done at higher elevations by pregnant woman with theses problems.

Snorkeling and scuba diving are examples of activities that take place at increased barometric pressures. When divers rise from such high pressures during the return to atmospheric pressure, potential tissue damage can occur if the ascent occurs too quickly. This is often referred to as the bends and is felt to be secondary to nitrogen escape from cells. It is unclear how the bends affects the developing fetus, and current recommendations are to avoid scuba diving or snorkeling below the water's surface during pregnancy.

The effects of exercise on fetal growth appear to show that strenuous exercise may lead to delivery of infants that are 300 to 500 grams smaller and that maternal weight gain is less than in nonexercising pregnant women.[26–28] Whether the lower birth weight is detrimental to the health of either the mother or the newborn has not been elucidated. If a pregnant woman is involved in hard toil or prolonged standing or is nutritionally deficient, then strenuous exercise may have an increased negative effect on fetal growth.[165] The latter study also found that women who were physically active had a lower chance of delivering prematurely. These studies demonstrate that the relationship between exercise and fetal growth needs to be researched further.

The practice of exercise in gestation diabetes has been addressed and appears to offer a therapeutic option for diabetic individuals. Gestational diabetes occurs in 4% to 7% of normal pregnancies, and although diet and insulin therapy have been utilized, exercise has been studied as an alternative method for treating such women. Both diabetic and nondiabetic populations respond similarly to exercise during pregnancy.[5,6,18,81] The latter studies also demonstrated that carbohydrate tolerance is improved and the need for insulin is reduced when exercise is used therapeutically in gestational diabetics. As a side benefit, no adverse effects on the woman or the fetus were demonstrated in the exercise regimens used in these studies.

CONCLUSIONS

Exercise certainly has beneficial effects for women, and these transcend pregnancy. Certain precautions should be taken and recommendations should be individualized as the physician takes into account the level of fitness present in the patient prior to pregnancy. Various exercise modalities are available that can be a welcome part of the pregnancy process, enabling a woman to have an active pregnancy, enjoy the positive effects of exercise, and perhaps improve the well-being of the newborn. General well-being, control over weight gain during pregnancy, and increased exercise tolerance can all be the positive results of a well-designed exercise program. A complete history and physical exam, including an exercise history, should be performed to ensure a healthy pregnancy. As long as the two are utilized adequately, inclusion of an exercise program is likely to be safe and beneficial for most women.

NUTRITION

The general area of sports nutrition is covered in greater detail in a separate chapter, but the nutritional needs of the female athlete may be somewhat different from those of the male athlete. This stems not only from different nutritional concerns and maturational requirements but also from the perspective of total caloric intake. If total caloric intake is adequate, then nutritional intake usually is as well, with the possible exception of iron. Societal influences have made constant dieting commonplace for females, and athletes appear to be at an increased risk. Numerous studies have demonstrated the poor eating behavior of athletes in general, and specifically of female athletes. The main issues to consider in the female athlete include total general caloric intake and specific intake of protein, fat, calcium, and iron.

In order to sustain optimal athletic performance, both adequate caloric intake and optimal nutritional intake are necessary. Ideally, individuals should consist of 6 to 10 grams of carbohydrate per kg body weight,[32] 0.8 to 1.5 grams of protein/kg,[57] and the rest of the calories from fat. This usually translates to a diet made of 60% to 70% carbohydrate, 10% to 15% protein, and 25% to 30% fat. More recent recommendations have increased the protein intake to 20% to 25% and decreased the fat intake to 10% to 15%. "Theoretically, women who eat more than 1200–1500 calories from a variety of wholesome foods can obtain most nutrients necessary for top athletic performance (with the possible exception of iron)."[30] Therefore, when making recommendations to athletes, practitioners should emphasize that proper food selection, and not supplementation, constitutes the ideal form of nutrition.

Iron Deficiency and Anemia

Iron deficiency in adolescent athletes has been examined and reviewed.[7,141,145,169] Although anemia may not be present, iron deficiency or decreased iron stores can be present in as many as 9.5% to 57% of young athletes depending on the study.[125,126,142,147,156] Increases in plasma volume also occur, ranging from 6% to 25%.[7] Female athletes are at increased risk for iron deficiency,[31] and decreases in ferritin levels during training have also been demonstrated.[40,142,146] Girls, more so than boys, have been shown to take in significantly less than the 18 mg per day recommended daily allowance (RDA).[56,125,127,148] The etiology of iron deficiency anemia in the athlete can be due to different mechanisms, and a systematic approach should be taken. There may be increased loss of iron due to hemolysis with hemoglobinuria,[125,161] gastrointestinal losses,[164] and loss of iron through excessive sweating.[17] Female athletes are at increased risk of iron deficiency due also to the increased iron loss that occurs with menses. Correction of anemia has been shown to improve performance.[62,130,147] Therapy of iron deficiency should include instruction on intake of iron-rich foods along with vitamin C and supplementation if necessary as an adjunct.

Calcium Intake

Inadequate calcium intake is also common in female athletes, and this is of particular concern given the risks of the female triad discussed earlier and the importance of calcium in bone density acquisition. Various studies have demonstrated that female athletes take in less than two-thirds of the RDA of calcium as follows: 40% of gymnast,[100] 51% of cross-country runners,[85] and 42% of ballet dancers.[50] Since peak bone mass is met early in life, adequate calcium intake throughout life, but especially during early childhood and adolescence, is essential to ensure bone health. The young athlete should be given to understand the importance of consuming adequate calcium.

Fat and Total Caloric Intake

Total caloric intake is a concern for the female athlete, and again, several studies have demonstrated that many athletes do not consume adequate calories to meet their physical need.[50,100] Because of the societal pressure to be thin, there are special demands on female athletes that often lead them to exercise excessively, yet also to continue to restrict their intake. Many athletes feel they can eat only if they have exercised, and they often underestimate what their caloric intake should be. In addition, in their misguided attempt to eat healthily, athletes may restrict fat intake such that the fat-soluble vitamins are also at risk for being deficient. Potential risks inherent in consuming a diet that contains less than 10% fat include low energy intake and low levels of protein, iron, zinc, and vitamin E. Deficiencies have also been noted of zinc, magnesium, folate, and vitamin B_6,[50,100] as well as of vitamins C,A, and B_{12}.[100] How these deficiencies affect performance or injury remains to be more clearly discerned.

MUSCULOSKELETAL ISSUES

In a consideration of the athletic woman, it is easy to recognize that menstrual dysfunction, eating disorders, and pregnancy are issues specifically important to evaluate. In recent years, along with the great advancements in training regimens and fitness levels, as well as the opportunities for girls and women to excel in sport, has come the understanding that certain musculoskeletal conditions pertain to the female athlete. No longer can such problems be attributed to inferior training or fitness. Certain musculoskeletal conditions are simply more common in women; for instance, the increased incidence of anterior cruciate injuries seen in women is worrisome. It is important that practitioners assess the female athlete's flexibility, ligamentous laxity, and sport-specific risks for injury and offer preventive rehabilitation to preclude injuries and improve athletic performance if possible.

Women have the same ability to gain strength and endurance of the musculoskeletal system as men do, although the absolute increase in muscle size is lower in women. When lean body mass is taken into account, women show the same strength gains in response to training.[105] Strength training can increase the ability of muscles, bones, ligaments, and musculotendinous connections to withstand stress, and it can increase power and endurance. An organized, supervised, and sport-specific strengthening program is safe and can optimize performance as well as help avoid associated injury.

There are musculoskeletal differences between the male and female bony pelvis, and these can be related to specific disorders. Women tend to have a wider pelvis, femoral neck anteversion, and varus at the hip and valgus at the knee. There is often compensatory external rotation of the tibial tubercle with pronation at the hindfoot.[152] This may lead to an increased Q angle—which is the angle formed by the intersection of a line drawn down the femoral shaft and a line drawn from the center of the patella to the tibial tubercle. The center of gravity in female athletes is also lower than in males: at 56.1% of height compared to 56.7%, respectively. This is believed to be secondary to the greater lower extremity length of men compared to women: 56% of height compared to 51.2%, respectively.[88]

CLINICAL PROBLEMS

Certain clinical problems appear more commonly in the female than in the male athlete; they include iliotibial friction syndrome, patellofemoral dysfunction, reflex sympathetic dystrophy, greater trochanteric bursitis, and, possibly, ankle and anterior cruciate ligament sprains.[25] Whether the foregoing clinical problems arise from differences between male and female biomechanics and musculoskeletal differences or whether there may be muscle imbalances or differences in the biomechanics of their jumping or running remains unclear. It will be very helpful to continue studies addressing the increased incidence of certain injuries in the female population. It may also be instructive to repeat past studies because as girls begin sports participation at a younger age and as the athleticism of young women increases, we are seeing differences in the kinds of injuries that occur.

Patellofemoral Dysfunction

An increased Q angle, when accompanied by genu recurvatum and genu valgum, can potentiate patellofemoral dysfunction (PFD), which can be thought of generally as a patellar tracking problem. PFD characteristically causes anterior knee pain, made worse with climbing or descending stairs or with sitting for a prolonged period of time. Individuals with PFD often have deficient vastus medialis obliquus musculature and/or tight vastus lateralis musculature, which, combined, can cause an abnormal tracking pattern of the patella. Assessing the orientation of the patella, both statically and with motion, is also very important in a determination of the biomechanics surrounding the patellofemoral joint. It is important to assess for the presence of an effusion, for the presence of a grade 2 effusion in the knee can adversely affect the strength of the quad complex by as much as 10% to 40% as measured by Cybex.[178] The presence of an effusion should expand the differential diagnosis to include meniscal lesions, ligamentious injury, articular surface defects, and osteochondral defects.

Strengthening of the vastus medialis obliquus (VMO) is one of the main treatment goals for PFD. Various taping techniques have been formulated to allow the patella to track more normally and to facilitate strengthening exercised for the VMO. Closed-chain kinetic exercises such as partial squats are excellent rehabilitative exercises. An individual can usually be partially unweighted by way of a harness attached by a pulley system to a weight. As the strengthening of the patellofemoral complex progresses, the individual can progress until able to lift one's own body weight and finally advance activity. Open-chain kinetic exercises such as knee extensions on a machine have lost favor because they are not sport-specific, but they may play a role in sports such as soccer and karate, which utilize open-chain activities.

Trochanteric Bursitis

Trochanteric bursitis is another common musculoskeletal problem faced by the female athlete. It may be secondary to the varus present at the hip, femoral neck anteversion, and tight iliotibial band (ITB) structures. In most situations, tight lateral structures compress the bursa and often irritate it with repetitive sliding over the greater trochanter. Occasionally, this can also be a cause of snapping hip, which is not usually associated with significant pain, and is explained by the ITB's repetitively crossing over the greater trochanter. In trochanteric bursitis, there is pain with passive as well as active leg abduction, but usually no pain with resisted abduction with the legs at neutral (unless there is concomitant tendinitis or a strain). Treatment with conservative measures such as oral nonsteroidal anti-inflammatory drugs, ice massage, ITB stretching, and, occasionally, phonophoresis or iontophoresis is usually sufficient, along with consideration of biomechanical and training pattern alterations. If this regimen is not successful, steroid injection into the bursa may be of benefit.

Some studies have shown that muscle imbalances in female athletes may put them at increased risk for injury. This may be of particular concern in sports that have a high incidence of lower extremity injuries. Knapik et al. found a higher incidence of lower extremity injuries in female collegiate athletes if there was also an imbalance in the athletes' muscle strength and flexibility. At 180° per second, a knee flexor/extensor ratio <0.75 was also associated with a higher incidence of injury.[89]

Anterior Cruciate Injuries

A disturbingly high number of anterior cruciate ligament (ACL) injuries have been occurring in athletic women.[181] In the National Collegiate Athletic Association (NCAA), for almost every sport there are more ACL injuries in women than men.[124] A 2-year study of NCAA athletes analyzed knee injuries in male and female soccer and basketball players. The data are summarized in Table 10 and demonstrates for both basketball and soccer play a significantly higher ACL injury rate in women compared to their male counterparts. The female basketball players had an ACL injury rate six times higher than the men's (0.3 vs 0.05); female soccer players had an ACL injury rate more than twice as high as the men's (0.29 vs 0.14). The 4-year data have not yet been reviewed, but they appear to follow the same trend. (personal communication, Elizabeth Arendt, Randall Dick). These statistics are alarming given the increased number of female participants, especially in these two sports.

Early beliefs held that women were less developed than men, thus constituting the sole reason for increased injuries. However, Ireland and Wall compared Olympic-caliber men and women basketball players and found that a higher incidence of injuries in the women compared to the men (53% vs. 13%, $p<0.0001$).[79] In addition, the severity of the injuries

TABLE 10. Knee Injuries in Collegiate Basketball and Soccer Athletes

Basketball (>400,000 A-E* for men and women)	Men	Women
Knee injuries (% all injuries)	12%	19%
Knee injuries requiring surgery (% all injuries)	20%	39%
Knee injury rate (per 1,000 A-E)	0.7	1.0
ACL injury rate (per 1,000) A-E)	0.05	0.3*
Soccer (>180,000 A-E for men and women)	**Men**	**Women**
Knee injuries (% all injuries)	16%	18%
Knee injuries requiring surgery (% all injuries)	15%	22%
Knee injury rate (per 1,000 A-E)	1.3	1.3
ACL injury rate (per 1,000 A-E)	0.14	0.29*

*ACL = anterior cruciate ligament; A-E = Ahtlete-exposure (defined as an athlete's participation in a practice or game).
**Significantly greater than M value ($p<0.05$).

and the need for surgery were also higher in women compared to men. These female athletes were elite, and thus one assumed they had good muscular development. Other theories explaining the increased incidence of ACL injury among females include muscle imbalances, trochlear groove size or configuration, biomechanical differences in jumping and landing technique, and malalignment differences. This area of research is very important, and it is hoped that preventive measures can be taken to decrease these often devastating injuries.

Upper Extremity Injuries

Upper extremity injuries do not differ significantly between male and female athletes, and they are less common than lower extremity injuries in both.[29,66,174] Despite the increase in sports participation by women and the increase in women's intensity of participation, there has not been an increase in the number of serious injuries that occur.[66] This may be explained by the growth of strengthening and conditioning programs and improved coaching and athletic trainer coverage that have accompanied those increases.[13]

PREVENTION

Practitioners must emphasize to athletes that the strengthening and conditioning program is essential in prevention of associated injuries and improvement of performance. Although it is difficult to substantiate with well-controlled studies, it seems hard to ignore that the better conditioned athletes are, the less likely they will get injured. Conditioning consists not only of aerobic and anaerobic conditioning but also of strengthening and flexibility training. The preparticipation examination is a good time to address strength deficits or imbalances, as well to create a sport-specific training program that can identify areas of specific concern. For example, in soccer, assessment of leg alignment and foot biomechanics and the athlete's participation in a strengthening program for the abdominals, back, knee, and ankle musculature can help prevent injuries. A conditioning program that emphasizes discontinuous running and sprints, along with endurance training, is beneficial for that soccer player, but may not be useful for a softball player. Many sport-specific drills can be devised that foster both the strengthening and conditioning of the athlete and that make them enjoyable. A program should be designed specifically for an individual and the sport the individual is involved in, and the physician can work closely with the coach and trainer to so identify it.

SUMMARY

It has been demonstrated that female athletes have a better and more positive body image than female nonathletes.[23] And exercise is important not only for general health, positive lifestyle behaviors, and positive self-image but also in the learning of such skills as goal setting, teamwork, commitment, and self-reliance. These skills are hard to master, and sport allows the young individual to learn them in a game situation. All of what young girls can glean from sport, however, should not overshadow problems that can prevent participation. The medical problems that a young female athlete may be at particular risk for such as poor nutrition, eating disorders, and amenorrhea need to be understood and recognized early so that they can be treated quickly. Education remains the cornerstone of understanding and early identification of these issues so that prevention of potentially irreversible consequences is possible. Female athletes should be encouraged to learn how their body functions, how exercise affects them, and how proper nutrition can improve their performance. In addition, the preparticipation examination can be utilized to identify athletes at risk and to screen for musculoskeletal problems, strength deficits, or imbalances that may also affect performance. The ultimate goal is to provide information such that the young female athlete can participate safely and establish healthy lifestyle behaviors that will remain with them throughout life.

REFERENCES

1. American College of Obstetricians and Gynecologists (ACOG) Technical Bulletin: Exercise During Pregnancy and the Postnatal Period. Washington, DC; ACOG, 1985.
2. Anderson TD: Exercise and sport in pregnancy. Midwife Health Visit Commun Nurse 22(8):275–278, 1986.
3. Arendt EA, Dick RW: Gender specific knee injury patterns in collegiate basketball and soccar athletes. National Collegiate Athletic Association: NCAA Injury Surveillance System, Overland Park, Kansas, NCAA, 1990–92.
4. Artal R: Exercise and Pregnancy. Clin Sports Med 11:363–377, 1992.
5. Artal R, Masaki D: Exercise in gestational diabetes. Pract Diabetol 8(2):7–14, 1989.
6. Artal R, Wiswill R, Romem Y: Hormonal responses to exercise in diabetic and nondiabetic pregnant patients. Diabetes 39(2):78:80, 1985.
7. Balaban EP: Sports anemia. Clin Sports Med 11:313–325, 1992.
8. Bale P, Nelson G: The effects of menstruation on performance of swimmers. Aust J Sci Med Sport 17:19–22, 1985.
9. Bemenn DA, Boileau RA, Bahr JM, et al: Effects of oral contraceptives on hormonal and metabolic responses during exercise. Med Sci Sports Exerc 24:434–441, 1991.
10. Berg K: Aerobic function in female athletes. Clin Sports Med 3:779–789, 1984.
11. Bonekat HW, Dombovy ML, Staats BA: Progesterone-induced changes in exercise performance and ventilatory response. Med Sci Sports Exerc 19:118–123, 1987.
12. Bonen A, Belcastro AN, Ling WY, et al: Profiles of selected hormones during menstrual cycles of teenage athletes. J Appl Physiol 50(3):545–551, 1981.
13. Bonen A, Keizer HA: Athletic menstrual cycle irregularity: Endocrine response to exercise and training. Physicians Sportsmed 12(8):78, 1984.
14. Boyden TW, Pamenter RS, Grosso D: Prolactin responses, menstrual cycles, and body composition of women runners. J Clin Endocrinol Metab 54:711, 1982.
15. Brooks-Gunn J, Burrow C, Warren MP: Attitudes toward eating and body weight in different groups of female adolesecent athletes. Int J Eat Disord 7:749, 1988.
16. Brown CH, Wilmore JH: The effects of maximal resistance training on the strength and body composition of women athletes. Med Sci Sports Exer 6:174, 1974.
17. Brune M, Magnusson B, Persson H, et al: Iron losses in sweat. Am J Clin Nutr 43:438–443, 1986.
18. Bung P, Artal R, Khodignian N, et al: Exercise in gestational diabetes: An optional therapeutic approach? Diabetes 40(Suppl 2):182–185, 1991.
19. Bunt JC:Metabolic actions of estradiol: Significance for acute and chronic exercise responses. Med Sci Sports Exerc 22:286–290, 1990
20. Bunt JC, Boileau RA, Bahr JM, et al: Sex and training differences in human growth hormone levels during prolonged exercise. J Appl Physiol 61:1796–1801, 1986.
21. Cann CE, Martin MC, Genant, et al: Decreased spinal mineral content in amenorrheic women. JAMA 251:626–629, 1984.
22. Carpenter AJ, Nunnely SA: Endogenous hormones subtly alter women's response to heat stress. J. Appl Physiol 65:2313–2317, 1989.
23. Chalip L, Villiger J, Duigan P: Sex role identity in a select sample of women field hockey players. Int J. Sport Psychol 11:240–248, 1980.
24. Chow R, Harrison JE, Notarius C: Effect of two randomized exercise programs on bone mass of healthy postmenopausal women. BMJ 295:1441–1444, 1987.
25. Ciullo JV: Lower extremity injuries. In Pearl AJ (ed): The Athletic Female. Champaign, IL, Human Kinetics, 1993.
26. Clapp JF III, Capeless EL: Neonatal morphometrics after endurance exercise during pregnancy. Am J Obstet Gynecol 163:1805–1811, 1990.
27. Clapp JF III, Dickstein S: Endurance exercise and pregnancy outcome. Med Sci Sports Exerc 16:556–562, 1984.
28. Clapp JF, III, Wesley M, Sleamaker RH: Thermoregulatory and metabolic responses to jogging prior to and during pregnancy. Med Sci Sports Exerc 19:124–130, 1987.
29. Clarke K, Buckley W: Women's injuries in collegiate sports. Am J Sports Med 8:187–191, 1980.
30. Clark N: Nutritional problems and training intensity, activity level, and athletic performance. In Pearl AJ (ed): The Athletic Female. Champaign, IL, Human Kinetics, 1993, pp 165–168.
31. Clement DB, Asmundson RC: Nutritional intake and hematological parameters in endurance runners. Physician Sportsmed 10:37, 1982.
32. Costill D: Carbohydrates for exercise: Dietary demands for optimal performance. Int J Sports Med. 9:1–18, 1988.
33. Cummings DC, Vickovic MM, Wall SR, et all: Defects in pulsatile LH release in normally menstruating runners. J Clin Endocrinol Metab 60:810–812, 1985
34. Cummings SR, Kelsey JL, Nevitt MC, et al: Epidemiology of osteoporosis and osteoporotic fractures. Epidemiol Rev 7:178, 1985.
35. Dalsky GP: Exercise: Its effect on bone mineral content. Clin Obstet Gynecol 30:820–831, 1987.
36. Dalsky GP: The role of exercise in the prevention of osteoporosis. Compr Ther 15:30–37, 1989.
37. DeBruyn-Prevost P, Masset C, Sturbois X: Physiological response from 18–25 years women to aerobic and anaerobic physical fitness tests at different periods during the menstrual cycle. J Sports Med 24:144–148, 1984.
38. DeSouza MJ, Maguire MS, Rubin K, et al: Effects of menstrual phase and amenorrhea on exercise reponses in runners. Med Sci Sports Exerc 22;575–580, 1990.
39. Dibrezzo R, Fort IL, Brown B: Relationships among strength, endurance, weight and body fat during three phases of the menstrual cycle. J Sports Med Phys Fitness 31:89–94, 1991.
40. Diehl KM, Lohman TG, Smith SC, et al: The effects of physical training in iron status of female field hockey players. Int J Sports Med 7:264–270, 1986.
41. Dink JH, Scheckter CB, Drinkwater BL, et al: Higher serum cortisol levels in exercise associated amenorrhea. Ann Intern Med 108:530, 1988.
42. Dombovy ML, Bonekat HW, Williams TJ, et al: Exercise performance and ventilatory response in the menstrual cycle. Med Sci Sports Exerc 19:111–117, 1987.
43. Doody KM, Carr BR: Amenorrhea. Obstet Gynecol Clin North Am 17:361–387, 1990.
44. Dressendorfer RH, Goodlin RC: Fetal heart rate reponse to maternal exercise testing. Phys Sports Med 8:91–94, 1980.
45. Drinkwater BL: Women and exercise: Physiological aspects. Exerc Sport Sci Rev 12:21, 1984.
46. Drinkwater BL Physiological response of women to exercise. Exerc Sports Rev 1:125–153, 1973.
47. Drinkwater BL, Bruemmer B, Chestnut CH III: Menstrual history as a determinant of current bone density in young athletes. JAMA 263:545, 1990.
48. Drinkwater BL, Nilson K, Chestnut CH III, et al: Bone mineral content of amenorrheic and eumenorrheic athletes. N Engl J Med 311:277, 1984.

49. Drinkwater BL, Nilson K, Ott S, et al: Bone mineral density after resumption of menses in amenorrheic athletes. JAMA 256:380, 1986
50. Druss RG: Body image and perfection of ballerinas: Comparison and contrast with anorexia nervosa. Gen Hosp Psychiatry 2:115, 1979.
51. Emans SJ, Grace E, Hoffer FA, et al: Estrogen deficiency in adolescents and yound adults: Impact on bone mineral content and effects of estrogen replacement therapy. Obstet Gynecol 76:585–592, 1990.
52. Ettinger B, Genant HK, Cann CE: Postmenopausal bone loss is prevented by treatment with low-dosage estrogen with calcium. Ann Intern Med 106:40–45, 1987.
53. Felson DT, Zhang Y, Hannan MT, et al: The effect of postmenopausal estrogen therapy on bone density in elderly women. N Engl J Med 329:1141–1146, 1993.
54. Fox EL, Mathews DK: The Physiological Basis of Physical Edcution and Athletics, 3rd ed. Philadelphia, Saunders College Publishing, 1981.
55. Flint MM, Drinkwater BL, Horvath SM: Effects of training on women's response to sub maximal exercise. Med Sci Sports Exer 6:89, 1974.
56. Fredrickson LA, Puhl JL, Runyan WS: Effects of training on indices of iron status of young female cross-country runners. Med Sci Sports Exerc 15:271, 1983.
57. Friedman J, Lemon P: Effect of chronic endurance exercise on retention of dietary protein. Int J Sports Med 10:118–123, 1989.
58. Frisch RE, Gotz-Welbergen AV, McArthur JW, et al: Delayed menarche and amenorrhea of college athletes in relation to age of onset of training. JAMA 246:1559–1563, 1981.
59. Frisch RE, Hall GH, Aoki TT et al: Metabolic, endocrine and reproductive changes of a woman channel swimmer. Metabolism 33:1106, 1984.
60. Frisch RE, McArthur JW:Menstrual cycles: Fatness as a determinant of minimum weight and height necessary for their maintenance or onset. Science 185:849, 1974.
61. Froberg K, Pederson PD: Sex differences in endurance capacity and metabolic response to prolonged, heavy exercise. Eur J Appl Physiol 52:446–450, 1984.
62. Gardner GW, Edgerton VR, Barnard RJ, et al: Cardiorespiratory, hematological and physical performance responses of anemic subjects to iron treatment. Am J Clin Nutr 29:982, 1975.
63. Garrick J, Requa R: Girls' sport injuries in high school athletics. JAMA 239:2245–2248, 1978.
64. Gilchrist NL: Bone density estimation. NZ Med J 101:260, 1988.
65. Gonzalez ER: Chronic anovulation may increase post menopausal breast cancer risk. JAMA 249:445–446, 1983.
66. Griffin LY: Upper extremity injuries. In Pearl AJ (ed): The Athletic Woman. Champaign, IL, Human Kinetics, 1993.
67. Hall JE: Females and physical activity. Curr Ther Sports Med:116, 1985.
68. Hatta H, Atomi Y, Shinohara S, et al: The effects of ovarian hormones on glucose and fatty acid oxidation during exercise in female ovariectomezed rats. Horm Metab Res 20:609–611, 1988.
69. Hauth JC, Gilstrap LC, Widmer M: Fetal heart rate reactivity before and during the third semester. Am J Obstet and Gynecol 142:545–547, 1982.
70. Hawlett TA, Tomlin S, Ngahfoong L, et al: Release of β-endorphin and metenkephalin during exercise in normal women: Response to training. BMJ 288:1950, 1984.
71. Herzog DB, Copeland PM: Eating disorders. N Engl J Med 313:295–303, 1985.
72. Herzog DB, Norman DK, Pepose M: Sexual conflict and eating disorders in 27 males. Am J Psychol 141:980–987, 1984.
73. Hessemer V, Bruck K: Influence of menstrual cycle on shivering skin blood flow and sweating responses measured at night. J Appl Physiol 59:1902–1910, 1985.
74. Hessemer V, Bruck K: Influence of menstrual cycle on thermoregulartory, metabolic, and heart rate repsonses to exercise at night. J App Physiol 59:1911–1917, 1985.
75. Higgs SL, Robertson LA. Cyclic variations in perceived exertion and physical work capacity in females. Can J App Sports Sciences 6:191–196, 1981.
76. Hopper JL, Seeman E: The bone density of female twins discordant for tobacco use. N Engl J Med 330;387–392, 1994.
77. Horvath SM, Drinkwater BL: Thermoregulation and the menstrual cycle. Aviat Space Environ Med 53:790–794, 1982.
78. Huisveld IA, Hospers JEH, Bernink MJ, et al: The effect of oral contraceptives and exercise on hemostatic and fibrinolytic mechanisms in trained women. Int J Sports Med 4:97–103, 1983.
79. Ireland ML, Wall C: Epidemiology and comparison of knee injuries in elite male and female United States basketball injuries. (abstract). Med Sci Sports Exerc S82, May 24, #491.
80. Jarski RW, Trippett DL: The risks and benefits of exercise during pregnancy. J Fam Pract 30:185–189, 1990.
81. Jojanovic-Peterson L, Durak EP, Peterson CM: Randomized trial of diet versus diet plus cardiovascular conditioning on glucose levels in gestational diabetes. Am J Obstet Gynecol 161:415–419, 1989.
82. Jurkowski JEH, Jones NL, Toews CJ: Effects of menstrual cycle on blood lactate, O_2 delivery and performance during exercise. J Appl Physiol 51:1493–1499, 1981.
83. Kadel NJ, Teitz CC, Kronmal RA: Stress fractures in ballet dancers. Am J Sports Med 20:445–449, 1992.
84. Kaiserauer S, Snyder AC, Sleeper M, et al: Nutritional, physiological, and menstrual status of distance runners. Med Sci Sports Exerc 21:120–125, 1989.
85. Kassenbaum S, et al: Nutrition, physiology and menstrual status of female distance runners. Med Sci Sports Exerc 21:2, 1989.
86. Katz VL, McMurray R, Goodwin WE, et al: Nonweight-bearing exercise during pregnancy on land and during immersion: A comparative sturdy. Am J Perinatol 7(3): 281–284, 1990.
87. Kilham L, Ferm VH: Exencephaly in fetal hamsters following exposure to hperthermia. Teratology 14:323–326, 1976.
88. Klafs CE, Lyon MJ: The Female Athlete. St. Louis, Mosby, 1988.
89. Knapik JJ, Bauman CL, Jones BH, et al: Preseason strength and flexibility imbalances associated with athletic injuries in female collegiate athletes. Am J Sports Med 19:76–81, 1991.
90. Lamon-Fava S, Fisher EC, Nelson ME: Effects of exercise and menstrual cycle status on plasma lipids, low density lipoprotein particle size and apolipoproteins. J Clin Encocrinol Metab 68:17–21, 1989.
91. LeBrun C: Effects of the Phases of the Menstrual Cycle and Oral Contraceptives on Athletic Performance. Presented at Medical and Orthopedic Issues of Active and Athletic Women. April 30, 1993, Penn State Unversity.
92. Lebrun CM: Effect of the different phases of the menstrual cycle and oral contraceptives on athletic performance. Sports Med 16:400–430, 1993.
93. Lebrun CM, McKenzie DC, Prior JC, et al: Effects of a triphasic oral contraceptive on athletic performance. Submitted for publication, 1995.
94. Lebrun CM, McKenzie DC, Prior JC, et al: Effects of menstrual cycle phase on athletic performance. Submitted for publication, 1995.
95. Same as Reference 128.
96. Lehtovirta P, Kuikka J, Pyorala T: Hemodynamic effects of oral contraceptives during exercise. Int J Gynecol Obstet 15:35–37, 1977.

97. Licata AA: Stress fractures in young athletic women: Case reports of unsuspected cortisol-induced osteoporosis. Med Sci Sports Exerc 24:955–957, 1992.
98. Lindberg JS, Fears WB, Hunt MM, et al: Exercise-induced amenorrhea and bone density. Ann Intern Med 101:647–648, 1984.
99. Littler WA, Bojorges-Bueno R, Banks J: Cardiovascular dynamics in women during the menstrual cycle and oral contraceptive therapy. Thorax 29:567–570, 1974.
100. Loosli A, Benson J, Gillian D: Nutrition habits and knowledge in competitive adolescent female gymnasts. Physician Sportsmed 14:8, 1986.
101: Lotgering FK, Van Doorn MB, Struijk PC, et al: Maximal aerobic exercise in pregnant women: Heart rate, O_2 consumption, CO_2 production, and ventilation. J Appl Physiol 70:1016–1023, 1991.
102. Loucks AB, Horvath SM: Athletic amenorrhea: A review. Med Sci Sports Exerc 17:45, 1985.
103. Lutter JM, Suchman S: Menstrual patterns in female runners. Physician Sportsmed 10(9):60, 1982.
104. Malina RM, Harper AB, Avent JJ, et al: Age at menarche in athletes and non-athletes. Med Sci Sport 5:11–13, 1973.
105. Malone TR, Sanders B: Strength training and the athletic female. In Pearl AJ (ed): The Athletic Female. Champaign, IL, Human Kinetics, 1993, pp 169–184.
106. Mansfield MJ, Emans SJ: Anorexia nervosa, athletics, and amenorrhea. Pediatr Clin North Am 36:533–549, 1989.
107. Marcus AD, McCulloch RG: Bone dynamics: Stress, strain and fracture. J Sports Sci 5:155–163, 1987.
108. Marcus R, Cann C, Madvig P, et al: Menstrual function and bone mass in elite women distance runners: Endocrine and metabolic features. Ann Intern Med 102:158–163, 1985.
109. Marcus R, Carter DR: The role of physical activity in bone mass regulation. Adv Sports Med Fitness 1:63–82, 1988.
110. Matute ML, Kalkjoff RL: Sex steroid influence on hepatic gluconeogenesis, and glycogen formation. Endocrinology 92:762–768, 1973.
111. McArthur JW, Bullen BA, Beitins IZ et al: Hypothalamic amenorrhea in runners of normal body composition. Endocr Res Commun 7:13, 1980.
112. McMurray RG, Hackney AC, Katz VL, et al: Pregnancy-induced changes in maximal oxygen uptake during swimming. J Appl Physio 71:1454–1459, 1991.
113. McMurray RG, Katz VL, Berry MJ, et al: Cardiovascular responses of pregnant women during aerobic exercise in water: A longitudinal study. Int J Sports Med 9:443–447, 1988.
114. McMurray RG, Mottola MF, Wolfe LA, et al: Recent advances in understanding maternal and fetal responses to exercise. Med Sci Sports Exerc 25:1305–1321, 1993.
115. McMurrary RG, Mottola MF, Wolfe LA, et al: Brief review: recent advances in understanding maternal and fetal responses to exercise. Med Sci Sport Exerc 25(12): 1305–1321, 1993.
116. McSherry JA: The diagnostic challenge of anorexia nervosa. Am Fam Physician 29:144, 1984.
117. Meilahn EN, Kuller LH, Mathews KA, et al: Potential for increasing high density lipoprotein cholesterol subfractions HDL2-C, HDL3-C and apolipoprotein A1 among middle-aged women. Prev Med 20:462–473, 1991.
118. Metka M, Holzer F, Heytmanek G et al: Hypergonadotropic hypogonadic amenorrhea (World Health Organization III) and osteoporosis. Fertil Steril 57;37–41, 1992.
118a. Moller-Nielson J, Hammar M: Women's soccer injuries in relation to the menstrual cycle and oral contraceptive use. Med Sci Sport Exerc 21:126–129, 1989.
119. Moore LG, McCullouogh RE, Weil JV: Increased hypoxic ventilatory response in pregnancy: Relationship to hormonal and metabolic changes. J Appl Physiol 62:158–163, 1987.
120. Morgan WP, Costill DL: Psychological characterization of the marathon runners. J Sports Med Phys Fitness 12:42, 1972.
121. Morton MJ, Paul NS, Compos GR, et al: Exercise dynamics in late gestation: Effects of physical training. Am J Obstet Gynecol 152:91–97, 1985.
122. Morton MJ, Paul MS, Metcalfe J: Exercise during pregnancy. Med Clin North Am 69:97–108, 1985.
123. Myburgh KH, Hutchins J, Fataar AB, et al: Low bone density is an etiologic factor for stress fractures in athletes. Ann Intern Med 113:754–759, 1990.
124. National Collegiate Athletic Association: NCAA injury surveillance system, Overland Park, Kansas, NCAA, 1991–1992.
125. Nickerson HJ, Holubets MC, Weiler BR, et al: Causes of iron deficiency in adolescent athletes. J Pediatr 114:657–663, 1989.
126. Nickerson HJ, Tripp AD: Iron deficiency in adolescent cross-country runners. Phys Sports Med 11:60–66, 1983.
127. Nickerson JH, Holubets M, Tripp AD, et al: Decreased iron stores in high school female runners. Am J Dis Child 139:1115, 1985.
128. Nicklas BJ, Hackney AC, Sharp RL: The menstrual cycle and exercise: Performance, muscle glycogen and substrate responses. Inter J Sports Med 10:264–269, 1989.
129. Notelovitz M, Zauner C, McKenzie L, et al: The effect of low-dose contraceptives on cardiorespiratory function, coagulation, and lipids in exercising young women: A preliminary report. Am J Obstet Gynecol 156:591–598, 1987.
130. Ohira Y, Edgerton VR, Gardner GW, et al: Work capacity, heart rate and blood lactate responses to iron treatement. Br J Haematol 41:365, 1979.
131. Otis CL: Exercise-associated amenorrhea. Clin Sports Med 11(2):351, 1992.
132. Petrofsky JS, Ledonne DM, Rinehart JS, et al: Isometric strength and endurance during the menstrual cycle. Eur J App Phys Occup Physiol 35:1–10, 1976.
133. Pivarnik JM, Lee W, Miller JF, et al: Alterations in plasma volume and protein during cycle exercise throughout pregnancy. Med Sci Sports Exerc 22:751–755, 1990.
134. Pivarnik JM, Lee W, Miller JF: Physiological and perceptual responses to cycle and treadmill exercise during pregnancy. Med Sci Sports Exerc 23:470–475, 1991.
135. Pivarnik JM, Marichal CJ, Spillman T, et al: Menstrual cycle phase affects temperature regulation during endurance exercise. J App Physiol 72:543–548, 1992.
136. Pollock ML, Miller JS Jr, Ribisl PM: Effect of fitness on aging. Physician Sportsmed 6:45, 1978.
137. Prior JC, et al: Spinal bone loss and ovulatory disturbances. N Engl J Med 323:1221, 1990.
138. Prior JC, Cameron K, Yuen BH, et al: Menstrual cycle changes with marathon training: Anovulation and short luteal phase. Can J Appl Sports Sci 7:173–177, 1982.
139. Putukian M: The female triad: Eating disorders, amenorrhea, and osteoporosis. Med Clin North Am 78:345–356, 1994.
140. Quadagno D, Faquin L, Lim G-N, et al: The menstrual cycle: Does it affect athletic performance? Physician Sportsmed 19:121–124, 1991.
141. Rauniker RA, Sabio H: Anemia in the adolescent athletes. Am J Dis Child 146:1201–1205, 1992.
142. Risser WL, Lee EJ, Poindexter HBW, et al: Iron deficiency in female athletes: Its prevalence and impact on performance. Med Sci Sports Exerc 20:116–121, 1988.
143. Robertson LA, Higgs LS: Menstrual cycle variations in physical work capacity, post-exercise blood lactate, and perceived exertion. Can J Appl Sports Sci 8:220, 1983.

144. Rosso P: A new chart to monitor weight gain during pregnancy. Am J. Clin Nutr 41:664–652, 1985.
145. Rowland TW: Iron deficiency in the young athlete. Pediatr Clin North Am 37:1153–1163, 1990.
146. Rowland TW, Black SA, Kelleher JF: Iron deficiency in adolescent endurance athletes. J Adolesc Health Care 8:322, 1987.
147. Rowland TW, Deisroth MA, Green GM, et al: The effect of iron therapy on the exercise capacity of nonanemic iron deficient adolescent runners. Am J Dis Child 142; 165, 1988.
148. Rowland TW, Kellehar JF: Iron deficiency in athletes: Insights from high school swimmers. Am J Dis Child 143:197, 1989.
149. Sady MA, Hayden BB, Sady SP, et al: Cardiovascular response to maximal exercise during pregnancy and at two and seven months postpartum. Am J Obstet Gynecol 162:1181–1185, 1990.
150. Sady SP, Carpenter MW, Sady MA, et al: Prediction of VO_2 max during cycle exercise in pregnancy women. J Appl Physiol 65:657–661, 1988.
151. Sady SP, Carpenter MW, Thomspon PD, et al: Cardiovascular response to cycle exercise during and after pregnancy. J Appl Physiol 66:336–341, 1989.
152. Sady SP, Freedson PS: Body composition and structural compositions of female and male athletes. Clin Sports Med 3:755–777, 1984.
153. Savard F, Palmer JE, Greenwood MRC: Effects of exercise training on regional adipose tissue metabolism in pregnant rats. Am J Phsiol 250:R837–844, 1986.
154. Schoene RB, Robertson HT, Pierson DJ, Peterson AP: Respiratory drives and exercise in menstrual cycles of athletic and nonathletic women. J Appl Physiol 50: 1300–1305, 1981.
155. Schwartz B, Cumming DC, Riordan E et al: Exercise-associated amenorrhea: A distinct entity? Am J Obstet Gynecol 141:662, 1981.
156. Selby GB, Eichner ER: Endurance swimming, intravascular hemolysis, anemia, and iron depletion: New perspective on athlete's anemia. Am J Med 81;791–794, 1986.
157. Shangold MM: How I manage exercise-related menstrual disturbances. Physician Sportsmed 14:113–120, 1986.
158. Shangold MM, Freeman R, et al: The relationship between long-distance running, plasma progesterone and luteal phase length. Fertil Steril 31:130, 1979.
159. Shangold MM, Levine HS: The effect of marathon training upon menstrual function. Am J Obstet Gynecol 143:862–869, 1982.
160. Shepard RJ, Davanagh T: The effects of training on the aging process. Physician Sportsmed 6:33, 1978.
161. Siegel AJ, Hennekens CH, Solomon HS, et al: Exercise-related hematuria. JAMA 241:391–392, 1979.
162. Smith EL, Gilligan: Mechanical forces and bone. Bone Miner Res 6:1399–173, 1989.)
163. Smith EL Jr, Reddan W, Smith PE: Physical activity and calcium modalities for bone mineral increase in aged women. Med Sci Sports Exerc 13:60–64, 1981.
164. Stewart JC, Ahlquist DA, McGill DB, et al: Gastrointestinal blood loss and anemia in runners. Ann Intern Med 100:843–845, 1984.
165. Tafari N, Naeye RL, Gobzie A: Effects of maternal undernutrition and heavy physical work during pregnancy on birth weight. Br J Obstet Gynaecol 87:222–226, 1980.
166. Tarnopolsky LJ, MacDougall JD, Atkinson SA: Gender differences in substrate for endurance exercise. J Appl Physiol 68:302–308, 1990.
166a. Veldhuis JD, Evans WS, Demers LM, et al: Altered neuroendocrine regulation of gonadotrophin secretion in women distance runners. J Clin Endocrinol Metab 61: 577–663, 1985.
167. Vellar OD: Changes in hemoglobin concentration and hematocit during the menstrual cycle. Acta Obste Gynecol Scand 53:243–246, 1974.
168. Warren MP: The effects of exercise on pubertal progression and reproductive function in girls. J Clin Endocrinol Metab 51:1150–1157, 1980.
169. Weaver CM, Rajaram S: Exercise and iron status. J Natr 122:782–787, 1992.
170. Wells CL, Horvath SM: Heat stress responses related to the menstrual cycle. J Appl Physiol 35:1–5, 1973.
171. Wenger NK: Coronary heart disease in women: Evolution of our knowledge. Presented at Medical and Orthopedic Issues in Active and Athletic Women, Seattle, WA, April 15–16, 1994.
172. White CM, Hergenroeder AC: Amenorrhea, osteopenia, and the female athlete. Pediatr Clin North Am 37:1125, 1990.
173. White J: Exercising for Two: What's safe for the active pregnant woman? Physician Sportsmed 20(5):179–186, 1992.
174. Whiteside P: Men's and women's injuries in comparable sports. Physician Sportsmed 8(3)130–140, 1980.
175. Wilmore JH, Brown CH: Physiological profiles of women distance runners. Med Sci Sports 6:178–181, 1974.
176. Wirth JC, Lohman TG: The relationship of static muscle function to use of oral contraceptives. Med Sci Sports Exerc 14:16–20, 1982.
177. Wolfe LA, Hall P, Webb KA, et al: Prescription of aerobic exercise during pregnancy. Sports Med 8:273–301, 1989.
178. Wood L, Ferrell WR, Baxendale RH: Pressures in normal and acutely distended knee joints and effects on quadriceps maximal voluntary contractions. Q J Exp Physiol 73:305–314, 1988.
179. Yeager KK: American College of Sports Medicine Ad Hoc Task Force on Women's Issues in Sports Medicine, June 1992.
180. Yeager KK, Agostini R, Nattiv A, Crinkwater B: The female athlete triad: Disordered eating, amenorrhea, osteoporosis (commentary). Med Sci Sports Exerc 25: 775, 1993.
181. Zelisko JA, Noble HB, Porter M: A comparison of men's and women's professional basketball injuries. Am J Sports Med 10;297–299, 1982.

9

Sports Psychiatry and Psychology

Todd P. Hendrickson, M.D.

Because 80% of patients with psychiatric conditions are treated by primary care specialists, psychiatric evaluation and assessment of the athlete must be regarded as integral to the primary care setting. Environmental catchment surveys have clearly shown the incidence of common psychiatric problems such as anxiety, depression, and substance abuse may be seen in up to 5–15% of people evaluated using the results of standardized mental status examinations. By understanding a few basic principles of psychiatric evaluation and assessment, it is hoped that the clinician can form psychiatric diagnoses in athletes and make clinical decisions regarding treatment plans for them. There is scant epidemiologic evidence to prove or disprove the thesis that there are any differences between psychiatric illness in the athletic setting compared to the general population. It is, however, the author's opinion based on clinical experience that psychiatric illness in the general population is similar to that in the athletic setting. This chapter attempts to elucidate some common tools used in evaluation and assessment of the athlete and, more important, demonstrate the use of a problem-based learning approach in understanding basic psychiatric issues that occur in the athletic setting.

EVALUATION AND ASSESSMENT

The principal features of the psychiatric evaluation are taking a psychiatric history and conducting the mental status examination. The ability to postulate symptoms based on results from the mental status examination gives the clinician an ability to cluster sets of symptoms into patterns to reveal a psychiatric diagnosis. In other words, as in the rest of medical care, history and examination reveal symptoms that can give a diagnosis, which then not only dictates treatment plans but also provides the clinician with an opportunity to develop a prognosis regarding the patient's problem. This is a key feature in the typical psychiatric evaluation.

USE OF THE BIOPSYCHOSOCIAL MODEL

When formulating diagnoses and treatments for patients with psychiatric illness, we use the biopsychosocial model.

1. Biological—includes medical history, current medical status, family history (especially of psychiatric illness), current physical skill level and development, and overall physiology of the athlete.
2. Psychological—includes the mental status examination, and ascertaining the patient's ability to participate in the evaluation process.
3. Social—includes analysis of the patient's athletic and non-athletic environment, i.e., social support systems, family dynamics, interpersonal relationships, substance abuse history, educational background, cultural background, childhood development, and successful and unsuccessful sport performance experiences.

All treatment plans should include therapeutic emphasis in each of these three areas; for example, pharmacological management in biological terms, psychotherapies in the psychological treatment plan, and social support systems as a part of the treatment plan.

Psychiatric diagnosis can now be coordinated with the use of the 1994 version of the Diagnostic and Statistical Manual, 4th edition (DSM-IV).

PSYCHIATRIC INTERVIEW

The psychiatric interview is an interaction between the patient and the physician designed to assess psychiatric status and to suggest treatment of an emotional or behavioral problem. The interview should be designed to allow patients to describe their perceptions of the difficulty. The physician then clarifies the chief complaint with help from the patient's history. In working with athletes, certain behavioral problems may actually be better evaluated in the performance setting, i.e., on the sports field. With the patient's permission, it may be extremely helpful to gather information from others such as sports physicians, coaches, family, and so forth. This can be a vitally important portion of the psychiatric interview. In performing a psychiatric evaluation, adequate time should be set aside for the interview. The physician ought to allot time to obtain the valuable information and to begin to develop a rapport or empathetic relationship with the patient. Because psychiatric symptoms can be difficult for an athlete to discuss with anyone, it is critically important to take a nonjudgmental approach, especially in initial interviews. The clinical interview may be diagnostic or therapeutic, but elements of both are often contained in these initial evaluations. Therapeutic interviews involve the use of psychotherapeutic techniques and should be intended to provide treatment in the form of support, reassurance, and exploration of the patient's history and current sources of stress.

Privacy and confidentiality are especially important for the athlete and great care should be taken to maintain this trusted relationship. Athletes may be ambivalent or embarrassed about discussing their symptoms with the clinician. It is further recommended that the purpose of the interview, i.e., psychiatric diagnosis, be clearly explained to the patient before the interview begins. The provision of a comfortable environment is obviously important for proper performance of the mental status examination. So it is advisable to use an office setting rather than the sports field for the interview.

The initial session should include history of the present condition as well as any previous experiences the athlete has had with psychiatric evaluation, diagnosis, or treatment. Information should include issues of past medication trials, length of medication trials, and types of therapy used in the past. The psychiatric history should also include family history, because we know that certain psychiatric illnesses such as depression and anxiety tend to run in families. The psychiatric history should always include a physical medical history as well, because it has been shown that organic illness may exacerbate psychiatric symptoms. In other words, psychiatric and medical histories should be seen as complementary. Table 1 gives an outline of a typical psychiatric history. It includes some factors of childhood development, including general issues of language and neurological development. Clinicians tend to hesitate asking questions about developmental history, but the answers may give important clues to the athlete's intellectual and social development.

TABLE 1. The Psychiatric History

Identifying Information
- Sociodemographic summary

Chief complaint

History of present illness
- Extended information about chief complaint
- Onset
- Duration/course
- Precipitants
- Exaggerating and alleviating factors

Psychiatric review of systems
- Psychological symptom inventory
- Review of major DSM-IV psychiatric diagnostic symptoms

Medical history

Individual and Family history of psychiatric disorders and treatment

Personal History
- Prenatal/birth history
- Childhood
- Adolescence
- Adulthood
  - Educational
  - Occupational
  - Interpersonal/Social
  - Sexual
  - Habits—alcohol, other drugs

Appropriate Use of Psychiatric Screening Questions

When comparing psychiatric illness to physical medical illness, symptoms of psychiatric illness may not always be easily apparent. The following indicators are helpful in detecting patients with a possibility of psychiatric illness.

1. A patient who is unresponsive to treatment in situations such treatments are usually effective
2. Multiple somatic, i.e., physical, complaints not accounted for by known medical conditions or symptoms outside the boundaries of known anatomy or physiology
3. Chaotic lifestyle, i.e., unstable relationships, substance abuse, and so forth
4. Doctor shopping, that is, a history of frequently changing doctors
5. Symptoms that seem to be related to stress or anxiety
6. Individual or family history of psychiatric illness

It should also be noted that the converse of the above is also applicable. For example, if a patient has definitive objective findings of physical illness or has a history of extreme emotional stability or the absence of any acute or chronic stressors that may have precipitated symptoms, one may be looking with a lower index of suspicion for psychiatric illness. Table 2 gives examples of psychiatric screening questions used in the primary care setting.

Mental Status Examination

The mental status examination (Table 3) is a systematic method to obtain psychological and be-

TABLE 2. Psychiatric Screening Questions for Patients in the Primary Care Setting

Depression
"Have you been feeling sad or depressed? Is this accompanied by trouble with sleep or appetite, low energy, or decreased interest in doing things? Do you have feelings of guilt or thoughts of harming yourself?"
Mania
"Do you feel on top of the world? Is this out of proportion to your usual self such that you talk more, don't need as much sleep, your thoughts race, or notice that your enthusiasm gets you into trouble?"
Psychosis
"Have you heard or seen things that others didn't? Do you feel that you have special powers? Have you felt that others were watching or following you? Have you received peculiar or special messages or felt that others knew or controlled your thoughts?"
Alcoholism
"Have others thought you had a drinking problem? Has drinking alcohol caused problems with friends or relatives, caused you to miss work or lose a job, resulted in arrest, or caused health problems? Do you use recreational drugs?"
Anxiety disorder
"Have you had trouble with nervousness, anxiety, or had a feeling like you are going to panic?"
Anorexia nervosa
"Do you take special measures to keep your weight at its current level?"

havioral data. This information is then integrated to determine the presence or absence of a formal psychiatric disease. The skilled interviewer gathers data regarding mental functioning as observed and elicited during the psychiatric interview. The patient's memory testing may be elicited by having the patient describe what is or is not known about the current presentation. Unusual behavior on the patient's part may also be observed in the initial impression that the clinician has of the patient, i.e., the patient's personal hygiene and cooperation during the interview. Affect is easily elicited by noting the patient's emotional responsiveness to the questions being asked. Specific cognitive evaluation, i.e., intellectual functioning and information processing, is obtained by specific questions relating to cognition, such as calculations, abstractions, and memory. Thought content is best assessed by asking patients questions regarding thought processes, including hallucinations and thoughts of suicide. For example, a patient who is having active psychotic symptoms secondary to the use of anabolic steroids may have perceptual distortion that other people are out to get him. This is known as a paranoid delusion, a fixed false belief. Insight and judgment are best determined by evaluating the patient's awareness of the situation and the ability to react responsibility.

Laboratory Testing

As part of the psychiatric evaluation, the clinician must appreciate the physical medical conditions that also have psychiatric manifestations. A general screening test for patients suspected of having psychiatric symptoms should always include a thyroid profile (hypothyroidism may resemble depression); a chemistry profile (hypoglycemia may cause confusion); electrolytes; and an ECG (arrhythmias leads to anxiety); and often a urine drug screen, (which is helpful in the patient's behavior suggests the probability of substance abuse). Laboratory testing should be left to the judgment of the clinician. It is important to avoid making a formal psychiatric diagnosis if a medical condition causes the psychiatric symptoms.

Psychological Testing

Psychological testing may be helpful in organizing an overall picture of the athlete, although it may not be indicated in all clinical cases. This testing can be extremely helpful when diagnostic issues are confusing, or when treatment is met with resistance or refractoriness.

Personality can be assessed through the use of the Minnesota Multiphasic Personality Inventory (MMPI), which helps to establish longstanding behavioral patterns and means of adaptation to life stressors. There are also other newer tools being tested to provide information about personality traits and their interaction with sport-specific situations.

TABLE 3. Mental Status Examination Outline

- Appearance, attitude, and behavior
  - Description of appearance and hygiene
  - Attitude toward examiner
  - Psychomotor activity
- Speech
- Mood and affect
  - Subjective and objective moods
  - Affect variability and appropriateness
  - Presence of anxiety
  - Assessment of suicidality
- Thought and Language
  - Production
  - Form
  - Current (Obsessions and Delusions)
- Perceptions
  - Hallucinations/Illusions
  - Depersonalization
  - Derealization
- Cognitive Function
  - Level of Consciousness
  - Orientation
  - Concentration
  - Memory
  - Intelligence
- Insight and Judgment

Assessment of the student athlete's mood may give valuable feedback about the athlete's personal feeling. The diagnosis of depressive illness in the student athlete is an extremely important aspect in assessing the student athlete's overall mental health because depression is one of the most common medical and mental health problems in our society. Assessment is done with the use of the Beck Depression Inventory (BDI), a scale that assesses the patient's neurovegetative symptoms of depression as well as the subjective sense of mood state. In addition, the Hamilton Depression Rating Scale (HDRS) can also be used. Another tool that has been used in the past is the Profile of Mood States (POMS).

Anxiety, which can be crippling to the athlete and may also deter performance capabilities, can be identified as well. In most cases, behavior is believed to be determined by the reciprocal interaction of personal traits and the characteristics of different situations. This can be especially helpful in understanding the anxiety-performance relationship. Several tools have been used to assess anxiety including the State/Trait Anxiety Inventory, the Sport Competition Anxiety Test (SCAT), and the Competitive State Anxiety Inventory (CSAI). These specific tests can provide clinical correlations to anxiety in several different sports problems including concentration, sleep disturbances, and the potential for injury.

The clinician can also evaluate stress, especially as it pertains to life skills stressors, through identifying causes using the Holmes-Rahe Scale. Subjective senses of stress are almost always perceived by the athlete as anxiety, but they may also include symptoms of depression as well as irritability.

Motivational assessment can be accomplished by the clinician through goal analysis and behavioral assessment. This is often best if done with the student athlete as well as others in the student athlete's environment—coaches, trainers, and medical staff.

If the clinician suspects that an athlete has a thought disorder, e.g., schizophrenia or a delusional disorder, several helpful tools exist including the previously mentioned MMPI, the Symptom Checklist-90 (SCL-90), and a Structured Clinical Interview (SCI).

PSYCHIATRIC DISORDERS

Diagnosis of illness is critical in the evaluation and treatment of athletes. Symptoms from the history and psychiatric evaluation are clustered together to form descriptions of psychiatric syndromes. It is important to keep these formulations simple and to consult with psychiatric colleagues should there be any question regarding diagnosis, because accurate diagnosis is crucial in formulating an effective treatment plan.

Affective Disorders

Major Depression

Major depression often has an insidious onset. The clinician may also find symptoms of subjective depression, loss of pleasure, suicidal thoughts, loss of appetite, sleep disturbance, self-reproach, lack of energy, dysphoria, and feelings of guilt. In children the clinician tens to see more somatic (physical) symptoms along with psychomotor agitation or restlessness. In adolescents, anorexia, weight loss, hypersomnia, and hopelessness are common findings.

Differential diagnosis includes substance abuse (especially cocaine withdrawal, sedative-hypnotic usage, and anabolic steroid use), anxiety, eating disorders, and organic illnesses that may predispose to depression, i.e., Cushing's syndrome and infectious mononucleosis, among others. Treatment for mental illnesses often include referral to psychiatric professionals, probably an appropriate management for a depressed patient. Other treatments include psychosocial therapies that may include individual, group, or family therapy. Pharmacotherapy (medication therapy) may also be used; it is especially indicated if the ability to function on a daily basis is significantly disturbed. Often a combination of medical therapy and psychotherapy is most effective to provide the quickest resolution of symptoms.

Adjustment Disorder

An adjustment disorder may be considered if the psychiatric symptoms (including symptoms of depression and anxiety) seem to be related to recent (within three months) psychosocial stressors. Adjustment disorders *must* be differentiated from major depression because adjustment disorders tend to respond better to psychotherapy than medication.

Situations specific to sports where the physician may see adjustment disorders include the period following athletic injury when depression, anxiety, and irritability are extremely common. Other situations include career termination, the death of a loved one, the loss of a relationship, demoted playing status, a change of coach, leaving high-school for college, loss of a big game, and anxiety regarding performance anxiety.

Chronic adjustment disorders may result from overuse and overtraining syndromes; common in patients who are experiencing burnout or in those athletes whose physical rehabilitation has failed to alleviate knee injuries and back injuries. These kinds of chronic adjustment disorders are often related to multiple somatic complaints as well as chronic pain.

The treatment for adjustment disorders includes psychosocial therapy, (either individually or in a group), which can be extremely helpful in this "reactive" depression through a support and nurturing. The clinician should allow time for transition because this clinical situation usually abates. As already noted, pharmacotherapy is rarely indicated for adjustment disorder, except in the case of the athlete who is experiencing significant sleep disorders. In such cases, a sedative hypnotic or a low-dose antidepressant may be used to remediate a sleep disturbance.

Dysthymic Disorder

The determining finding is a chronically depressed mood present during most of the day and occurring on more days than not for at least two years in adults and one year in children and adolescents. The severity of the mood disturbance, however, does not meet the criteria for major depression. In addition, poor self-esteem, hopelessness, pessimism, low energy, and social withdrawal are common. The athlete typically perceives a physical problem, and often there have been extensive medical workups for symptoms of fatigue, poor athletic performance, and trouble concentrating.

Differential Diagnosis. Substance Abuse (benzodiazepines, narcotics, CNS depressants), medical illness (hypothyroidism, mononucleosis, hyperglycemia, Cushing's syndrome), or chronic anxiety (generalized anxiety disorder).

Treatment. Pharmacotherapy for dysthymic disorder includes prescribing monoamine oxidase inhibitors (MAOIs), which may be more beneficial than tricyclic antidepressants. In addition, the newly introduced and well-tolerated serotonin specific reuptake inhibitors (SSRIs), i.e., fluoxetine and paroxetine; have also been effective in the treatment of dysthymia. Psychotherapy includes developing cognitive means of altering behavior—ways of thinking and behaving to replace faulty or negative attitudes about themselves, the world, and the future. Behavioral therapies focus the patient on specific goals to increase activity and to relax.

Organic Affective Disorder (Depression Secondary to Medical Illness or Medications)

Hypothyroidism (can also cause confusion and delirium)
Narcotic and benzodiazepine abuse
Anemia resulting from chronic disease
Cushing's syndrome
Infectious mononucleosis
Cardiomyopathy
Medication (metoclopramide [Reglan], corticosteroids, antiarrhythmics)
Treatment consists of changing or discontinuing the medication, and/or the treatment or both, prescribed for the underlying medical illness.

Bipolar Affective Disorder (Manic Depressive Illness)

Clinical Features. The hallmark feature is presence of mania or hypomania. Mania is defined as a clinical condition manifested in expansive, elevated, or irritable mood. Associated symptoms include hyperactivity, risk-taking behavior, pressured speech, racing thoughts, grandiosity (inflated self-esteem), decreased need or sleep and food, excessive distractibility, and occasionally delusional (psychotic) thinking. These periods of mood expansiveness are pervasive and may last from several days to several weeks and alternate with periods of depression. The depressive phase of bipolar affective disorder is identical to the vegetative depressive symptoms seen in major depression. This depression, however, is more often a "shut-down" depression.

Differential Diagnosis. Substance abuse, including mania resulting from cocaine abuse, schizophrenia, borderline personality disorder, and organic causes of mania (anabolic steroids, hyper-

TABLE 4. **Depressive Disorders**

	Adjustment Disorder	Dysthymia	Major Depressive Episode
Onset	Sudden	No identifiable onset (no history of sustained normal mood during adulthood)	Gradual onset (but period of normal functioning during adulthood can be identified)
Precipitating event	Always	None	Occasionally
Duration	Less than 6 months	At least 2 years	2 weeks to 2 years
Response to treatment	Good	Poor	Good

thyroidism) are common findings. Stabilization treatment of bipolar affective disorder includes the use of lithium carbonate and valproic acid, carbamazepine, and mood stabilizers are all usually essential in treating this illness. Pharmacological treatment must also take account of the depressed phase of the illness. Care must be taken, however, because there is evidence that recurrent use of antidepressants in manic depressive illness has some propensity for precipitating manic episodes. Mania can be effectively managed with use of either benzodiazepines or antipsychotic medications (e.g., haloperidol, thiothixene, and so forth).

Use of Antidepressant Medication in Athletes

That athletes can resist using a medication to treat their symptoms as control is a major issue for most competitive athletes. Careful use of the antidepressants is advised, however, because side effects often cause athletes to decide to discontinue the use of antidepressant medications.

Tricyclic Antidepressants. Classic tricyclic antidepressants such as amitriptyline and imipramine are particularly bothersome for athletes because they may cause concomitant symptoms of dry mouth, constipation, and an increased resting heart rate. The same medications may be sedating as well as causing orthostatic changes in blood pressure. For these reasons, the classic tricyclic antidepressants typically are not the first choice in treating depression in athletes. Amitriptyline and imipramine are, however, extremely useful for treating athletes who have components of both anxiety and depressive illness along with significant insomnia. Tricyclics can cause potential slowing of atrioventricular conduction, so that electrocardiograms should be done both before and during tricyclic antidepressant treatment. Nortriptyline is an extremely effective antidepressant to use in athletes for several reasons. It has fewer anticholineregic side effects and is relatively nonsedating. Also note that desipramine can be another tricyclic antidepressant that has fewer anticholinergic side effects and may be helpful in patients with depression and substance abuse, i.e., alcoholism and cocaine abuse.

Selective Serotonin Reuptake Inhibitors (SSRI). This fairly new class of medications is extremely popular among clinicians treating depression in athletes because of their relative specificity and lack of anticholinergic, antihistaminic, cardiotoxic effects, and, most importantly for some athletes, less associated weight gain. They also are easy to administer. Examples include fluoxetine (Prozac), paroxetine (Paxil), and sertraline (Zoloft). Serotonin-selective agents are effective in treating depression and obsessive compulsive symptoms in athletes with eating disorders (bulimia nervosa) and obsessive compulsive disorder.

Monoamine Oxidase Inhibitors. The MAOIs are not widely prescribed because of their potential to produce a hypertensive crisis if the athlete ingests a food rich in tyramine or takes a sympathomimetic drug. The side effect profile of some orthostatic blood pressures often deters clinicians from using MAOIs in the treatment of depression in athletes. They are the most underutilized effective pharmacological treatment against depression.

Psychostimulants. The use of psychostimulants in treating depression in athletes is usually contraindicated because psychostimulants are currently banned in most competitive athletic organizations. Professional athletes and olympic-level athletes should not be prescribed amphetamines.

Prognosis for the treatment of depression improves as patients are treated for a typical duration of 3–6 months with attempts of tapering medications after that period. Recent literature suggests a certain subgroup of depressed patients may indeed benefit from longer term treatment of antidepressant therapy, i.e., greater than 1 year's duration. This is, however, extremely variable and should be based on patient compliance and symptom resolution.

Anxiety Disorders

Anxiety is best characterized by subjective feelings of anticipation, dread, apprehension, or a sense of impending disaster associated with varying degrees of autonomic arousal and reactivity. Anxiety can lead to changes in behavior, thus playing an important role in learning and adaptation. This factor may be particularly pertinent in the athletic environment because it relates to athletic performance. The specific psychiatric syndromes of anxiety include:

Generalized Anxiety

The patient with generalized anxiety has an unrealistic or excessive worry about various life circumstances. In addition, there are typically symptoms of motor tension (trembling, restlessness, easy fatigability), and symptoms of autonomic hyperactivity (shortness of breath, dry mouth, sweating). There may also be symptoms of vigilance and scanning, such as an athlete who is "edgy".

Differential diagnosis includes organic causes of anxiety, including hyperthyroidism, hypertension, caffeinism, unstable angina, and substance abuse. Particular substances include stimulants and alcohol withdrawal. In addition, the clinician must rule out major depression and adjustment disorders because these depressive illnesses are also present with anxiety.

The treatment for anxiety includes both pharmacological and nonpharmacological methods. The benzodiazepine class of medications are the treatment of choice for most anxiety disorders, especially generalized anxiety disorder and panic disorder. Tolerance can develop to the sedative effects, but not to the anxiolytic properties. These medications do have addictive properties, especially in their additive effects when taken with alcohol use. Commonly, combined treatment of benzodiazepines with antidepressant therapy is effective for most anxiety disorders. Nonpharmacological measures include behavioral therapies, i.e., systemic desensitization, relaxation training, and biofeedback. In addition, individual psychotherapy may also be particularly important for a student athlete with specific psychosocial stressors that may cause an anxious state: these include psychodynamic therapy and cognitive behavioral therapy, that is, identification of irrational beliefs and thoughts. One of the best things a clinician can do is to provide an empathetic environment for the student athlete to discuss the student's anxiety, because this often produces therapeutic benefit.

Obsessive Compulsive Disorder (OCD)

OCD is characterized by recurrent obsessions and compulsions with near-magical thinking. Obsessions are thoughts or images that are involuntary, intrusive, and anxiety provoking. They often have a sexual, violent, or derogatory connotation, and provoke severe anxiety. These symptoms are almost always troublesome to the patient. Compulsions refer to impulses to perform a variety of stereotyped behaviors or rituals that serve to reduce anxiety or get rid of obsessions. The patient usually experiences a sense of relief upon completing the compulsive act. The diagnosis of OCD should be made when these symptoms cause marked distress to the individual or interfere with social or occupational functioning. Many competitive athletes have obsessive compulsive personalities, but unless the ritualistic behaviors cause dysfunction, these traits are not considered a disorder. Symptoms of OCD usually begin in childhood and young adulthood with marked variability and dysfunction.

Differential diagnosis includes schizophrenia, major depression, exercise addiction, compulsive gambling, and substance abuse, especially alcohol and cocaine. OCD must be differentiated from obsessive compulsive personality.

Treatment issues may be complex and difficult, and often these patients are best referred to a psychiatrist. Psychosocial treatments include behavioral therapy using exposure, modeling, and response prevention, with careful attention to thought-stopping techniques. Although supportive psychotherapy may be helpful, it usually does not help the patient deal with the problematic ritualistic behavior. Pharmacotherapy includes antidepressants, especially the serotonergic class of antidepressants, i.e., fluoxetine, clomipramine, and imipramine. Other medications that have recently been studied for OCD therapy but remain in clinical trial include paroxetine and sertraline. The MAOIs phenelzinesulfate (Nardil) and tranylcypromine (Parnate) have also been tried. Antianxiety medications may also be helpful for the obsessive compulsive patient who has extreme autonomic arousal.

Panic Disorder

Panic as a symptom is usually a subjective feeling more powerful than normally experienced. Panic has a sudden onset without a clear precipitant and is generally associated with physical symptoms of autonomic nervous system activation. Panic has a catastrophic quality not present in more general forms of anxiety. Individuals with this disorder have a sense of impending doom and may think they are going to die. Disorientation can be seen. Symptoms of panic may last from a few minutes to a few hours. Panic disorder with agoraphobia includes full-blown panic symptoms with a fear of being in places or situations from which escape might be difficult (or embarrassing), or in which help may not be available in the event of a panic attack. Common trigger situations for the student athlete include being outside the home alone, being in a crowd—especially in a stadium situation, or traveling by bus, train, or car. Panic may also be seen in the athlete who is fearful of travel away from home.

Differential diagnosis includes organic precipitants of panic attack including cardiac arrythmias, hypoglycemia (seen in athletes with restricted diets), vertigo, drug and alcohol abuse, hypochondriasis, generalized anxiety disorder, and performance anxiety. The clinician must also be careful to rule out hyperthyroidism as a cause of panic attacks. In addition, the clinician must do electrocardiographic testing because a fairly high association of mitral valve prolapse (8 to 20%) exists in patients with panic disorder. In fact, mitral valve prolapse and panic disorder may coexist and be treated not only for the cardiac condition but also for the panic disorder. Treatment includes pharmacotherapy based on the severity of the attack, the frequency of attacks, and the amount of dysfunction. Medications may be especially helpful for patients with prominent depressive symptoms; these medications include antidepressants, specifically MAOIs, imipramine and fluoxetine. Benzodiazepines, especially alprazolam

(Xanax), are most helpful because of their rapid onset; this can be useful early in treatment when psychosocial dysfunction is greatest. In certain situations, beta-blockers (propranolol) have been used for panic attacks. They are contraindicated in athletes with asthma, however, and are relatively contraindicated in athletes with heart disease, especially conduction abnormalities and diabetes, because beta-blockers may mask hypoglycemia. Also important is psychosocial therapy which usually deals with supportive and insight-oriented therapy to help the athlete deal with the psychosocial complications of panic attacks. Exposure therapies are also helpful in dealing with the athletes' fear and avoidance behavior.

Phobias are more common in athletes than one might think. A phobic athlete's panic attack is always related to a particular situation that is either feared or avoided. In contrast, the panic attacks of panic disorder often are spontaneous and not necessarily related to a phobic stimulus. There are several types of phobias. Agoraphobia, the fear of being alone in public situations, may occur when athletes leave home, for example.

Treatment for agoraphobia usually includes psychosocial therapy, primarily behavioral therapy issues of exposure treatment (systematic desensitization), and cognitive therapy (identifying irrational beliefs and thoughts). Psychotherapy may be facilitated by use of relaxation therapy to help decrease the patient's overall physiological arousal. Support groups and family therapy have also been known to be effective. If agoraphobia presents with specific panic attacks, benzodiazepine therapy may be indicated as it is in panic disorder. Long-term treatment with benzodiazepines in agoraphobia should be avoided.

Another type of phobia is social. Athletes may have specific fears, such as a fear of speaking in public, whereas others may have more general fears of being embarrassed, humiliated, scrutinized, or unable to perform in public or social situations, or most common, when athletes are being competitively judged. They key to the diagnosis is that the anxiety increases as the individual approaches a situation that may be avoided or can be endured only with extreme anxiety. In sports situations, the anxiety is usually displayed as tremulousness or speaking inappropriately while in the feared competitive environment.

Pharmacotherapy for social phobia includes the benzodiazepines, i.e., the anxiolytics, and the beta-blockers, (e.g., propranolol). Long-term treatment of the social phobias may be facilitated by the use of antidepressants including serotonin-specific agents and also the MAOIs. Beta-blockers are banned in international competition in certain sports such as the biathlon. Psychosocial therapy for the social phobias includes desensitization through gradual exposure to the anxiety-provoking situation. Use of an anxiety hierarchy is essential. If there are underlying emotional problems that precipitate social phobias, psychotherapy may be helpful.

Simple phobias usually start in childhood and are quite common. They involve a persistent fear of a circumscribed stimulus (object or situation) other than the fear of having a panic attack (as in panic disorder), or a humiliation in social situations (as in social phobia). Exposure to the stimulus produces an immediate anxiety response. The object or situation is usually avoided, and this avoidant behavior becomes more and more disruptive to the person's normal routine. Simple phobias are best treated with psychosocial therapies such as desensitization and exposure therapy. An insight-oriented approach showing the phobia as unrealistic may also be helpful.

Post-Traumatic Stress Disorder (PTSD)

PTSD is defined as the temporal relationship between a recognizable traumatic event and the development of symptoms that result in impairment of psychological, social, and physical function. Stressors involved are generally outside the range of normal experience (rape, sexual abuse, assault, traffic accidents, natural disasters, among others). There is an increasing emphasis, however, on the nature of extraordinary athletic injuries, including back and knee injuries, as a definable cause of PTSD in athletes. The clinician will see several different disturbances, including a re-experiencing of the traumatic event in the form of either nightmares or flashbacks. In addition, a numbing of general responsiveness is also noted, with a tendency toward being easily startled. Persistent symptoms of increased arousal are noted, especially with activation of the autonomic nervous system (tachycardia, dry mouth, constipation). In the athlete, it is not unusual to see symptoms of physiological reactivity (increased arousal) upon exposure to events that symbolize an aspect of the traumatic event. For example, an athlete with a serious knee injury may have extreme physiological arousal, and an exaggerated startle response when re-exposed to someone's brushing up against the athlete's knee. This symbolism of contact may be enough to precipitate extreme physiological symptoms of anxiety seen in PTSD. In addition to an exaggerated startle response, irritable and, at times, oppositional behavior may be exhibited. This may be the first sign of an athlete who is having difficulty following a traumatic event.

Differential diagnosis for PTSD includes adjustment disorder, substance abuse, and panic disorder.

Treatment issues for PTSD often include the necessity of decreasing physiological arousal, often best facilitated with a low dose of benzodiazepine.

For nightmares, flashbacks, and sleep disturbance, antidepressant therapy with particular attention to the tricyclic antidepressants and serotonergic antidepressants are extremely useful. Psychosocial therapies are similar to those seen in other anxiety disorders where group therapy (injury rehabilitation groups) can be extremely helpful, as well as individual therapy focusing on eventual re-exposure to the stimulus that may have precipitated the post-traumatic stress. In other words, a clinical decision will need to be made at some point in regard to the athlete's re-exposure to the athletic event if this is where the trauma occurred. This process can take several weeks to months, and the clinician must show great patience in working with the athlete who has this significant anxiety disorder.

Pharmacotherapy of Anxiety Disorders

The use of benzodiazepine treatment, i.e., anxiolytics, should be done only after careful consideration. The benzodiazepines are an extremely helpful class of medications that may significantly reduce anxiety, but side effects such as sedation, short-term memory loss, and slowed coordination may be particularly bothersome for athletes. These medications may produce intoxication and this fact should be carefully considered before prescription. Benzodiazepines should be used as therapy only in specific circumstances:

Generalized Anxiety Disorder. Use of medications such as lorazepam (Ativan), alprazolam (Xanax), and the longer-acting clonazepam (Klonopin) is extremely helpful for treatment of generalized anxiety disorder. Adjunctive use of antidepressant therapy such as imipramine or the serotonergic reuptake inhibitors are often helpful.

Panic Disorder. Pharmacotherapy with benzodiazepines for panic disorder is extremely helpful, although evidence suggests that medication use does not effectively treat the agoraphobia as manifested in panic disorder. This factor is best treated by psychotherapy and behavioral management.

Post-traumatic Stress Disorder. PTSD in athletes, especially following traumatic injury, is effectively treated with benzodiazepine therapy, because decreasing anxiety may help with pain management, insomnia, and a decrease in irritability. In this particular situation, benzodiazepines should be used for a short period, i.e., 2–4 weeks. If symptoms persist longer than this, antidepressant medication may be more helpful. In other anxiety disorders, such as stress-related anxiety, which is extremely common in athletes, and phobias—including social phobias (performance anxiety)—do not *always* respond to benzodiazepine therapy. Often in these types of anxiety disorders chemical dependence and tolerance may become an issue. It is therefore recommended that the use of benzodiazepines be restricted to the above specific anxiety disorders.

Antidepressant Medication. Tricyclic antidepressants such as imipramine have a long track record in successfully treating anxieties such as panic disorder and generalized anxiety disorder. Often MAOIs such as phenelzene sulfate (Nardil) and tranylcypromine sulfate (Parnate) are first-line choices for treatment of athletes with panic disorder. These are underutilized. In addition, recent evidence suggests use of SSRIs, i.e., fluoxetine (Prozac) and paroxetine (Paxil), may be extremely helpful in the treatment of both generalized anxiety disorder and panic disorder.

Psychotic Illness

Psychosis is not common in athletic populations. Psychotic symptoms are described as fixed, false beliefs. In other words, the patient is not in touch with reality. Common syndromes in this category include schizophrenia, manic depressive psychosis, and major depression with psychosis. Psychotic symptoms may also include paranoid delusions and paranoid thinking. From my clinical experience, the most common psychotic symptoms seen in athletes are those associated with major depressive illness, as anywhere from 10–15% of depressed patients may have delusional thinking. This should be carefully evaluated when diagnosing depression in an athlete. The clinician should also be aware of psychosis in athletic populations that is secondary to substance abuse, namely abuse of psychostimulants and hallucinogenics. Such symptoms are typically short-lived and dose-related. Although schizophrenia is not uncommon, schizophrenic illnesses can be precipitated by extreme psychosocial stressors, including psychosocial stressors incurred during or after athletic competition. Athletes who experience psychotic symptoms are typically referred to psychiatric specialists in consultation with the primary care physician. Symptoms include looseness of association, disorganized thought processes, paranoid thinking, and extreme social and interpersonal isolation, typically with decreased self-hygiene. The onset is usually insidious, over a period of weeks to months. Organic causes of psychosis may include substance abuse, namely amphetamines and psychostimulants, hyperthyroidism, the hyperglycemia of diabetes mellitus, steroid therapy including corticosteroid therapy, and anabolic steroid use.

The typical treatment for psychotic illness includes the use of antipsychotic medications such as haloperidol (Haldol); thiothxene (Navane), and thioridazine (Melaril) or treatment of the underlying medical condition causing psychosis.

Personality Disorders

Every individual has a personality or certain personality traits to distinguish that person from others. This is, of course, not to say that everyone has a personality disorder. Personality traits are enduring patterns of perceiving, relating to, and thinking about the environment and oneself, and are exhibited in a wide range of important social and personal contexts. Personality disorders become evident when these traits become inflexible and maladaptive, and cause either significant impairment in social or occupational functioning or subjective distress. Usually this maladaptive behavior is evident by adolescence or young adulthood.

Most personality disorders can be grouped into three different areas.

The personality disorders characterized by oddness or eccentricity include paranoid, schizoid, and schizotypic personality disorders. Whereas these personality disorders often include unusual thoughts as well as behavior, they do not include psychosis. Typically, these personality disorder patients are loners, aloof and resistant to having relationships with other people. Care must be taken with these patients to legitimize their need for privacy and individualism and to avoid confrontation unless absolutely necessary. Clear boundaries and roles, especially in the athlete, are important when dealing with a paranoid personality.

The dramatic, emotional personalities include histrionic, narcissistic, antisocial, and borderline. These patients tend to have an exaggerated response to stressful situations, and thus often tax the clinician's patience and time. The histrionic patient has exaggerated mannerisms and often employees seduction as a means to express their need for relationships. Care should be taken to be professional and courteous but not be become involved in the patient's excessive clinging. The narcissistic patient has an exaggerated sense of self-importance and often sees himself as the center of the universe. These patients may be demanding, erratic in their behavior, and sometimes hostile. They usually have a great difficulty handling close relationships, especially with coaches, medical staff, and other athletes as well as training staff. The narcissistic patient's sense of self-esteem must be bolstered by professional, honest, courteous, non-patronizing behavior. Confrontations can exacerbate the narcissistic person's sense of integrity. The antisocial patient frequently gets into trouble with the law, abuses drugs and alcohol, and generally speaking has little regard for the welfare of others. Such patients are challenging to work with because their sense of autonomy is derived from self-satisfaction. Treat these patients with respect, but with clear boundaries as to what is acceptable and unacceptable behavior. The borderline patient provides a unique perspective for the clinician in dealing with frustration because these patients are prone to self-injurious behavior, chemical dependency, and hostile-dependent relationships with caretakers. The borderline patient has a very fragile ego and is prone to misinterpretation and misunderstanding. Direct descriptions of roles for the student athlete with a borderline personality disorder are important, because these patients have a tendency to play one person against another. Team management of athletic problems is the rule here. A psychotherapeutic relationship with a mental health professional is often extremely helpful.

The last category of personality disorders include those whose primary signs involve anxiety and fear. These include avoidant, dependent, passive-aggressive and compulsive personality disorders. Generally speaking, these patients have very precarious relationships with others and can be manipulative, especially in regard to the management of athletic injury. Care must be taken to be direct and honest, with a reassuring approach, yet careful not to develop pathologically dependent relationships with these student athletes. Encouragement of the athlete to develop independent skills is important, as is developing self-esteem.

When dealing with personality disorders in athletes, the manifestations of a personality disorder often develop under such stress as is typical in the athletic environment. Several different stressors generally cause the clinician to become aware of the student with a personality disorder. These stressors include athletic injury, where a patient sabotages rehabilitation by overworking or missing appointments. Second, consistently poor performance with resultant worry, i.e., acting out behavior at practice, not obeying rules, getting into fights, back-stabbing comments to other teammates, and not listening, can be a significant symptom of a patient with a passive-aggressive, borderline, or antisocial personality. Another stressor that may precipitate symptoms of a personality disorder include demotion in playing status or situations that an athlete cannot control. This often raises anxiety significantly and the patient will attempt to defend against this anxiety in keeping with their personality. All athletes have individual personalities, which is not to say that all athletes have personality disorders. The clinician must be comfortable with the different types of personalities, the way athletes use these individual personalities to defend against anxiety, and to be able to work *with,* rather than *against,* the athlete to help them deal with stressful situations. If the clinician can take the time to understand where the athlete is coming from and work with their personality, he or she may be able to avoid many unnecessary confrontations and problematic relationships with the student athlete.

REFERENCES

1. Alderman RB: Psychological Behavior in Sport. Philadelphia, W.B. Saunders Co., 1974.
2. Frost RB: Psychological Concepts Applied to Physical Education and Coaching. Reading, MA, Addison-Wesley Publishing Company, 1971.
3. Orlick T: In Pursuit of Excellence. Champaign, IL, Human Kinetics Publishers, Inc., 1980.
4. Suinn RM: Psychology in Sports: Methods and Applications. Burgess Publishing Co., 1980.
5. Williams JM (ed): Applied Sport Psychology. Palo Alto, CA, Mayfield Publishing Company, 1986.

10

Eating Disorders in Athletes

Ann C. Grandjean, Ed. D.
Glenda R. Woscyna, M.S., R.D.
Jaime S. Ruud, M.S., R.D.

Eating disorders are not a new phenomenon. Accounts of self-inflicted starvation and weight loss date back to the Middle Ages, and accounts of emphasis on slimness in Ancient Egypt, Greece, and Rome also can be found. The Romans are known for designing the vomitorium, a site where vomiting was used as a method of weight control after gorging.[7,48]

What is new is a greater awareness of eating disorders among athletes, with a proliferation in recent years in interest, research, and publications related to this problem. Case studies illustrate the intense emotional distress many athletes have regarding food, body weight, and body image.[51] Although the incidence of eating disorders in athletes is not well defined, it appears to occur more often in sports that emphasize leanness.[6,8,10,42,43,46] Dancers and gymnasts are the most frequently studied sport groups, followed by figure skaters and runners. Eating disorders, however, are not limited to these sports. Pathogenic weight control practices also have been reported in female swimmers[5,17] and softball players.[49]

While eating disorders can affect both male and female athletes, research shows that it is more prevalent among females. Results of a survey administered to NCAA athletic programs indicate that 15 of 17 women's sport categories reported at least one incidence of an eating disorder compared with 11 of 20 men's sport categories.[14]

It is speculated that females are at greater risk for developing eating problems for several reasons. Society places more pressure on females than on males to be thin, which is exemplified by the fact that even adolescent girls who are underweight for height are dieting to combat their fears of becoming obese.[30,37] Studies show that, for many girls, weight and dieting concerns emerge between the ages of 9 and 11.[30,36]

Another factor in the development of abnormal eating behaviors in young women relates to the family environment.[28,33] According to Johnson et al.,[28] there is remarkable consistency in the descriptions of parents of anorexics. Mothers are reportedly domineering, overprotective, and critical, while fathers are passive, submissive, emotionally insensitive, and withdrawn. Additionally, alcoholism, sexual abuse, physical abuse, and financial problems may also be present in families of anorexics.[28]

In female athletes, pressures from coaches and parents to reduce body size for competition as well as attitudes about body image may encourage disordered eating practices. Thus, it is important for coaches, physicians and other professionals working with young female athletes to evaluate eating attitudes and habits and be aware of the warning signs that are associated with inappropriate eating behaviors.

DEFINITIONS

Eating disorder refers to a distorted pattern of thought and behavior about food. While this term conventionally refers to anorexia nervosa or bulimia nervosa, it has also been applied to chronic overeating or binge eating that results in a weight greater than that which was biologically intended.

Anorexia nervosa is self-imposed starvation in an obsessive effort to lose weight and achieve thinness (Table 1).[3] The anorexic individual often looks malnourished due to the extreme thinness. However, when looking in a mirror, anorexics perceive themselves as fat. A common behavior in anorexia is a constant preoccupation with and discussion of weight, food, and dieting. Everything related to food or weight becomes highly emotional. To increase weight loss, anorexics may engage in exces-

TABLE 1. Diagnostic Criteria for Anorexia Nervosa

A. Refusal to maintain body weight at or above a minimally normal weight for age and height (e.g., weight loss leading to maintenance of body weight less than 85% of that expected: or failure to make expected weight gain during period of growth, leading to body weight less than 85% of that expected).
B. Intense fear of gaining weight or becoming fat, even though underweight.
C. Disturbance in the way in which one's body weight or shape is experienced, undue influence of body weight or shape on self-evaluation, or denial of the seriousness of the current low body weight.
D. In postmenarcheal females, amenorrhea, i.e., the absence of at least three consecutive menstrual cycles. (A woman is considered to have amenorrhea if her periods occur only following hormone, e.g., estrogen, administration.)

Specify type:

Restricting Type: during the current episode of Anorexia Nervosa, the person has not regularly engaged in binge-eating or purging behavior (i.e., self-induced vomiting or the misuse of laxatives, diuretics, or enemas)

Binge-Eating/Purging Type: during the current episode of Anorexia Nervosa, the person has regularly engaged in binge-eating or purging behavior (i.e., self-induced vomiting or the misuse of laxatives, diuretics, or enemas)

Adapted from Diagnostic and Statistical Manual of Mental Disorders IV. Washington, DC, American Psychiatric Association, 1994.

sive exercise regimens. As weight loss continues, they often become depressed, withdrawn, irritable, and show a lack of interest in social activities.

Anorexia nervosa includes significant weight loss, body distortion and, in 30 to 50 percent of cases, bulimic behaviors. As recently as 20 years ago, anorexia was considered rare. It is currently estimated to occur in 0.5–1.0% of the adolescent and young adult woman population. Incidence in males is estimated at 1/10 of the occurrence in females. Of anorexics who have received treatment, long-term outcome data reveal a mortality of 6%.[24]

Bulimia nervosa is identified as recurring binge eating, usually followed by purging (Table 2).[3] The bulimic usually appears within normal weight range, but may experience weight fluctuations greater than 10 pounds. Vomiting, laxative abuse, and intense exercise are purging methods often used to relieve guilt and avoid weight gain. The person with bulimia binges to cope with or avoid emotional stress. All too often, bulimia emerges in the midst of strenuous dieting efforts due to dissatisfaction with body shape and weight. When hunger or the desire for certain foods becomes overpowering, a binge occurs. The binge/purge cycle becomes repetitive to the point where it can no longer be controlled or stopped. As the cycle continues, feelings of depression and low self-esteem increase.

The term "bulimia nervosa" was first used in 1976 to describe this pattern of purging to lose weight and did not appear in the Diagnostic and Statistical Manual for Mental Disorders until 1980. Incidence is estimated at 4–5% of the adolescent and young adult female population.[3]

INCIDENCE AMONG ATHLETES

Reports of the incidence of eating disorders vary with sport and the diagnostic tool used to measure eating disorders. The Eating Attitudes Test (EAT) and the Eating Disorder Inventory (EDI) are the measures frequently use. The EAT is a 40-item measure of eating and dieting behaviors and attitudes associated with eating disorders.[20] The EDI is a 64-item, self-report, multi-scale measure designed to assess a broad range of psychological and behavioral traits common in person with anorexia nervosa or bulimia.[22] Both of these measures are standardized self-report instruments with demonstrated reliability and validity.

Some investigators, however, have developed their own surveys or questionnaires specifically for use with athletes. For example, Rosen and Hough[42] and Dummer et al.[17] administered the Michigan State University (MSU) Weight Control Survey to groups of young female gymnasts and male and female swimmers, respectively. The MSU survey is a

TABLE 2. Diagnostic Criteria for Bulmia Nervosa

A. Recurrent episodes of binge-eating. An episode of binge eating is characterized by both of the following:
   (1) eating, in a discrete period of time (e.g., within any 2-hour period), an amount of food that is definitely larger than most people would eat during a similar period of time and under similar circumstances
   (2) a sense of lack of control over eating during the episode (e.g., a feeling that one cannot stop eating or control what or how much one is eating)
B. Recurrent inappropriate compensatory behavior in order to prevent weight gain, such as self-induced vomiting; misuse of laxatives, diuretics, enemas, or other medications; fasting; or excessive exercise.
C. The binge eating and inappropriate compensatory behaviors both occur, on average, at least twice a week for 3 months.
D. Self-evaluation is unduly influenced by body shape and weight.
E. The distrubance does not occur exclusively during episodes of Anorexia Nervosa.

Specify type:

Purging Type: during the current episode of Bulimia Nervosa, the person has regularly engaged in self-induced vomiting or the misuse of laxatives, diuretics, or enemas

Nonpurging Type: during the current episode of Bulimia Nervosa, the person has used other inappropriate compensatory behaviors, such as fasting or excessive exercise, but has not regularly engaged in self-induced vomiting or the misuse of laxatives, diuretics, or enemas

Adapted from Diagnostic and Statistical Manual of Mental Disorders IV. Washington DC, American Psychiatric Association, 1994.

three-part survey of weight-control behaviors developed for athletes to identify factors associated with use of pathogenic weight-control measures. Rosen and Hough[42] reported that 62% of female gymnasts were using at least one form of pathogenic weight control. In the study by Dummer et al,[17] 15.4% of female (n=487) and 3.6% of male swimmers (n=468) used pathogenic weight-control techniques.

Burckes-Miller and Black[9] surveyed 695 male and female athletes from 22 midwestern colleges and universities. The authors developed a four-page, 41-item questionnaire using DSM-III-R criteria. Twenty-one athletes (3%) met the criteria for anorexia and 195 (21.5%) for bulimia.

In the studies of female ballet dancers, 6–33% were at risk for anorexia nervosa.[8,18,21] Kurtzman et al. [32] reported that, overall, dancers had the highest prevalence of anorexia nervosa symptoms when compared with other groups of university female students. Similarly, Brooks-Gunn et al.[8] concluded that ballet dancers showed more restraint when eating than did skaters or swimmers. All of these studies employed either the EDI or the EAT.

Using the Bulimia Test-Revised (BULIT-R),[50] a 36-item, self-report measure based on the diagnostic criteria of DSM-III-R, Petrie and Stoever[41] determined the prevalence of bulimia nervosa and pathogenic weight control behaviors among 218 female gymnasts. Results showed that approximately 4% of the gymnasts were classified as bulimic.

Compared with female swimmers, however, the gymnasts studied by Benson et.al.[4] showed fewer tendencies towards eating disorders, 11% vs. 1%. Elite-level gymnasts reported being more satisfied with their bodies and less concerned about weight than nonelite gymnasts.[25] However, according to Weight and Noakes,[52] elite distance runners are more likely than nonelite distance runners to show physical and psychological features of anorexia nervosa. They used the EAT and EDI as a measure of the incidence of anorexia nervosa in 125 female distance runners (marathon, elite marathon, cross-country, and control). The highest percentage of abnormal EAT scores (>30) occurred in the elite marathon and cross-country groups.

The prevalence of eating disorder–related symptoms may be greater than the prevalence of eating disorders.[32] Schotte and Stunkard[44] surveyed 1,965 university students and found that although binge eating and self-induced vomiting are common among college women, clinically significant bulimia, as described in DSM-IV, is not.

IDENTIFYING AN ATHLETE WITH AN EATING DISORDER

There is a distinct difference between being thin and having anorexia nervosa, as well as between vomiting to reach a mandatory weight and having bulimia. Abnormal eating behaviors do not automatically signal an eating disorder. In fact, normalized eating habits and weight gain after season usually indicate that the athlete does not have an eating disorder. However, assessment is indicated if an athlete exhibits the following warning signs.

Warning Signs for Anorexia Nervosa[38]

- Dramatic loss in weight
- Preoccupation with food, calories, and weight
- Constantly wearing baggy or layered clothing
- Relentless, excessive exercise
- Mood swings
- Avoiding food-related social activities

Warning Signs for Bulimia Nervosa[38]

- Noticeable weight loss or gain
- Excessive concern about weight
- Bathroom visits after meals
- Depressive moods
- Strict dieting followed by binges
- Increasing criticism of one's body

Warning signs that the team physician or sports nutritionist may not be exposed to, but may be detected by teammates, coaches, and trainers include food wrappers in the locker room, sneaking food from the training table, and complaining frequently of constipation. Clues that a serious problem is present are emotional instability and withdrawal from social relationships.[34] Unusual eating patterns alone are not sufficient for diagnosis of an eating disorder, and only suggest that evaluation by a professional trained in the area of eating disorders is indicated.

While few researchers have compared athletes and nonathletes in terms of behavioral and psychological traits associated with eating disorders, Taub and Blinde[49] did find significant differences on two of the eight subscales of the Eating Disorder Inventory (EDI). The athletes they studied were more likely to be perfectionists and to engage in uncontrollable overeating than nonathletes. The athletes, however, also reported higher self-esteem scores. In a survey by Borgen and Corbin,[6] compared with nonathletes, athletes scored higher on drive for thinness, bulimia, body dissatisfaction, perfectionism subscales.

MEDICAL COMPLICATIONS OF ANOREXIA AND BULIMIA

Anorexia

Athletes with eating disorders are susceptible to significant medical complications that can be life threatening. Palla and Litt[40] reported that adolescents with anorexia or bulimia exhibited derangement in every organ system evaluated. Cardiovascular abnormalities were frequent, including bradycardia, prolonged corrected QT intervals, dysrhythmias, and marked orthostatic pulse and BP instability. Hypothermia, with temperatures less than 35.5° C (95.9°F), was common. Electrolyte imbalances occurred in patients who vomited or purged. Hypokalemia was most common, but hypocalcemia and hypophosphatemia also were noted. The reported abnormalities were secondary to malnutrition or to the methods used to achieve weight loss. However, symptoms were rarely present and were typically denied by the patients.

General Medical Signs and Symptoms of Anorexia Nervosa[51]

- Amenorrhea
- Gastrointestinal problems
- Cardiac arrhythmias
- Hypotension
- Hypothermia
- Dehydration and electrolyte complications

Amenorrhea is one of the diagnostic criteria for anorexia. In a study of adolescents with anorexia nervosa and bulimia nervosa,[40] all anorexic patients had primary or secondary amenorrhea. A total of 22% of bulimic patients had secondary amenorrhea, with menstrual irregularity being more common among bulimic patients at lower weights.

Among athletes in general, the prevalence of amenorrhea varies depending on sport groups. In a study of 226 elite athletes, gymnasts had the highest incidence of amenorrhea (71%), followed by lightweight rowers (46%) and runners (45%).[53]

There is a high incidence of amenorrhea and irregular menstrual cycles in ballet dancers.[11,13] Thirty-three percent of the university and professional dancers studied by Benson et al.[5] experienced abnormal or absent cycles. In another study of 89 young professional ballet dancers, 15% reported secondary amenorrhea and 30% reported irregular cycles.[19]

Johnson et al.[27] believe anorexics are aware of their menstrual threshold and strive to maintain themselves below it. They speculate that self-starvation, low body weight, and excessive exercise, all of which inhibit menstruation, are the tools used to manage pubertal demands and maintain internal control.

Amenorrhea is not a harmless alteration of endocrine status. It is associated with decreased bone mineral content of the lumbar spine,[16,39] a greater incidence of scoliosis among adolescents, and a greater incidence of stress fractures.[12,26,35] Although the long-term consequences of amenorrhea are unknown, a major concern is osteoporosis, as extended periods of amenorrhea can lead to irreversible bone loss.[15]

The Female Athlete Triad

Physicians who attend female athletes should be cognizant of the relationship between eating disorders, amenorrhea, and osteoporosis. A panel of experts convened in 1992 has labeled this triad of disorders "the female athlete triad".[56] Young women who are driven to excel in their chosen sport may develop an eating disorder, osteoporosis, and amenorrhea. As a result, these athletes tend to have lower bone mass and may be at increased risk of stress fractures. Each of these disorders, individually or collectively, can affect an athlete's health and performance.

All young female athletes should be considered at risk. However, factors that apparently increase an athlete's risk of developing one or more of the triad disorders include the pressure to excel and the constant focus on achieving or maintaining "ideal" body weight and/or "optimal" body fat.[56]

Some physicians believe that amenorrhea is the most obvious sign of an athlete who may be suffering from the triad.[45] Unfortunately, amenorrhea is a symptom of which the coach or trainer may not be aware. Thus, as part of the preparticipation exam, the physician should obtain a menstrual history, including the age of menstruation, frequency and duration of the cycles, last period, and any hormonal therapy the athlete may be taking.[56]

Bulimia

Several features of anorexia nervosa are also seen in bulimia. However, the primary characteristic—emaciation—is not present. Most bulimics are of normal weight. One study[11] reported the most common physical symptoms of bulimics include swelling of hands and feet, abdominal fullness, fatigue, headache, and nausea.

The most serious medical consequences, fluid and electrolyte imbalances, result from vomiting.[47] Enamel erosion and swollen parotid glands are also symptoms of bulimia. Abuse of diuretics and laxatives can also lead to dehydration and electrolyte abnormalities, resulting in loss of muscular strength and endurance.

General Medical Signs and Symptoms of Bulimia Nervosa[51]

- Menstrual irregularities
- Dental and gum disease
- Swollen parotid glands
- Gastrointestinal problems
- Electrolyte abnormalities and dehydration

IS ATHLETICS TO BLAME?

The sport environment is often identified as a cause of an eating disorder. Fingers are pointed at coaches, weigh-ins, imposed weight restrictions, and activities that are a normal part of athletics. However, the word "cause" is inappropriate. An eating disorder is a symptom of underlying distress. It is first a coping mechanism and then becomes an additional problem. The athlete who has an eating disorder will also have a history of low self-esteem and difficulty with problem-solving and coping with stress.

It is possible, however, for an eating disorder to be "triggered" by a single event or by comments from a person who is close to the athlete. Coaches, trainers, and teammates are significant people in athletes' lives and, as a result, have the power to be helpful or harmful. An off-handed remark can become deeply imbedded in the mind of a potential anorexic or bulimic. Rosen and Hough[42] reported that 75% of the gymnasts who were told by their coaches that they were too heavy resorted to dangerous weight control measures to lose weight. Young athletes may need only one or two suggestions about reducing body fat before they begin pathogenic eating behaviors.[57]

Athletes who have developed eating disorders often refer to traumatic experiences involving weigh-ins. Coaches may weigh team members and hold them responsible for a certain weight. The risk of triggering an eating disorder increases when weigh-ins result in unrealistic weight goals, browbeating or ridiculing, or excessive pressure on the athlete.

REFERRAL

While athletic trainers, coaches, sports nutritionists, and others who work with athletes can identify symptoms that may indicate risk, a diagnosis can be made only by a physician or professional with expertise in eating disorders, and preferably an eating disorders specialist who has worked with athletes. It is extremely important for schools, clubs, and organizations to have a system in place to identify athletes at risk, obtain documentation that a problem exists, and for securing treatment. There is no perfect system, and the exact procedure will vary with each case.

The athletic trainer is often the person to whom the athlete turns regarding an eating problem or after diagnosis. The athlete may resist seeing a psychologist or other professional because of denial and reluctance to reveal disorganized thoughts and feelings. Although the eating-disordered athlete may insist that the eating problem/weight problem can be solved with the help of only the athletic trainer or nutritionist, it is imperative that the athlete be referred to a professional who can effectively deal with the psychological aspects of eating disorders.

Many universities and colleges have student health centers or counseling centers with qualified professionals. Medical centers and some hospitals also provide assessment, counseling, and education for anorexia, bulimia, and compulsive overeating. If these services are not available, the Anorexia Nervosa & Related Eating Disorders (ANRE) maintains a referral list of over 2,000 professionals across the United States who have experience in treating individuals with eating disorders.

TREATMENT

Eating disorders are now accepted as having psychological, physiologic, and social components.[31] Treatment must therefore address each of these areas. The complex multifactorial nature of anorexia and bulimia requires an interdisciplinary team consisting of a physician, psychologist, and nutritionist (RD).[3] The physician monitors the athlete's medical condition and supervises overall treatment. The psychologist focuses on family and peer relationships as well as body image and eating disordered behavior. The nutritionist addresses diet and weight issues, disordered eating patterns, and co-facilitates body image group therapy. Figure 1 illustrates the interdisciplinary focus of nutrition education/counseling and psychotherapy in the treatment process.[54]

The professionals providing treatment need to work closely together so the messages communicated to the athlete are consistent. They also should have experience with and an appreciation for athletes and the sport environment. Thompson and Sherman[51] write: "To athletes . . . the sport world is very real. They may have trained for years in preparation to perform their sport. For many, their sport is their whole life, and being an athlete is who they are."

Most guidelines for the treatment of eating disorders have been developed based on clinical experience with nonathletes. There may be inherent differences in the treatment of athletes. For example, prohibiting exercise is sometimes used as a treatment component. This eliminates the potential to abuse exercise as a form of purging, helps in weight restoration, and balances caloric intake within healthful energy expenditures. However, such limitations may not be appropriate for athletes.

According to Johnson and Tobin,[29] one of the first issues likely to arise in treating an athlete is how the treatment plan will affect the athlete's training and performance schedule. Restrictive eating or excessive exercise may be directly related to the athlete's performance expectations.[29]

Weight gain is a priority in treatment because many of the presenting symptoms of an eating disorder are secondary to starvation. This condition must be reversed before the athlete can benefit from psychotherapy or nutrition counseling.[23] A weight gain of 1 to 1.5 kg (2 to 3 lbs) per week is promoted until the athlete achieves the goal weight. The goal weight

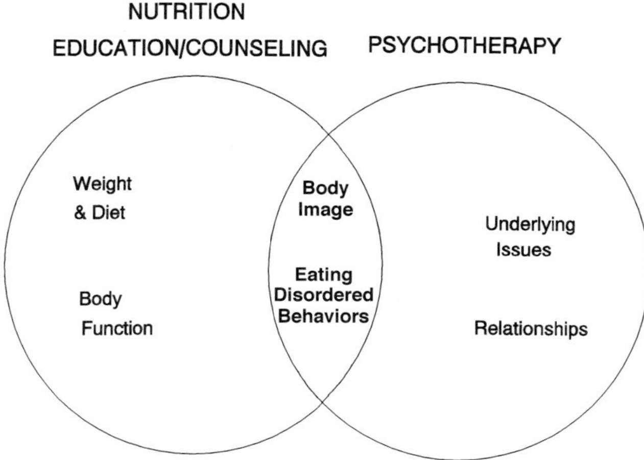

FIGURE 1. Interrelationship between nutritionists and psychotherapists in treating elements of eating disorders.[54]

should be based on height/weight tables, growth charts, and personal history, with the knowledge that many athletes weigh more than nonathletes.

Outpatient treatment is always preferred and generally is successful in treating normal weight patients with bulimia nervosa. Indications for inpatient care include emaciation, acute psychological stress, medical complications, and lack of progress in outpatient care.[55]

During the first several weeks or months of treatment, most patients devote a staggering amount of emotional energy to food and fear of fatness. The Eating Disorder Program at the University of Nebraska Medical Center, as a part of the nutrition education and counseling process, uses a series of structured activities (e.g., drawings, collages, poems) to help patients express their food and weight-related fears. Patients draw a picture of the images that appear in their minds when the nutritionist suggests, for example, they have a "hamburger and fries." The drawings reveal the intense anxiety, fear, and conflict patients have about food and weight issues. Using the visuals or drawings, patients begin to effectively verbalize their emotions relating to food.

PREVENTION

Physicians, athletic trainers, coaches, and others who work closely with athletes need to be informed about eating disorders—what they are, how to recognize the warning signs, what to do if a problem is suspected, and what treatment options are available. Being prepared to handle the situation when it is suspected that an athlete has a problem reduces the stress and assures that the athlete will receive the appropriate support and treatment.

Preparticipation exams provide an opportunity to determine the athlete's health status and to screen for possible eating disorders. One important component of the pre-exam is the medical and dietary history. Physicians should question athletes about their eating habits. If the physician detects concerns about weight control, nutrition counseling is advised. Early detection and intervention are important to the athlete's health and performance. Be aware, however, that athletes with anorexia or bulimia may be reluctant to discuss their eating habits or provide a reliable dietary history.

Physicians and those working with athletes may be more effective if they understand eating behavior within the sport environment. More research is needed to identify predictors for adolescent athletes who later develop anorexia and bulimia. Eating disorders may be prevented if early warning signs are recognized and if athletes are provided with realistic expectations about body weight, body image, and athletic performance.

REFERENCES

1. Abraham SF, Beumont PJV: How patients describe bulimia binge eating. Psychol Med 12:625-635, 1982.
2. Position of the American Dietetic Association: Nutrition intervention in the treatment of anorexia nervosa and bulimia nervosa. J Am Diet Assoc 88:68-71, 1988.
3. American Psychiatric Association: Diagnostic and Statistical Manual of Mental Disorders III-R, Washington, DC, 1987.
4. Benson JE, Alleman Y, Theintz GE, Howald H: Eating problems and calorie intake levels in Swiss adolescent athletes. Int J Sports Med 11:249-252, 1990.
5. Benson JE, Geiger CJ, Eiserman PA, Wardlaw GM: Relationship between nutrient intake, body mass index, menstrual function, and ballet injury. J Am Diet Assoc 89:58-64, 1989.
6. Borgen JS, Corbin CB: Eating disorders among female athletes. Physician Sportsmed 15(2):89-95, 1987.
7. Boskind-White M, White WC: Bulimarexia: A historical-sociocultural perspective. In Brownell KD, Foreyt JP (eds): Handbook of Eating Disorders. New York, Basic Books, 1986, pp 354-366.
8. Brooks-Gunn J, Warren MP, Hamilton LH: The relation of eating problems and amenorrhea in ballet dancers. Med Sci Sports Exerc 19:41-44, 1987.
9. Burckes-Miller ME, Black DR: Male and female college athletes: Prevalence of anorexia nervosa and bulimia nervosa. Athletic Training 23:137-140, 1988.

10. Calabrese LH: Nutritional and medical aspects of gymnastics. Clin Sports Med 4:23-30, 1985.
11. Calabrese LH, Kirkendall DT, Floyd M, et al: Menstrual abnormalities, nutritional patterns, and body composition in female classical ballet dancers. Physician Sportsmed 11:86-98, 1983.
12. Cann CE, Martin MC, Genant HK, Jaffe RB: Decreased spinal mineral content in amenorrheic women. JAMA 251:626, 1984.
13. Cohen JL, Potosnak L, Frank O, Baker H: A nutritional and hematologic assessment of elite ballet dancers. Physician Sportsmed 13:43, 1985.
14. Dick RW: Eating disorders in NCAA athletic programs. Athletic Training 26:136-140, 1991.
15. Drinkwater BL, Bruemner B, Chesnut CH: Menstrual history as a determinant of current bone density in young athletes. JAMA 263:545-548, 1990.
16. Drinkwater BL, Nilson K, Chesnut CH, et al: Bone mineral content of amenorrheic and eumenorrheic athletes. N Engl J Med 311:277-281, 1984.
17. Dummer GM, Rosen LW, Heuser WW, et al: Pathogenic weight-control behaviors of young competitive swimmers. Physician Sportsmed 15:75-84, 1987.
18. Evers CL: Dietary intake and symptoms of anorexia nervosa in female university dancers. J Am Diet Assoc 87:66-68, 1987.
19. Frisch RE, Wyshak G, Vincent L: Delayed menarche and amenorrhea in ballet dancers. N Engl J Med 303:17, 1980.
20. Garner DM, Garfinkel PE: The Eating Attitudes Test: An index of the symptoms of anorexia nervosa. Psychol Med 9:273-279, 1979.
21. Garner DM, Garfinkel PE: Socio-cultural factors in the development of anorexia nervosa. Psychol Med 10:647-656, 1980.
22. Garner DM, Olmstead MP, Polivy J: Development and validation of a multidimensional eating disorder inventory for anorexia nervosa and bulimia. Int J Eat Disord 2 (2):15-34, 1983.
23. Garner D, Rockert W, Olmsted M, et al:Psychoeducational principles in the treatment of bulimia and anorexia nervosa. In Garner D, Garfield P (eds): Handbook of Psychotherapy for Anorexia Nervosa and Bulimia. New York: Guilford Press, 1985, pp 530-541.
24. Halmi KA: Ten year study: Anorexia nervosa. Keynote address presented at the Tenth National Conference on Eating Disorders, Columbus, OH, November 1991.
25. Harris MB, Greco D: Weight control and weight concern in competitive female gymnasts. J Sport Exerc Psychol 12: 427, 1990.
26. Howat PM, Carbo ML, Mills GQ, Wozniak P: The influence of diet, body fat, menstrual cycling, and activity upon the bone density of females. J Am Diet Assoc 89:1305, 1989.
27. Johnson MD: Tailoring the preparticipation exam to female athletes. Physician Sportsmed 20(7):61-72, 1992.
28. Johnson CL, Sansone RA, Chewning M: Good reasons why young women would develop anorexia nervosa: The adaptive context. Pediatr Ann 21:731-737, 1992.
29. Johnson C, Tobin DL: The diagnosis and treatment of anorexia nervosa and bulimia among athletes. Athletic Training 26:119-128, 191.
30. Koff E, Rierdan J: Perceptions of weight and attitudes toward eating in early adolescent girls. J Adolesc Health 12:307-312, 1991.
31 Krey SH, Palmer K, Porcelli KA: Eating disorders: The clinical dietitian's changing role. J Am Diet Assoc 89:41-42, 1989.
32. Kurtzman FD, Yager J, Landsverk J, et al: Eating disorders among selected female student populations at UCLA. J Am Diet Assoc 89:45-50, 1989.
33. Larson BJ: Relationship of family communication patterns to Eating Disorder Inventory scores in adolescent girls. J Am Diet Assoc 91:1065-1067, 1991.
34. Mallick MJ, Whipple TW, Huerta E: Behavioral and psychological traits of weight-conscious teenagers: A comparison of eating-disordered patients and high- and low-risk groups. Adolescence 22:157-168, 1987.
35. Marcus R, Cann C, Madvig P, et al: Menstrual function and bone mass in elite women distance runners. Ann Intern Med 102:158-163, 1985.
36. Mellin LM, Irwin CE, Scully S: Prevalence of disordered eating in girls: A survey of middle-class children. J Am Diet Assoc 92:851-853, 1992.
37. Moses N, Banilivy MM, Lifshitz F: Fear of obesity among adolescent girls. Pediatrics 83:393-398, 1989.
38. National Collegiate Athletic Association: Nutrition and Eating Disorders Series. Three-part video series. Overland Park, KS, NCAA 1990.
39. Nelson ME, Fisher EC, Catsos PD, et al: Diet and bone status in amenorrheic runners. Am J Clin Nutr 43:910, 1986.
40. Palla B, Litt IF: Medical complications of eating disorders in adolescents. Pediatrics 81:613-623, 1988.
41. Petrie TA, Stoever S: The incidence of bulimia nervosa and pathogenic weight control behaviors in female collegiate gymnasts. Res Q Exerc Sport 64:238-241, 1993.
42. Rosen LW, Hough DO: Pathogenic weight-control behaviors of female college gymnasts. Phys Sportsmed 16(9): 141-144, 1988.
43. Rucinski A: Relationship of body image and dietary intake of competitive ice skaters. J Am Diet Assoc 89:98-100, 1989.
44. Schotte DE, Stunkard AJ: Bulimia vs. bulimic behaviors on a college campus. JAMA 258:1213-1215, 1987.
45. Skolnick AA: "Female athlete triad" risk for women. JAMA 270:921-923, 1993.
46. Steen SN, McKinney S: Nutrition assessment of college wrestlers. Physician Sportsmed 14:100-116, 1986.
47. Stephenson JN: Medical consequences and complications of anorexia nervosa and bulimia nervosa in female athletes. Athletic Training 26:130-135, 1991.
48. Strober M: Anorexia nervosa: History and psychological concepts. In Brownell KD, Foreyt JP (eds): Handbook of Eating Disorders. New York, Basic Books, 1986, pp 231-246.
49. Taub DE, Blinde EM: Eating disorders among adolescent female athletes: Influence of athletic participation and sport team membership. Adolescence 27:833-848, 1992.
50. Thelen MH, Farmer J, Wonderlich S, Smith M: A revision of the Bulimia Test: The BULIT-R. Pyschological assessment. J Consult Clin Psychol 3:119-124, 1991.
51. Thompson RA, Sherman RT (eds): Helping Athletes with Eating Disorders. Champaign, IL, Human Kinetics, 1993.
52. Weight LM, Noakes TD: Is running an analog of anorexia? A survey of the incidence of eating disorders in female distance runners. Med Sci Sports Exerc 119:213-217, 1987.
53. Wolman RL, Harries MG: Menstrual abnormalities in elite athletes. Clin Sports Med 1:95, 1989.
54. Woscyna G: Nutritional aspects of eating disorders: Nutrition education and counseling as a component of treatment. Athletic Training 26:144, 1991.
55. Woscyna G, Madison J: Treatment of anorexia nervosa and bulimia nervosa: Outcome data and nutritionist's role. Presented at the 71st Annual Meeting of the American Dietetic Association. San Francisco, CA, October 6, 1988.
56. Yeager KK, Agostini R, Nattiv A, Drinkwater B: The female athlete triad: Disordered eating, amenorrhea, osteoporosis. Med Sci Sports Exerc 25:775-777, 1993.
57. Zucker P, Avener J, Bayder S, et al: Eating disorders in young athletes. Physician Sportsmed 13:88-106, 1985.

11

The Athletic Heart Syndrome

Loren A. Crown, M.D.
Wm. MacMillan Rodney, M.D.
Timothy P. Huston, M.D.

Since the turn of the century, it has been recognized that athletes trained for endurance performance have larger hearts than nonathletes.[12] Not infrequently these apparently healthy performers are found to possess murmurs, extracardiac sounds, and conduction abnormalities.[10] It is also noted that athletes trained for strength performance are found to have thicker myocardium, but not overall cardiac enlargement.[1,21] In daily practice, primary care physicians encounter both youthful and more mature individuals of both genders with these findings as the public has increasingly adopted values of health and fitness. Early in the history of this syndrome it was believed that these cardiovascular changes represented nascient heart disease, but it is now recognized that the conditioned myocardium represents a successful and healthy adaption to physiological demands.[22]

It is the purpose of this chapter to provide an understanding of the physiologic and morphologic changes occurring in what is now called athletic heart syndrome (AHS) and also to describe the clinical findings that accompany them so that appropriate management strategies can result, thus preventing unnecessary expenditure of resources or incurrence of emotional damage to the patient.

EFFECTS OF CONDITIONING

The Aerobic Athlete

The aerobic athlete is also known as the performance, dynamic, endurance, or isotonic conditioned athlete. Increased conditioning by such athletes in response to sustained aerobic loads leads to numerous physiologic and morphologic changes that allow them to deliver a greater amount of oxygenated blood to muscular tissues, which more efficiently utilizes it, thus enabling greater work to be done. The greatest amount of work able to be done by the body is known by many labels, including maximized oxygen uptake, functional aerobic capacity, and maximum work capability, and is commonly expressed as VO_2 max. It is related to and affected by a large number of variables, which interact to produce changes that in the athlete increase performance and efficiency, but in the nonathlete might be signs of organic heart disease.

VO_2 max is directly proportional to cardiac output (CO), which is the product of heart rate (HR) and stroke volume (SV); to tissue oxygen extraction; and to peripheral vascular resistance. It is also related to total blood volume, which is increased in aerobic athletes. In addition, it is dependent on the increased parasympathetic tone and the decreased level of circulating catecholamines. The subsequent bradycardia allows both a lengthened diastolic filling time, which increases stroke volume, and improved coronary circulation, which is predominantly a diastolic phenomenon.[2] Peripheral resistance, while potentially a factor, seems to be unpredictable in its response to endurance training and is not considered an important factor in AHS. Enhancement of tissue oxygen extraction occurs as the result of an increased number of intracellular mitochondria and the formation of new capillaries in the muscles;[8] these tissue changes alone may be responsible for half of the increase in VO_2 max seen in the aerobic-trained athlete, but they are difficult to quantify clinically.[1]

On the other hand, the maximum CO may increase by a similar magnitude proportional to changes in the HR and SV. Because there is no change in the maximum HR between the sedentary and the athletic individual, it may be assumed that it is the SV that has been adjusted.[21] Also, because minute-to-minute alterations in SV are physiologically difficult, it can be predicted that the HR will be the primary adjustment made. Finally, because at suboptimal work loads oxygen consumption is nearly the same for both groups, it will be necessary for the HR of the athlete to be considerably slower than the counterpart at any level of activity, especially at rest.[1]

SV can change either by alteration of the ejection fraction or by a change in the left ventricular end diastolic (LVED) volume. Evidence is conclusive that it is the latter.[6] In order to accommodate for the increased LVED volume, and the subsequent distention, there is a proportional increase in left ventricular (LV) chamber size, LV mass, and LV wall thickness.[30] This allows for the required SV augmentation without compromising ventricular compliance and also permits adherence to the law of LaPlace, which requires an appropriate increase in wall thickness to relieve the stress of the volume overload.[14,30] Though the LV wall thickness is greater in the aerobic-trained individual than in the sedentary, 98.3% of healthy athletic dimensions fall in the normal range.[27] The increased LV mass to lean body mass (LBM) ratio is greater in the endurance-trained athlete than in controls and is proportional to the enhanced VO_2 max that results from conditioning.[19] There are concomitant structural enlargements in the right ventricle (RV) and both atria.[10] Taken together, the altered configuration of the athlete's heart is labeled eccentric hypertrophy, and a summary of the changes are found in Figure 1.

The Anaerobic Athlete

The anaerobic athlete is also known as the strength, weight, static, or isometric conditioned athlete. Increased conditioning of anaerobic athletes leads to changes that produce a different type of LV appearance and function. These individuals do not require an increase in VO_2max, but instead, their cardiovascular system is subject to tremendous pressure stress (i.e., blood pressures of up to 320/250).[15] The increased wall thickness is a response to this stimulus and results in a symmetrically thickened muscle without increased chamber volume. Therefore, no increase results in LVED volume, SV, or CO. In addition, there neither a change in HR nor alteration in diastolic compliance.[26] Strength training may lead to left ventricular hypertrophy. The LV cardiac mass to LBM ratio remains unchanged because concomitant with the increase in myocardium, there is a proportional increase in skeletal muscle, as distinct from the aerobic athlete.[10] These isometric athletes develop what is termed a concentrically hypertrophied heart.[30]

The Hypertrophic Cardiomyopathic Individual

Hypertrophic cardiomyopathy was formerly known as idiopathic hypertrophic subaortic stenosis and also as hypertrophic obstructive cardiomyopathy. In the familial condition, there is increased

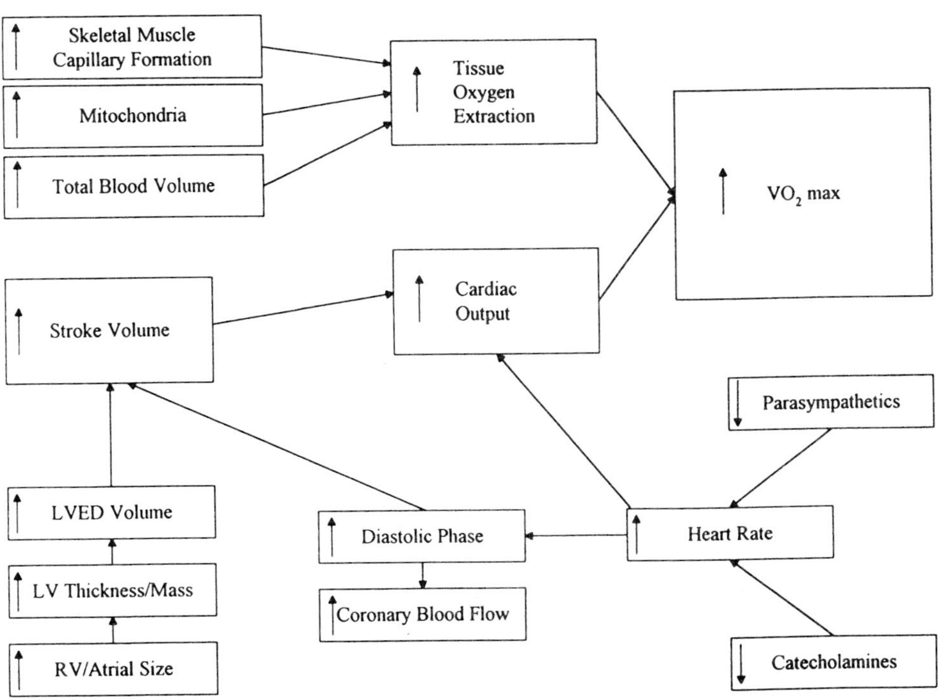

FIGURE 1. Physiologic changes in the eccentrically hypertrophied athletic heart.

wall thickness, which occurs in an unpredictable manner, though asymmetrical septal hypertrophy is most frequent. This is due to markedly defective and disorganized myocardial formation on both a cellular and an end organ basis. The encroachment of myocardial tissue into the left ventricle compromises SV and impedes outflow. Catecholamine levels and HRs are increased in an attempt to compensate for the decrease in CO. There are both inflow restriction and outflow obstruction, including interference with systolic mitral valve motion, and ultimately areas of localized hypertrophy may serve as arrhythmoganic foci.[17]

The Chronic Heart Failure Individual

Changes occurring in unhealthy individuals with chronic pressure or volume overload states that produce either enlargement or hypertrophy are associated with such manifest stigmata of clinical disease in such different contexts from those seen in the athlete exam that an unlikely confusion with AHS would ensue, and so they will not be discussed further herein.

Table 1 summarizes differences between the hearts of aerobic, anaerobic, hypertrophic cardiomyopathic (HCM), and congestive heart failure individuals; Figure 2 illustrates schematically the configurations of each type.

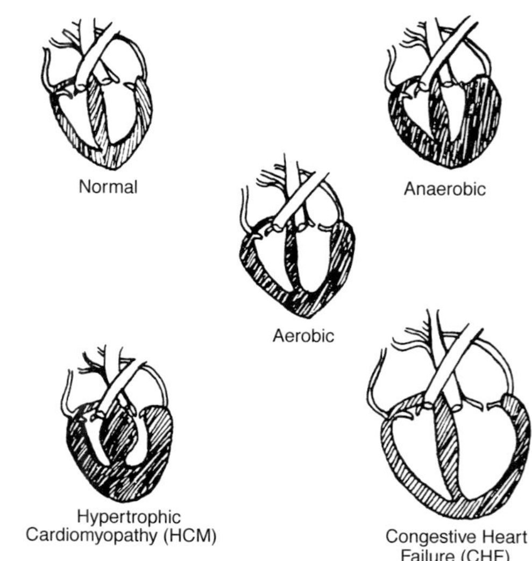

FIGURE 2. Schematic representation of cardiac configuration.

EVALUATION

History

The health history taken during the examination of an athlete should include the following topics pertaining to the cardiovascular system (which may of course overlap with evaluation of other body-organ systems): history of chronic/recurrent illnesses, surgeries, hospitalizations, medication usage; history of heart problems, murmurs, blood pressure elevation, family members' dying younger than 40 years of age of causes other than accidents or younger than 55 years of age of cardiac problems or heart attacks; and history of chest pain, palpitations, dyspnea, or syncope with exertion.[9] The questions optimally will be on a printed form to be signed by the athlete (and the parent if the patient is a minor). The medicolegal and ethical aspects of documentation will be appreciated by most clinicians; it is unlikely that the conditioned individual with AHS will answer in the affirmative to any of the aforementioned topics. High-yield prognostic indicators for sudden death include a positive family history of early cardiac demise, as well as palpitations, exertional syncope, and/or dyspnea in the athlete.[17]

Table 1. **Summary of Comparisons**

↑Greater than average —No change from ↓ Less than average	Aerobic	Anaerobic	HCM	CHF
VO_2 max	↑	—	↓	↓
HR	↓	—	↑	↑
CO(max)	↑	—	↓	↓
SV	↑	—	↓	↓
LVED volume	↑	—	↓	↑
LV wall thickness	↑	↑	↑	↓↑
LV compliance	—	—	↓	↓
LV Mass/LBM	↑	—	↑	— or ↑
Reversibility to normal status	Restoration to baseline within days/weeks of cessation of training		Minimal or no restoration to baseline despite major medical or surgical intervention	

CHF = chronic heart failure, HCM = hypertrophic cardiomyopathy.

Physical

The physical exam of the athlete is most frequently entirely normal. In the dynamic athlete one might note a large pulse amplitude as well as a diffuse LV impulse. Ventricular gallops and soft systolic murmurs are commonly heard; midsystolic murmurs have been noted in 30–50% of conditioned athletes. The murmurs are nonradiating, ejection-type grade I and II, beginning after the first and ending before the second sound with a crescendo-decrescendo profile; are best heard at the lower left sternal border; and decrease on standing up or performing the Valsalva maneuver.[28,29] It should be recalled that most children have murmurs at some time and that nearly all of this type are nonpathologic.[28] The individual who has a systolic ejection murmur that increases on Valsalva manuever and who has a positive family cardiac history and/or symptoms involving chest pain, syncope, dyspnea, or palpations must be further evaluated. Third heart sounds are audible in 20–60% of conditioned athletes and are completely benign. Fourth heart sounds are frequently detected phonocardiographically but are not usually heard during the physical exam. When audible, an S_4 gallop requires further study to eliminate pathology.[29] The pulse is often bradycardiac at rest but normal after exertion. In the context of the examination of an asymptomatic, healthy, conditioned athlete, a midsystolic murmur, a gallop, and/or a bradycardia is not likely to signal cardiac disease. In the individual with HCM, there may be a palpable LV impulse that may be double pulsus biferiens and a harsh systolic murmur at the lower left sternal border radiating to the apex, which decreases on squatting and increases on standing or in response to a Valsalva maneuver.[17,28]

Electrocardiography

The most common rhythm disturbance in dynamic athletes is sinus bradycardia, with a prevalence frequently exceeding 50% in several large studies.[5,24,25] The etiology may be due to a combination of intrinsic cardiac conditioning and to either an increase in vagal or a decrease in sympathetic tone. There is marked sinus arrhythmia in 13.5–69% of performance-trained athletes.[5,20]

A wandering pacemaker may be found in about 20% of cases.[10] Ectopic atrial and junctional rhythms—anticipated from the theory of excess vagal tone—are reported in 7–20% of conditional individuals.[10,31] After sinus bradycardia and arrhythmia, atrioventricular (AV) blocks are the next most common, with first-degree blocks occurring in up to one-third of endurance-trained athletes[2]. Type I second-degree AV block occurs during intensive training; it disappears shortly after cessation of training in up to 10% of cases.[18,23] Reports mention rare occasions of type II second-degree AV blocks and of third-degree AV blocks, and the relationship to AHS is not clear. By contrast, the individual with HCM is more likely to have ventricular tachycardia and couplets, premature ventricular contractions, premature atrial contractions, atrial fibrillation, and/or atrial tachycardia, especially when searched for by Holter testing.[3] Table 2 summarizes the frequency of such rhythm disturbances follows.[11]

There are additional variations that occur in the electrocardiograms (EKGs) of conditioned athletes that differ from those of the general population; they are typically ST and T-wave aberrancies. The most common is the early repolarization pattern consisting of ST-segment elevation associated with J-point elevation and peaked T waves; a pattern of juvenile T-wave inversion in V_1–V_3 may be seen about 10% of the time.[10,21] Also noted are ST-segment depression with a depressed J-point and T-wave inversion in the lateral chest leads. The frequency of ST-segment changes varies, but it appears to directly relate to the level of conditioning and diminishes when training ceases; in general, the more highly trained the athlete, the more likely that ST-T-wave changes will be found.[13]

The most striking alteration in the EKG of an endurance-trained athlete consists of the large voltages. Increases in the p-wave and especially the LV amplitudes are found routinely; RV increases are not as frequent. Less voltage elevation is seen in the static-trained athlete. Finally, minor conduction defects usually taking the form of incomplete right bundle branch block may be found in more than 50% of conditioned athletes.[10]

TABLE 2. Frequencies of Rhythm Disturbances on Resting Electrocardiograms of the General Population and Athletes

Arrhythmia	General Population (%)	Athletes (%)
Sinus bradycardia	23.7	50–85
Sinus arrhythmia	2.4–20	13.5–69
Wandering atrial pacemaker	—	7.4–19
First-degree block	0.65	6-33
Second-degree block		
Mobitz I	0.003	0.125–10
Mobitz II	0.003	Not reported
Third-degree block	0.0002	0.017
Nodal rhythm	0.06	0.031–7.0
Ventricular pre-excitation	0.1–0.15	0.15–2.5
Atrial fibrillation	0.004	0–0.63

From Huston TP, Puffer JC, Rodney WM: The athletic heart syndrome. N Engl J Med 313:24-32, 1985, with permission.

TABLE 3. **Summary of Changes Seen Clinically in the Athletic Exam**

	Aerobic	**Anaerobic**	**HCM**	**Sedentary Normal**
History				
Family	—	—	Sudden death < 40 Cardiac death < 55	—
Review of Systems	—	—	Syncope Palpitations Dyspnea Chest pain	—
Physical				
Palpation	↑ Cardiac impulse	↑ Cardiac impulse	↑ Cardiac impulse (often double) Cartoid pulsus biferiens	—
Auscultation	SEM(↓ Valsalva) S_3 gallop	SEM (↓ Valsalva)	SEM (↑ Valsalva) S_4 Gallop	SEM(↓ Valsalva)
ECG				
Rhythm	Sinus arrhythmia and bradycardia, PAC's Wandering atrial/junctional pacemaker, 10AV/block 2° AV type I	Sinus arrhythmia Sinus bradycardia	PAC's Atrial fib/flutter/tach PVC's, couplets V tach	Sinus arrhythmia Sinus bradycardia
Patterns	Increased voltage Early repolarization ST↑ ↓ J point ↑ T ↓ R B B B	Increased voltage	Increased voltage p mitrale Q in I, AVL, V-6 ST↓ T ↓	—
Chest x-ray	Upper limit of normal	—	Increased or normal	—
ECHO				
LV wall thickness	Upper limit of normal	Upper limit of normal	Asymmetric increased	—
MRI				
LV mass	Eccentric increase	Concentric increase	Asymmetric increase	—

Radiographic Studies

Chest films often reveal a slightly enlarged heart with a globular silhouette.[21] Cardiothoracic ratios greater than 0.5 are found in less than a quarter of those studied, yet on the average, the heart of the conditioned athlete is generally larger than those of sedentary controls.[10]

Echocardiography

Echocardiographic studies of conditioned athletes indicate that eccentric hypertrophy of the LV rarely overlaps with the dimensions commonly accepted for HCM and usually does not exceed those of the normal population.[3] In a study of nearly a thousand elite endurance-trained athletes, including aerobic and anaerobic performers, only 1.7% had LV thickness that extended into the range minimally compatible with the diagnosis of HCM(>13 mm), none exceeded 16 mm, and the median was 9.7 mm[27] Of those exceeding the cutoff point—a total of 16— all were Olympic-level performers, 94% were rowers or canoeists, none had any familial or personal cardiac history or symptoms, all had smooth-contoured hypertrophy (rather than the marked irregularity found in HCM), and all showed immediate reversal of enlargement back into the normal range upon deconditioning.[27]

Magnetic Resonance Imaging

Studies of endurance athletes by means of magnetic resonance imaging techniques have consistently found increases in LV mass of 26–37% compared to controls; these increases have persisted regardless of adjustments for body weight, surface area, or lean body mass.[19] The increases in LV mass in endurance athletes parallels the other observed increases in LVED volume, mean wall thickness, and VO_2 max in both sexes when compared to sedentary controls.[30] Again, the increase in aerobic athletes is eccentric rather than concentric as in the case of anaerobic athletes.

MANAGEMENT

In the tertiary care context, an individual with a systolic murmur, an S_3 gallop, increased voltages plus ST changes on EKG, and a thickened LV wall on echo would merit consideration for a diagnosis of HCM. But in a primary care setting where athletic exams are being performed, AHS is a more likely diagnosis. Consideration of the patient's lack of symptoms (especially syncope, dyspnea, or chest pain on exertion), negative family history of sudden premature death, and the relative bradycardia present when increased cardiac output is required helps to reduce ambiguity and aids in distinguishing AHS in an athlete presenting for evaluation from that of an individual with a pathologic heart condition. In a similar fashion, a ventricular gallop with an unusual degree of ventricular dilation might simulate a pathologically failing heart in an elderly individual; yet, in a conditioned senior, excellent ventricular function and performance capacity would argue against myocardial disorder. Usually, the context, the history, and the physical exam are sufficient for a diagnosis of AHS, only occasionally will further testing be required, and rarely will consultation be needed.

But when confronted by an athletic patient who may also have a positive family cardiac history, increased personal risk factors, and/or recent significant symptoms of chest pain, palpitations, dyspnea, or syncope, the clinician should not hesitate to request additional studies including exercise testing, echocardiography, or even angiography. Sudden cardiac events do occur even in the well-conditioned athlete such as Jim Fixx, late guru of runners; tennis great Arthur Ashe, victim of a myocardial infarction in his 30s; the legendary "Pistol" Pete Marovich; and more recently, Hank Gathers, whose demise triggered renewed interest in the athlete at risk.[22,32] The furor surrounding the collapse and subsequent death of Celtic star Reggie Lewis in mid-1993 again has thrust the issue to the forefront of sports medicine. Terminal events in such circumstances are most often attributable to cardiomyopathies or coronary artery disease.[4,7,16] The annual mortality rate for youths involved in athletics is very small—approximately a dozen per year in the United States—and is estimated at about 1 per 200,000 at risk.[7,17]

CONCLUSION

In summary, the process of athletic conditioning produces physiological changes that allow maximum cardiac output to occur with enhanced efficiency. Approximately 20 million youths participate in physical education and athletic programs in this country, as do an even larger number of older individuals involved in self-directed exercise programs, so the clinician will encounter numerous patients of either sex and of varying age who will present with more AHS. Improved diagnostics, especially in ultrasound, make possible more rapid and more accurate assessments in athletes with unusual findings yet allow the clinician to avoid ordering unnecessary curtailment of activity as well as to avoid patients' development of crippled cardiac syndrome.[29] An understanding of AHS permits reassurance and conservative management of those in whom it is encountered.

REFERENCES

1. Appenseller O: Sports Medicine, 3rd ed. Baltimore, Urban and Schwarzenberg, 1988.
2. Berkow R: The Merck Manual, 16th ed. Rahway, NJ, Merck Research Laboratories, 1992.
3. Bethesda Conference 16: Cardiovascular abnormalities in the athlete: recommendations regarding eligibility for competition. J Am Coll Cardiol 6:1185-1232, 1985.
4. Chillag S, Bates M, Voltin R, et al: Sudden death: Myocardial infarction in a runner with normal coronary arteries. Physician Sportsmed 18(3):89-94, 1990.
5. Cohen JL, Gupta PK, Lichstein E, et al: The heart of a dancer: Noninvasive cardiac evaluation of professional ballet dancers. AM J Cardiol 45:959-965, 1980.
6. Crawford MH, Petru MA, Robinowitz C: Effect of isotonic exercise training on left ventricular volume during upright exercise. Circulation 72:1237-1243, 1985.
7. Epstein SE, Maron BJ, Roberts WC: Causes of sudden death in competitive athletes. J Am Coll Card 7: 204-214, 1986.
8. Gollnick PD, Saltin B: Significance of skeletal muscle oxidative enzyme enhancement with endurance training. Clin Physiol 2:1-12, 1982.
9. Hulse E, Strong WB: Preparticipation evaluation for athletics. Pediatr Rev 9:173-182, 1987.
10. Hurst JW: Medicine for the Practicing Physician, 3rd ed. Stoneham, MA, Butterworth, 1992.
11. Huston TP, Puffer JC, Rodney WM: The athletic heart syndrome. N Engl J Med 313:24-32, 1985.
12. Jokl E: Sudden Death of Athletes. Springfield, IL, Charles C Thomas, 1985.
13. Kosunen K, Pakarinen A, Kuoppasalmi K, et al: Cardiovascular function and the renin-angiotensin-aldosterone system in long distance runners during various training periods. Scand J Clin Lab Invest 40:429-435, 1980.
14. Levine BD, Lane LD, Buckey JC: Left ventricular pressure-volume and Frank Starling relations in endurance athletes. Circulation 84:1016-1023, 1991.
15. MacDougall JD, Tuxen D, Sale DG, et al: Arterial blood pressure response to heavy resistance exercise. J Appl Physiol 58:785-790, 1985.
16. Maron BJ: Sudden death in young athletes. Circulation 62: 218-229, 1980.
17. McCaffrey FM, Braden DS, Strong WB: Sudden cardiac death in young athletes. Am J Dis Child 145:177-183, 1991.
18. Meytes I, Koplinsky E, Yahini JH, et al: Wenckeback A-V block: A frequent problem following heavy physical training. Am Heart J 90:426-430, 1975.
19. Milliken MC, Stray-Gundersen J, Peshock RM, et al: Left ventricular mass as determinted by magnetic resonance imaging in male endurance athletes. Am J Cardiol 62: 301–305, 1988.
20. Minamitani K, Miyagawa M, Konco M, et al: The electrocardiogram of professional cyclists. In Lubich T, Venerando A (eds): Sports Cardiology. Bologna, Aulo Gaggi, 1980, pp 315-25.
21. Mitchell JH: How to recognize "athlete's heart." Physician Sportsmed 20(8):87-94, 1992.
22. Munnings F: The death of Hank Gathers: A legacy of confusion. Physician Sportsmed 18(5):97-102, 1990.
23. Nakamoto K: Electrocardiograms of 25 marathon runners before and after 100-meter dash. Jpn Circ J 33:105-128, 1969.
24. Parker MB, Londeree BR, Cupp GV, et al: The noninvasive cardiac evaluation of long distance runners. Chest 73: 376-381, 1978.

25. Paulsen W, Boughner D, Ko P, et al: Left ventricular function in marathon runners: Echocardiographic assessment. J Appl Physiol 51:881-886, 1981.
26. Pearson AC, Schiff M, Mrosek D, et al: Left ventricular diastolic function in weight lifters. Am J Cardiol 58:1254-1259, 1986.
27. Pelliccia A, Maron BJ, Spataro A: The upper limit of physiologic cardiac hypertrophy in highly trained elite athletes. N Engl J Med 324:295-301, 1991.
28. Pipe AL, VanCamp SP: Heart murmur in a football player with a normal ECG. Physician Sportsmed 18:93-98, 1990.
29. Plieger KL, Strong WB: Screening for heart murmurs. Physician Sportsmed 20(10):71-81, 1992.
30. Riley-Hagen M, Pechock RM, Stray-Gundersen J, et al: Left ventricular dimensions and mass using magnetic resonance imaging in female endurance athletes. Am J Cardiol 69:1067-1074, 1992.
31. Roeske WR, O'Rourke RA, Klein A, et al: Noninvasive evaluation of ventricular hypertrophy in professional athletes. Circulation 53:286-292, 1976.
32. Sadaniantz A, Clapton MA, Sturner WQ, et al: Sudden death immediately after a record setting athletic performance. Am J Cardiol 63:375, 1989.
33. Strong WB, Steed D: Cardiovascular evaluation of the young athlete. Pediatr Clin North Am 29: 1325-1339, 1982.

12

The Hypertensive Athlete

Jeffrey L. Tanji, M.D.
Morris B. Mellion, M.D.

Nearly 20 to 25% of the adult American population is afflicted with high blood pressure,[2] a proven risk factor for both coronary artery disease and stroke. Hypertension is one of the more common medical problems associated with athletes and active individuals. This chapter focuses on hemodynamics and cardiovascular physiology, diagnostic categories of hypertension, and approaches to the management of hypertension, addressing both nonpharmacologic and pharmacologic therapies.

PHYSIOLOGY OF HYPERTENSION

We assume that Fick's law (pressure = flow × resistance) adequately describes the cardiovascular system that establishes the environment for hypertension. This equation, translated to the language of the heart and vessels, is BP=CO ×TPR (blood pressure is equivalent to cardiac output times total peripheral resistance).

BORDERLINE HYPERTENSION

Transiently elevated blood pressures in a normotensive person often precede the later development of hypertension. This "borderline" or "high normal" hypertension is the earliest known stage of hypertension. Other terms such as "latent" or "labile" hypertension are also associated with this condition. Early studies by Lund-Johanssen demonstrated that elevated blood pressures in young persons with borderline hypertension are physiologically associated with elevated cardiac output and normal total peripheral resistance.[16] While the mechanism for this physiologic relationship is unclear, associated pathophysiologic markers include increased serum catecholamine levels and increased serum renin levels.[5,9]

ESTABLISHED HYPERTENSION

Repeated spikes of elevated blood pressure may result in anatomic changes such as the hypertrophy of peripheral arterioles and arteries associated with established hypertension. At this established stage, cardia output decreases while total peripheral resistance increases. Beyond this stage, central changes in the circulation are marked by the presence of left ventricular hypertrophy. End-stage hypertensive disease may be characterized by a cardiac output that can no longer keep up with the body's physiologic demands. Congestive heart failure, peripheral edema, hypertensive nephropathy, and hypertensive retinopathy complicate long-standing hypertension.

BLOOD PRESSURE RESPONSE TO DYNAMIC EXERCISE

With dynamic exercise, the peripheral musculature increases the demand for oxygen to the heart and circulation as measured by an increased VO_2 (VO_2 is the measurement of the body's ability to uptake and metabolize oxygen). Cardiac output during dynamic exercise increases in response to stroke volume times heart rate.

While it is established that both systolic and diastolic blood pressure increase linearly in response to moderate-to high-intensity exercise (70–95% of VO_2 max), [27] a newer understanding of this relationship is recognized at lower levels of exercise intensity.[25,28,29] At low-intensity exercise in both normotensive and hypertensive subjects (exercise between 60 to 70% of VO_2 max), total peripheral resistance decreases and cardiac output increases very slightly, resulting in a transient and temporary decrease in mean blood pressure, a slight decrease in diastolic blood pressure, and a modest increase in systolic blood pressure. As exercise intensity increases beyond this level, both systolic and diastolic blood pressure increase linearly. At maximal exercise, systolic blood pressure and diastolic blood pressures peak. The clinical significance of the lowering of diastolic blood pressure with low-to-moderate-intensity exercise is that this level of repeated exercise may be optimal for long-term blood pressure control among mild hypertensives.[9] Immediately post-exercise, diastolic pressure drops significantly while systolic pressure remains elevated, and this dramatically increased pulse pressure meets the peripheral skeletal demand for oxygen.

The hypertensive person is characterized by elevations in both systolic and diastolic blood pressures at any level of work load, and by a dramatically increased systolic blood pressure measurement immediately post-exercise. While many absolute criteria for a hypertensive response to exercise are used, a systolic blood pressure above 200 mmHG immediately post-exercise is accepted as standard.[23]

Left ventricular hypertrophy in the athletic heart syndrome is distinctly different from left ventricular hypertrophy associated with the presence of long-standing hypertension.[3] In pathophysiologic left ventricular hypertrophy associated with hypertension, the left ventricle is both dilated (increased chamber diameter) as well as hypertrophied (increased wall thickness). In physiologic left ventricular hypertrophy associated with the normal athlete who participates in aerobic endurance sport, the left ventricular enlargement is primarily dilatation with only slightly increased wall thickness. This physiologic enlargement may be entirely reversible with as little as two months of physical inactivity.

BLOOD PRESSURE RESPONSE TO STATIC EXERCISE

In contrast to dynamic exercise, static exercise such as isometrics (weightlifting) is associated with a dramatic increase in both systolic and diastolic blood pressures. In one classic study, systolic pressure increased in excess of 300 mmHg, while diastolic pressure increased in excess of 200 mmHg in young normotensive athletes performing maximal leg presses.[17] Many sports which combine static and dynamic components of exercise, such as volleyball or basketball, may increase both left ventricular wall thickness and chamber diameter.

ADVICE FOR EXERCISING HYPERTENSIVES

Among hypertensive athletes, isotonic, isometric, and static exercise can result in marked blood pressure elevations. These individuals must be counseled carefully in the participation of their given sport to not allow blood pressure values to elevate to dangerously high levels.

Blood pressure can increase dramatically with dynamic exercise but less than with static exercise. Blood pressure, therefore, ought to be monitored on a regular basis during a new training program for hypertensives or with a change in intensity in training program.

Athletes with hypertension do not shunt blood to the skin as effectively as normotensives. This phenomenon may result in a precipitous increase in core temperature and exercise in the heat, particularly dangerous for the hypertensive because of the inability to dissipate heat through the peripheral shunting of circulation.[6] Exercising hypertensives should be familiarized with the symptoms of dehydration and heat illness.

THE DIAGNOSIS OF HYPERTENSION

Hypertension is defined by the fifth report of the Joint National Committee on the Detection Evaluation and Treatment of High Blood Pressure using the following criteria.[12] Normal blood pressures are values below 130 mmHg systolic and 85 mmHg diastolic. High normal values are a systolic pressure between 130 and 139 mmHg and a diastolic pressure between 85 and 89 mmHg. Hypertension is categorized into four stages.

Stage 1: Systolic between 140 and 159 mmHg, and a diastolic between 90 and 99 mm Hg.
Stage 2: Systolic between 160 and 179 mmHg, and a diastolic between 100 and 109 mm Hg.
Stage 3: Systolic between 180 to 209 mmHg, and a diastolic between 100 and 119 mm Hg.
Stage 4: Systolic above or equal to 210 mmHg, and a diastolic pressure above or equal to 120 mmHg.

Cross sectional studies of hypertensives show that early, or labile, hypertension is usually associated with an increase in isolated systolic blood pressure, particularly in response to exercise. Studies reveal that an exaggerated blood pressure elevation with dynamic exercise is primarily due to an increase in cardiac output with a normal total peripheral resistance. Several studies of young persons with labile blood pressures demonstrate that this exaggerated response to exercise can be predictive of the future development of hypertension.[11,24,32] As a person with hypertension ages, diastolic blood pressure slowly begins to increase. Consistently elevated diastolic pressures place patients at risk for the sequelae of hypertension, including coronary artery disease, stroke, and renal disease. What is particularly problematic about these three conditions is that 70% of all patients with known coronary artery disease present with sudden death or with a myocardial infarction. Further, early renal damage may be insidious and not necessarily associated with an increase in serum creatinine or BUN during blood testing. These facts fuel the search for effective screening tools to diagnose hypertension.

It is recommended that blood pressure values be checked every two years, and a recheck in one year for individuals with high-normal blood pressures. Guidelines also recommend a recheck within two months in persons with Stage 1 hypertension, an evaluation or referral for care within one month for individuals with Stage 2 hypertension, evaluation or referral for individuals within one week for Stage 3 hypertension, and immediate evaluation for individuals with Stage 4 hypertension.[12]

NONPHARMACOLOGIC MANAGEMENT OF HYPERTENSION

Nonpharmacologic strategies for the treatment of hypertension remain the cornerstone for initial effective management. These strategies have very few side effects and are generally accepted as significant interventions even when augmented by pharmacologic management. Although directly unrelated to hypertension, cigarette smoking is a risk factor for coronary artery disease and, therefore, avoidance of tobacco is indicated in patients with hypertension. Weight reduction reduces blood pressure in a significant number of hypertensives who are above 10% of ideal body weight. Obesity increases intravascular volume, which consequently increases cardiac output and blood pressure. Elevated norepinephrine levels are also associated with obesity, and they increase total peripheral resistance and blood pressure. Reduction in blood pressure consequently may occur early during a weight loss program, often with as modest a loss as 10 pounds. Further, weight loss in hypertensive patients augments the effects of antihypertensive agents. Moderation of alcohol intake must also be considered as a major nonpharmacologic intervention.

Limitation of dietary sodium is another useful measure. Current goals for hypertensives limit sodium intake to 2 grams per day or less. Approximately one third of all individuals and two thirds of African Americans with hypertension are salt-sensitive. High dietary potassium intake may protect against the development of hypertension and has been demonstrated to clearly lower blood pressure in the hypokalemic patient. Increasing dietary calcium intake, while controversial, has been proposed as a dietary measure in the reduction of blood pressure for hypertensives. Increasing magnesium intake has been loosely associated with decrease in blood pressure; this has been the least well studied of the previously discussed measures.

Exercise as Treatment

Regular aerobic physical activity clearly lowers blood pressure in patients who have mild hypertension. Currently over 40 randomized clinical trials attest that aerobic exercise programs are effective in significantly lowering resting blood pressures.[27] Because several studies counter that high-intensity exercise did not reduce blood pressure in hypertensive people, some investigators feel that low- to moderate-intensity exercise, such as walking, may optimize the blood-pressure–lowering effects of aerobic exercise. Current recommendations for aerobic exercise consist of a walking program of 30–45 minutes a day, 5–6 days a week, and an exercise intensity of 50–70% of predicted maximal heart rate (60–80% of VO_2 max).[1]

In discussing exercise as a treatment for hypertension it is important to draw several distinctions. Acute versus chronic exercise and moderate- versus high-intensity exercise arise as two of the most salient points. During acute aerobic exercise, or a single bout, an elevation of both systolic and diastolic blood pressures is generally followed by a 2–4 hour period of a relative decrease below baseline values of resting blood pressures.[31] This observation has been termed "post-exercise hypotension" and may be mediated by the release of endogenous opioids.[26] The higher the intensity of exercise, the greater the reduction in post-exercise blood pressure. The antihypertensive effect of chronic aerobic exercise may not be explained by the additive effects of these bouts of acute exercise, because of the discrepancy in optimal exercise intensity. Moderate-intensity exercise scheduled regularly is emerging as the optimal type of exercise for hypertensives. Initially presented by Tipton[28] and Urata,[29] both animal and human studies demonstrate that moderate (50–70% of maximal heart rate) exercise optimally lowers blood pressure in hypertensives. The mechanism for this has been discussed under the section on dynamic exercise.

The Deadly Quartet

One major advance in the pathophysiology of hypertension that has emerged in the past decade, is the deadly quartet (also called syndrome X), the association of hypertension, type II diabetes mellitus, obesity and hypertriglyceridemia, associated with increased peripheral insulin resistance, hyperinsulinemia and elevated serum catecholamines.[14,21] Hyperinsulinemia results in elevation in blood pressure through an increase in sympathetic tone by the stimulation of catecholamines, increased aldosterone levels resulting in increased fluid retention and sodium retention, increased reabsorption of sodium by tubules in the kidneys, and proliferation of the endothelium and smooth muscles of peripheral arterioles. Particularly appealing about the insulin hypothesis is that nonpharmacologic therapy such as weight reduction and aerobic exercise can decrease blood pressure independent of pharmacologic therapies, which may improve one and worsen another cardiac risk factor. For example, while the use of a diuretic may improve blood pressure in an individual with hypertension, type II diabetes mellitus can be exacerbated by hyperglycemia. Similarly the use of insulin therapy in the type II diabetic can further worsen or exacerbate blood pressure by increasing serum insulin levels in the already insulin-resistant state.

PHARMACOLOGIC TREATMENT OF HYPERTENSION

When nonpharmacologic therapy, including lifestyle modification, fails the use of a pharmacologic agent in addition to such lifestyle modifications is indicated. Diuretics and beta-blockers are now the preferred agents for initial therapy,[12] because of cost and because large epidemiologic studies have demonstrated a reduction in morbidity and mortality using these two agents. However, in the hypertensive athlete, there are several critical issues which may not make them agents of choice.

Diuretics

Diuretics decrease plasma volume transiently, decrease cardiac output through decreasing stoke volume, and consequently decrease blood pressure. Newer recommendations advocate very small doses of diuretics (such as 12.5 mg to 25 mg of hydrochlorothiazide). These agents may be particularly useful in individuals who are salt sensitive, but they can deplete both sodium and potassium, which can provoke dysrhythmias in individuals prone to hypokalemia. Further, diuretics which lead to dehydration can impair thermoregulation and the effective peripheral shunting of the central circulation under heat stress. Because of these considerations, diuretics may not be the initial drug of choice for the exercising athlete with high blood pressure.

Beta-Blockers

There are numerous beta-blockers, but all have several major concerns. All beta-blocking agents, notably nonselective beta blockers, can potentially reduce exercise tolerance.[15] The effect of a beta-blocker is to decrease myocardial contractility and heart rate, to increase coronary profusion, and to decrease myocardial oxygen demand. Nonselective beta blockers used in well-trained subjects result in a greater drop in maximal oxygen uptake than do beta-blockers in untrained subjects. Perceived exertion increases and absolute workloads are limited in the exercising individual on beta blockers because of both central and peripheral factors. Centrally, these agents have both negative inotropic and chronotropic effects. Peripherally, nonselective beta-blockers attenuate glycogenolysis, reducing energy substrate and promoting fatigue during endurance activity. Further, during exercise, beta-blockers may provoke an increase in serum potassium through mechanisms that are not well understood.[4] Serum potassium, therefore, needs to be closely monitored in physically active patients who take beta-blockers. Thermoregulation can also be impaired with the use of beta blockers by a reduction of peripheral blood flow to the skin, or by an indirect reflex vasoconstriction of peripheral arterioles as a result of decreased left ventricular contractility.[7,8] Athletes who are prescribed beta-blockers should be aware of the signs and symptoms of hyperthermia. Selective beta-blocking agents, however, can be used effectively in exercising hypertensives. Current data suggests that selective beta-blockers are not contraindicated in the exercising hypertensive.[4]

ACE Inhibitors

Angiotensin converting enzyme (ACE) inhibitors block the conversion of angiotensin I to angiotensin II and block vasoconstriction and, therefore, reduce total peripheral resistance. This agent also works by decreasing sodium retention stimulated by angiotensin II. These agents, although more expensive than diuretics and beta-blockers, are excellent for hypertensive patients who exercise. Side effects are minimal and do not appear to interfere with maximal exercise capacity or result in an increase in perceived exertion during exercise. Several studies have documented significant efficacy in managing high blood pressure with ACE inhibitors without a decrease in VO_2 max, increased rate of perceived exertion, or decrease in maximal heart rate.[10,30,34]

Calcium Channel Blockers

Calcium channel blockers reduce blood pressure by lowering calcium concentration in vascular smooth muscle cells with a consequent result in decrease in total peripheral resistance.[19,20,22,23] Like ACE inhibitors, calcium channel blockers are excellent for exercising adults. Although some calcium antagonists, particularly verapamil, are noted for decreasing left ventricular contractility as a part of their effect, the use of these agents does not seem to result in a decrease in functional capacity as may occur with beta-blockers. Alpha-2 receptor blockers selectively block alpha-1 arteriolar smooth muscle receptors and decrease total peripheral resistance. These agents normalize central hemodynamics both at rest and during exercise.[16,18] They are effective in controlling hypertension in the exercising person and have very few side effects. Occasionally, an exaggerated hypotensive response with the first dose can be noted and this response should therefore be monitored.

Other Agents

Combined alpha- and beta-blockers demonstrate both a decrease in heart rate as well as decrease in total peripheral resistance. Beta effects outweigh the alpha effects and can result in the decrease in cardiac output and a decrease in total peripheral resistance for a significant period. Again, the considerations which limit the use of beta-blockers, such as increased rate of perceived exertion and decreased heart capacity, need to be monitored in the exercising hypertensive.

The African American Athlete

The prevalence of hypertension, and overall morbidity and mortality at all levels of hypertension, among African Americans is greater than in the overall population. This relationship is true not only for Americans, but also for blacks compared with whites living in Brazil as well as Africa.[13] There is earlier onset of disease, more rapid progression, and less optimal control of blood pressure. Possibly, various defects in sodium transport associated with a low serum renin level are the pathophysiology behind these differences. African Americans have been highly responsive to diuretic agents for the control of blood pressure and may represent a special population where these agents may be considered. The cautions expressed about diuretics above should be communicated with the athlete. Calcium channel blockers have been used with success in this population as well.

REFERENCES

1. American College of Sports Medicine: Position statement on the recommended quantity and quality of exercise, Indianapolis, 1993.
2. American Heart Association: Heart Facts. Dallas, American Heart Association, 1988.
3. Bryan G, Ward A, Rippe JM: Athletic heart syndrome. Clin Sports Med 11:259-272, 1992.
4. Carlsson E, Fellenius E, Lundborg P, et al: Beta-adrenoreceptor blockers, plasma potassium and exercise. Lancet 2(8086):424-425, 1978.
5. Duncan JJ, Farr JE, Upton SJ, et al: The effects of aerobic exercise on plasma catecholamines and blood pressure in patients with mild essential hypertension. JAMA 254: 2609-2613, 1985.
6. Gordon NF: Effective selective and nonselective beta adrenoreceptor blockade on thermoregulation during prolonged exercise in heat. Am J Cardiol 55:74D-78D, 1985.
7. Gordon NF, Krager PE, VanRensburg JP, et al: Effect of beta-adrenoreceptor blockade on thermoregulation during prolonged exercise. J Appl Physiol 58:899-906, 1985.
8. Gordon NF, VanRensburg JP, Russell HM, et al: Effective beta-adrenoreceptor blockade and calcium antagonism, alone and in combination in thermoregulation during prolonged exercise. Int J Sports Med 8(1):1-5, 1987.
9. Hagberg JM, Goldring D, Heath GW: Effect of exercise on plasma catecholamines and hemodynamics during rest, submaximal exercise and orthostatic stress. Clin Physiol 4:117-124, 1984.
10. Heald JF, Bulpitt CJ, Fletcher AE: Angiotensin converting enzyme inhibitors and the quality of life: The European trial. J Hypertens 3:S91-S94, 1985.
11. Jette M, Landry F, Sidney K, et al: Exaggerated blood pressure response to exercise in the detection of hypertension. J Cardiopulmon Rehabil 8:171-177, 1988.
12. Joint National Committee on Detection, Evaluation and Treatment of High Blood Pressure: Fifth Report of the Joint National Committee on Detection, Evaluation and Treatment of High Blood Pressure. Bethesda National Institutes of Health, NIH publication No. 73-1088, 1993, p 4.
13. Kaplan NM: Clinical Hypertension, 5th ed. Baltimore, Williams & Wilkins, 1990, p 14–15.
14. Kaplan NM: The deadly quartet: Upper body obesity, glucose intolerance, hyperglyceridemia and hypertension. Arch Intern Med 149:1514-1520, 1989.
15. Kaplan NM, Alderman MH, Flamenbaum W, et al: Guidelines for treatment of hypertension. Am J Hypertens 2: 75-77, 1989.
16. Lund-Johanssen P, Onvik P, Haugland H: Acute and chronic hemodynamic effects of doxazocin in hypertension at rest and during exercise. Br J Clin Pharmacol 21: 45S-54S, 1986.
17. MacDougall JD, Tuxen D, Sale DG, et al: Arterial blood pressure response to heavy resistance exercise. J Appl Physiol 58:785-790, 1985.
18. Monsalve P, Vera O, Acuna FP, et al: Echocardiographic assessment of doxazosin on left ventricular mass in patients with essential hypertension. Am Heart J 121:156-361, 1991.
19. Myburgh DP, Gordon NF: Comparison of diltiazem and atenolol in young physically active men with a central hypertension. Am J Cardiol 60:1092-1095, 1987.
20. Pool PE, Seagren SC, Salel AF: Effects of diltiazem on serum lipids, exercise performance and blood pressure: A randomized double blind placebo controlled evaluation for systemic hypertension. Am J Cardiol 56: 91H-96H, 1985.
21. Reaven GM: Insulin resistance, hyperinsulinemia and hypertriglyceridemia in the etiology and clinical course of hypertension. Am J Med 90(Suppl 2A):7A-12S, 1991.
22. Szlacheic J, Hirsch AT, Tuba JF, et al: Diltiazem v Propranolol in essential hypertension: Responses of rest and exercise, blood pressure and effects on exercise capacity. Am J Cardiol 59:393-399, 1987.
23. Tanji JL: Exercise and the hypertensive athlete. Clin Sports Med 11:291-302, 1992.
24. Tanji JL, Champlin JJ, Wong GY, et al: Blood pressure recovery curves after submaximal exercise: A predictor of

hypertension at 10 year follow up. Am J Hypertens 2:135-138, 1989.

25. Tanji JL, Smith RE, Bernauer EM, et al: Acute diastolic blood pressure lowering effects of mild to moderate intensity exercise. In press.
26. Thoren P, Floras JS, Hoffmann P, Seals D: Endorphins and exercise: Physiological mechanisms and clinical implications. Med Sci Sports Exerc 22:417-428, 1990.
27. Tipton CM. Exercise, training and hypertension: An update. Exerc Sport Sci Rev 19:547-505, 1991.
28. Tipton CM, Matthes RD, Marcus KD, et al: Influence of exercise intensity, age and medication on resting systolic blood pressure of SHR populations. J Appl Physiol 55:1304-1310, 1983.
29. Urata H, Tanabe Y, Kiyonaga A, et al: Antihypertensive volume-depleting effects of mild exercise on essential hypertension. Hypertension 9:245-252, 1987.
30. Veterans Administration Cooperative Study Group on Antihypertensive Agents: Low-dose Captopril for the treatment of mild to moderate hypertension: Result of the fourteen week trial. Arch Intern Med 144; 1947-1953, 1984.
31. Wilcox RG, Bennett T, Brown AM, MacDonald IA: Is exercise good for high blood pressure? Br Med J 285:767-769, 1982.
32. Wilson NV, Meyer BM: Early prediction of hypertension using exercise blood pressure. Prev Med 10: 61-68, 1981.
33. Yamakado T, Onishi N, Kondo S, et al: Effects of diltiazem on cardiovascular responses during exercise in systemic hypertension in comparison with propranolol. Am J Cardiol 52: 1023-1027, 1983.
34. Yodfat Y, Fiedel J, Bloom DS: Captopril as a replacement for multiple therapy and hypertension: A controlled study. J Hypertens 3:S155-S158, 1985.

13

Guidelines for Physically Active Diabetics

Kris E. Berg, Ed.D.

Exercise has been a part of diabetic management for many years. In comparison to insulin, oral hypoglycemic medications, and diet, however, exercise has typically received little emphasis. It is only recently that diabetes education has included detailed information regarding exercise.

Although the acute effects of exercise on diabetics are well understood, the chronic effects have not been investigated thoroughly.[7] In theory, physical activity can have a number of benefits for people with type 1 and type 2 diabetes, and probably for this reason current medical expertise supports the role of exercise in the management of diabetes,[8,18] The American Diabetes Association cites the specific enhancement of blood glucose (BG) management in type 2 patients, whereas this benefit is stated to be less likely to occur in most people with type 1 diabetes.

TYPES OF DIABETES

The characteristics of the two types of diabetes are summarized in Table 1.[5] Approximately 90 percent of the 12 million diabetics in the United States have type 2 or non-insulin-dependent diabetes mellitus. Exercise probably has a more consistent effect on improving the medical status of those in this majority group than those in the type 1 group. Although people with type 2 diabetes are prone to hypoglycemia if taking oral hypoglycemic medication or insulin, they are not prone to ketosis. In addition, with exercise, some type 2 diabetics may be able to control their blood sugar without oral medication or insulin, particularly if they lose weight.

BENEFITS OF EXERCISE

Consistent maintenance of BG levels reasonably close to normal may reverse the sequelae of poorly controlled diabetes such as retinopathy, nephropathy, microangiopathy, and neuropathy. Furthermore, current research data suggest that the state of the BG is probably a key determinant of when and how severely these sequelae occur. Because exercise typically causes the BG to drop in controlled diabetics of both types, it is a useful adjunct to the insulin or medication-diet regimen.

Exercise of the proper type, intensity, duration, and frequency has the same training effect in diabetics as in nondiabetics, if reasonable BG control is maintained and if a reasonable level of health exists so that the vigor and duration of exercise sessions are comparable.[10,16] For these reasons, exercise appears to offer a number of advantages for people with diabetes in terms of general health as well as in diabetes management specifically.

With today's availability of equipment that measures BG at home, diabetics should find it easier and safer to exercise. A daily record of BG test results enables both the patient and the physician to keep track of progress in BG control. Periodic measures of glycosylated hemoglobin (Hb_{AIC}) can also substantiate BG control for the previous 4–6 weeks. With such indices of diabetic management, the value of exercise in glucose control can be determined in patients.

Table 2 summarizes the physical, physiological, and psychological benefits that can accrue in properly regulated and properly exercised diabetics. Details are available elsewhere in the literature.[6]

EXERCISE GUIDELINES

BG should be measured before and after exercise. Diabetics perform best during exercise when BG is normal to moderately elevated and some insulin is in the blood. This facilitates normal substrate utilization rather than an exaggerated use of protein and fat. In moderate and vigorous exercise, limited use of glycogen and glucose impairs performance. Exercising when BG is below normal is dangerous, and a reasonable intensity of effort cannot be maintained long enough to provide a training effect. Conversely, exercise with BG levels above

TABLE 1. Characteristics of Type 1 and Type 2 Diabetes

Characteristics	Type 1 or Insulin Dependent	Type 2 or Noninsulin Dependent
Former terminology	Juvenile onset	Adult onset
Age at onset	Usually before 20	Usually after 40
Family history	Infrequent	Frequent
Appearance of symptoms	Rapid	Slow
Use of insulin	Always	Common but not always required
Production of insulin by pancreas	Absent or greatly reduced	Usually normal or elevated
Proneness to ketoacidosis	Prone	Not prone; rarely occurs
Body fatness	Usually normal or lean	Often obese

From Berg, K: Diabetic's Guide to Health and Fitness. Champaign, IL, Human Kinetics, 1986, p 16, with permission.

about 250 mg/dl tends to further elevate BG as well as possibly lead to ketosis. When BG reaches this threshold level, the lack of insulin stimulates the liver to release glucose via glycogenolysis. However, the tissues have a limited capacity to take in glucose, and, consequently, the longer the relative lack of insulin occurs, the greater the rise in BG.

TABLE 2. Summary of Chronic Training Effects in Healthy, Well-Controlled Diabetics

1. Improved circulorespiratory fitness
   - Greater maximal minute ventilation and frequency
   - Capacity for greater workload before heavy breathing occurs (i.e., a rise in ventilation or lactate threshold)
   - Greater maximal stroke volume, cardiac output, and oxygen pulse
   - Less strain on heart at the same submaximal workload (i.e., lower pressure-rate product due to reduction in exercise heart rate and blood pressure)
2. Improved ability for tissues to use oxygen
   - Greater volume of mitochondria
   - Greater activity of mitochondrial enzymes
   - More myoglobin
   - Enhanced use of fat versus glycogen as a source of muscular energy, which increases the capacity for prolonged exercise and allows a more vigorous work pace to be sustained
3. Greater muscular fitness; increased strength, muscle mass, muscle endurance, and power
4. Increased joint range of motion
5. Reduced risk factors for cardiovascular disease
   - Less body fat
   - Drop in blood pressure
   - Reduced cholesterol and triglyceride
   - Improved lipoprotein profile: greater HDL, greater HDL-to-total-cholesterol ratio, less LDL
   - Increased maximum oxygen uptake
   - Increased fibrinolysis
   - Reduced clotting
   - Reduced uric acid
   - Better ability to tolerate stress
   - Increased joie de vivre
6. Improved blood sugar control
7. Reduced likelihood of hypoglycemia during exercise due to greater fat utilization and increased liver and muscle glycogen
8. Reduced insulin or oral medication to regulate blood glucose
9. Increased self-concept and self-image

HDL = high-density lipoprotein, LDL = low-density lipoprotein.

Low blood insulin levels also stimulate the breakdown of fat through lipolysis. A rise in several hormones including the catecholamines, cortisol, growth hormone, and glucagon add to the effects of insulin shortage and enhance the rise in ketones and glucose. Type 1 diabetics are particularly prone to these effects. The liver converts some of the fatty acids to ketones, leading to ketoacidosis. Severe disturbance in acid-base balance, dehydration, and loss of electrolytes make for a serious state that may necessitate hospitalization. Consequently, exercising diabetics should have a functional level of insulin in the blood to prevent those changes. Assessment of BG before exercise is essential for this reason, particularly in type 1 patients.

Table 3 describes guidelines for making decisions regarding food intake before exercise. The BG level prior to exercise determines whether or not food is needed beforehand. Many type 2 diabetics need to lose weight; consequently, it is important that they use exercise as a means of taking less medication rather than eating more. Insulin reactions actually occur more frequently in the hours after exercise rather than during activity—probably because of the increased insulin sensitivity of muscle tissue, increased muscle glycogen resynthesis,

TABLE 3. Guidelines for Preexercise Snack

If BG exceeds 250 mg/dl, do not exercise: take __________ units of rapid-acting insulin and postpone exercise until later in the day. Check ketone level of urine.

If BG is 200–250 mg/dl, no snack is needed. If duration exceeds 30–45 minutes, assess BG again. If BG is below 200, see next step.

If BG is 120–199, consume 15 grams of CHO (one CHO exchange). For exercise beyond 30 minutes, consume 15 grams CHO per half hour. If BG is less than 120, consume 30 grams of CHO (two CHO exchanges). Beyond 30 minutes, consume 15 grams of CHO per half hour.

BG = blood glucose, CHO = carbohydrate.

and the small but long lasting rise in metabolism in the hours after exercise. Patients should understand the importance of monitoring ketones when BG exceeds 250 mg/dl and that the presence of ketones contraindicates exercise.

Skyler and associates recommend striving to keep BG in the range of 60–130 mg/dl before meals, 140–180 mg/dl 1 hour after meals, and 120–150 mg/dl 2 hours after meals.[17] If the blood sugar remains reasonably close to these values, a diabetic can be considered well controlled.

Exercise should be done about an hour after a meal whenever possible. This will minimize the occurrence of insulin reactions. Insulin reactions are most likely to occur late in the interval between meals or at the time of a scheduled snack. If one's schedule dictates exercise at such times, a snack before exercise can provide the energy needed. As stated previously, a BG test before exercise followed by one after the exercise session will indicate if enough or too many calories of the right type were consumed. The snack should be composed largely of carbohydrates, which can be digested and assimilated rapidly. These processes take 2–3 hours for fats and proteins, and they are therefore of no value in a typical 30- to 40-minute exercise bout. Furthermore, the rise in BG from fat and protein will not occur until well after the exercise is completed, which may produce an unexplained or unanticipated rise in postexercise BG.

Insulin or oral medication will typically need to be reduced when an exercise program is started. In the first several months of an exercise program, a 20–40% reduction is typical.[3] Additional reductions may not be needed, because one of the results of aerobic or endurance training is increased utilization of fat[12,15] and increased storage of muscle and liver glycogen.[9] Furthermore, because exercise and fat loss increase insulin sensitivity, less insulin or medication is needed. Consequently, whereas increased energy expenditure from exercise and increased insulin sensitivity reduce the requirement for insulin or medication, the increased fat utilization during exercise maintains the need for some medication. Thus, an exercise program has a limited effect in reducing the insulin or medication requirement in type 1 patients.

Skyler et al. suggest an insulin dosage for type 1 diabetics in the range of 0.5–1.0 units/kg of body weight.[17] However, highly active diabetics are often below that range, particularly during days of prolonged activity.[4]

On days of normal activity, many diabetics do not reduce their insulin.[12] This would be expected if the activity has been performed consistently for several months. Also, if exercise is a customary part of each day, no alteration in insulin or oral medication is needed.

The degree to which a typical exercise session reduces blood sugar should be tested. If diabetics err, it is all too common that they allow the BG to be elevated too high. Because most diabetics starting an exercise program fear insulin reaction, they exaggerate the amount of food eaten in a preexercise snack of they reduce their insulin or medication excessively. By measuring BG before and after exercise, patients may realize that though activity reduces BG if an adequate amount of insulin or medication has been taken, it will not commonly drop the glucose to the point of hypoglycemia. Fear of that occurrence may be alleviated by having the patient carry dextrose or candy during exercise.

During prolonged exercise such as running a marathon, backpacking, or playing in a daylong athletic tournament, carbohydrate should be consumed every 20–30 minutes. In addition, for patients using insulin, the dosage of intermediate (e.g., NPH, lente) or long-lasting insulin (e.g., ultralente) should be decreased about 50%,[11] but some insulin will be needed to maintain normal metabolism in type 1 patients.[8]

Athletes should measure their blood sugar before practice and particularly before games. All athletes get anxious and nervous before competition, and the symptoms mimic those of insulin reaction (e.g., tremor, perspiration, nervousness). Checking the BG allows distinguishability between nervousness and insulin reaction. Also, the stress associated with the pregame conditions will elevate the BG. If the athlete eats something as a treatment for symptoms of "false" insulin reaction, blood sugar may rise to the point where optimal performance is compromised. Ketosis may be produced in a type 1 diabetic. High-intensity exercise, due to increased sympathoadrenal activation, often leads to a rise in BG in diabetic athletes. Runners, for example, using interval training at intensities equal to or even surpassing VO_2 max often note this disturbing phenomenon. The surge in BG, however, typically subsides within several hours. The tricky question then arises as to whether or not to administer a bolus of regular insulin to counteract the elevated BG. Because of the heightened insulin sensitivity, glycogen resynthesis, and metabolic rate, supplemental insulin may well lead to hypoglycemia several hours later. For this reason, if supplemental insulin is used, the dosage should be smaller than when not associated with exercise. Furthermore, BG should be monitored at least once within 90 minutes after the insulin has been administered to determine the magnitude of change in BG.

The insulin injection site should be selected according to the type of exercise performed. The absorption of insulin into the blood is enhanced by an increase in local circulation.[18] This brings the injected insulin(s) to a peak effect sooner than normal, which would tend to lower the BG faster. To avoid the hypoglycemia possibly produced from this effect, diabetics using insulin should not use the thigh as an injection site before walking, running, cycling, aerobic dance, or other leg-predominant forms of exercise. Similarly, the arm or shoulder should not be used as an injection site before activities such as rowing, weight training, and calisthenics. Concern about injection site has been simplified somewhat by the observation that the most consistent absorption rates of insulin occur when injected into the abdomen. Generally, the farther from the heart, the slower the absorption and the longer time to peak insulin action. Most diabetics striving for optimal BG management are probably advised to use the abdomen as the preferred site. If this location is used and exercise follows at a similar time on a daily basis, the summative effects of insulin, food, and exercise will become well understood. Consequently, for most diabetics using insulin, the injection site may not be particularly critical so long as a consistent pattern is established with insulin, food, and exercise.

Diabetics should be wary of insulin reaction after extensive exercise at night and the following day. After a diabetic spends a day hunting, backpacking, or raking leaves, the glycogen level in the active muscles can be very low. This may be particularly true for type 1 patients who are poorly insulinized and hence store less muscle glycogen. Many of the carbohydrate calories ingested on the following day will be taken up by the skeletal muscles in order to synthesize glycogen. Furthermore, the rate of metabolism is elevated for hours after vigorous, prolonged exercise.[14] Consequently, the BG may have a tendency to be lower than expected the day after extensive exercise. There is also a tendency for nighttime insulin reactions to occur for the same reasons. If the BG is not normally measured before retiring, it should be during those times of unusual physical activity. Extra monitoring is the only means of preventing serious episodes of hypoglycemia. Some patients find that a small reduction of insulin the day after the activity reduces hypoglycemic episodes.

The main goal of people with type 2 diabetes should be to lose weight. Reduction of body fat and increased physical activity independently improve insulin sensitivity. Consequently, in some type 2 diabetics, insulin production may become adequate to normalize their metabolism without oral medication or with less medication.

Research indicates that exercise can be effective in fat loss if two criteria are met: first, exercise must be taken at least three times weekly; second, in each session at least 300 kcal must be expended.[1] To achieve that level of energy expenditure, most people should aim to reach a level of exercise intensity that is moderate, often just meeting, or even below, the level necessary for a cardiorespiratory training effect to occur. Inactivity and an associated obesity typify the majority of people with type 2 diabetes, so their relative lack of fitness will typically not allow burning 300 kcal per session unless the exercise intensity is low to moderate.

A cardiorespiratory or aerobic training effect threshold occurs at 40–50% of a person's maximum oxygen uptake. This is equivalent to about 55–65% of the maximum heart rate (maximum heart rate can be estimated by the equation 220 minus age in years). This threshold heart rate can be a training goal for the inactive, overweight diabetic, but if used at the onset of an exercise program, the intensity of the work may be perceived by the patient as too high. A useful adjunct to the heart rate concept and perhaps a more valid indicator regarding the physiological strain imposed by exercise is the concept of the talk test (the talk test is failed if one is unable to converse while physically active because of labored breathing). When their breathing is moderate and not labored, most people perceive the workload to be acceptable and are able to sustain continuous exercise for at least 15–20 minutes. Over several weeks of increasing the duration of each exercise session, most people will be able to tolerate a duration of exercise that allows expending 300 or more kcal.

Thus, exercise duration, rather than intensity, is the key training variable for each exercise session. Nearly any activity that uses the legs predominantly involves adequate muscle mass to expend the required 300 kcal. Depending on the work rate and body weight, approximately 30–60 minutes of exercise are needed by people of low to moderate fitness levels to expend this amount of energy. However, as the level of fitness improves and body weight is slowly decreased, speed of movement increases and more kcal can be expended each minute. For example, a person weighting 160 pounds expends about 3 kcal per minute when walking 1 mile in 30 minutes. Walking the mile in 15 minutes, however, would expend about 7.9 kcal per minute. If that 160-pound individual walked 30 minutes at this rate, 237 kcal would be expended. A 10-minutes-per-mile jog pace, however, expends 10 kcal each minute, or 300 kcal for a 30-minute session.[19]

Type 1 diabetics can gain weight with improved glucose control and exercise. When BG is elevated, it indicates an inadequate level of insulin or medication. That elevation retards glucose uptake by the tissues and the synthesis of glycogen. Because glycogen formation is accompanied by water storage, the poorly regulated diabetic stores less glycogen and water and tends to be chronically dehydrated. Inadequate insulin also slows the uptake of amino acids, which may interfere with the normal rate of protein synthesis and maintenance of skeletal muscle mass.

A shortage of insulin stimulates lipolysis (the breakdown of fat) and inhibits fat synthesis by decreasing the rate of glucose uptake into the adipose tissue to produce triglyceride. Consequently, the sum of these effects is that the diabetic with chronically elevated BG loses glycogen, body water, protein, and fat. For type 2 diabetics, this weight loss coincides with their most important exercise goal: to lose weight. However, it occurs at the expense of healthy tissue and body water. Some diabetics may purposely overeat, recognizing that a weight loss ensues when many calories are eliminated by the kidneys. Obviously, this practice should be discouraged.

Most type 1 diabetics are lean or of normal body weight. Young males commonly wish to gain lean tissue. Progressive resistance exercise is effective in producing muscle hypertrophy in diabetics as well as nondiabetics, but a second factor promoting weight gain for diabetics is BG management. Tight control minimizes water, fat, and protein loss and helps to maximize the building and maintenance of muscle weight. For some patients, this realization may encourage stricter dietary management and BG control.

CONTRAINDICATIONS FOR EXERCISE

Metabolic control must be established before an exercise program is started. As previously stated, if exercise occurs with a lack of insulin in the blood, the BG will rise during exercise and ketosis may develop. Newly diagnosed diabetics or those who are not reasonably well controlled should not begin an exercise program. First priority should be to achieve a fairly stable relationship between food intake and insulin or medication. Once a balance is demonstrated by acceptable BG data, only then should the third variable, exercise, be introduced. For some diabetics, this special clearance for exercise may aid in the motivation to use a home glucose monitoring kit and to discipline their eating habits to achieve good BG control.

An exercise electrocardiogram is usually warranted for diabetics older than age 40 or if the duration of diabetes has exceeded 25 years. Diabetics are at two to three times the risk for heart and large-artery disease than are nondiabetics. Consequently, a functional test of their circulation and exercise capacity should be administered. The results of the test are useful in deciding if their exercise program should be supervised (e.g., cardiac rehabilitation program) and for the writing of an exercise prescription.

Exercise that causes trauma to the feet should be avoided in patients with limited peripheral nerve and blood vessel function. One of the common sites of vascular insufficiency and peripheral sensory neuropathy is the feet. Patients with these disabilities may injure their feet without realizing the damage. For those with limited peripheral circulation, injuries are slow to heal and infection is more likely to be a problem. Activities such as jogging, martial arts, and diving place considerable trauma on the feet. For the same reasons, diabetics are advised to avoid not wearing shoes and socks; to examine their feet for blisters, corns, and bunions regularly; and to keep the feet well lubricated.

Patients with retinopathy should avoid strenuous activity, which may induce hemorrhage. Contact sports, jumping, scuba diving, weight training, and hanging inverted are not recommended for that reason. The greater the rise in blood pressure, the more likely episodes of hemorrhaging are. Consequently, limits may need to be set even on nonjarring aerobic exercise such as cycling and swimming.

SUMMARY

People with diabetes should consistently use exercise in a judicious manner as a basic part of their overall management program. Exercise has a number of physical, physiological, and psychological benefits, many of which may directly or indirectly affect BG and consequently patients' long-term health. With appropriate use of home/field glucose monitoring devices, most diabetics can and should be regularly active. Pubescent and adolescent diabetics can be active in competitive sports. As a matter of fact, for many adolescent diabetics, participation in sports may end the common stigma that they are physically limited. Furthermore, regular exercise may motivate some diabetics to maintain better BG control because of the impact on their capacity to exercise.

REFERENCES

1. American College of Sports Medicine: Guidelines for Exercise Testing and Prescription, 3rd ed. Philadelphia, Lea & Febiger, 1986.
2. American Diabetes Association: Exercise and NIDDM. Diabetes Care 13:785–789, 1990.
3. A Round Table: Diabetes and exercise. Physician Sportsmed 7:49–64, 1979.
4. Berg K: Blood glucose regulation in an insulin-dependent diabetic backpacker. Physician Sportsmed 11:101–104, 1983.
5. Berg K: Diabetic's Guide to Health and Fitness. Champaign, IL, Human Kinetics, 1986.
6. Berg K: Metabolic disease: diabetes mellitus. In Seefeldt V (ed): Physical Activity and Human Well Being. Reston, VA, American Alliance of Health, Physical Education, Recreation and Dance, 1986.

7. Berger M: Metabolic diseases and exercise performance. In Knuttgen HG, Voge JA, Poortman J (eds): Biochemistry of Exercise: International Series on Sports Sciences, Vol. 13. Champaign, IL, Human Kinetics, 1983.
8. Berger M, Berchtold P, Cuppers JJ, et al: Metabolic and hormonal effects of muscular exercise in juvenile type diabetics. Diabetologica 13:355–65, 1977.
9. Bergstrom J, Hermansen L, Saltin B: Diet, muscle glycogen and physical performance. Acta Physiol Scand 71:140–150, 1967.
10. Costill DL, Cleary P, Fink WJ, et al: Training adaptations in skeletal muscle of juvenile diabetics. Diabetes 28:812–822, 1979.
11. Etzwiler DD: When the diabetic wants to be an athlete. Physician Sportsmed 2:45–50, 1974.
12. Felig P, J Wahren: Amino acid metabolism in exercising man. J Clin Invest 50:2703–2714, 1971.
13. Flood T: Who's running? Forecast, March–April 1979, p 22.
14. Hagberg JM, Mullin JP, Nagle FJ: Effect of work intensity and duration in recovery O_2. J Appl Physiol 48:540–544, 1980.
15. Hagenfeldt L, Wahren J: Metabolism of free fatty acids and ketone bodies in skeletal muscle. In Pernow B, Saltin B (eds): Muscle metabolism during exercise. New York, Plenum Press, 1971.
16. Larsson Y, Persson B, Sterky G, Thoren C: Functional adaptation to vigorous training and exercise in diabetic and nondiabetic adolescents. J Appl Physiol 19:629–635, 1964.
17. Skyler J, Skyler D, O'Sullivan M: Algorithms for adjustment of insulin dosage by patients who monitor blood glucose. Diabetes Care 4:311–318, 1981.
18. Vranic M, Berger M: Exercise and diabetes mellitus. Diabetes 28:147–163, 1979.
19. Wilmore JH: Sensible Fitness. Champaign, IL, Leisure Press, 1986.

14

"Exercise-Induced" Asthma and Related Problems

Roger H. Kobayashi, M.D.
Morris B. Mellion, M.D.

EXERCISE-INDUCED ASTHMA

Exercise-induced asthma (EIA) is a common disease that can affect even world-class competitors. Until the 1972 Summer Olympic Games, however, when United States swimmer Rick DeMont had his gold medal rescinded following detection of traces of the antiasthmatic drug ephedrine in his urine, most were unaware of its significance. As a result of this unfortunate incident, athletes in this country were screened for asthma, and, in the XXIII Summer Olympics in Los Angeles, 41 of the 67 asthmatic American athletes participating won medals. That asthmatic athletes did well in the highly polluted air of Los Angeles serves as encouragement to all individuals with asthma who would like to participate in physical activity. Indeed more recently, Olympic champions such as Greg Louganis and Nancy Hogshead have won multiple gold medals despite having significant asthma.

The Chinese have known since antiquity that exercise could bring about an asthma attack. In the West, Aretaeus of Cappadocia described this phenomenon in the second century AD. In the 17th century, the English physician Thomas Willis provided a classical description of exercise-induced asthma. Nevertheless, despite awareness of this condition for over 20 centuries, the mechanisms of asthma, particularly EIA, remain unknown.[37,64]

During exercise, the bronchioles dilate and cause an increase in pulmonary function. In the post exercise period, however, pulmonary function decreases, slightly in normal individuals but significantly in asthmatics. After exercising for 5–10 minutes, patients with EIA experience a decrease of 15% or more in their lung function tests.[6,93] These individuals may be unaware of bronchospasm, experiencing only shortness of breath, coughing, chest pain, or tightness. Adults frequently think that they are "out of shape" whereas in children, coughing and lack of endurance may result in avoidance of vigorous play. This situation may go on for months or years before being recognized as EIA. Even when the examining physician suggests asthma, there is often denial or rejection of this diagnosis by the patient or patient's parents.

EIA occurs in as many as 80–90% of known asthmatics[1,37] and in 40–50% of persons with allergic rhinitis without any previous history of asthma.[25] In the general population, numerous studies have shown that 10% of high school and college athletes, randomly tested, have EIA (Fig. 1). Risk factors which should alert the physician or coach to look for EIA are shown in Table. 1

Definition

EIA is described as a transient increase in airway resistance following 6–8 minutes of vigorous exercise.[7,18,38] More precisely it is defined as a 15% or more decrease in forced expiratory volume in 1 second (FEV_1) or peak exploratory flow rate (PEFR) occurring maximally at 3–15 minutes postexercise.[1,37] A decrease of 20% or less is classified as mild disease, a 20–40% decrease is moderately severe, and 40% or more severe.[28]

Several important factors determine the severity of EIA: (1) the type of exercise, (2) the strenuousness of the exercise, (3) the conditions under which the exercise is occurring (Table 2), and (4) the duration of the exercise. Generally, the more vigorous and prolonged the exercise, the more severe the bronchospasm. Exercising in cold, dry air or where allergens, irritants, or air pollutants are present will significantly aggravate EIA. A concurrent viral in-

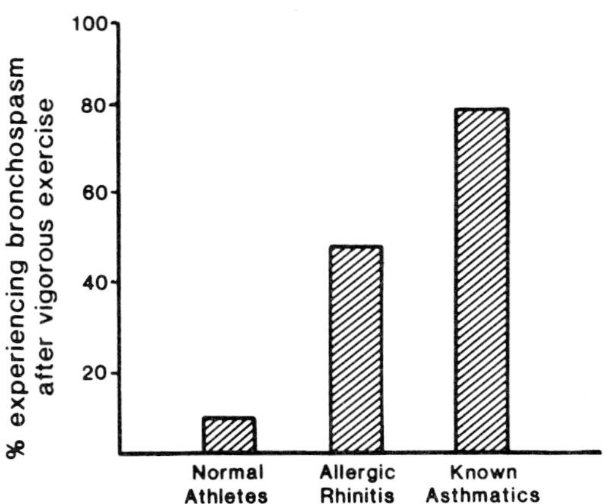

FIGURE 1. Incidence of exercise-induced bronchospasm.

TABLE 1. Athletes at Risk for Exercise-Induced Asthma

Those known to have asthma
Those with allergic rhinitis (hay fever)
Those with a family history of asthma
Those with frequent chest symptoms, i.e., coughing, congestion
Those with viral bronchitis
One out of every 10 members on your team

TABLE 2. Stimuli Which Contribute to Attacks of Exercise-Induced Asthma

Exercise
Cold
Low humidity
Pollutants:
Allergens
Dust
Irritants
Automobile exhaust and commercial pollutants, especially: SO_2, NO_2, O_3
Respiratory infections
Fatigue
Emotional stress
Athletic overtraining

fection will increase the likelihood of inducing EIA. These factors combine to exceed the individual's threshold for EIA (Fig. 2).

Mechanisms

In the early 1970s, it was generally held that EIA resulted from mediator-release through a mechanism provoked by exercise. This view was particularly attractive, because cromolyn sodium, an inhibitor of mediator-release attenuated EIA worked if given before exercise, but was ineffective if given after exercise in the wheezing patient (i.e., presumably after mediators have been released). It was difficult to explain, however, why certain kinds of strenuous exercise, such as swimming, failed to cause asthma.

Early studies suggested that breathing humidified air decreased the severity of EIA,[2,6] thus helping to explain how swimming might be less likely to cause bronchospasm. Subsequently, McFadden and colleagues published a series of articles indicating a correlation between the amount of respiratory heat loss and the severity of asthma.[64] It appeared that heat loss was the important factor, whether induced by hyperventilation from exercise or by hyperventilation alone.[23,24] On the other hand, several studies have indicated that EIA can occur even when there is no respiratory heat loss.[8,9,42] Careful studies by Anderson and associates, as well as others, suggest that it may be relative water loss with resultant hyperosmolarity in the respiratory epithelial fluid that

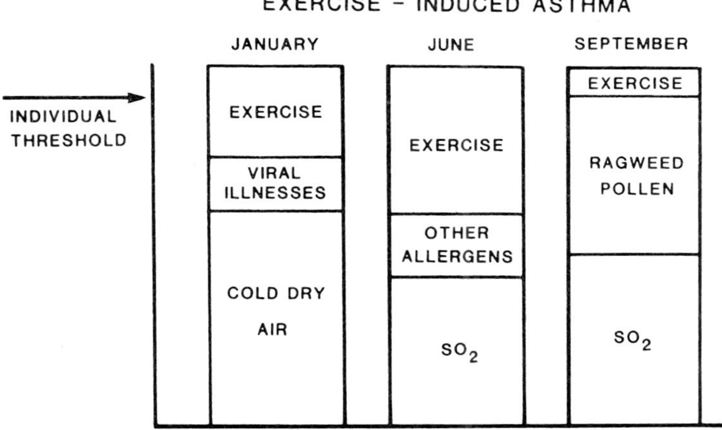

FIGURE 2. Relative contribution to exercise-induced bronchospasm (EIB) in an individual who has EIB and ragweed hay fever.

initiates bronchospasm[2,3,4,5,89] rather than heat loss. More recently, McFadden's group have suggested that airway rewarming with vascular dilatation can lead to airway obstruction.[65,66]

As it is with the three blind men, each describing the elephant only by the part he is touching, so it is with EIA. Recently, there has been tremendous refocusing of interest back to mediator release. Histamine and neutrophil chemotactic factor (NCF) release have been studied extensively in EIA and have been shown to play an important role.[57,58,59] Other anti-inflammatory mediators that can be released following vigorous exercise or hyperventilation include eosinophil chemotactic factor of anaphylaxis (ECF-A), the leukotrienes (LTC_4, LTD_4, LTE_4), formerly known collectively as slow-reacting substance of anaphylaxis, and platelet-activating factor (PAF).[41,60,68] Many of these mediators may be responsible for late-phase asthma, that is, bronchospasm occurring 4 to 8 hours after challenge (Fig. 3).[12] Finally, there may be cholinergic influence either centrally mediated or in response to local inflammation (Table 3).[41,101] Where does this leave us? Dr. Simon Godfrey, a highly respected asthma researcher from Jerusalem, has some practical advice: "What this all means for the asthmatic athlete is probably that he/she should try to avoid exercising in cold, dry conditions and should choose swimming rather than skiing as the preferred sport."[38] Physicians caring for athletes, however, must develop treatment strategies that are appropriate no matter what the chosen sport.

Testing

Testing for EIA should be considered in any athlete with a prior history of childhood asthma, chronic cough, present or past history of chest problems, and allergies. Pulmonary function tests (PFTs) should be within 80% of predicted normal levels before exercise challenge.[28] Medications for treating asthma should be withheld for 8–24 hours, depending on the drug. Beta-agonist and theo-

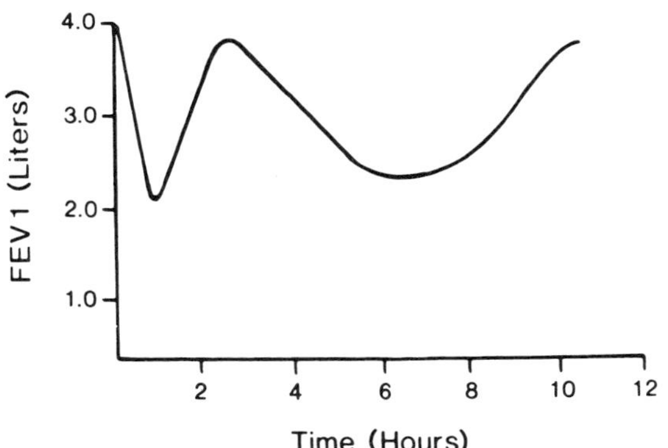

FIGURE 3. Early and late-phase bronchospasm.

TABLE 3. Mechanisms of Exercise-Induced Asthma

Early Reactions
Respiratory water loss—resulting in changes in epithelial cell osmolarity
Temperature change—airway cooling
Cholinergic response—neurological, inflammatory
Mediator release—histamine
Reactive hyperemia from rapid rewarming
Late Reaction—Mast-Cell Degranulation
Neutrophil chemotactic factor
Eosinophil chemotactic factor
Leukotrienes (LTC_4, LTD_4, LTE_4)

phylline should be withheld for 8 hours with regular acting preparations or 12 to 24 hours with sustained-release preparations. Cromolyn sodium should not be used for 24 hours, and cholinergic antagonists 8 hours. Steroid preparations can be used unless the patient is also being studied for the presence of late-phase asthma. Certain antihistamines such as astemizole, terfenadine, or loratadine may have mild antiasthma properties and are best avoided prior to testing.

Equipment necessary for testing depends on the setting and resources available. If a pulmonary function laboratory is available, then a treadmill or cycloergometer is used. Because EIA induces both large and small airway disease, several different pulmonary function parameters may be used including forced expiratory flow $(FEF)_{25-75}$, FEV_1, or PEFR. These may be measured on a spirometer or in the case of PEFR, a peak flow meter. Electrocardiographic (ECG) monitoring may be advisable for those at risk, and a cardiotachometer makes monitoring the heart rate simpler. Equipment and drugs necessary to treat cardiac and pulmonary complications should be readily available and patients with known heart disease should be tested very cautiously. The equipment used for these standardized exercise challenge tests is expensive and cumbersome. For formal testing, the workload must be strenuous, continuous, and at least 6–8 minutes in duration. A nose clip is used to induce breathing through the mouth, and the workload is adjusted to 80–85% of the patient's predicted work capacity or to a heart rate of 90% of predicted maximum values.[28] A cycloergometer is much cheaper and less cumbersome than a treadmill. From a practical standpoint, the subject is coached to achieve a heart rate between 170 and 200/min (220 minus the age in years) and to maintain this rate for 6–8 minutes. After baseline pulmonary functions are obtained, strenuous exercise is sustained for 6–8 minutes and then subsequent PFT are obtained every 5 minutes for 20–30 minutes; generally the greatest fall in PFT is observed at 10 minutes after exercise. Results are expressed as a percentage decrease:

$$\% \text{ decrease} = \frac{\text{Baseline PFT} - \text{lowest PFT value after exercise} \times 100}{\text{Baseline PFT}}$$

A decrease of 15% or more is considered a positive challenge. Ideally, because EIA is enhanced in cold air with low humidity, testing should not be done in a room with high temperature and humidity. To determine the protective effect of certain drugs, PFT is measured before the drug is administered and again just before exercise. The patient is then exercised and the results are compared to the nondrug treated measurements.

In an office, elaborate equipment is often neither available nor affordable. Nevertheless, it may be still possible to determine whether exercise provokes bronchospasm. A baseline PFT, obtained by an office spirometer or peak flow meter, and a resting heart rate are recorded. The patient is then made to run around the building or up and down flights of stairs in an attempt to sustain a heart rate of 170–200 beats per minute continually for 6–8 minutes. PFTs are then measured every 5 minutes over a 20–30-minute period. Although this is neither ideal nor standardized, an indication of whether bronchospasm is induced or not *can* be determined. More importantly, testing does not cost the typical $200–$400 charged by many pulmonary function laboratories.

An extension of laboratory or office testing is to measure lung function changes on the playing fields. A peak flow meter or portable spirometer may be used to monitor obstructive lung changes under actual sporting conditions, either in practice or in actual competition. The advantage of this setting is that it is inexpensive, it duplicates the actual "field" conditions, and it permits the assessment of drug effectiveness.

Several cautions must be kept in mind when performing exercise-pulmonary testing:

1. Avoid doing more than one or two challenges a day on the same subject as "refractoriness" may follow successive periods of exercise.
2. Certain patients may not experience EIA when challenged under warm, humid conditions and may experience EIA only under cold, dry conditions.
3. Additionally, others may have significant EIA only when exposed concurrently to air pollutants, allergens, or other pulmonary irritants. Testing these individuals under office or laboratory conditions may not provoke bronchospasm, thus leading to the erroneous conclusion that EIA is not present. Several challenges may be necessary before EIA can be effectively excluded.
4. Clearly, patients at risk for cardiac problems or those who are taking beta-blockers should be tested with extreme caution, if at all. Fatalities have been reported in individuals exercising while taking beta-blockers.[85]
5. Elaborate and sophisticated laboratory studies cannot substitute for a careful, thoughtful medical history and examination by an astute physician.

Pharmacologic Therapy

Among the many drugs used in the treatment and prevention of EIA (Table 4), beta-2-specific agonists are the most effective.[69] These include albuterol, terbutaline, bitolterol, and salmeterol. Other beta-2-specific agents are available in Europe and other countries but not in the United States, including fenoterol and rimiterol.

Other sympathomimetic agents used in asthma with effectivness include metaproterenol, isoetharine, isoproterenol, ephedrine and epinephrine. Most of these drugs are familiar and time-honored in the treatment of asthma.

Albuterol (Ventolin, Proventil), terbutaline (Brethaire, Bricanyl), pirbuterol (Maxair) and bitolterol (Tornalate) are administered by aerosol 10 to 60 minutes before exercise. When administered correctly, they may effectively inhibit bronchospasm for as long as 3 to 6 hours.[51,55,69,80] Salmeterol, a recently available beta-agonist, may inhibit EIA for as long as 9 to 12 hours,[40,47,73] but has a slower onset of action. Delivery by metered-dose inhalers (MDI), or nebulizer, result in more rapid onset of action, fewer side effects, and greater effectiveness when compared with oral administration.[70,92] Usually 2 puffs by MDI are sufficient, although as many as 4 to 6 puffs may be even more effective. When using the oral form, it is advisable to take the drug at least 1 hour before exercise, because the onset of action is delayed by slower intestinal absorption. Although less effective, the long-acting oral beta-ag-

TABLE 4. Drugs Effective Against Exercise-Induced Asthma

Most Effective
•Albuterol
•Pirbuterol
•Terbutaline
•Bitolterol
Effective
•Cromolyn
•Nedocromil
•Metaproterenol
•Theophylline
•Salmeterol
Effective in Preventing Late-phase Asthma
•Cromolyn
•Nedocromil
•Inhaled steroids

onists are convenient and some athletes prefer this over the inhalers (which may be less convenient); tremors and tachycardia can be a problem, however.

Cromolyn sodium given a few minutes before exercise protects as many as 70% of patients with EIA, possibly by preventing mast-cell degranulation and inhibiting mediator release.[50,53] It is not as effective as the beta-2-specific agonists,[16,82] however, and the duration of action is not as long. Further, because it does not cause bronchodilation, baseline PFTs are not improved. It is as effective as theophylline and is more effective than atropine and ketotifen. Cromolyn has the added advantage of being effective against late reaction asthma and of having virtually no known side effects. It was previously thought that the Spinhaler delivery system with its lactose powder capsule was less effective because of the irritant effect of lactose on the airways; however, several investigators have shown no difference between cromolyn delivered by Spinhaler and cromolyn delivered by nonlactose-containing MDI.[20]

Nedocromil sodium (Tilade), a structurally different compound from cromolyn sodium has been found to share similar characteristics.[10,15] It appears to stabilize mast-cell membranes, inhibit mediator release, inhibit some of the activities of inflammatory mediators, and inhibit neuropeptide release from sensory nerves. It is provided in a pressurized MDI that releases 2 mg per accentuation.The usual dose is 4 mg (2 puffs) 2–4 times/day. Nedocromil sodium blocks both early and late-phase asthma and has been shown to be as effective or slightly more effective than cromolyn sodium in clinical settings. It has been moderately effective in EIA.[54,86]

Theophylline, although not as widely used as in the past, has been shown to be effective in preventing EIA.[11,26,29,30,33,78,99,100] Although less effective than inhaled beta-2-specific agonists,[56] sustained use of theophylline may be more effective than taking a single dose before exercise.[30] Chronic use of theophylline appears to exert a potent prophylactic effect,[9] and more recent data suggest an anti-inflammatory effect as well.[72,76,99] There is a correlative effect between serum theophylline levels and the degree of bronchodilation;[59] therefore, Weinberger argues for maintaining a serum theophylline level between 10 and 20 μg/ml.[99] More recent data indicate that lower levels, i.e., 5 to 15 μg/ml, are effective and may avoid some of the side effects.[31] Occasionally, it may be beneficial to combine theophylline with a beta-2-specific agonist.[46,56,97] The combination of these two agents may increase side effects or have potentially dangerous cardiotoxicity,[27] particularly under conditions of hypoxia. Therefore, appropriate caution should be exercised. A search for effective, but safer, xanthine drugs is under way.[74,75]

Atropine and ipratropium bromide have been studied with conflicting results in EIA,[14,19,79,96] although they are now generally felt to be moderately effective agents.[101] Ipratropium is preferred to atropine because the side effects are fewer. Onset of action is between 1 and 2 hours and the duration of protection is about 3–5 hours. At present, its use is somewhat limited in EIA, because it requires a near-normal baseline PFT.

Inhaled steroids are not useful in EIA, although they may prevent late-phase asthma.[43] Inhaled steroids, such as beclomethasone, triamcinolone, and budesonide, are useful in chronic, moderately severe asthma where airway inflammation and hyperreactivity are prevalent.

Treatment must be kept simple and convenient, and the number of medications used must be minimized. It is unrealistic to expect a busy student or athlete to use three or more inhalers because this would be highly inconvenient. From a practical standpoint, often the long-acting beta-agonists such as salmeterol or bitolterol may be useful because they afford long-term (8–12 hours) protection. Shorter-acting agents such as cromolyn (2 hours' effective duration) are often impractical.

New and Experimental Drugs

Many other drugs have been evaluated (Table 5). Several cromolyn-like drugs have been studied extensively but thus far have been disappointing in clinical trials. Anti-inflammatory-histamine agents have also been investigated, with ketotifen showing some positive effect. Calcium antagonists such as nifedipine, taken in 20-mg doses 30 minutes before exercise, may afford limited protection.[17,21] Diltiazem, PY108-068, and other calcium channel blockers have also been evaluated in EIA, but none has demonstrated major clinical benefit. Other agents such as antiplatelet-activating factor medications, leukotriene inhibitors, and antiinflammatory drugs are being extensively investigated.[13] Inhibitors of arachidonic acid metabolism and leukotriene C_4 or leukotriene D_4 blockers and receptor antagnoists appear to have the greatest clinical potential. Zileuton blocks leukotriene production by inhibiting arachidonic acid metabolism and the 5-lipoxygenase pathway. This compound has been shown to be effective in bronchospasm on by cold, dry air hyperventilation.[44] Another agent, MK-571, a highly selective leukotriene D_4 receptor antagonist, has a bronchodilating effect and also is effective against EIA.[36,63] Significant liver enzyme abnormalities resulted in cessation of clinical studies, however. Studies on related compounds are under way. Other leukotriene D_4 receptor antagonists such as ICI204, 219 (Accolate),[32] Ly171, 883,[45] and SKF104, 353[81]

TABLE 5. New or Experimental Agents

Cromolyn-like Agents	
Proxicromil	Mildly effective in asthma and exercise-induced asthma; investigation suspended when malignancies occurred in long-term animal studies.
Doxantrazole	More active than cromolyn in vitro but ineffective in clinical asthma and exercise-induced asthma.
Fenprinast	Investigational dosages indicated drug was ineffective; higher dosage ranges are now being studied.
Cromolyn-like Activity with Different Chemical Structure	
Lodoxamide	In aerosol form, somewhat effective. Orally, effective but significant side effects.
Bufrolin	300 times more potent than cromolyn in vitro but only slightly effective in clinical studies.
Nivimedone	25 to 30 times more potent than cromolyn sodium in vitro; only slightly effective clinically.
Anti-inflammatory/Antihistamine	
Tiaramide	Anti-inflammatory agent with anti-asthma properties; clinical studies indicated effectiveness; however studies in the U.S. were suspended when seizures occurred in several patients.
Ketotifen-oral antihistamines	5000 times more potent than cromolyn in vitro. In clinical trials, effectiveness appears to be comparable to theophylline and cromolyn. Effectiveness with exercise-induced asthma is unclear.
Azatadine (Trinalin)	Antihistamine and in vitro inhibitor of mediator release. However, the high dosages required to prevent exercise-induced bronchospasm and are associated with considerable side effects.
Calcium Channel Blockers	
Verapamil/Nifedipine	Studies suggest some protection against exercise-induced bronchospasm but without bronchodilatory effect.
Irratropium Bromide	Quaternary derivative of atropine. Effective in asthma, particularly bronchitic asthma; however, results in preventing exercise-induced asthma are controversial.
Steroids	
Budesonide-Steroid Aerosol	Some protection after prolonged treatment.
Leukotriene Receptor Antagonists	
Zileuton	5-lipoxygenase inhibitor. Useful in asthma and cold, dry air-induced bronchospasm.
Ly171, 883	Leukotriene D_4 receptor antagonist. Beneficial in asthma and in cold dry air-induced bronchospasm.
MK-571	Potent, highly selective leukotriene D_4 receptor antagonist. Effective in bronchial asthma and in exercise-induced asthma. However, studies have been halted because of liver abnormalities.
ICI204, 219 (Accolate)	Oral leukotriene D_4 receptor antagonist. Effective in allergen and exercise-induced asthma.
SKF104, 353	Inhaled agent; effective in exercise-induced asthma and perhaps in some aspirin-induced bronchospasm.

have shown effectiveness in preventing bronchospasm induced by cold-air hyperventilation or exercise. Further studies are required before these agents receive indications and are released by the Food and Drug Administration. For an overview of nontraditional agents used in the treatment of asthma, see the review by Furukawa.[35]

Permitted and "Banned" Drugs

The experience of Rick DeMont, the U.S. swimmer disqualified in 1972 Olympics, was sad. Any athlete competing on an organized level should check carefully with the appropriate governing boards as to which drugs used in the treatment of asthma are acceptable. Before the 1993–1994 school year, the National Collegiate Athletic Association (NCAA) maintained a long list of banned substances contained in common medications used to treat asthma and allergic rhinitis. Since then, any legitimate medication prescribed by a physician for asthma and allergic rhinitis has been permitted, with the exception that the beta-2-agonists are permitted by aerosol only. Tables 6 and 7 list drugs approved and banned

TABLE 6. Therapeutic Agents for Exercise-induced Asthma Acceptable to the International Olympic Committee Medical Commission

Atropine sulfate
Caffeine*
Corticosteroids**
Cromolyn sodium
  Methylxanthines-theophylline
  Sympathomimetic amines (beta-2-specific aerosols only)**

*Caffeine is a *weak* bronchodilator, which is banned if urinary concentration >15 μg/ml for NCAA and >12 μg/ml for Olympic competition.
**Requires letter from team physician.

TABLE 8. Drugs That Might Be Used by the Asthmatic Athlete That Are Banned from Use during Competition

All sympathomimetic amines (except albuterol and terbutaline aerosols)
  Includes virtually all oral decongestants and many topical decongestants for the eyes
Opiate analgesics and antitussives (nonopiates are acceptable, e.g., dextromethorphan, diphenhydramine)

by the International Olympic Committee. Table 7 includes a list of banned antiasthmatic drugs and Table 8 lists banned drugs that might be inadvertently taken by the athlete. Particular care must be focused on antiallergic agents because many can be obtained over-the-counter in ubiquitous "cold" preparations. Table 8 lists other banned drugs that might be prescribed for the asthmatic athlete. Not infrequently, asthmatics have persistent coughing and some widely available cough medications, such as PennTuss or Dimetapp with Codeine, may be used without the athlete's knowing they contain drugs that may cause disqualification.

Nonpharmacologic Modalities

Conditioning. Although there are documented reports of exercise conditioning prescribed for asthma as far back as the 1500s,[62] unfortunately most physicians do not encourage exercise programs for asthmatics. Certainly, increased physical fitness results in a reduced ventilation rate during exercise; earlier reports suggest that increased physical conditioning decreases the requirement for antiasthmatic medications, decreases the frequency and severity of asthma, and reduces work and school absences.[33,48,77] In a Norwegian study, bicycling challenge before and after training significantly decreased EIA.[34] More recent studies have shown that even children with chronic, severe asthma can engage in strenuous, long-distance exercise without adverse effects provided they receive the proper medications. Nevertheless, highly strenuous exercise can provoke EIA even in the well-conditioned athlete,[91] so physicians should exercise good clinical judgment.

Inducing "Refractoriness" by Short Bursts of Activity. Short bursts of repeated physical activity can decrease EIA.[67,71,91] Schnall and Landau reported that seven 30-second periods of running, separated by short intervals of rest, appeared to protect their small patient sample.[84] Subjects appear to be "protected" from EIA for 1–3 hours.

Other Protective Maneuvers. Long-distance running may permit athletes to "run though" their EIA.[95] Whether this is true refractoriness or merely enhanced endurance remains unknown.[84] Nevertheless, some asthmatic athletes tolerate running long distances, and this effect may be due to endogenous catecholamine release during exercise. Although it is important for all athletes to warm up before engaging in vigorous exercise, it is especially important for asthmatic individuals. Each session should begin with a warm-up period of 10 to 15 minutes of stretching exercises and calisthenics. Likewise, following vigorous exercise the asthmatic athlete should "warm down" for about 10 minutes.[33,49,61]

A well-planned conditioning program of increasing intensity should be devised for each asthmatic athlete. The training program should allow the athlete to exercise different muscle groups, with particular focus on strengthening the upper body musculature. Breathing exercises may be beneficial with emphasis on breathing in a slow, deep, rhythmic pattern to allow more efficient air flow and relaxation. Hyperventilation should be avoided. The athlete should be encouraged to breathe through the nose whenever possible because the filtering and warming effects caused by the nasal passage may lower the risk of EIA;[90] with increasing workload, however, mouth-breathing is invariably necessary to meet metabolic requirements. Patients with nasal

TABLE 7. Sympathomimetic Amines Banned or Permitted in Olympic Competition

BANNED
  Adrenaline (epinephrine)
  Ephedrine
  Isoetharine
  Isoproterenol
  Metaproterenol
  Bitolterol
  Salmeterol
  Fenoterol*
  Rimiterol*

PERMITTED (With a letter from team physician)**
  Albuterol (Aerosol only)
  Terbutaline (Aerosol only)

*Not currently available in the United States.
**The NCAA allows any legitimately approved asthma medication provided it is prescribed by a licensed physician.

obstruction from allergic rhinitis tend to breathe through the mouth, thus negating the air-conditioning effects of the nasal passages. Wearing a surgical mask to warm and humidify the air around the mouth may help to prevent EIA.[83] When possible, athletes should avoid exercising vigorously in cold, dry, polluted air.

While athletes should be encouraged to choose activities that they enjoy, certain sports such as tennis, swimming, baseball, or volleyball, which are associated with short exercise bursts, may be much better tolerated. Activities that require prolonged, vigorous exercise, such as long-distance running, competitive bicycling, downhill or cross-country skiing, ice skating, soccer, and basketball, are often poorly tolerated. Nonetheless, with proper conditioning, "warm-up" periods, and repetitive short exercise bursts to induce a "refractory" period, along with appropriate pharmacotherapy, the athlete may be able to participate in these vigorous activities on a competitive level. It is important for the physician, coaching staff, and affected athletes to work together.

EXERCISE-INDUCED ANAPHYLAXIS

Exercise-induced anaphylaxis (EIAna), although uncommon, can be frightening and potentially fatal. I recall a 30-year-old laboratory technician who nearly expired on two occasions but was fortunately given epinephrine by his wife, who happened to be a nurse. Not all cases are as dramatic; however, the following example demonstrates that this can be a frightening experience.

> A 16-year-old active girl went out on a tennis date after dinner with a boy whom she wanted to impress. After several minutes of exercise, she began feeling warm and itchy, and noticed an erythematous rash with some urticaria. She was too embarrassed to say anything and continued playing. She then began to have facial swelling and a choking sensation. Nevertheless, because she wanted to make a favorable impression, she continued to play. Subsequently, she had difficulty breathing, felt faint, and her face became increasingly swollen. Reason prevailed, and she was taken to the emergency room where the pediatrician on call gave her epinephrine, intravenous steroids, and antihistamines. Over the next 24 hours, her symptoms gradually abated. On questioning, she had experienced two less-severe episodes while in gymnastics class during the previous 2 years. She could not remember whether she had eaten shortly before the exercise periods, and she had engaged in similar activities previously without precipitating these symptoms.

Exercise-induced anaphylaxis was recognized in the past, however, it was only clearly described as a syndrome by Sheffer and Austen in 1980.[87] It is an unpredictable and potentially life-threatening reaction consisting of erythema, pruritus, urticaria, angioedema, laryngospasm, and hypotension (Table 9). In one series, 32% of patients lost consciousness.[98] In addition, patients may experience gastrointestinal symptoms, including cramping, nausea, vomiting, and diarrhea, and possibly headaches.

Risk Factors

There are several risk factors for EIAna, but symptoms may come on unexpectedly and conditions that brought on the first attack may not precipitate other attacks. Exercising shortly after eating has been associated with EIAna. For reasons that are not clear, celery has been implicated in several cases.[52] Whether this represents a cross-reactivity with celery antigen and ragweed antigen remains to be proved. Prior consumption of shellfish, cabbage, peaches, caffeine, wheat products, ethanol, and aspirin has been associated with EIAna. Intensity of exercise also appears to be an important factor: the likelihood and severity of symptoms vary directly with exercise intensity.[88] Jogging is the most common inciting activity, but racquet sports, bicycling, skiing, walking, and other activities have also precipitated attacks. A positive personal or family history of allergies may be present in some patients. Weather conditions may also play a factor. Unlike EIA, EIAna is associated more commonly with hot, humid weather conditions.

TABLE 9. **Exercise-induced Anaphylaxis**

SIGNS AND SYMPTOMS
- Generalized pruritus
- Generalized urticaria
- Angioedema (face, palms of the hands, soles of the feet)
- Upper respiratory tract symptoms
- Choking and difficulty swallowing
- Gastrointestinal symptoms, cramping, nausea, diarrhea
- Headaches

RISK FACTORS (Factors are unproven)
- Positive personal or family history of allergies
- Food consumed—shellfish, celery, aspirin
- Weather conditions—seem more common with hot, humid weather conditions
- Intensity of exercise—appears to be worse with highly vigorous exercise

PREVENTION/PRECAUTIONS
- Reduction in intensity of exertion
- Avoidance of exercise on hot, humid days
- Avoid eating before exercise
- Immediate availability of an individual capable of treating anaphylaxis

MEDICATIONS
- Pretreatment with antihistamines partially effective
- Pretreatment with beta adrenergic agents and theophylline compounds of unproven benefit

Prevention and Therapy

It is somewhat difficult to treat an condition with a cause not clearly defined, the attacks of which may be sporadic. Nevertheless, in those athletes with a previous attack of EIAna, it is advisable to avoid eating before exercise and also to avoid exercising under hot, humid conditions. Because intensity of exertion appears to be related to the severity of symptoms, less intense exercise may be advisable. Ingestion of aspirin and other nonsteroidal anti-inflammatory agents should be avoided before exercise. Clearly if warmth and itching occur, especially on the palms and soles, the athlete should stop exercising immediately. Athletes with a history of EIAna should not exercise alone and should advise their companion that an attack might occur and what first aid measures to be taken if one does. An Epi-Pen or Ana-kit should be available, and the individual and companion should know how to administer these medications.

Anecdotally, pretreatment with certain antihistamines has been partially effective, however, preadministration of theophylline or beta-adrenergic compounds has not been shown to be beneficial.[95]

Appropriate, rapid treatment of anaphylaxis is mandatory. Subcutaneous epinephrine should be given immediately and antihistamines such as diphenhydramine or hydroxyzine should be given. Steroids and intravenous fluids can also be given if warranted. Distinction must be made from other exercise-associated severe events such as myocardial infarction and arrhythmias, cerebral vascular accidents, "heat stroke," and syncope.

CHOLINERGIC URTICARIA

Cholinergic urticaria or generalized heat urticaria is a syndrome characterized by generalized, small, urticarial papules occurring after a warm bath, shower, exercise, or with increased body temperature. These lesions typically occur as small papules on the upper thorax and neck and spread downwards to involve the entire body. Generalized, systemic reactions such as abdominal pain, syncope, or wheezing are rare. Cholinergic reactions (lacrimation, salivation, diarrhea) may be observed. Risk factors include heat and increased humidity. The mechanisms are unclear; however a neurogenic reflex has been hypothesized. Mediator release, including histamine and neutrophil chemotactic factor, has been observed. Although this is an annoying problem, the best treatment is preventing exposure to heat and humidity. Antihistamines may prevent cholinergic urticaria or at least decrease the incidence. Therapy includes hydroxyzine (at a dose of 25–200 mg per day in divided doses) or cyproheptadine (at a dose of 4–20 mg/day in 2 or 3 divided doses).[22,39]

SUMMARY

Exercise-induced asthma is both very common and under-diagnosed. Symptoms encountered may not necessarily relate to those classically associated with asthma, such as wheezing. Awareness and proper recognition by the physician and coach can enable proper treatment of this entity. Appropriate conditioning, warming up, inducing "refractoriness," engaging in sports that are less likely to provoke EIA, and aggressive use of appropriate medications will allow athletes to enjoy sports and compete effectively. Exercise-induced anaphylaxis is being described more frequently. Appropriate recognition and precautions are necessary.

Acknowledgments. The secretarial assistance of Lucinda Gillette was greatly appreciated.

REFERENCES

1. Anderson SD: Current concepts of exercise-induced asthma. Allergy 38:289–302, 1983.
2. Anderson SD: Is there a unifying hypothesis for exercise-induced asthma? J Allergy Clin Immunol 73:660–665, 1984.
3. Anderson SD, Daviskas E: The airway microvasculature and exercise-induced asthma. Thorax 47:748–758, 1992.
4. Anderson SD, Schoeffel RE, Follet R: Sensitivity to heat and water loss at rest and during exercise in asthma patients. Eur J Respir Dis 63:459–71, 1982.
5. Anderson SD, Schoeffel RE: Respiratory heat loss and water loss during exercise in patients with asthma. Eur J Respir Dis 63:472–480, 1982.
6. Anderson SD, Silverman M, Konig P, et al: Exercise-induced asthma. Br J Dis Chest 69:1–39, 1975.
7. Bar-Yishay E, Godfrey S: Mechanisms of exercise-induced asthma. Lung 162:195–204, 1984.
8. Ben-Dov I: Refractory period after exercise-induced asthma unexplained by respiratory heat loss. Am Rev Respir Dis 125:530–34, 1982.
9. Ben Dov I, Bar-Yishay E, Godfrey S: Exercise-induced asthma without respiratory heat loss. Thorax 37:730–31, 1982.
10. Bernstein JA, Bernstein IL: Cromolyn and nedocromil: Novel anti-allergy drugs. Immunol Allergy Clin North Am 13:891–902, 1993.
11. Bierman CW, Shapiro GG, Pierson We, et al: Acute and chronic theophylline therapy in exercise-induced asthma. Pediatrics 60:845, 1977.
12. Bierman CW, Spiro SG, Petheram I: Characterization of the late response in exercise-induced asthma. J Allergy Clin Immunol 74:701–06, 1984.
13. Bjornsdottir US, Bush RK: Leukotriene antagonists and inhibitors. Immunol Allergy Clin North Am 13:861–890, 1993.
14. Borut TC, Tashkin DP, Fischer TJ, et al: Comparison of aerosolized atropine sulfate and SCH 1000 on exercise-induced asthma in children. J Allergy Clin Immunol 60:127–33, 1977.
15. Brogden RN, Sorkn EM: Nedocromil sodium: An updated review of its pharmacological properties and therapeutic efficacy in asthma. Drugs 45:639–715, 1993.

16. Broulet L, Turcotte H, Tennino S: Comparison of efficacy of salbuterol, ipratropium and cromolyn in the prevention of bronchospasm induced by exercise and hyperosmolar challenge. J Allergy Clin Immunol 83:882–887, 1989.
17. Cerrina J, Denjean A, Alexandre G, et al: Inhibition of exercise-induced asthma by a calcium antagonist, nifedipine. Am Rev Respir Dis 123:156–160, 1981.
18. Chan-Yeung MM, Vyas MN, Grzybowski S: Exercise-induced asthma. Am Rev Respir Dis 104:915–23, 1971.
19. Chan-Yeung M: The effect of ScH 1000 and disodium cromoglycate on exercise-induced asthma. Chest 71:320–23, 1977.
20. Corkey C, Mindorff C, Levison H, Newth C: Comparison of three different preparations of disodium cromoglycate in the prevention of exercise-induced asthma. Am Rev Respir Dis 125:623–26, 1982.
21. Corris PA, Nariman S, Gibson GH: Nifedipine in the prevention of asthma induced by exercise in histamine. Am Rev Respir Dis 128:991–92, 1983.
22. Daman L, Lieberman P, Ganier M, et al. Heat localized urticaria. J Allergy Clin Immunol 61:273, 1978.
23. Deal EC, McFadden ER, Ingram RH, Jaeger JJ: Hyperpnea and heat flux. J Appl Physiol 46:476–82, 1979.
24. Deal EC, McFadden ER, Ingram RH, Jaeger JJ: Esophageal temperature during exercise in asthmatic and non-asthmatic subjects. J Appl Physiol 46:484–90, 1979.
25. DeCotiis BA, Braman SS, Corrao WM: Pulmonary function studies and the prevalence of bronchial hyperreactivity in patients with allergic rhinitis. Am Rev Respir Dis 122: 64, 1980 (abstract).
26. Dusdieker L, Green M, Smith G, et al: Comparison of orally administered metaproterenol and theophylline in the control of chronic asthma. J Pediatr 101:281–87, 1982.
27. Eggleston PA, Beasley PP, Kindley RT: The effects of oral doses of theophylline and fenoterol on exercise-induced asthma. Chest 79:399–405, 1981.
28. Eggleston PA: Methods of exercise challenge. J Allergy Clin Immunol 73:666–69, 1984.
29. Ekwo E, Weinberger MM: Evaluation of a program for the pharmacologic management of children with asthma. J Allergy Clin Immunol 61:240, 1978.
30. Ellis EF: Inhibition of exercise-induced asthma by theophylline. J Allergy Clin Immunol 73:690–692, 1984.
31. Fairshter RD, Busse WW: Theophylline: How much is enough? J Allergy Clin Immunol 77:646–651, 1986.
32. Finnerty JP, Wood-Baker R, Thompson H, et al: Role of leukotrienes in exercise-induced asthma. Am Rev Respir Dis 145:746–753, 1992.
33. Fitch KD, Morton AR, Blanksby BA: Effects of swimming training on children with asthma. Arch Dis Child 51: 190–94, 1976.
34. Fitch TK: Sport, physical activity and the asthmatic In Oseid S, Edwards AM (eds): The Asthmatic Child in Play and Sport. London, Pitman Press, 1983, p 249.
35. Furukawa CT: Other pharmacologic agents that may effect bronchial hyperreactivity. J Allergy Clin Immunol 73: 693–98, 1984.
36. Gaddy JN, Margolskee D: Bronchodilator with a potent and selective leukotriene D_4 receptor antagonist (MK-571) in patients with asthma. Am Rev Respir Dis 146:358–362, 1992.
37. Godfrey S: Exercise-induced asthma. Allergy 33:299–37, 1978.
38. Godfrey S: Introduction. Symposium on special problems in management of allergic athletes. J Allergy Clin Immunol 73:630–33, 1984.
39. Grant JA, Findley SR, Theuson DO, et al: Local heat associated urticaria/ angioedema: Evidence for histamine release without complement activation. J Allergy Clin Immunol 67:75, 1981.
40. Green CP, Price JF: Prevention of exercise-induced asthma by inhaled salmeterol xinafoate. Arch Dis Child 67:1014–1016, 1992.
41. Gross NJ, Skorodin MS: Anticholinergic, antimucarinic bronchodilators. Am Rev Respir Dis 129:856–70, 1984.
42. Hahn AG, Anderson SD, Morton AR, et al: A reinterpretation of the effect of temperature and water content of inspired air in exercise-induced asthma. Am Rev Respir Dis 130:575–79, 1984.
43. Henriksen JM, Dahl R: Effects of inhaled budesonide alone and in combination with low-dose terbutaline in children with exercise-induced asthma. Am Rev Respir Dis 128: 993, 1983.
44. Isreal E, Demarkerian R, Rosenberg M, et al: The effects of 5-lipoxygenase inhibitor on asthma induced by cold, dry air. N Engl N Med 323:1740–1745, 1990.
45. Isreal E, Juniper EF, Callaghan JR, et al: Effect of leukotriene antagonist LY171883 on cold-air induced bronchoconstriction in asthmatics. Am Rev Respir Dis 140:1348–1351, 1989.
46. Joad JP, Ahrens RC, Lindgren SD, Weinberger MD: Relative efficacy of maintenance therapy with theophylline, inhaled albuterol and the combination for chronic asthma. J Allergy Clin Immunol 79:78–85, 1987.
47. Johnson M, Butchers PR, Coleman RA, et al: The pharmacology of salmeterol. Life Sci 52:2131–2143, 1993.
48. Johnson WR, Buskirk ER (eds): Science and Medicine of Exercise in Sports, 2nd ed. New York, Harper and Row, 1980, p. 125.
49. Jones RV, Williams H, Zarabbi V, et al: The use of training programs in asthmatic children. In Oseid S, Edwards AM, eds: The Asthmatic Child in Sport and Play. London, Pitman Press, 1983, p 312.
50. Katz HR, Stevens RL, Austen KF: Heterogeneity of mammalian mast cells differentiated in vivo and in vitro. J Allergy Clin Immunol 76:250–59, 1985.
51. Kettlehut BV, Kobayashi RH, Kobayashi AD: Pharmacologic management of asthma in infants and young children. Nebr Med J 71:295, 1986.
52. Kidd JM, Cohen SH, Sosman AJ, Fink, JN: Food-dependent exercise-induced anaphylaxis. J Allergy Clin Immunol Abstr 71:407–11, 1983.
53. Konig P: The use of cromolyn in the management of hyperreactive airways and exercise. J Allergy Clin Immunol 73:686–89, 1984.
54. Konig P, Hordvik NL, Kreutz C: The preventive affect and duration of action of nedocromil sodium and chromolyn sodium in exercise-induced asthma in adults. J Allergy Clin Immunol 79:64–68, 1987.
55. Kraan J, Koeter GH, Mark T, et al: Changes in bronchial hyperreactivity induced by four weeks of treatment with anti-asthmatic drugs in patients with allergic asthma: A comparison between budesonide and terbutaline. J Allergy Clin Immunol 76:628, 1985.
56. Lee HS, Evans HE: Albuterol by aerosol and orally administered theophylline in asthmatic children. J Pediatr 101: 632–35, 1982.
57. Lee TH, Nagy L, Nagakura T, et al: Identification and partial characterization of an exercise-induced neutrophil chemotactic factor in bronchial asthma. J Clin Invest 69:889–99, 1982.
58. Lee TH, Nagakura T, Papageorgiou N, et al: Exercise-induced late asthmatic reactions with neutrophil chemotactic activity. N Engl J Med 308:1502–05, 1983.
59. Lee TH, Nagakura T, Papageorgiou N, et al: Mediators in exercise-induced asthma. J Allergy Clin Immunol 73: 634–39, 1984.
60. Lewis RA, Robin JL: Arachidonic acid derivatives as mediators of asthma. J Allergy Clin Immunol 76:259–64, 1985.

61. Lilker ES, Manicatide M, O'Hara W, Lasachuk K: Exercise-induced asthma is prevented by warm-down. Am Rev Respir Dis 131:A48, 1985.
62. Major RH: A note of history of asthma. In Underwood EA (ed): Science, Medicine and History. London, University Press, 1953, p 522.
63. Manning PJ, Watson RM, Margolskee DJ, et al: Inhibition of exercise-induced bronchoconstriction by MK-571, a potent leukotriene D_4 receptor antagonist. N Engl J Med 323:1736–1739, 1990.
64. McFadden ER, Ingram RH: Exercise-induced asthma: Observations on the initiating stimulus. N Engl J Med 301: 763–69, 1979.
65. McFadden ER: Hypothesis: Exercise-induced asthma as a vascular phenomenon. Lancet 335:880, 1990.
66. McFadden ER, Gilbert IA: Asthma. N Engl J Med 327: 1928–1933, 1992.
67. McNeill RS, Nairn JR, Millar JS, et al: Exercise-induced asthma. Q J Med 35:55–67, 1966.
68. Nadel JA: Inflammation and asthma. J Allergy Clin Immunol 73:651, 1984.
69. Nelson HS: Beta adrenergic agonists. Chest 82:33 S, 1982.
70. Newhouse MT, Delovich MB: Control of asthma by aerosols. N Engl J Med 315:870–74, 1986.
71. Orenstein DM, Reed ME, Grogan FT, Crawford LV: Exercise conditioning in children with asthma. J Pediatr 106:556–60, 1985.
72. Pauwels R: New aspects of the therapeutic potential of theophylline in asthma. J Allergy Clin Immunol 83:548–551, 1989.
73. Pearlman DS, Chervinsky P, LaForce C, et al. A comparison of salmeterol with albuterol in the treatment of mild to moderate asthma. N Engl J Med 327:1420–1425, 1992.
74. Persson, CG: Overview of effects of theophylline. J Allergy Clin Immunol 78:780–87, 1986.
75. Persson CG: Development of safer xanthine drugs for treatment of obstructive airways. J Allergy Clin Immunol 78:817, 1986.
76. Persson CGA: Choline xanthines as airway anti-inflammatory drugs. J Allergy Clin Immunol 81:615–619, 1988.
77. Petersen KH, McElhenney TR: Effects of a physical fitness program upon asthmatic boys. Pediatrics 35:295–99, 1965.
78. Polack J, Kiechel F, Cooper D, et al: Relationship of serum theophylline concentration of inhibition of exercise-induced asthma in comparison with cromolyn. Pediatrics 60:840, 1977.
79. Poppius H, Salorinne Y: Comparative trial of salbutamol and an anticholinergic drug. SCH 1000, in prevention of exercise-induced asthma. Scand J Respir Dis 54:142, 1973.
80. Reed CE: Adrenergic bronchodilators: Pharmacology and toxicology. J Allergy Clin Immunol 76:335–41, 1985.
81. Robushchi M, Riva E, Fuccella LM, et al: Prevention of exercise-induced asthma by a new leukotriene antagonist (SKF104353), a double-blind study vs. chromoglycate and placebo. Am Rev Respir Dis 145:1285–1290, 1992.
82. Rohr A, Siegel SC, Katz RM, et al: A comparison of inhaled albuterol and cromolyn in the prophylaxis of exercise-induced asthma. Ann Allergy 59:107–112, 1987.
83. Schachter EN, Lach E, Lee M: The protective effect of a cold weather mask on exercise-induced asthma. Ann Allergy 46:12–16, 1981.
84. Schnall RP, Landau R: Protective effects of repeated short sprints in exercise-induced asthma. Thorax 35:828–832, 1980.
85. Schwartz S, Davies S, Juers JA: Life-threatening cold and exercise-induced asthma potentiated by the administration of propranolol. Chest 73:100–101, 1980.
86. Shaw RJ, Kay AB: Nedocromil, a mucosal and connective tissue mast cell stabilizer inhibits exercise-induced asthma. Br J Dis Chest 49:385–388, 1985.
87. Sheffer AL, Austen KF: Exercise-induced anaphylaxis. J Allergy Clin Immunol 66:106–11, 1980.
88. Sheffer AL, Austen KF: Exercise-induced anaphylaxis. J Allergy Clin Immunol 73:699–703, 1984.
89. Sheppard D, Eschenbacher WL: Respiratory water loss as a stimulus to exercise-induced bronchoconstriction. J Allergy Clin Immunol 73:640–42, 1984.
90. Shturman-Ellstein R, Zeballos RJ, Buckley JM, et al: The beneficial effect of nasal breathing on exercise-induced bronchoconstriction. Am Rev Respir Dis 118:65–73, 1978.
91. Siegel SC: Summary. International symposium on special problems of allergic athletes. J Allergy Clin Immunol 73:745–48, 1984.
92. Sly RM: Beta adrenergic drugs in the management of asthma in athletes. J Allergy Clin Immunol 73:680–85, 1984.
93. Smith SB: Exercise-induced asthma: Diagnostic clues with recommendations for treatment. Postgrad Med 77:42–45, 1985.
94. Songsiride V, Busse WW: Exercise-induced anaphylaxis. Clin Allergy 13:317–21, 1983.
95. Sterns DR, McFadden ER, Breslin FJ, Ingram RH: Reanalysis of the refractory period in exertional asthma. J Appl Physiol 50:503–08, 1981.
96. Tinkelman DG, Cavanaugh MJ, Cooper DM: Inhibition of exercise-induced bronchospasm by atropine. Am Rev Respir Dis 114:87–94, 1976.
97. Vandewalker ML, Kray KT, Weber RW, et al: Addition of terbutaline to optimal theophylline therapy. Chest 90: 198–203, 1986.
98. Wade JP, Liang MH, Sheffer AL: EIA: Epidemiologic observation. Prog Clin Biol Res 297:175, 1989.
99. Weinberger M, Hendeles L: Theophylline use: An overview. J Allergy Clin Immunol 76:277–84, 1985.
100. Weinberger MM: Theophylline. Immunol Allergy Clin North Am 10(3):559, 1990.
101. Yeung R, Nolan GM, Levison H: Comparison of the effects of inhaled SCH 1000 and fenoterol on exercise-induced asthma in children. Pediatrics 66:109–14, 1980.

15

Medical Syndromes Unique to Athletes

Morris B. Mellion, M.D.
J. B. Ketner, M.D.

There are several medical syndromes that are rare, or even nonexistent, in people who do not exercise regularly or intensively. These syndromes may be perplexing to physicians who have only cursory experience with athletes. The patients who are affected are "different" in that they maintain an extremely active, physically intense lifestyle. This chapter focuses on nine areas that encompass many of the more common athletic syndromes.

OVERTRAINING

There is a well-documented, but poorly understood, syndrome in which the training program of the athlete exceeds the body's physiological and psychological limits and the individual's whole system seems to break down as a result. This is a major setback in both performance and general well-being which takes weeks, and sometimes months, of rest to resolve. This problem results from a short- to medium-term, often massive, increase in training volume or intensity over a previously substantial baseline. It is not merely the result of a few days of *overdoing it.*

The term overtraining refers to an imbalance between exercise and recovery in which the athlete's training program goes beyond the body's physiological and psychological limits, causing fatigue and reduced functional capacity.[33,41,57] "Proper training loads bring about a degree of fatigue which temporarily lowers the functional ability of the athlete. The adaptation to the training stimulus essentially is achieved through the recovery process which not only entails a renewal of the energy sources, but may regenerate such sources beyond the original level."[41] This process involves using "overload" to obtain "super compensation," or "over compensation." If the amount of overload is too great or if the periods of rest between training sessions are too short, the athlete encounters training overloads while still fatigued and unrecovered. Instead of super compensation, the result is overtraining.[41] Although repeated overload and recovery are necessary to increase the functional capacity of the athlete, it is often difficult to attain the proper balance between exercise and recovery. As the overtraining syndrome has been accepted as a diagnosis in sports medicine, certain terms have been developed to describe its components.

> "*Overload training* is the process of stressing an individual to provide a stimulus for adaptation and supercompensation. This includes increasing training volume and/or intensity beyond what the athlete is accustomed to.
>
> *Training fatigue,* or acute fatigue, is the normal response that is experienced following one or several days of heavy training associated with an overload stimulus.
>
> *Overtraining* is the process of training at abnormally high levels of volume or intensity. According to some authorities, this term also includes performance decrements accompanying this stressful training process.
>
> *Overreaching* is a form of overtraining that follows short-term intensive training. It is sometimes a planned phase of a periodized training program. The symptoms of overreaching can be reversed by a longer than normal regeneration period.
>
> *Overtraining syndrome* or staleness refers to the final stage in a proposed continuum of increasingly severe chronic fatigue states that develop as a result of overtraining.This syndrome includes the many symptoms associated with overtraining, including decreased performance.
>
> *Muscular overstrain* is acute tissue damage induced by a single intensive training session that exceeds the muscular stress tolerance. This generally occurs after single or repeated bouts of excessive exercise that result

in damage to muscle fibers. Muscular overstrain does not always accompany overreaching or overtraining."[57]

Van Borselen et al. suggest that there is a continuum of overtraining symptoms beginning with acute fatigue and progressing with overload to overreaching and a full blown overtraining or "staleness" syndrome.[57] Figure 1 is a modification of their concept. Continued overload during a period of training fatigue may lead to overreaching. A further continuance of the overload may produce the full overtraining syndrome. Clearly, early recognition of this process allows intervention at less serious stages of the continuum.[36]

Overtraining or "staleness" is a multisystem problem the pathophysiology of which is only partly understood. The athlete feels "run down" and tired and experiences sleep difficulty and loss of appetite. Resting heart rate and heart-rate recovery time after exercise increase. The athlete loses weight and notes a heavy-legged feeling when exercising. Muscle pain is common[18] and performance suffers, often dramatically. Illnesses and injuries are common in this setting.[2,3,18,33,41] There is a great variation in symptoms among individuals, and few athletes exhibit all the potential aspects of the syndrome.[33,36] Table 1 lists common psychological, physiological, and performance problems in athletes who overtrain.

Although overtraining involves virtually every system in the athlete's body, several aspects are more prominent. They include the cardiovascular and neuroendocrine systems, psychological state, and the effect of load and extreme overload on the muscles themselves.

TABLE 1. Common Problems In Overtrained Athletes*

Psychological
- Fatigue[2,18,21,58]
- Apathy (loss of motivation)[2,21,33,58]
- Sleep difficulty[2,3,5,18,21,33,41,57]
- Loss of appetite[3,5,18,21,33,41,57,58]
- Depression[5,18,21,36,41,43,58]
- Irritation and restlessness[3,18,21,33,57,58]
- Emotional lability[5,6,21,57]
- Reduced concentration or focus[21,41,58]
- Loss of confidence[18]

Physiological
- Increased basal heart rate[5,18,21,33]
- Increased resting blood pressure[21,33,57]
- Weight loss (fluid, body fat, and possibly muscle mass)[2,3,5,18,21,33,57,58]
- Chronic muscle soreness[5,18,36,57]
- Heavy feeling in legs[2,5]
- Gastrointestinal disturbance[2,5,21,41]
- Lymphadenopathy[2,5,21]
- Frequent illness and infection[2,5,21,33,41,57]
- Frequent overuse injuries[2,33,57]
- Poor healing of overuse injuries[3,21]
- Increase evening fluid intake[2,3,21]
- Postural hypotension[5,33]

Performance-Related
- Intolerance to training[3,21,33]
- Decreased maximum work output[2,3,5,6,18,21,33,36,41,57]
  - Speed
  - Endurance
  - Power
- Increased heart rate, ventilation, and blood lactate at a given load[5,21,57]
- Prolonged heart-rate recovery time[5,21,41]
- Prolonged reaction time[21,41]
- Prolonged general recovery from exercise[3,21]
- Increased perceived exertion at a given workload[43,58]
- Decreased maximum plasma lactate during exercise[21,33]
- Decreased coordination[21,41,57]

Cardiovascular Aspects

The hallmark of overtraining is an increased basal resting heart rate. Most highly trained endurance athletes will have an early morning basal heart rate of 50 beats per minute or lower. This phenomenon is known as "athletic bradycardia." It is caused by an increased parasympathetic activity due to athletic conditioning.[19,30] Athletes who monitor their resting pulse immediately upon awakening each morning often note the remarkable consistency of this measurement for a given training state. As fitness improves, the basal heart rate decreases but as the athlete experiences even incipient overtraining, the rate may increase.[3,18,28] Rises of 5 beats/min are suggestive of overtraining, and increases of 10 beats/min are considered almost diagnostic.[2,18] Anecdotal information from some athletes with very consistent basal heart rate indicates

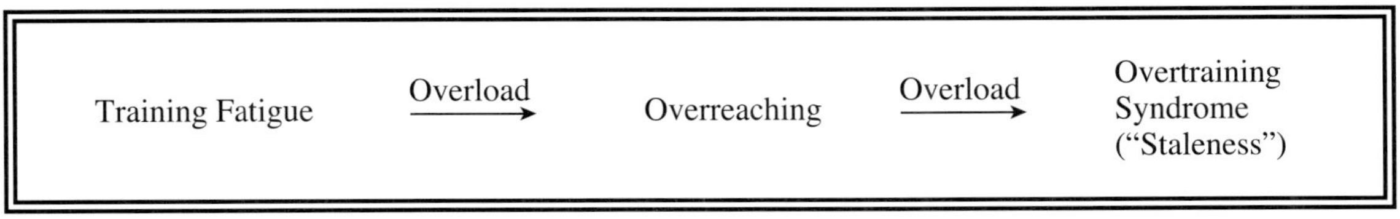

Training Fatigue —Overload→ Overreaching —Overload→ Overtraining Syndrome ("Staleness")

FIGURE 1. Continuum of overtraining symptoms. (Modified from van Borselen F, Vos NH, Fry AC, Kraemer WJ. The role of aerobic exercise in overtraining. NSCA Journal 14:74–79, 1992.)

that they become concerned with changes as small as two beats/min. Some authors suggest that sleeping heart rate may be a more sensitive measure.[28] On the other hand, there are some athletes who develop the overtraining syndrome without a rise in resting heart rate.

Two mechanisms have been implicated in the cardiovascular aspect of the overtraining syndrome, left ventricular fatigue and decreased blood volume. Several studies have demonstrated a decrease in stroke volume in athletes performing extremely long-distance runs or major triathlons.[4,15,48] Two of these studies identified decreases in the fractional shortening of cardiac muscle during systole which the authors felt suggested a decrease in myocardial contractility or "cardiac fatigue."[15,48] A report of two athletes completing a 90-km race with clinical signs of left ventricular failure and hemoptysis also suggested progressive impairment of myocardial contractility during prolonged exercise.[42]

In addition to the contractile state of the ventricular myocardium, the other major factor in stroke volume is blood volume.[7,8,18] Endurance exercise training causes the expansion of blood volume. This effect is caused by both plasma volume expansion and increased red blood cell (RBC) mass.[7] Studies of the effect of detraining on athletes demonstrate an early drop in blood volume primarily due to a decrease in plasma volume.[13,27,46] The fluid loss noted, which is so common in overtrained athletes, is likely to reflect a major drop in baseline plasma volume. Moreover, because there is a well established relationship between changes in intravascular plasma volume and changes in plasma protein content,[7,24] the loss of body mass, including muscle mass, may effect the amount of intravascular plasma protein.

Hormonal Aspects

Hypothalamic dysfunction has been identified as possible cause in the overtraining syndrome. In a comparison of four overtrained athletes with five asymptomatic marathoners, the overtrained athletes demonstrated impaired plasma cortisol, adrenocorticotropic hormone (ACTH), growth hormone, and prolactin responses to insulin induced hypoglycemia.[2] Recent research has identified reduced pituitary beta-endorphin response to corticotropin releasing hormone in overtrained athletes.[29]

Several studies demonstrate decreased testosterone levels in overtrained runners, cyclists, and rowers.[14,17,23,52,55] The decline in testosterone, often accompanied by elevations of cortisol,[14,31,37,56] suggest catabolic activity with consequent decrease in muscle mass. A 30% decline in the testosterone: cortisol ratio has been suggested as a criterion for overtraining.[1] Weight loss in overtrained athletes may be in part due to this anabolic to catabolic shift. Catecholamines have also been implicated in overtraining. Nocturnal catecholamine release was reduced in studies of overtrained cyclists, runners, and soccer players.[35,38] By contrast, exercise-related and daytime catecholamine levels were elevated in studies of highly stressed and overtrained athletes.[26,34,40,50,53]

Muscle Aspects

A muscle overuse syndrome has been identified in long-distance runners pushing their mileage and themselves to new limit. Serum creatine kinase is elevated, and muscle circumference is decreased, with no accompanying drop in estimated body fat.[16] This syndrome, known as delayed-onset muscle soreness (DOMS), is discussed later in this chapter. It clearly could be a component of the overtraining syndrome.

Some athletes may develop chronic muscle fatigue by failing to consume adequate carbohydrate to match the energy demands of increased training. In a study of 12 highly trained male swimmers who doubled their training distance for 10 consecutive days, 4 swimmers were unable to tolerate the increased training demands and, consequently, swam at significantly slower speeds during the training sessions. These 4 swimmers had significantly reduced muscle glycogen levels caused by relatively low carbohydrate intake.[10] Other investigators have also identified the protective role of carbohydrate intake in overreaching.[20] Clearly, a markedly increased training demand warrants a parallel increase in nutritional intake.[20]

Psychological Aspects

Major increases in training volume at high intensity have been shown to increase fatigue, depression, anger, and global mood disturbance as measured with the Profile of Mood States (POMS). There is a concurrent reduction in the athlete's general sense of well-being and an increase in both overall and local ratings of perceived exertion (RPE) for a given exercise load.[44,45,49,57,58] Morgan et al.[43] have demonstrated that mood state disturbances increase "in a dose response manner" to increased training load and decrease similarly with reduced training load. They suggest that monitoring mood state using the POMS is a potential method of preventing the overtraining syndrome.[43]

Identification and Treatment

In order to prevent and detect the overtraining syndrome, the athlete's physical and emotional status should be observed and monitored. Data should be collected on a long-term basis and compared to previous measurements of the same athlete.[3,21,33]

Particularly useful parameters in detecting potential or incipient overtraining include (1) decreased performance; (2) weight loss; (3) increased resting or sleeping heart rate; (4) decline in general health status; (5) increased thirst and evening fluid intake; and (6) poor sleep or a later time to bed.[3,5,21,33,36,41] Occasionally, however, overtraining may cause decreased performance with few, if any, other objective findings.[6,20,54]

To prevent overtraining, the coach should balance and individualize workouts.[33] Each athlete is an individual with a unique tolerance for stress and unique capacity for regeneration. Coaches should recognize other sources of stress in the athlete's life and adjust training work loads accordingly.[5,33] The athlete's training regimen should be broken into short cycles of heavy workloads followed by appropriate rest periods for regeneration.[22,33,39] Athletes should follow a training schedule and not react to performance slumps or to periods of feeling particularly good by increasing the intensity or volume of workouts.[3,9]

As noted above, the POMS can be a valuable tool for monitoring mood disturbance and incipient overtraining syndrome.[39,43,58] The POMS can be paired with RPEs[39] and the values followed over time.

There is no good single marker for overtraining; however, when the syndrome reaches the point that there is a sudden decrease in performance combined with an intolerance to training, intervention is necessary. The treatment for incipient overtraining syndrome is to cut back training volume. There is an abundant literature on detraining which demonstrates that major cuts can be made in frequency and duration while maintaining performance.[11,12,25,46,47] In fact, "tapering" training over a period of 2 weeks before competition may produce marked gains in muscle power and maximum performance.[11,12] For the athlete who is merely overreaching a 3- to 5-day rest may be all that is necessary.[33] Once the overtraining syndrome has reached its full dimensions, there may be no choice but for the athlete to break off from serious training for a period of several weeks to months.[3,5,33,36,58] One study of overtrained athletes actually demonstrates an increase in performance after 3 to 5 weeks without training.[32]

REFERENCES

1. Adlercreutz H, Harkonen M, Kuoppasalmi K, et al: Effect of training on plasma anabolic and catabolic steroid hormones and their response during physical exercise. Int J Sports Med 7(Suppl):27–28, 1986.
2. Barron JL, Noakes TD, Levy W, et al: Hypothalamic dysfunction in overtrained athletes. J Clin Endocrinol Metab 60:803–806, 1985.
3. Brown RL, Frederick EC, Falsetti HL, et al: Overtraining of athletes. Physician Sportsmed 11:93–110, 1983.
4. Bruce RA, Kusumi F, Culver BH, Butler J: Cardiac limitation to maximal oxygen transport and changes in components after jogging across the United States. J Appl Physiol 39:958–964, 1975.
5. Budgett R: Overtraining syndrome. Br J Sports Med 24: 231–236, 1990.
6. Callister R, Callister RJ, Fleck SJ, Dudley GA: Physiological and performance responses to overtraining in elite judo athletes. Med Sci Sports Exerc 22:816–824, 1990.
7. Convertino VA: Blood volume: its adaptation to endurance training. Med Sci Sports Exerc 23:1338–1348, 1991.
8. Convertino VA, Keil LC, Greenleaf JE: Plasma volume, renin, and vasopressin responses to graded exercise after training. J Appl Physiol 54:508–514, 1983.
9. Costill DL. Detection of overtraining. Sports Med Dig 8:4–5, 1986.
10. Costill DL, Flynn MG, Kirwan JP, et al: Effects of repeated days of intensified training on muscle glycogen and swimming performance. Med Sci Sports Exerc 20:289–254, 1988.
11. Costill DL, King DS, Thomas R, Hargreaves M: Effects of reduced cross training on muscular power in swimmers. Physician Sportsmed 13(2):94–101, 1985.
12. Costill DL, Thomas R, Robergs A, et al: Adaptations to swimming training: Influence of training volume. Med Sci Sports Exerc 23:371–377, 1991.
13. Coyle EF, Hemmert MK, Coggan AR: Effects of detraining on cardiovascular responses to exercise: role of blood volume. J Appl Physiol 60:95–99, 1986.
14. deVries W, Koppeschaar H, Verstappen P, et al: Changes in basal plasma levels of testosterone, cortisol, albumin and SHBG in professional cyclists. Med Sci Sports Exerc 24(Suppl):S166, 1992.
15. Douglas PS, O'Toole ML, Hiller, WDB, et al: Cardiac fatigue after prolonged exercise. Circulation 76:1206–1213, 1987.
16. Dressendorfer RH, Wade CE: The muscular overuse syndrome in long-distance runners. Physician Sportsmed 11:116–130, 1983.
17. Dressendorfer RH, Wade CE, Iverson D: Decreased plasma testosterone in overtrained runners. Med Sci Sports Exerc 19(Suppl):S10, 1987.
18. Dressendorfer RH, Wade CE, Scaff JH: Increased morning heart rate in runners: A valid sign of overtraining? Physician Sportsmed 13:77–86, 1985.
19. Frick MH, Elovainio RO, Somer T. The mechanism of bradycardia evoked by physical training. Cardiologia 51:46–54, 1967.
20. Fry RW, Lawrence SR, Morton AR, et al: Monitoring training stress in endurance sports using biological parameters. Clin J Sports Med 3:6–13, 1993.
21. Fry RW, Morton AR, Keast D: Overtraining in athletes: An update. Sports Med 12:32–65, 1991.
22. Fry RW, Morton AR, Keast D: Periodisation and the prevention of overtraining. Can J Sport Sci 17:241–248, 1992.
23. Griffith RO, Dressendorfer RH, Fullbright CD, Wade CE: Testicular function during exhaustive endurance training. Physician Sportsmed 18:54–64, 1990.
24. Harrison MH: Effects of thermal stress and exercise on blood volume in humans Physiol Rev 65:149–209, 1985.
25. Hickson RC, Rosenkoetter MA: Reduced training frequencies and maintenance of increased aerobic power. Med Sci Sports Exerc 13:13–16, 1981.
26. Hooper SL, Mackinnon LT, Gordon RD, Bachmann AW: Hormonal responses of elite swimmers to overtraining. Med Sci Sports Exerc 25:741–747, 1993.
27. Houmard JA. Impact of reduced training on performance in endurance athletes. Sports Med 12:380–393, 1991.
28. Jeukendrup AE, Hesselink MKC, Snyder AC, et al: Physiological changes in male competitive cyclists after two

weeks of intensified training. Int J Sports Med 13:534–541, 1992.
29. Keizer HA, Platen P, Koppeschaar H: Blunted β-endorphin responses to corticotropin releasing hormone and exercise after exhaustive training. Int J Sports Med 12:97, 1991.
30. Kenney WL: Parasympathetic control of resting heart rate: relationship to aerobic power. Med Sci Sports Exerc 4:451–455, 1985.
31. Kirwan JP, Costill DL, Flynn MG, et al: Physiological responses to successive days of intense training in competitive swimmers. Med Sci Sports Exerc 20:255–259, 1988.
32. Koutedakis Y, Budgett R, Faulmann L: Rest in underperforming elite competitors. Br J Sports Med 24:248–252(a), 1990.
33. Kuipers H, Keizer HA: Overtraining in elite athletes: Review and directions for the future. Sports Med 6:79–92, 1988.
34. Lehmann M, Baumgartl P, Wiesenack C, et al: Training-overtraining: influence of a defined increase in training volume vs. training intensity on performance, catecholamines and some metabolic parameters in experienced middle- and long-distance runners. Eur J Appl Physiol 64:169–177, 1992.
35. Lehmann M, Dickhuth HH, Gendrrisch G, et al: Training—overtraining: A prospective, experimental study with experienced middle- and long-distance runners. Int J Sports Med 12:444–452, 1991.
36. Lehmann M, Foster C, Keul J: Overtraining in endurance athletes: A brief review. Med Sci Sports Exerc 25: 854–862, 1993.
37. Lehmann M, Gastmann U, Petersen KG, et al: Training—overtraining: performance, and hormone levels, after a defined increase in training volume *versus* intensity in experienced middle- and long-distance runners. Br J Sports Med 26:233–242, 1992.
38. Lehmann M, Schnee W, Scheu R, et al: Decreased nocturnal catecholamine excretion: Parameter for an overtraining syndrome in athletes? Int J Sports Med 13:236–242, 1992.
39. Levin S: Overtraining causes Olympic-sized problems. Physician Sportsmed 19:112–118, 1991.
40. Liederbach M, Gleim GW, Nicholas JA: Monitoring training status in professional ballet dancers. J Sports Med Phys Fitness 32:187–95, 1992.
41. Ludin P: The monitoring of recovery in endurance athletes. NSCA Journal 7:41–42, 1985.
42. McKechnie JK, Leary WP, Noakes TD, et al: Acute pulmonary oedema in two athletes during a 90-km running race. S Afr Med J 56:261–265, 1979.
43. Morgan WP, Brown DR, Raglin JS, et al: Psychological monitoring of overtraining and staleness. Br J Sports Med 21:107–114, 1987.
44. Morgan WP, Costill DL, Flynn MG, et al: Mood disturbance following increased training in swimmers. Med Sci Sports Exerc 20:408–414, 1988.
45. Morgan WP, O'Connor PJ, Sparling PB, Pate RR: Psychological characterization of the elite female distance runner. Int J Sports Med 8(Suppl):124–131, 1987.
46. Neufer PD: The effect of detraining and reduced training on the physiological adaptations to aerobic exercise training. Sports Med 8:302–321, 1989.
47. Neufer PD, Costill DL, Fielding RA, et al: Effect of reduced training on muscular strength and endurance in competitive swimmers. Med Sci Sports Exerc 19:486–490, 1987.
48. Niemela KO, Palatsi IJ, Ikaheimo MJ, et al: Evidence of impaired left ventricular performance after an uninterrrupted competitive 24 hours run. Circulation 3:350–356, 1984.
49. O'Connor PJ, Morgan WP, Raglin JS: Psychobiologic effects of 3 d of increased training in female and male swimmers. Med Sci Sports Exerc 23:1055–1061, 1991.
50. Pestel RG, Hurley DM, Vandongen R: Biochemical and hormonal changes during a 1000 km ultramarathon. Clin Exp Pharmacol Physiol 16:353–361, 1989.
51. Raglin JS, Morgan WP, O'Connor PJ: Changes in mood states during training in female and male college swimmers. Int J Sports Med 12:585–589, 1991.
52. Roberts AC, McClure RD, Weiner RI, Brooks GA: The effects of overtraining on reproductive variables in trained men vs. controls. Med Sci Sports Exerc 22(Suppl):S21, 1990.
53. Sagnol M, Claustre J, Pequignor JM, et al: Catecholamies and fuels after van ultralong run: Persistent changes after 24-h recovery. Int J Sports Med 10:202–206, 1989.
54. Seifert JG, Snyder AC, Welsh R, Dennis K: The effects of a 17 day road race series on indices of overtraining. Med Sci Sports Exerc 24(Suppl):S95, 1992.
55. Urhausen A, Kullmer T, Kindermann W: A 7-week follow-up study of the behavior of testosterone and cortisol during the competition period in rowers. Eur J Appl Physiol 56:528–533, 1987.
56. Uusitalo A, Ruska H, Vaananen I, et al: Overtraining in young male skiers during an intensified training period. Med Sci Sports Exerc 25(Suppl):S172, 1993.
57. van Borselen F, Vos NH, Fry AC, Kraemer WJ: The role of anaerobic exercise in overtraining. NSCA Journal 14: 74–79, 1992.
58. Veale DMW: Psychological aspects of staleness and dependence on exercise. Int J Sports Med 12(Suppl 1):S19–S22, 1991.

DELAYED-ONSET MUSCLE SORENESS

Delayed-onset muscle soreness (DOMS) is a muscular overuse syndrome that occurs in athletes either initiating and unaccustomed to exercise or experiencing an extremely great increase of an exercise that they had been performing at a more modest level.

DOMS is characterized by severe muscle soreness and swelling accompanied by elevated creatine kinase (CK) levels peaking 2–3 days after the inciting exercise.[4,5] The degree of soreness is generally directly proportional to the exercise intensity and adversely proportional to the individual's fitness.[6]

DOMS is commonly caused by unaccustomed eccentric exercise;[9,17,20] however, it may be triggered simply by a huge increase in training volume.[15] Because in eccentric contractions, in which the muscle elongates during contraction, fewer muscle fibers are recruited, the stress on each individual fiber is greater.[2,4,9,19] When the stress on the fiber exceeds its tensile limit, damage and a secondary inflammatory response ensue.[3,12,19,20] Interestingly, a bout of eccentric exercise, even if it results in DOMS, may protect against subsequent episodes of DOMS.[4,5,8,9,20]

Until DOMS has abated, the athlete typically has reduced muscle glycogen,[16] increased oxygen uptake requirements,[23] decreased shock absorption ability,[10] altered gait,[11] and reduced economy of movement.[20] Attempts to treat DOMS have been frustrating. Light exercise may provide temporary pain relief, but the pain returns after the exercise is complete.[1] Transcutaneous electric nerve stimulation (TENS)[6] and ultrasound[13] may reduce the discomfort. Most studies of nonsteroidal anti-inflammatory drugs (NSAIDs) in DOMS have shown little benefit.[7,8,21] A single study has shown that ibuprofen used prophylactically decreases perceived muscle soreness.[12] Cryotherapy[14,18] and stretching[22] have been ineffective treatments.

There are lessons to be learned from our knowledge of DOMS. First, the syndrome can be avoided by a graduated training program. Second, when DOMS occurs, the athlete should allow adequate time for muscle recovery. Third, athletes may use their ability to adapt to DOMS in training. One authority recommends the use of sport-specific eccentric exercises every 4 weeks to prevent subsequent bouts of DOMS.[20]

REFERENCES

1. Armstrong RB: Mechanisms of exercise-induced delayed onset muscular soreness: a brief review. Med Sci Sports Exerc 16:529–538, 1984.
2. Armstrong RB: Muscle damage and endurance events. Sports Med 1986;3:370–381.
3. Armstrong RB, Warren GL, Warren JA: Mechanisms of exercise-induced muscle fibre injury. Sports Med 12:184–207, 1991.
4. Clarkson PM, Nosaka K, Braun B: Muscle function after exercise-induced muscle damage and rapid adaptation. Med Sci Sports Exerc 24:512–520, 1992.
5. Cleak MJ, Eston RG: Delayed onset muscle soreness: Mechanisms and management. J Sports Sci 10:325–341, 1992.
6. Denegar CR, Perrin DH: Effect of transcutaneous electrical nerve stimulation, cold, and a combination treatment on pain, decreased range of motion, and strength loss associated with delayed onset muscle soreness. J Athletic Training 27:200–206, 1992.
7. Donnelly AE, Maughan RJ, Whiting PH: Effects of ibuprofen on exercise-induced muscle soreness and indices of muscle damage. Br J Sports Med 24:191–195, 1990.
8. Donnelly AE, McCormick K, Maughan RJ, et al: Effects of a non-steroidal anti-inflammatory drug on delayed onset muscle soreness and indices of damage. Brit J Sports Med 22:35–38, 1988.
9. Ebbeling CB, Clarkson PM: Exercise-induced muscle damage and adaptation. Sports Med 7:207–234, 1989.
10. Hamill J, Freedson PS, Clarkson PM, Braun B: Muscle soreness during running: Biomechanical and physiological considerations. Int J Sport Biomech 7:125–137, 1991.
11. Harris C, Wilcox A, Smith G, et al: The effect of delayed onset muscular soreness (DOMS) on running kinematics. Med Sci Sports Exerc 22(Suppl):S34, 1990.
12. Hasson SM, Daniels JC, Divine JG, et al: Effect of ibuprofen use on muscle soreness, damage, and performance: A preliminary investigation. Med Sci Sports Exerc 25:9–17, 1993.
13. Hasson SM, Mundorf R, Barnes WS, Williams JH: Effect of ultrasound on muscle soreness and performance. Med Sci Sports Exerc 21(Suppl):S90, 1989.
14. Isabell WK, Durrant E, Myrer W, Anderson S: The effects of ice massage, ice massage with exercise, and exercise on the prevention and treatment of delayed onset muscle soreness. J Athletic Training 27:208–217, 1992.
15. O'Connor PJ, Morgan WP, Raglin JS: Psychobiologic effect of 3 d of increased training in female and male swimmers. Med Sci Sports Exerc 23:1055–1061, 1991.
16. O'Reilly K, Warhol MJ, Fielding RA, et al: Eccentric exercise-induced muscle damage impairs muscle glycogen repletion. J Appl Physiol 63:252–256, 1987.
17. Scifres JC, Martin DT, Thomas DP: Velocity of eccentric contraction affects the magnitude of delayed-onset muscle soreness (DOMS). Med Sci Sports Exerc 24:S142, 1992.
18. Scifres JC, Oceanak JA, Martin DT, et al: Effects of cold whirlpool treatment on delayed onset muscle soreness following eccentric exercise. Med Sci Sports Exerc 25:S133, 1993.
19. Smith LL: Acute inflammation: The underlying mechanism in delayed onset muscle soreness? Med Sci Sports Exerc 3:542–551, 1991.
20. Smith LL: Causes of delayed onset muscle soreness and the impact on athletic performance: A review. J Appl Sport Sci Res 6:135–141, 1992.
21. Wells JM, Smith LL, Holbert D, et al: The effect of indomethacin on delayed onset muscle soreness (DOMS) and markers of muscle damage and acute inflammation. Med Sci Sports Exerc 24(Suppl):S142, 1992.
22. Wessel J, Wan A: Effect of stretching on the intensity of delayed-onset muscle soreness. Clin J Sport Med 4:83–87, 1994.
23. Wilcox A, Climstein M, Quinn C, Lawson L: The effects of delayed onset muscle soreness (DOMS) on running economy. Med Sci Sports Exerc 21(Suppl):S90, 1989.

"RUNNER'S HIGH" AND EXERCISE ADDICTION

> "Then, some time into the second hour comes the spooky time. Colors are bright and beautiful. Water sparkles, clouds breathe, and my body, swimming, detaches from the earth. A loving contentment invades the basement of my mind, and thoughts bubble up without trials. I find the place I need to live if I am going to live."[12]

Mandell's description of "the second second wind" is a literary example of what many call "the runner's high." Runner's high has been described as "a euphoria"[4] or state of "general relaxation"[13] often experienced late in a long, slow-distance run, and sometimes after the run, by well-conditioned athletes who typically run more than 20 miles weekly. It has also been described as "a lifting a spirits and a feeling of harmony with one's surroundings.[20] In one survey, 69% of 424 American runners have experienced a "high period," and this group reported that an average of 44% of their runs elicited a "high."[4] Similar results were found in a group of 44 male Hong Kong long-distance runners.[5]

Causes

Although there are no well-proven explanations for runner's high at present, there are several hypotheses. Morgan has presented three theoretical bases of runner's high,[14] and Wagemaker and Goldstein a fourth.[20]

Distraction Hypothesis. The distraction hypothesis proposes that distraction from stressful stimuli produces the affective changes associated with exercise. The exercise itself merely serves as a distraction from the stressors in the runner's life.[14]

Monamine Hypothesis. The monamine hypothesis is based on the observation that exercise stimulates increased production of norepinephrine and increased brain uptake of this neurotransmitter, thereby producing an elevated affect. Serotonin may also be involved in this process.[14]

Endorphin Hypothesis. The endorphin hypothesis suggests that endogenous morphine-like compounds elevate mood and reduce pain. In 1974, Hughes discovered two pentapeptides, which would become known as enkaphalins, each of which functioned "as an endogenous mediator at central morphine receptor sites."[9] Two years later, a larger peptide called beta endorphin was shown to have the same type of activity on naturally occurring opiate receptors in the brain.[8] These three compounds and several others with similar effects have become collectively known as endorphins. In 1980, Pargman and Baker suggested that enkaphalins may be the causative factor in runner's high.[16] The same year, Appenzeller and associates demonstrated a relationship between intense endurance exercise and serum beta endorphin levels.[1] This finding initiated speculation about whether the increased beta endorphin production might cause "behavioral alterations" such as the runner's high.

Right Brain/Left Brain Hypothesis. The right brain/left brain hypothesis is based on the typical functional division between the two sides of the brain. The left brain ordinarily performs "verbal thinking," which is analytical, and the right brain performs "image thinking," which is much more free-form. Wagemaker and Goldstein noted that in mentally fatigued or emotionally upset individuals, most electroencephalographic (EEG) activity takes place on the right side of the brain. When tired or stressed, individuals may find it difficult to perform verbal or analytical thinking using the left side of the brain. Called right-left confusion, this phenomenon represents "the inability to change from image thinking on the right side to verbal thinking on the left side of the brain."[20] In five subjects with right-left confusion by EEG, jogging for 25–35 minutes reversed the phenomenon, eliminating right-left confusion and allowing an appropriate switch from image to verbal thinking. They proposed this phenomenon as a possible explanation for runner's high.[20]

EXERCISE ADDICTION

Exercise addiction has become a well-recognized syndrome in runners and other endurance athletes. There are three generally recognized criteria for an addictive substance or activity: (1) the substance or activity produces pleasurable emotions which lead to continued administration, (2) tolerance develops, and (3) withdrawal signs appear on cessation and are relieved or prevented by the substance or activity.

As already noted in the section on runner's high, runners and other endurance athletes can experience this pleasurable emotion. Moreover, a more general "affective beneficence" has been attributed to vigorous physical activity.[14]

Tolerance develops to running and other exercise when it used as a means of feeling good. Over time, it takes more and more exercise in order to feel good. Ultimately, it may take even a greater amount of exercise to prevent feeling bad. Endurance exercise, particularly running, may start as a means of improving health, controlling weight, and obtaining social benefit; but eventually it can become an end in itself. When the habitual exerciser fails to exercise, he or she may experience a level of depression far worse than any negative effect present before starting the exercise program.[3]

A broad range of "withdrawal" symptoms is experienced by habitual runners and other habitual endurance athletes who stop exercising. These include anxiety, restlessness, sleep disturbance, irritability, nervousness, guilt, muscle twitching, and a bloated feeling.[15] These symptoms, as well as a commonly experienced negative affect, can be relieved by reinstituting the exercise activity at the same or increased level.

Glasser was the first to associate the concept of addiction with exercise. He identified running and meditation as forms of an attainable "positive addiction" that may "strengthen us and make our lives more satisfying."[7] Unfortunately, not all people with exercise addiction have such a positive experience. Glasser envisioned the addiction process as being an extension of normal behavior: exercise or meditation would replace dysfunctional or self-defeating behaviors in the individual's life.

Morgan, on the other hand, has identified a syndrome of "negative addiction" in which the compulsion to exercise becomes a distortion of normal behavior. He noted a progression that occurs as a formerly sedentary individual becomes a runner and enjoys many of the positive psychological changes that take place. "At this time, daily exercise can become as much a part of the jogger's life as cigarettes for the pack-a-day smoker, alcohol for the alcoholic, and heroin for the mainliner."[15] He pointed out three signals that indicate that the addictive process is developing negatively: less attention to family and other close personal relationships, less concern with external issues such as achievements at work, and a pattern in which "feeling good becomes more important than anything else." The ultimate test of whether someone has an exercise addiction is how he or she responds when told to stop exercising because of a medical condition.[15]

Yates has described "obligatory runners" and compared them to anorexics.[22,23,24] Although some other research had demonstrated significant evidence of depression[2] and body image distortion[21] in habitual runners, habitual runners are less psychopathologic than anorexics.

Yates' obligatory runner may be described as "a person who is *not* about to *not* run." Typically the obligatory runner became committed to running at a time of anxiety, depression, or identity crisis. Whereas the anorexic is more likely to be a younger female, the obligatory runner generally is usually a somewhat older male with a ritualistic preoccupation with running. He minimizes or denies pain and injury and continues to run. Inadequate levels or lack of exercise produces anger and depression.[23] The obligatory runner has a series of characteristics in common with anorexics. Both are generally from upper middle class backgrounds and are high achievers with a competitive nature. Common shared personality characteristics include discomfort with anger, restlessness, tolerance of physical discomfort, introversion, social isolationism, obsessive rumination, and tendency to depression. Both maintain a "the leaner the better" notion of body image. They diet meticulously and deny emaciation.[22]

Yates suggests that the obligatory runner exhibits some of the psychological sequelae of a semi-starvation state resulting from prolonged caloric restriction combined with increased energy expenditure. Citing the work of Keyes on the biology of starvation, he notes that "when normal persons are starved, they become seclusive, somber, constricted, and compulsive."[22]

Anorexia athletica is a relatively new term that is used broadly to describe an anorexia in which the primary means of reducing weight is compulsive exercise, often coupled with reduced nutritional intake. Several case reports have associated obligate running with anorexic symptoms in both men and women.[10,11,17] Although there are some proposed criteria for anorexia athletica in the nutrition literature,[19] they do not place the emphasis on the intense exercise which typifies the general usage of the term. The nutritional deficit in the face of high energy expenditure has been documented for a group of 19- to 30-year-old women with anorexia athletica.[18]

The information regarding exercise addiction is growing, but the research in the area is extremely confused because of a lack of a commonly accepted set of diagnostic criteria. DeCoverley Veale has proposed a set of diagnostic criteria to identify exercise dependence[6], which is presented in Table 2. Future research on exercise addiction is more likely to elucidate this phenomenon and provide guidance for prevention and management.

TABLE 2. Proposed Diagnostic Criteria for "Exercise Dependence"

(A) Narrowing of repertoire leading to a stereotyped pattern of exercise with a regular schedule once or more daily.
(B) Salience with the individual giving increasing priority over other activities to maintaining the pattern of exercise.
(C) Increased tolerance to the amount of exercise performed over the years.
(D) Withdrawal symptoms related to a disorder of mood following the cessation of the exercise schedule.
(E) Relief or avoidance of withdrawal symptoms by further exercise.
(F) Subjective awareness of a compulsion to exercise.
(G) Rapid reinstatement of the previous pattern of exercise and withdrawal symptoms after a period of abstinence.

Associated Features

(H) *Either* the individual continues to exercise despite a serious physical disorder known to be caused, aggravated, or prolonged by exercise and is advised as such by a health professional, *or* the individual has arguments or difficulties with his partner, family, friends, or in his occupational environment.
(I) Self-inflicted loss of weight by dieting as a means towards improving performance.

From De Coverley Veale DM: Exercise dependence. Br J Addict 82:735–740, 1987, with permission.

Physicians who see large numbers of athletes are likely to have many patients with exercise addiction. They may be particularly difficult to evaluate and treat. Yates has provided guidance in the form of a series of questions to ask the injured athlete suspected of compulsive behavior (Table 3).[22]

TABLE 3. What to Ask the Injured Athlete Suspected of Compulsive Behavior

- How do you feel about being inactive while your injury repairs?
- What would it take for you not to engage in your sport?
- What else in life is as gratifying as your sport?
- How much time do you spend thinking about the sport compared with work and family?
- How much time do you spend alone?
- How exacting is your training schedule?
- How strictly do you manage your diet?
- After you eat more than you should, do you exercise to get rid of calories?
- What other diet methods do you use (diet pills, diuretics, vomiting, laxatives?)
- Are you satisfied with your performance?
- How are you trying to improve it?

From Yates A: Understanding and helping the compulsive athlete. J Musculoskel Med 9(3):45–59, 1992, with permission.

Management of exercise addition may be even more challenging than diagnosis. The individual may be resistant to therapy. Confrontation techniques commonly used to pressure alcoholics into treatment may be useful to initiate therapy. Exercise addicts can consume so much therapeutic energy that a combination of individual, group, and support group therapy may be optimal.

REFERENCES

1. Appenzellar D, Standefer J, Appenzeller J, Atkinson, R: Neurology of endurance training. V. endorphins (abstract). Neurology 30:418–419, 1980.
2. Blumenthal JA, O'Toole LC, Chang JL: Is running an analogue to anorexia nervosa? An empirical study of obligatory running and anorexia nervosa. JAMA 252: 520–523, 1984.
3. Blumethal JA, Rose S, Chang JL: Anorexia nervosa and exercise: Implications from recent findings. Sports Med 2:237–247, 1985.
4. Callen KE: Mental and emotional aspects of long-distance running. Psychosomatics 24:133–141, 1983.
5. Chan DW, Lai B: Psychological aspects of long-distance running among Chinese male runners in Hong Kong. Int J Psychosom 37:30–34, 1990.
6. DeCoverley Veale DM: Exercise dependence. Br J Addict 82:735–740, 1987.
7. Glasser W: Positive Addiction. New York, Harper and Row, 1976.
8. Goldstein A: Opioid peptides (endorphins) in pituitary and brain. Science 193:1081–1086, 1976.
9. Hughes J, Smith TW, Kosterlitz: Identification of two related pentapeptides from the brain with potent opiate agonist activity. Nature 258:577–579, 1975.
10. Katz JL: Long-distance running, anorexia nervosa, and bulimia: A report of two cases. Comp Psych 27:74–78, 1986.
11. Lyons HA, Cromey R: Compulsive jogging: Exercise dependence and associated disorder of eating. Ulster Med J 58:100–102, 1989.
12. Mandell AJ: The second second wind. In Sachs MH, Sachs ML (eds): Psychology of Running. Champaign, IL, Human Kinetics, 1981, pp 211–223.
13. Masters KS: Hypnotic susceptibility, cognitive dissociation, and runner's high in a sample of marathon runners. Am J Clin Hypn 34:193–201, 1992.
14. Morgan WP: Affective beneficence of vigorous physical activity. Med Sci Sports Exerc 17:94–100, 1985.
15. Morgan WP: Negative addiction in runners. Physician Sportsmed 7(2):56–70, 1979.
16. Pargman D, Baker MC: Running high: Enkephalin indicted. J Drug Issues 3:341–350, 1980.
17. Roberts WO, Elliot DL: Malnutrition in a compulsive runner: A case conference. Med Sci Sports Exerc 23:513–516, 1991.
18. Sundgot-Borgen J: Nutrient intake of female elite athletes suffering from eating disorders. Int J Sport Nutr 3: 431–442, 1993.
19. Sundgot-Borgen J: Prevalence of eating disorders in female elite athletes. In J Sport Nutr 3:29–40, 1993.
20. Wagemaker Jr. H, Goldstein L: The runner's high. J Sports Med 20:227–229, 1980.
21. Wheeler GD, Wall SR, Belcastro AN, et al: Are anorexic tendencies prevalent in the habitual runner? Br J Sports Med 20:77–81, 1986.
22. Yates A: Understanding and helping the compulsive athlete. J Musculoskel Med 9(3):45–59, 1992.
23. Yates A, Leehey K, Shisslak CM: Running–an analogue of anorexia? N Engl J Med 308:251–255, 1983.
24. Yates A, Shisslak C, Crago M, Allender J: Overcommitment to sport: Is there a relationship to the eating disorders? Clin J Sport Med 4:39–46, 1994.

ANEMIA, "PSEUDOANEMIA," AND IRON DEFICIENCY

As athletes have become increasingly aware that anemia and possibly even iron deficiency alone can affect performance, especially in endurance training and competition, the burden has fallen upon physicians to understand, evaluate, and treat a group of imperfectly understood problems currently lumped together under the heading of "sports anemia." In daily practice, there is a hazy area in the decision-making process about whether a borderline hemoglobin or hematocrit warrants a work-up for anemia and subsequent treatment. The situation is more difficult in athletes, because what *appears* to be true anemia may not be anemia at all, but rather "pseudoanemia," and what appears to be normal hematologic status may be rather significant iron deficiency.

This section will (1) discuss the "pseudoanemia" of sports; (2) identify the common mechanisms causing the true anemia in the athlete; (3) attempt to clarify the role of iron deficiency, with or without anemia, in athletic performance; and (4) suggest a therapeutic plan for these problems.

Athletic Pseudoanemia

Intensive endurance exercise conditioning causing major increases in plasma volume[3,6,13,28,29,44,62] as well as in total RBC mass and total body hemoglobin.[3,6,13,28,62] Because the increase in plasma volume exceeds the increments of RBC and hemoglobin production, the standard hematologic measures of RBC count, serum hemoglobin, and packed RBC volume (hematocrit) may appear depressed.[6,19,25,28,62] Plasma volume in well-conditioned runners has been shown to exceed that in nonrunners by as much as 31%, whereas total RBC mass and total body hemoglobin have been documented to be 18% and 20% higher in runners than controls, respectively. Plasma volume begins to increase right at the onset of the increased training load.[28,29] The increase in RBC mass may not be evident until 4 weeks or more after the increase in training has occurred.[28] One study has actually demonstrated minimal impairment through respiratory gas exchange and acid base balance after early increments in training have produced a hypervolemia, but before the RBC mass has expanded.[29]

Some authors have called this phenomenon "sports anemia;"[9,19,25,66,22,35,36,66] but because others have used the same term to describe a broader range of anemias in athletes, it may be clearer to call it "athletic pseudoanemia."[61,62] In a study of 12 male runners in a 20-day 312-mile road race, hemoglobin fell from 16.0 to 13.4 dL, RBCs from 5.17 to 4.36 million/mm^3, and hematocrit from 47.7% to 40.7%, with no concurrent drop in running performance.[19] Another study demonstrated that when a group of cross-country runners decreased their running mileage, their hemoglobin and hematocrit levels rose toward pre-season levels.[25] A study elevating both male and female athletes for athletic "psuedoanemia" found the phenomenon in male athletes but not female athletes.[62]

Is the dilutional effect of plasma volume expansion in the blood a functional adaptation to exercise training that improves performance? The answer to this question remains unclear. Crowell and Smith suggested that the most efficient oxygen delivery to tissue takes place when the hematocrits is 40%; at this level there would be a compromise between the oxygen-carrying capacity of the blood and the vascular resistance to increasing blood viscosity.[15] Recent studies on blood doping (blood boosting), however, demonstrate increased performance in response to RBC transfusions, which raised the hematocrit well above the 40% level.[5,64]

Athletic "pseudoanemia" is a benign condition requiring no medical management. Iron, vitamin B_{12}, and folate supplementation have no effect on it.[7,31,32,34,37,40,54] The problem for the physician is to differentiate it from true anemia, which does require therapy and monitoring.

Iron Deficiency in the Athlete

Although athletes are subject to all of the anemias that afflict other populations, the specific anemia problem related to exercise is one of iron deficiency. In a study of 52 elite Canadian distance runners, 29% of men and 82% of women were iron deficient.[10] Numerous other studies demonstrate deficient iron stores in both male and female endurance athletes and ballet dancers.[20,32,35,36,37,40,41,42,47,50,65] Most of these studies are performed without comparison to nonathletic controls. Several recent studies using nonathletic controls suggest that iron-store deficiencies are similar in comparable groups of athletes and nonathletes.[1,49,53,55]

Research has shown that iron deficiency in athletes results from a combination of : (1) insufficient iron intake, (2) inadequate iron reabsorption, and (3) accelerated iron loss.[39] The recommended dietary allowance (RDA) of iron is 10 mg/day for men and 15 mg/day for women.[24] The average iron content of Western diets is 5 to 6 mg/1000 kcal; hence, assuming normal rates of iron absorption and loss, the average man requires a 1700–2000-kcal diet and the average women, a 2500–3000-kcal diet to obtain adequate iron intake without supplementation. Endurance athletes, especially women, often fall below these dietary levels.[8,9,11,21,39,63] Additionally, there is evidence of an iron absorption defect as well. The rate of radioactive iron absorption in a study of iron-depleted runners was only half that seen in the control group of iron-depleted blood donors.[20]

Endurance athletes lose more iron than their sedentary counterparts. Basal iron loss in urine, stool, sweat, skin and hair is estimated at 0.5 to 1.0 mg/day with an additional 0.5 mg/day average additional loss due to menstruation. Measured loss in the cohort of eight long-distance runners followed for 2 years with radioactive iron studies averaged 2 mg/day.[20] This increase is multifactorial. Intense exercise can waste iron by microscopic or gross hematuria, hemoglobinuria, and myoglobinuria.[17,21,33,57] (See also section on Proteinuria, Hematuria, and "Athletic Pseudonephritis.") Several studies have demonstrated that profuse sweating can cause up to 1 mg/day iron loss,[30,48,60] although a more recent study suggests that the iron loss in sweat may make only a marginal contribution to total body iron losses.[4] Microscopic or frank gastrointestinal bleeding, common in runners, can produce additional iron loss.[38,41,52,59] (See also section on Diarrhea and Gastrointestinal Bleeding in Runners.) In female athletes, these athletic losses may be compounded by normal menstrual loss. Additionally, many athletes, particularly female athletes, may start training with already reduced iron stores. The result may be a significantly elevated iron requirement for athletes to maintain an equilibrium.

Diagnosis of Iron Deficiency and Iron Deficiency Anemia

A staging system is commonly employed to elucidate the relationship of iron deficiency to the development of clinical anemia (Table 4).[9,14,42,47,51] Stage 1, "prelatent" iron deficiency, is characterized by markedly diminished or absent bone marrow iron stores. Erythropoiesis occurs in stage 1, but the RBCs may be iron deficient. The diagnosis is generally made by measuring serum ferritin, which correlates with the body's iron stores. Levels below 12 ng/ml suggest absent bone marrow iron, but higher levels may also correspond to significant depletion in athletes, since heavy training may elevate serum ferritin levels spuriously.[9] One study demonstrates that pairing serum ferritin levels with RBC ferritin levels increases the specificity of the test.[2] Several authorities suggest that more than one index of iron deficiency should be examined in order to establish the diagnosis in ultraendurance athletes.[45,46,61] Their conclusion was also suggested in earlier work by Magnusson et al.[35]

TABLE 4. Stages of Iron Deficiency*

Stage	Characteristic	Serum Ferritin	Serum Iron	Binding Capacity	Transferrin Saturation	Hemoglobin	Bone Marrow Iron Stores
1. Prelatent	Marrow iron depletion	↓	N	N	N	N	0-trace
2. Latent	Serum iron depletion with iron-deficient erythropoiesis	↓	↓	↑	↓	N-low N	0
3. Manifest	Iron deficiency anemia	↓	↓	↑	↓	↓	0

*Adapted from Clement DB, Sawchuk LL: Iron status and sports performance. Sports Med 1:65–74, 1984; Cook J: Clinical evaluation of iron deficiency. Semin Hematol 19:6–18, 1982; Parr RB, Bachman LA, Moss RA: Iron deficiency in female athletes. Physician Sportsmed 12:81–86, 1984; Risser WL, Risser JNH: Iron deficiency in adolescents and young adults. Physician Sportsmed 18(12):87–101, 1990.

An accurate measure of iron stores in athletes by serum ferritin levels in athletes is difficult because of a shift of iron from the marrow to the liver. Haptoglobin binds the free hemoglobin that is released by footstrike and exertional hemolysis.[21,36,49] Circulating haptoglobin-hemoglobin complexes are taken up by hepatocytes, and iron stored in the liver in this manner is not measured by serum ferritin.[36,49]

Stage 2 is "latent" iron deficiency. Serum iron stores are depleted, and hemoglobin and other RBC parameters may be reduced but within the normal range. As serum iron levels drop, total iron binding capacity increases reactively; transferrin saturation is decreased as well. Transferrin saturation below 16% indicates too low an iron store available to the developing RBC for normal erythropoiesis.[14] Erythropoiesis continues or is slowed in stage 2, and the RBCs are iron-deficient.

Stage 3 is "manifest" iron deficiency characterized by anemia. Hemoglobin drops below 12 g/100 ml in women and 14 g/100 ml in men.[12] In black athletes, the diagnosis of anemia is slightly more difficult, because the normal hemoglobin level in black children and adults is 1 g/100 ml lower than in their white counterparts, and this difference is not accounted for by dietary or socioeconomic considerations.[26,27] Red blood cell count, hematocrit, and RBC indices may reflect the severity of the anemia.

Effects of Iron Deficiency, with and without Anemia, on Performance

Hemoglobin is the freight car of the body's oxygen transport system. A major reduction in hemoglobin will produce an obvious diminution of muscle function, particularly when the athlete is attempting to exercise at a maximal level. The body can compensate for mild anemia at submaximal loads by increasing ventilation and cardiac output, and by increasing RBC levels of 2,3-diphosphoglycerate, which, in turn, enhances oxygen release from hemoglobin to the tissues. A point is reached at which the anemia is so severe or the work demand is so high that the compensating mechanisms are no longer adequate and performance is diminished.

In the absence of clinical anemia, iron deficiency may theoretically affect maximum performance levels. Iron is a basic component of myoglobin, which transports and stores oxygen in muscle, and of cytochrome C, which is necessary for oxidative metabolism. Both have been found to be depleted in iron-deficient rats,[23] and treatment with iron is therapeutic.[16,18] Iron deficiency without anemia has been shown to diminish oxidative metabolism in humans, necessitating more energy production by less efficient muscle anaerobic metabolism and causing accumulation of lactate in the blood.[43,56] Similarly, in laboratory animals, it dramatically reduces exercise time to exhaustion.[23] On the other hand, several recent clinical studies failed to show significant performance reduction due to nonanemic iron deficiency.[7,22,31,32,34,37,40]

Treatment

In most situations of established iron deficiency in athletes, dietary iron is unlikely to provide adequate replacement. This source of iron should not be overlooked, because ferrous (Fe^{++}) heme-iron contained in red meat, poultry, and fish, is much more readily absorbed than ferric (Fe^{+++}) nonheme-iron, found in nonmeat foods and iron supplements. Indeed, a small amount of meat in the diet appears to enhance the absorption of nonheme iron from other sources.[39] Ascorbic acid supplementation is also well known to enhance nonheme iron absorption.[10] Ascorbic acid works by reducing Fe^{+++} to Fe^{++}, and antacids negate this effect.[39] Vegetarian athletes are particularly at risk for reduced iron absorption due to the lack of heme-iron in their dietary intake.[58]

Oral iron supplementation should be given in the form of ferrous salt, yielding approximately 65 mg of elemental iron one to three times daily, depending on the severity of the deficiency. Typically, one to two doses daily are adequate for the anemia and iron deficiency seen in athletes. The most commonly used preparations are ferrous sulfate, fumarate, and gluconate. Absorption is better on an empty stomach. Gastrointestinal side effects are less common with fumarate and gluconate, and are less frequently when the dose is small at first and gradually increased. Ascorbic acid in 250-mg doses may be given concurrently with the iron; commercial preparations are available that combine this absorption enhancer with iron in a single dose.

This discussion is not complete without mention of overtreatment with iron. As athletes, coaches, and trainers have become increasingly aware of the importance of iron for performance, many athletes have started taking large, and often excessive, doses of iron without a physician's supervision. Hemochromatosis from iron supplementation is a rare but real complication. Athletes of Mediterranean heritage should be screened for thalassemia, and black athletes should be evaluated for sickle-cell disease before iron therapy is instituted.

REFERENCES

1. Balaban EP, Cox JV, Snell P, et al: The frequency of anemia and iron deficiency in the runner. Med Sci Sports Exerc 21:643–648, 1989.
2. Balaban EP, Cox JV, Vaughan RH, et al: Iron deficiency in the runner as determined by a direct cell ferritin measurement. Med Sci Sports Exerc 20(2 Suppl):S78, 1988.
3. Brotherhood J, Brozovic B, Pugh LGC: Haematological status of middle- and long-distance runners. Clin Sci Mol Med 48:139–145, 1975.
4. Brune M, Magnusson B, Persson H, Hallberg L: Iron losses in sweat. Am J Clin Nutr 43:438–443, 1986.
5. Buick FJ, Gledhill N, Force AB, et al: Effect of induced erythrocythemia on aerobic work capacity. J Appl Physiol 48:636–642, 1980.
6. Bunch TW: Blood test abnormalities in runners. Mayo Clin Proc 55:113–117, 1980.
7. Celsing F, Blombstrand E, Werner B, et al: Effects of iron deficiency on endurance and muscle enzyme activity in man. Med Sci Sports Exerc 18:156–161, 1986.
8. Clement DB, Asmundson RC: Nutritional intake and hematological parameters in endurance runners. Phys Sportsmed 10(3):37–43, 1982.
9. Clement DB, Sawchuk LL: Iron status and sports performance. Sports Med 1:65–74, 1984.
10. Clydesdale FM: Physiochemical determinants of iron bioavailability. Food Technol 37:133–138, 1983.
11. Cohen JL, Potosnak L, Frank O, Baker H: A nutritional and hematologic assessment of elite ballet dancers. Physician Sportsmed 13(5):43–49,54 1985.
12. Committee on Iron Deficiency: Iron deficiency in the United States. JAMA 203:119–124, 1968.
13. Convertino VA, Brock PJ, Keil LC, et al: Exercise training-induced hypervolemia: Role of plasma albumin, renin, and vasopressin. J Appl Physiol 48:665–669, 1980.
14. Cook J: Clinical evaluation of iron deficiency. Semin Hematol 19:6–18, 1982.
15. Crowell JW, Smith EE: Determination of the optimal hematocrit. J Appl Physiol 22:501–504, 1967.
16. Dallman PR, Schwartz HC: Myoglobin and cytochrome response during repair of iron deficiency in the rat. J Clin Invest 44:1631–1638, 1965.
17. Davidson RJL: March or exertional haemoglobinuria. Semin Hematol 6:150–161, 1969.
18. Davies KJA, Maguire JJ, Brooks GA, et al: Muscle mitochondrial bioenergetics, oxygen supply, and work capacity during dietary iron deficiency and repletion. Am J Physiol 242:E418–E427, 1982.
19. Dressendorfer RH, Wade CE, Amsterdam EA: Development of pseudoanemia in marathon runners during a 20-day road race. JAMA 246:1215–1218, 1981.
20. Ehn L, Carlmark B, Hoglund S: Iron status in athletes involved in intense physical activity. Med Sci Sports Exerc 12:61–64, 1980.
21. Eichner ER: Runner's macrocytosis: A clue to footstrike hemolysis. Am J Med 78:321–325, 1985.
22. Eichner ER: Sports anemia, iron supplements, and blood doping. Med Sci Sports Exerc. 24(9 Suppl):S315–S318, 1992.
23. Finch CA, Miller LR, Inamdar AR, et al: Iron deficiency in the rat: Physiological and biomechanical studies of muscle dysfunction. J Clin Invest 58:447–453, 1976.
24. Food and Nutrition Board Committee on Dietary Allowances, National Research Council: Recommended Dietary Allowances, 10th Ed. Washington, DC, National Academy Press, 1989.
25. Frederickson LA, Puhl J, Runyan WS: Effects of training on indices of iron status of young female cross country runners. Med Sci Sports Exerc 15:271–276, 1983.
26. Garn SM, Ryan AS, Owen GM, Abraham S: Income matched black-white hemoglobin differences after correction for low transferrin saturations. Am J Clin Nutr 34:1645–1647, 1981.
27. Garn SM, Smith NJ, Clark DC: Lifelong differences in hemoglobin levels between blacks and whites. J Natl Med Assoc 67:91–96, 1975.
28. Green H, Coates J, Sutton J, Jones S: Time course changes in blood volume and hematology during extreme endurance training. Med Sci Sports Exerc 20(2 Suppl): S13, 1988.
29. Green HJ, Hughson RL, Thomson JA, Sharratt MT. Supramaximal exercise after training-induced hypervolemia. I. Gas exchange and acid-base balance. J Appl Physiol 62:1944–1953, 1987.
30. Green R, Charlton R, Seftel H, et al: Body iron excretion in man: A collaborative study. Am J Med 45:336–353, 1968.
31. Hegenauer J, Strause L, Saltman P, et al: Transitory hematologic effects of moderate exercise are not influenced by iron supplementation. Eur J Appl Physiol 52:57–61, 1983.
32. Klingshirn LA, Pate RR, Bourque SP, et al: Effect of iron supplementation on endurance capacity in iron-depleted female runners. Med Sci Sports Exerc 24:819–824, 1992.
33. Knochel JP, Schlein EM: On the mechanism of rhabdomyolysis in potassium depletion. J Clin Invest 51:1750–1758, 1972.
34. Lamanca J, Haymes E: Effects of dietary iron supplementation on endurance. Med Sci Sports Exerc 21(2 Suppl): S77, 1989.
35. Magnusson B, Hallberg L, Rossander L, Swolin B: Iron metabolism and "sports anemia." I. A study of several iron parameters in elite runners with differences in iron status. Acta Med Scand 216:149–55, 1984.
36. Magnusson B, Hallberg L, Rossander L, Swolin B: Iron metabolism and "sports anemia." II. A hematological com-

parison of elite runners and control subjects. Acta Med Scand 216:157–64, 1984.
37. Matter M, Stittfall T, Graves J, et al: The effect of iron and folate therapy on maximal exercise performance in female marathon runners with iron and folate deficiency. Clin Sci 72:415–422, 1987.
38. McMahon LF, Ryan MJ, Larson D, Fisher RL: Occult gastrointestinal blood loss in marathon runners. Ann Intern Med 100:846–847, 1984.
39. Newhouse IJ, Clement DB: Iron status in athletes: An update. Sports Med 5:337–352, 1988.
40. Newhouse IJ, Clement DB, Taunton JE, McKenzie DC: The effects of prelatent/latent iron deficiency on physical work capacity. Med Sci Sports Exerc 21:263–268, 1989.
41. Nickerson HJ, Holubets MC, Weiler BR, et al: Causes of iron deficiency in adolescent athletes. J Pediatr 114: 657–663, 1989.
42. Nickerson HJ, Tripp AD: Iron deficiency in adolescent cross-country runners. Physician Sportsmed 11(6):60–66, 1983.
43. Ohira Y, Edgerton VR, Gardner GW, et al: Work capacity, heart rate, and blood lactate responses to iron treatment. Br J Haematol 41:365–372, 1979.
44. Oscai LB, Williams BT, Hertig BA: Effect of exercise on blood volume. J Appl Physiol 24:622–624, 1968.
45. O'Toole ML, Iwane H, Douglas PS, Hiller WDB: Estimates of iron sufficiency in ultraendurance triathletes. Med Sci Sports Exerc 21(2 Suppl):S78, 1989.
46. O'Toole ML, Iwane H, Douglas PS, et al: Iron status in ultraendurance triathletes. Physician Sportsmed 12(17): 90–102, 1989.
47. Parr RB, Bachman LA, Moss RA: Iron deficiency in female athletes. Physician Sportsmed 12(4):81–86, 1984.
48. Paulev P-E, Jordal R, Pedersen NS: Dermal excretion of iron in intensely training athletes. Clin Chim Acta 127: 19–27, 1983.
49. Resina A, Gatteschi L, Giamberardino MA, et al: Hematological comparison of iron status in trained top-level soccer players and control subjects. Int J Sports Med 12:453–56, 1991.
50. Risser WL, Lee EJ, Poindexter HBW, et al: Iron deficiency in female athletes: Its prevalence and impact on performance. Med Sci Sports Exerc 20:116–121, 1988.
51. Risser WL, Risser JMH: Iron deficiency in adolescents and young adults. Physician Sportsmed 18(12):87–101, 1990.
52. Robertson JD, Maughan RJ, Davidson RJL: Faecal blood loss in response to exercise. BMJ 295(6593):303–305, 1987.
53. Rowland TW: Iron deficiency in the young athlete. Pediatr Clin North Am 37:1153–1163, 1990.
54. Rowland TW, Deisroth MB, Green GM, Kelleher JF: The effect of iron therapy on the exercise capacity of nonanemic iron-deficient adolescent runners. Am J Dis Child 142:165–169, 1988.
55. Rowland TW, Stagg L, Kelleher JF: Iron deficiency in adolescent girls. Are athletes at increased risk? J Adolesc Health 12:22–25, 1991.
56. Schoene RB, Escourrou P, Robertson HT, et al: Iron repletion decreases maximum exercise lactate concentrations in female athletes with minimal iron-deficiency anemia. J Lab Clin Med 102:306–312, 1983.
57. Siegel AJ, Hennekens CH, Solomon HS, Van Boeckel B: Exercise-related hematuria: findings in a group of marathon runners. JAMA 241:391–392, 1979.
58. Snyder AC, Dvorak LL, Roepke JB: Influence of dietary iron source on measures of iron status among female runners. Med Sci Sports Exerc 21:7–10, 1989.
59. Stewart JG, Ahlquist DA, McGill DB, et al: Gastrointestinal blood loss and anemia in runners. Ann Intern Med 100:843–845, 1984.
60. Vellar OD: Studies on sweat losses of nutrients. I. Iron content of whole body sweat and its association with other sweat constituents, serum iron levels, hematological indices, body surface area and sweat rate. Scand J Clin Lab Invest 21:157–167, 1968.
61. Weight LM: "Sports anaemia" Does it exist? Sports Med 16:1–4, 1993.
62. Weight LM, Darge BL, Jacobs P: Athletes' pseudoanaemia. Eur J Appl Physiol 62:358–362, 1991.
63. Weight LM, Jacobs P, Noakes TD: Dietary iron deficiency and sports anaemia. Br J Nutr 68:253–260, 1992.
64. Williams MH, Wesseldine S, Somma T, Schuster R: The effect of induced erythrocythemia upon 5-mile treadmill run time. Med Sci Sports Exerc 13:169–175, 1981.
65. Wishnitzer R, Vorst E, Berrebi A: Bone marrow iron depression in competitive distance runners. Int J Sports Med 4:27–30, 1983.
66. Yoshimura H: Anemia during physical training (sports anemia). Nutr Rev 28:251–253, 1970.

PROTEINURIA, HEMATURIA, AND "ATHLETIC PSEUDONEPHRITIS"

Over one hundred years ago, von Luebe reported finding protein in the urine of 14 of 119 soldiers who had just undergone strenuous exercise, whereas there was no protein in the early morning specimens from the same men.[8,38] In 1910, Barach found protein, red blood cells, and hyaline and granular casts in the urine of marathon runners.[4] In 1956, Gardner identified protein, RBCs, and a wide variety of cellular and granular casts in the urine of a group of 47 football players and correlated the incidence of these findings with the increasing intensity of physical activity. Noting that the urine in healthy athletes would clear after "a few days of less strenuous activity," he proposed the term "athletic psuedonephritis" to distinguish this transient phenomenon in the athlete from the urinary findings of glomerulonephritis.[22]

Effects of Exercise on Renal Function

Exercise may reduce renal blood flow, the extent of which varies with the intensity of exercise. Research has shown that moderate exercise (50% of the individual's maximum aerobic capacity) may lower renal blood flow nearly 30%, whereas strenuous exercise may lower it as much as 75%. These changes appear within the first 10 minutes of exercise. Both the afferent and efferent arterioles of the renal glomeruli constrict in response to sympathetic nervous system stimuli and the increased circulating levels of epinephrine and norepinephrine related to the exercise load. Second, the glomerular filtration rate decreases during exertion as well, although not to the same extent. An intense exercise load may reduce the glomerular filtration rate by up to 50% of the resting value. Hydration level is also an important determinant of glomerular filtration rate; intense exercise increases circulating levels of plasma anti-diuretic hormone, thus decreasing urine flow and conserving plasma volume.[9,37]

"Athletic Pseudonephritis"

It is now well established that strenuous exercise produces increased excretion of protein, red and white blood cells, and both cellular and noncellular renal tubular casts in a variety of contact and noncontact sports.[2,4,6,7,19,22,37,48] These findings are transient and will disappear if the athlete rests for one to several days.[2,7,22,31,37,48] Recent studies have demonstrated that the majority of urinary sediment findings in "athletic pseudonephritis" are renal in origin.[7,19,31,37,49] It appears that the kidney responds to the reduced renal blood flow with increased glomeruler permeability and decreased renal tubulus reabsorption of protein.[30,37,39,40,42,43,44] One hypothesis is that the renal vasoconstriction in response to the exercise load causes many glomeruli to stop functioning. After exercise, when these glomeruli resume their function, they may leak protein and, presumably, blood cells.[37,49] The urinary sediment findings correlate with the intensity of the exercise.[2,22,37,49] and the state of hydration[37,45] and the interaction between these.[27]

Postexercise Proteinuria

Strenuous exercise has been documented to increase urinary protein in runners,[1,34,44] swimmers,[40] cyclists,[34,43] triathletes,[42] rowers,[43] and judo competitors,[13] but not in weightlifters.[28] Increased proteinuria is not simply an exaggeration of normal physiological urinary protein excretion. Proteinuria following prolonged light exercise appears to be caused by a combination of increased glomerular permeability[9,34,38,40,42,44] and decreased renal tubular reabsorption of protein in intense shortterm exercise.[38,39,40] Similar postexercise proteinuria patterns exist in childhood and adolescence.[29,41] In triathlon, the highest level of proteinuria occurs during swimming.[42,25] Exercise-induced proteinuria may be attenuated by indomethacin, suggesting a role for prostaglandins in this process.[35]

Exertional Hemolysis and Hemoglobinuria

In 1881, Fleischer described recurrent hemoglobinuria induced in a soldier by marching.[11] Since then, abundant evidence has linked exertion with intravascular hemolysis.[12,16,17,18,23,24,36,46,47] Early writings developed the concept that footstrikes on a hard surface can destroy RBCs.[11] If the amount of hemoglobin release exceeds the capacity of serum haptoglobin to bind and transport it to the liver for recycling, free hemoglobin may be excreted in the urine, coloring it red to brown-black. Evidence for hemolysis includes reduced plasma haptoglobin,[3,10–12,14,17,36,46,47] mild reticulocytosis,[3,12,17] and mild macrocytosis.[3,17]

Footstrike hemolysis has been described in recreational[12] and competitive runners, triathletes,[36] and aerobic dancers.[46] The degree of hemolysis varies with surface hardness,[11,17,46] shoe shock absorbency,[11,17] distance and intensity,[17,36] aerobic dance technique and duration,[46] and the athlete's size and weight. With modern running shoes, severe hemolysis is rare.

Not all exertional hemolysis is caused by footstrike. Hemolysis has been correlated with exertion in swimmers, but the pathophysiology has not yet been elucidated.[47]

Early reports suggested that the hemoglobin lost from exertional hemolysis could contribute significantly to anemia in athletes, but more recent research and analysis suggest that the resulting diminution of iron stores may be negligible.[3,14,17,46] In marginally iron sufficient athletes, however, particularly menstruating athletes, the hemolysis-induced hemoglobinuria may cause enough iron loss to reduce competitive performance levels.[3,17]

Gross Hematuria

A separate syndrome of gross hematuria in runners has been well documented. It consists of grossly bloody urination, occasionally without warning symptoms, but sometimes preceded by urinary frequency and tenesmus. Painless blood clots as large as 0.5×1.0 cm have been reported. Evaluation with excretory urograms has been consistently negative. Cystoscopic examinations have varied with the interval between symptoms and examination. Early cystoscopies have revealed localized bladder contusions with loss of bladder epithelium and the presence of fibrinous exudates. The syndrome has been identified in both male and female runners. Early urinalysis will show RBCs. This syndrome is also benign, and all urinary findings disappear within a few days.[5,9,20,21] It is important to remember that hematuria may result from acute or chronic renal trauma.[32]

Urinary Screening

Traditionally, preparticipation athletic screening has included urine testing by dipstick for protein, blood, and glucose. A recent study demonstrated that in 701 high school students undergoing athletic screening, 40 had proteinuria and one glycosuria. Repeat testing with first-voided morning specimens revealed normal urine in all students, and a glucose tolerance test was normal in the student with glycosuria.[26] Consequently, routine urinary screening is no longer recommended.[15,33]

If a urinalysis is obtained for other reasons, and an athlete has abnormal sediment, it may be necessary that the athlete rest completely for several days before the urinary findings revert to normal. In some individuals, even a small amount of exercise may produce an abnormal urine.

REFERENCES

1. Alvarez C, Mir J, Obaya S, Fragoso M: Hematuria and microalbuminuria after a 100 kilometer race. Am J Sports Med 15:609–611, 1987.
2. Alyea EP, Parish HH: Renal response to exercise-urinary findings. JAMA 167:807–813, 1958.
3. Balaban EP: Sports anemia. Clin Sports Med 11:313–325, 1992.
4. Barach JH: Physiological and pathological effects of severe exertion (marathon race) on the circulatory and renal systems. Arch Intern Med 5:382–405, 1910.
5. Blacklock NJ: Bladder trauma in the long-distance runner: "10,000 meters haematuria." Br J Urol 49:129–132, 1977.
6. Boileau M, Fuchs E, Barry JM, Hodges CV: Stress hematuria: Athletic pseudonephritis in marathoners. Urology 15:471–474, 1980.
7. Campanacci L, Faccini L, Englaro E, et al: Exercise-induced proteinuria. Contrib Nephrol 26:31–41, 1981.
8. Castenfors J: Renal function during prolonged exercise. Ann N Y Acad Sci 301:151–159, 1977.
9. Cianflocco AJ: Renal complications of exercise. Clin Sports Med 11:437–451, 1992.
10. Davidson RJL: Exertional haemoglobinuria: a report on three cases with studies on the haemolytic mechanism. J Clin Pathol 17:536–540, 1964.
11. Davidson RJL: March or exertional haemoglobinuria. Semin Hematol 6:150–161, 1969.
12. Deitrick RW: Intravascular haemolysis in the recreational runner. Br J Sports Med 25:183–187, 1991.
13. DeMeersman RE, Wilkerson JE. Judo Nephropathy: Trauma versus non-trauma. J Trauma 22:150–152, 1982.
14. Diehl LF, Butler WM, Ferguson EW, Schoomaker EB: Intravascular hemolysis in marathon runners. Clin Res 30:314A, 1982.
15. Dyment PG (ed.): Sports Medicine: Health Care for Young Athletes, 2nd ed. Elk Grove Village, IL, American Academy of Pediatrics, 1991.
16. Eichner ER: The anemias of athletes. Physician Sportsmed 14(9):122–130, 1986.
17. Eichner ER: Runner's macrocytosis: a clue to footstrike hemolysis. Am J Med 78:321–325, 1985.
18. Eichner ER: Sports anemia, iron supplements and blood doping. Med Sci Sports Exerc 24(9 Suppl):S315–S318, 1992.
19. Fassett RG, Owen JE, Fairly J, et al: Urinary red-cell morphology during exercise. Br Med J 285:1455–1457, 1982.
20. Fred HL: More on grossly bloody urine of runners. Arch Intern Med 138:1610–1611, 1978.
21. Fred HL, Natelson EA: Grossly bloody urine of runners. South Med J 70:1394–1396, 1977.
22. Gardner KD: "Athletic pseudonephritis"-alteration of urine sediment by athletic competition. JAMA 161:1613–1617, 1956.
23. Gilligan DR, Altschule MD, Katersky EM: Physiological intravascular hemolysis of exercise. Hemoglobinemia and hemoglobinuria following cross-country runs. J Clin Invest 22:859–869, 1943.
24. Gilligan DR, Blumgart HL: March hemoglobinuria. Medicine 20:341–395, 1941.
25. Glace B, Gleim G, Constantini N, et al: The effect of exercise sequence on proteinuria during a triathlon. Med Sci Sports Exerc 25(5Suppl):S35, 1993.
26. Goldberg B, Saraniti A, Witman P, et al: Pre-participation sports assessment—an objective lesson. Pediatrics 66: 736–745, 1980.
27. Helzer-Julin MJ, Latin RW, Mellion MB, et al: The effect of exercise intensity and hydration on athletic pseudonephritis. J Sports Med Phys Fitness 28:324–329, 1988.
28. Hickson JF, Wolinsky I, Rodriguez GP, et al: Failure of weight training to affect urinary indices of protein metabolism in men. Med Sci Sports Exerc 18:563–567, 1986.
29. Houser MT, Jahn MF, Kobayashi A, Walburn J: Assessment of urinary protein excretion in the adolescent: Effect of body position and exercise. J Pediatr 109:556–561, 1986.
30. Javitt NB, Miller AT: Mechanism of exercise proteinuria. J Appl Physiol 4:834–839, 1952.
31. Kincaid-Smith P: Haematuria and exercise-related haematuria. Br Med J 285:1595–1597, 1982.
32. Kleiman AH: Renal trauma in sports. W J Surg Obstet Gynecol 69:331–340, 1961.
33. Lombardo J, Robinson J, Smith D: Preparticipation physical evaluation, Kansas City, MO, American Academy of Family Physicians, American Academy of Pediatrics, American Medical Society for Sports Medicine, American Orthopaedic Society for Sports Medicine, American Osteopathic Academy of Sports Medicine, 1992.
34. Miller PD, Goldfab AH, Kroll MH, et al: Comparative effects of submaximal cycling and running on urinary protein excretion. Med Sci Sports Exerc 21(2Suppl):S106, 1989.
35. Mittleman KD, Zambraski EJ: Exercise-induced proteinuria is attenuated by indomethacin. Med Sci Sports Exerc 24:1069–1074, 1992.
36. O'Toole ML, Hiller DB, Roalstad MS, Douglas PS: Hemolysis during triathlon races: its relation to race distance. Med Sci Sports Exerc 20:272–275, 1988.
37. Poortmans JR: Exercise and renal function. Sports Med 1:125–153, 1984.
38. Poortmans JR: Postexercise proteinuria in humans. JAMA 253:236–240, 1985.
39. Poortmans JR, Brauman H, Staroukine M, et al: Indirect evidence of golmerular/tubular mixed-type postexercise proteinuria in healthy humans. Am J Physiol 254:F277–F283, 1988.
40. Poortmans JR, Engels M-F, Sellier M, Leclercq R: Urine protein excretion and swimming events. Med Sci Sports Exerc 23:831–835, 1991.
41. Poortmans JR, Geudvert C, Schorochoff P, et al: Postexercise proteinuria in childhood and adolescence. Med Sci Sports Exerc 25(5Suppl):S19, 1993.
42. Poortmans JR, Jeannaud J, Vertongen F, et al: Renal responses to exercise in triathlon athletes. Med Sci Sports Exerc 24(5Suppl):S43, 1992.
43. Poortmans JR, Jourdain M, Heyters C, Reardon FD: Postexercise proteinuria in rowers. Can J Sport Sci 15: 126–130, 1990.
44. Poortmans JR, Labilloy D: The influence of work intensity on postexercise proteinuria. Eur J Appl Physiol 57:260–263, 1988.
45. Riess RW: Athletic hematuria and related phenomena. J Sports Med Phys Fitness 19:381–388, 1979.
46. Schwellnus MP, Penfold GK, Cilliers JF, et al: Intravascular hemolysis in aerobic dancing: the role of floor surface and type of routine. Physician Sportsmed 17(8):55–67, 1989.
47. Selby GB, Eichner ER: Endurance swimming, intravascular hemolysis, anemia, and iron depletion. Am J Med 81:791–794, 1986.

48. Siegel AJ, Hennekens CH, Solomon HS, van Boeckel B: Exercise-related hematuria: findings in a group of marathon runners. JAMA 241:391–392, 1979.
49. White HL, Rolf D: Effects of exercise and of some other influences on the renal circulation in man. Am J Physiol 152:505–516, 1948.

DIARRHEA AND GASTROINTESTINAL BLEEDING IN RUNNERS

Few groups of athletes spend more time discussing their bowel function than serious runners. This phenomenon is not some bizarre fixation but the result of a common problem known as "runner's trots." One survey demonstrated that 30% of runners have experienced this difficulty, and 12% of these noted frank rectal bleeding.[15] For some runners, this diarrhea may be incapacitating. Among runners with rectal bleeding, many report significant, sometimes frightening, amounts of blood loss with these episodes. At least one study found that as few as 25% of runners with hematochezia seek medical evaluation.[11]

Several theories exist regarding the causes of runner's diarrhea and gastrointestinal (GI) bleeding. The principal hypotheses reviewed here include increased GI motility, ischemia, and mechanical factors unique to running. When analyzing the data, it appears that there may not be a single unifying hypothesis: these problems may be multifactorial.

Runner's Diarrhea

Several studies have examined the prevalence of runner's diarrhea. The most common symptom was the urge to defecate, found in 30–42% of respondents, whereas diarrhea associated with running ranged from 14–30%.[9,15,19,23,26] A direct relationship exists between severity of symptoms and level of physical exertion.[8,15,19,23,26] Interestingly, diarrhea is much more commonly associated with running than with other activities that have similar physical demands.

Increased Gastrointestinal Motility

Altered gastrointestinal motility is a frequently proposed mechanism for runner's diarrhea. Priebe and Priebe found that 30% of 425 participants in a 10-km race experienced runner's diarrhea. Two-thirds of this group provided a description of their diarrhea that was consistent with a disorder of GI motility such as functional bowel syndrome. Indeed 15% of these subjects reported having irritable bowel syndrome when not running. Of these runners, 13% had known lactose intolerance, and 33% were on high-fiber diets. The authors also found anecdotal evidence of reduced diarrhea frequency in those using antimotility agents, and they concluded altered GI motility associated with intensive running was the cause of the diarrhea.[15] Further support for this explanation is provided by evidence that concentrations of motilin and other GI regulatory peptides rise during prolonged running.[21]

Gastrointestinal Bleeding.

GI bleeding is a well-documented phenomenon in endurance runners. Several studies of runners have documented GI blood loss after competitions ranging from 10 km to 100 miles,[2,3,4,7,11,12,15,20,24] with one demonstrating GI bleeding in 9 of 41 marathon runners.[24] It is likely that almost all runners will develop heme-positive stools if they exert themselves hard enough or long enough. Baska and colleagues demonstrated fecal hemoglobin loss in 85% of participants in an ultramarathon (100 miles),[2] and several other studies have suggested that GI bleeding correlates with effort intensity.[3,4,7,12] Up to 2% of runners may experience grossly bloody stools,[9] although the majority of bleeding is occult.[22]

Mesenteric Ischemia

There is evidence that mesenteric ischemia associated with running is the cause of GI bleeding and possibly runner's diarrhea as well. Studies have demonstrated that splanchnic blood flow may decrease by as much as 80% with strenuous exercise.[5] It is postulated that this relative gut ischemia during running leads to malabsorption and focal areas of necrosis or ulceration. Heer et al. presented the case of a 34-year old runner with bloody diarrhea. Colonscopy revealed hemorrhagic lesions throughout the colon and histologic examination was consistent with ischemic colitis. Subsequently, the patient's superior mesenteric artery blood flow was found to be decreased by 30% during treadmill exercise.[8] Several other studies have documented ischemic lesions in both the stomach and colon following intensive endurance running.[4,8,13,24] The shunting of blood away from the mesenteric circulation may be compounded by the elevations in core body temperature and dehydration that many competitive runners routinely experience.[4] Two studies found a positive correlation between percentage of body weight lost and severity of lower GI symptoms.[16,17]

Mechanical Factors

The lower incidence of diarrhea and GI bleeding in other endurance sports such as cycling[6,25] has led to the idea that mechanical factors unique to running may contribute to both runner's diarrhea and GI bleeding. In a study demonstrating that running produces much more abdominal vibration than bicycling, the authors suggested that the vibratory forces lead to GI dysfunction.[18] Others theorize that the shearing force of the diaphragm on the gastric fundus may be sufficient to produce mucosal lesions in the stomach, the most common site of documented GI bleeding.[14] One study verified erosive and hemorrhagic gastric lesions on endoscopy in symptomatic runners; studies performed more than 48 hours after competition were unremarkable.[24] It appears that damage, whatever its cause, may be transient.

Prevention and Treatment

A careful history focusing on factors such as recent changes in mileage or effort, travel history, dietary habits and preexisting GI problems is the cornerstone of evaluation. Stool studies, including occult blood, white blood cell count, ova and parasite, and culture, guided by the history, may be appropriate. Patients with frank GI bleeding or chronic occult bleeding require prompt and thorough evaluation.[10]

Managing runner's diarrhea and GI bleeding may be challenging because precise etiologic factors have not been identified. In addition, many athletes are unwilling to reduce their workouts or switch sports to help alleviate their problem. The diagnosis of functional bowel syndrome should be entertained when it is consistent with the history. These patients may benefit from dietary manipulation. Judicious use of prophylactic antimotility agents, such as loperamide, may also prove helpful.

If the dietary history shows that the athlete consumes a high-fiber diet, as is common in competitive runners, a trial of fiber reduction may prove beneficial. Conversely, an increase in fiber may help to solidify the gut contents in runners who include little or no fiber in their diet yet still experience "runner's trots."

Runners with bloody diarrhea or heme-positive stools may benefit from some of the measures described above. Because ischemia likely plays a pivotal role in these patients, adequate hydration in between hard workouts or races is critical. These athletes should also take fluids in smaller quantities and at more frequent intervals while running. H_2 blockers are quite useful in treating upper GI complaints and at least one study indicates that they may be of benefit in preventing running associated GI bleeding.[1]

A maneuver that frequently has been successful is cutting back training and competition 20–40% in both mileage and intensity and then building them back up slowly. Crosstraining provides an excellent way to maintain cardiovascular fitness while decreasing the likelihood of lower GI complaints. Runners should also be encouraged to defecate prior to their workout if possible. A light meal or brief jog a few hours before competition may help stimulate the gastrocolic reflex and thus help prevent diarrhea.

Diarrhea and GI bleeding are surprisingly common. Although the causes remain controversial, theories regarding etiology provide logical bases for evaluation and treatment. Various strategies are available to the clinician and athlete that can provide relief from these troubling ailments.

REFERENCES

1. Baska RS, Moses FM, Deuster PA: Cimetidine reduces running-associated gastrointestinal bleeding: A prospective observation. Dig Dis Sci 35:956–960, 1990.
2. Baska RS, Moses FM, Graeber G, Kearney G: Gastrointestinal bleeding during an ultramarathon. Dig Dis Sci 35:276–279, 1990.
3. Buckman MT: Gastrointestinal bleeding in long distance runners. Ann Intern Med 101:127–128, 1984.
4. Cantwell JD: Gastrointestinal disorders in runners. JAMA 246:1404–1405, 1981.
5. Clausen JP: Effect of physical training on cardiovascular adjustments to exercise in man. Physiol Rev 57:779–815, 1977.
6. Dobbs TW, Atkins M, Ratliff R, Eichner ER: Gastrointestinal bleeding in competitive cyclists. Med Sci Sport Exerc 20(Suppl):S78, 1988.
7. Fogoros RN: "Runner's trots": Gastrointestinal disturbances in runners. JAMA 243:1743–1744, 1980.
8. Heer M, Repond F, Hany A, et al: Acute ischemic colitis in a female long distance runner. Gut 28:896–899, 1987.
9. Keefe EB, Lowe DK, Goss JR, Wayne R: Gastrointestinal symptoms of marathon runners. West J Med 141: 481–484, 1984.
10. Larson DC, Fisher R: Management of exercise-induced gastrointestinal problems. Physician Sportsmed 15(9):112–126, 1987.
11. McCabe ME, Peura DA, Kadakia SC, et al: Gastrointestinal blood loss associated with running a marathon. Dig Dis Sci 31:1229–1232, 1986.
12. McMahon LF, Ryan MJ, Larson D, Fisher RL: Occult gastrointestinal blood loss in marathon runners. Ann Intern Med 100:846–847, 1984.
13. Moses FM, Brewer TG, Peura DA: Running-associated proximal hemorrhagic colitis. Ann Intern Med 108:385–386, 1988.
14. Moses F: The effect of exercise on the gastrointestinal tract. Sports Med 9:159–172, 1990.
15. Priebe WM, Priebe JA: Runner's diarrhea—prevalence and clinical symptomatology. Am J Gastroenterol 79:827–828, 1984.
16. Rehrer NJ, Janssen GM, Brouns F, et al: Fluid intake and gastrointestinal problems in runners competing in a 25-km race and a marathon. Int J Sports Med 10(Suppl): 22–25, 1989.
17. Rehrer NJ, Beckers EJ, Brouns F, et al: Effects of dehydration on gastric emptying and gastrointestinal distress while running. Med Sci Sports Exerc 22:790–795, 1990.
18. Rehrer NJ, Meijer GA: Biomechanical vibration of the abdominal region during running and bicycling. J Sports Med Phys Fitness 31:231–234, 1991.
19. Riddoch C, Trinick T: Gastrointestinal disturbances in marathon runners. Br J Sports Med 22:71–74, 1988.
20. Stewart JG, Ahlquist DA, McGill DB, et al: Gastrointestinal blood loss and anemia in runners. Ann Intern Med 100:843–845, 1984.

21. Sullivan SN, Champion MC, Chrisofides ND, et al: Gastrointestinal regulatory peptide responses in long-distance runners. Physician Sportsmed 12:77–82, 1984.
22. Sullivan S: Gastrointestinal bleeding in distance runners. Sports Med 3:1–3, 1986.
23. Sullivan SN: Exercise-associated symptoms in triathletes. Physician Sportsmed 15:105–108, 1987.
24. Schwartz AE, Vanagunas A, Kamel PL: Endoscopy to evaluate gastrointestinal bleeding in marathon runners. Ann Intern Med 113:632–633, 1990.
25. Wilhite J, Mellion MB: Occult gastrointestinal bleeding in endurance cyclists. Physician Sportsmed 18:75–78, 1990.
26. Worobetz LJ, Gerrard DF: Gastrointestinal symptoms during exercise in enduro athletes: Prevalence and speculations on the etiology. NZ Med J 98:644–646, 1985.

INGUINAL HERNIAS IN ATHLETES

Both inguinal hernias and groin strains are common in athletes and may be difficult to differentiate. Moreover, the two conditions may coexist. Athletic programs now commonly utilize weight lifting in their training, and even junior high school athletes may routinely lift hundreds of pounds. Hernias are often seen in football and soccer players, and other athletes as well. These athletes may present with severe, insidious-onset groin pain and a normal musculoskeletal examination. A rehabilitation trial for suspected "groin pull" may have been unsuccessful.

It may be extremely difficult to detect hernias by physical examination.[1] In the male athlete with an inguinal hernia, examination may be normal or there may be only an increased impulse to palpation at the inguinal ring. In both male and female athletes there may not be appreciable bulge over the inguinal ligament with Valsalva maneuver. Often athletes with occult inguinal hernias have seen several physicians and are frustrated by a lack of adequate diagnosis and treatment.

Imaging

Herniography has been available since the early 1970s and remains the preferred diagnostic standard.[2] Nonionic radiopaque contrast medium is injected into the peritoneal cavity under fluoroscopy, and the patient is then examined radiographically on a tilt table. Valsalva maneuver causes dye to flow into the hernial sac.[3] The procedure has a low false-positive rate, and complications are rare.[2]

Herniography often demonstrates hernias undetected by physical examination. Smedberg et al. evaluated 78 athletes with groin pain, including 23 with bilateral symptoms. Only 8 of the 101 symptomatic sides demonstrated a palpable hernia on physical examination. Herniography revealed hernias in 85 of the 101 symptomatic sides and 27 of the 55 asymptomatic sides as well. In the study, 53 went on to surgery, including 10 who underwent bilateral herniorrhaphy. Operative findings correlated well with herniography. The surprising finding in this group was that 55% of the hernias in athletes under 30 were direct, in contrast to previous reports in the 4–10% range for this general age group. Surgical repair resolved symptoms in the majority of patients. Of the 19 groin sides that did not respond to surgery, later diagnoses revealed chronic tenoperiostitis of the adductor muscle group in 13, prostatitis in 2, hip joint arthritis in 1, and no clear diagnosis in the remaining 3.[1] Other investigators have found similar comorbidity rates in patients with groin pain and on that basis recommended a multidisciplinary approach in refractory cases.[4]

Herniography, CT scanning and ultrasound may be complementary in the evaluation of athletes with suspected inguinal hernia.[2] Ultrasonography and CT demonstrate the precise location and extent of the muscular defect, which helps in planning the type of surgical repair.[5] Ultrasonography is particularly well suited for patients with a history of contrast dye allergy. Herniography, on the other hand, is superior in diagnosing hernias that are slender and not filled with bowel.[2] Therefore, in patients in whom an inguinal hernia is suspected clinically but the physical examination is equivocal or negative, herniography is currently the preferred procedure for diagnosis.[2] Because ultrasound is noninvasive and less expensive, however, it is a reasonable test to consider first when an experienced ultrasonographer is available. Some authorities predict that as clinical experience grows, MRI will prove useful in the investigation of groin pain and inguinal hernia.[6]

Treatment

Once diagnosed, symptomatic hernias should be repaired. Many athletes, however, prefer to continue their competitive season and to delay repair. This may be more appropriate if the hernia is asymptomatic, in which case participation may be allowed with regular evaluation to detect any progression. If an athlete continues to play in spite of an asymptomatic or mildly symptomatic inguinal hernia, the discussion about willingness to assume the risks of potential hernia incarceration should be well documented.

Following traditional herniorrhaphy for indirect inguinal hernias, athletes are often kept out of contact sports for several weeks. Recently, laparoscopic hernia repair has dramatically shortened the recovery time for hernia repair; in properly selected cases, it may allow athletes to return to contact sports in as little as 10 days.[7]

In summary, inguinal hernia is a common cause of groin pain in athletes. Thorough history and physical examination form the diagnostic foundation. Herniography continues to be effective in diagnosing inguinal hernias in cases where the diagnosis is suspected but the physical examination is unremarkable. Ultrasound and CT are noninvasive techniques that may be extremely useful. They may also provide information about the anterior abdominal wall and femoral hernias. Surgical repair is effective treatment, and the advent of laparoscopic herniorrhaphy has shortened postoperative convalescence. In refractory cases, the comorbidity of other disorders may warrant further evaluation and treatment following herniorrhaphy.

REFERENCES

1. Smedberg SGG, Broome AEA, Gullmo A, Roos H: Herniography in athletes with groin pain. Am J Surg 149:378–382, 1985.
2. Van den Berg JC, Strijk SP: Groin hernia: role of herniography. Radiology 184:191–194, 1992.
3. Gulimo A, Broome A, Smedberg S: Herniography. Surg Clin North Am 64:229–244, 1984.
4. Ekberg O, Persson N, Abrahamsson P, et al: Longstanding groin pain in athletes. A multidisciplinary approach. Sports Med 6:56–61, 1988.
5. Yeh HC, Lehr-Janus C, Cohen B, Rabinowitz J: Ultrasonography and CT of abdominal and inguinal hernias. J Clin Ultrasound 12:479–486, 1984.
6. Taylor DC, Meyers WC, Moylan JA, et al: Abdominal musculature abnormalities as a cause of groin pain in athletes. Inguinal hernias and pubalgia. Am J Sports Med 19: 239–242, 1991.
7. Rich BSE, Hough DO, Monroe JS, Nogle S: Inguinal mass in a college football player: A case study. Med Sci Sports Exerc 25(3):318–320, 1993.

THORACIC OUTLET SYNDROME AND EFFORT THROMBOSIS

Thoracic outlet syndrome and its sequela, effort thrombosis, can occur in athletes in relation to the exertion of their sport, as a result of weight/training, or as a response to trauma. It is important to recognize these syndromes because both can impair or stop athletic performance, and because the latter can also result in long-term disability if not properly diagnosed and treated.

Thoracic Outlet Syndrome

The thoracic outlet is the space through which the subclavian artery and the brachial plexus pass en route to the axilla. Its bony boundaries are the clavicle, scapula, and first rib. The pectoralis minor, the scalenus anticus, and scalenus medius muscles further define this space. Typically, the neurovascular bundle passes between the scalenus anticus and medius. Numerous motions of the shoulder, particularly those involving depression of the shoulder or hyperabduction of the arm, will exert pressure on the neurovascular bundle. Anatomical variants, including a cervical rib, an abnormal first rib, or congenital hypertrophy of the scalenus muscles may cause severe pressure on the nerves and artery passing through the thoracic outlet. Additionally, exercise may induce scalenus anticus hypertrophy, which will result in the same problem. Thoracic outlet syndrome occurs when the compression is great enough to produce symptoms.

The patient generally experiences burning, numbness, and tingling in a variable distribution in the upper extremity. Pain in the upper extremity may imitate a variety of athletic overuse syndromes. Weakness and sensory deficits may occur. Adson's maneuver and the hyperflexion-abduction test may be positive. It is beyond the scope of this discussion to describe the variety of physical examination, laboratory, and radiographic procedures that may be used to diagnose thoracic outlet syndrome.

Thoracic outlet syndrome has been reported in relationship to swimming, throwing sports, rowing, and weight training.[3,8,23] It has also been documented in the left arm of concert string players.[19] Personal experience indicates that minor levels of thoracic outlet syndrome are not uncommon. While definitive treatment for these problems is surgical, a trial of physical therapy is generally warranted first.[4,12,13,20,22]

Effort Thrombosis

Effort thrombosis is a common variant of the thoracic outlet syndrome in which the subclavian or axillary vein becomes acutely thrombosed. It is also called Paget-Schroetter syndrome after the authors who wrote two descriptions over 100 years ago. Generally, the venous injury is the result of activity combined with anomalous external compression of the vein between a hypertrophied scalene or subclavius tendon and the first rib.[15,17,21] Although effort thrombosis was initially thought to be a spontaneous problem, an underlying chronic venous compressive anomaly has been identified in recent years.[15] It typically occurs in physically active males between the ages of 15 and 40 and physically active females between the ages of 20 and 50. The right (dominant) arm is much more commonly involved than the left. Onset is generally abrupt and may follow either a bout of heavy exercise or trauma within 24 hours.

The pathophysiology is multifactorial and follows Virchow's well-known thrombosis triad: stasis, vessel wall damage, and hypercoagulability.[21]

Stasis is caused by chronic compression and stricture of the axillary-subclavian vein by a hypertrophied scalene or subclavius tendon and the first rib.[15,21] Additional evidence for neurovascular compression at the thoracic outlet comes from documentation of positive clinical tests for arterial compression in 27 (82%) of a series of 33 patients with effort thrombosis.[15] The thrombosis is generally the result of an intimal tear of the axillary vein caused by forceful hyperabduction and external rotation of the shoulder, stretching the axillary vein.[2,21] It has been postulated that during a sudden effort with simultaneous tightening of the subclavius tendon and the anterior scalene muscle, the vein gets pinched between these structures, causing the intimal tear.[18] A local hypercoaguability has been implicated as the result of the stress of exercise.[21] Oral contraceptives,[2,17] and dehydration in athletes such as wrestlers trying to "make weight,"[17] have also been implicated.

Effort thrombosis has been most commonly reported in baseball, gymnastics, tennis, and weightlifting, all sports in which the arm is forcefully loaded in a hyperabducted, externally rotated position.[2]

The syndrome initially presents as pain and swelling of the involved extremity. A prominent pattern of venous distension and dilated superficial collateral veins develops over the upper arm, shoulder, neck and thorax. The extremity may take on a blue or a mottled violaceous discoloration. Both the venous pattern and the discoloration are more prominent when the individual attempts to exercise the extremity. A tender "cord" is often palpable along the course of the axillary vein. Accompanying neurologic and arterial insufficiency symptoms related to thoracic outlet syndrome have been reported as well. The diagnosis is clinical, but confirmation is made by venogram.[1,2,6,7,15–17,21,25] Color Doppler ultrasonography has been used increasingly to identify effort thrombosis.[11,14] It is not quite as accurate as venography,[11] but it may have a significant role in the follow-up evaluation.[11,14]

The traditional treatment of effort thrombosis, rest, and anticoagulation resulted in 68% to 75% chronic problems, consisting of residual pain, swelling, and weakness.[1,5,6,7,25] In many patients, the residual symptoms are caused by persistent occlusion of the subclavian and axillary veins, where recanalization has not taken place.[7] Many cases of reocclusion have also been noted.[10,18,24] Consequently, several surgical authorities have advocated early thrombectomy and repair of the anatomic cause of the venous compression.[1,7,18,24] Others have shown some success in correcting the etiologic anatomic problem later on in those patients with persistent disability.[5,9,15] With the advent of fibrinolytic therapy for the lysis of intravascular clots, early diagnosis of effort thrombosis is even more important. Using this technique, the thrombus may be lysed percutaneously. Because of the high rate of recurrence and sequelae of effort thrombosis, definitive treatment of the underlying thoracic outlet syndrome should then be seriously considered.[10,15,18,24,25]

REFERENCES

1. Adams JT, De Weese JA: "Effort" thrombosis of the axillary and subclavian veins. J Trauma 11:923–930, 1971.
2. Aquino BC, Barone EJ: "Effort" thrombosis of the axillary and subclavian vein associated with cervical rib and oral contraceptives in a young woman athlete. J Am Board Fam Pract 2:208–211, 1989.
3. Baker CL, Liu SH: Neurovascular injuries to the shoulder. J Orthop Sports Phys Ther 18:360–364, 1993.
4. Britt LP: Nonoperative treatment of the thoracic outlet syndrome symptoms. Clin Orthop 51:45–48, 1967.
5. Campbell CB, Chandler JG, Tegtmeyer CJ, Bernstein EF: Axillary, subclavian, and brachiocephalic vein obstruction. Surgery 82:816–826, 1977.
6. Crowell DL: Effort thrombosis of the subclavian and axillary veins: Review of the literature and case report with two-year follow-up with venography. Ann Intern Med 52:1337–1343, 1960.
7. Drapanas T, Curran WL: Thrombectomy in the treatment of "effort" thrombosis of the axillary and subclavian veins. J Trauma 6:107–119, 1966.
8. Frankel SA, Hirata I: The scalenus anticus syndrome and competitive swimming: Report of two cases. JAMA 215: 1796–1798, 1971.
9. Glass BA: Their relationship of axillary venous thrombosis to the thoracic outlet compression syndrome. Ann Thorac Surg 19:613–621, 1975.
10. Grassi CJ, Bettmann MA: Effort thrombosis: Role of interventional therapy. Cardiovasc Intervent Radiol 13:317–322, 1990.
11. Grassi CJ, Polak JF: Axillary and subclavian venous thrombosis: Follow-up evaluation with color doppler flow US and venography. Radiology 175:651–654, 1990.
12. Karas SE: Thoracic outlet syndrome. Clin Sports Med 9: 297–310, 1990.
13. Kenny RA, Traynor GB, Withington D, Keegan DJ: Thoracic outlet syndrome: A useful exercise treatment option. Am J Surg 165:282–284, 1993.
14. Longley DG, Finlay DE, Letourneau JG: Sonography of the upper extremity and jugular veins. Am J Radiol 160:957–962, 1993.
15. Machleder HI: Effort thrombosis of the axillosubclavian vein: A disabling vascular disorder. Compr Ther 17:18–24, 1991.
16. Matas R: Primary thrombosis of the axillary vein caused by strain: report of a case with comments on diagnosis, pathology, and treatment of this lesion in its medico-legal relations. Am J Surg 24:642–666, 1934.
17. Medler RG, McQueen DA: Effort thrombosis in a young wrestler. J Bone Joint Surg 75-A:1071–1073, 1993.
18. Molina JE: Surgery for effort thrombosis of the subclavian vein. J Thorac Cardiovasc Surg 103:341–6, 1992.
19. Roos DB: Thoracic outlet syndromes: Symptoms, diagnosis, anatomy and surgical treatment. Med Probl Perform Art 1:90–93, 1986.

20. Roy S, Irvin R: Sports medicine: Prevention, Evaluation, Management, and Rehabilitation. Englewood Cliffs, NJ, Prentice-Hall, 1983, pp 189–191.
21. Skerker RS, Flandry FC: Case presentation: Painless arm swelling in a high school football player. Med Sci Sports Exerc 24(11):1185–1189, 1992.
22. Smith KF: The thoracic outlet syndrome: A protocol for treatment. J Orthop Sports Phys Ther 1:89–99, 1979.
23. Strukel RJ, Garrick JG: Thoracic outlet compression in athletes: A report of four cases. Am J Sports Med 6:35–39, 1978.
24. Thompson RW, Schneider PA, Nelken NA, et al. Circumferential venolysis and paraclavicular thoracic outlet decompression for "effort thrombosis" of the subclavian vein. J Vasc Surg 16:723–32, 1992.
25. Vogel CM, Jensen JE: "Effort" thrombosis of the subclavian vein in a competitive swimmer. Am J Sports Med 13:269–272, 1985.

EXERCISE-INDUCED HEADACHES

Few data indicate that athletes are more or less prone to having headaches than nonathletes. There are, however, headache syndromes brought on by exercise that may be perplexing to physicians diagnostically as well as frightening to patients. Most of these headache syndromes are benign, but it is often difficult to sort them out from more severe underlying organic problems. In a landmark study, Rooke followed 103 patients diagnosed as having "benign exertional headache" for 3 or more years after the diagnosis was made. In 10 of these patients, significant intracranial lesions were found, including three Arnold-Chiari deformities, two cases of platybasia, one basilar impression, one chronic and one acute subdural hematoma, and two brain tumors. Of the patients, 16 had hypertension (150/100 or greater), but their elevated blood pressure elevation was not considered to be the cause of their headaches.[28] Exercise-induced headaches may also be a manifestation of ischemic heart disease.[33]

Patients presenting with headaches induced by exercise or exertion require a careful history and physical examination and consideration for appropriate imaging and laboratory evaluation as well as neurology or cardiology consultation. CT or MRI of both the head and neck may be necessary to rule out basilar skull malformations.

Benign Exertional Headache

Benign exertional headache is a brief, generally bilateral, and throbbing headache precipitated by sports and other activities that involve a sudden, marked expenditure of energy.[5,13] It usually lasts about 5 minutes, but it may be followed by a dull posterior or suboccipital headache, which lasts for a day.[5] Some reports describe headaches of several hours' duration without indicating whether such headaches follow this pattern.[7] Benign exertional headache is not associated with other neurologic signs or symptoms or with any systemic disorder.[5,13] Lifetime prevalence in an epidemiologic survey of 1,000 adults aged 25 to 64 was 1%.[27]

Headache location is variable but is more often occipital than frontal. The headache pattern for each patient, however, is generally consistent. Increased physical effort or head movement may intensify the headache. Vomiting is uncharacteristic and may suggest an underlying organic pathology.[29]

The causes of benign exertional headache are unclear, but exertion that involves a Valsalva maneuver appears to be the common characteristic of triggering activities.[10,29,31] The resulting intrathoracic pressure is transmitted to the venous sinuses,[10,29,31] but the actual headache initiating mechanism is not well defined.[29] A single case study has demonstrated segmental cerebral artery vasoconstriction, but the potential role of vasospasm in benign exertional headache has not been well studied.[31]

These headaches are associated with a variety of sports, but weightlifting[5] and swimming[14,18,23] are particularly common. Patients with benign exertional headaches may also have headaches associated with other maneuvers, which involve increased intrathoracic pressure, such as coughing, sneezing, bending, defecating, and attaining sexual orgasm.[1,3,9,17,18,23,29,30,31]

Indomethacin has been the most effective treatment and prophylaxis for this problem.[7,9] A broader range of NSAIDs, including naproxen, ketoprofen, fenoprofen, calcium, and salsalate, are also effective.[7]

Acute-Effort Migraine

Acute-effort migraine is a unilateral throbbing retro-orbital headache that occurs a few minutes after extremely intense exercise. It is generally preceded by an aura consisting of scintillating scotomata and occasional lateral visual field cuts. It is usually accompanied by nausea and frequently by vomiting and photophobia. Hemiplegic variants are common. The duration is generally a few minutes to an hour, but many of these syndromes will persist for several hours. These headaches are less common in highly conditioned athletes, but many of them were seen in internationally competitive athletes at the Mexico City Olympics, held at an altitude of 7,800 feet.[1,3,21] Treatment is generally not necessary, but standard therapies for classical migraine have been tried in cases of more prolonged or frequent headaches. Prevention techniques include increasing the athlete's conditioning level and avoiding intense exercise when poorly acclimated at high altitude. One detailed case report demonstrates that a long, gradual warmup in a highly competitive swimmer prevented her headaches.[19]

Vascular Headaches with Prolonged Exercise

A third common syndrome is a vascular headache that comes on more gradually after prolonged low-intensity exercise, such as running or swimming. It is characterized by intense throbbing pain, either unilateral or bilateral, and variable in location. It is generally not preceded by a scotoma nor focal neurological signs. Accompanying nausea is common, but vomiting is rare. This type of headache may last from one to many hours. It is commonly seen in the poorly conditioned athlete, and it is often associated with exercise in the heat, dehydration, hypoglycemia, exercise by the poorly acclimated athlete at high altitude, and antecedent alcohol consumption. Treatment consists of analgesics, especially the NSAIDs, and treatment of associated conditions. Preventive measures include increasing the level of conditioning and avoiding the associated situations that make the athlete susceptible.[1,3]

Migraine Precipitated by Minor Head Trauma

A migraine syndrome known as "footballer's migraine" occurs a few minutes after minor head trauma, following which the athlete remains conscious. It is a unilateral, throbbing, retro-orbital headache, preceded or accompanied by scintillating scotomata and other visual disturbances. Paresthesias and hemiplegic symptoms are common, as are nausea, vomiting, and photophobia. These headaches may last from a few hours to 2 days.[2,3,5,6,11,12,16,22] The athlete may have a personal or family history of migraine.[5] This problem may be recurrent. Because it may be difficult to distinguish the first episode from severe neurologic damage, CT or MRI and observation are warranted initially.[5] These headaches should not be confused with the migraine syndrome, which develops following more severe trauma and which appears weeks to months after blunt head trauma.[4] Migraine precipitated by minor head trauma may be managed with standard treatments for classical or hemiplegic migraine. There are not enough data available about whether various forms of migraine prophylaxis will work for athletes with these headaches. This problem has caused some serious athletes to give up participation.[8]

Weightlifter's Headache

There is a syndrome of headache in weightlifters and other people doing resistance forms of exercise which differs from benign exertional headache. It comes on suddenly while straining to lift. The headache is typically occipital and upper cervical but may extend to the parietal areas. It is a severe, steady, burning or "boring" headache. It lasts for days to many weeks and subsides gradually. The etiology is unclear, but it is possibly a form of cervical ligament strain. The treatment is rest; although there is no mention of physical therapy in the literature, it seems appropriate to start the athlete on a neck rehabilitation program. This type of headache may be recurrent and may necessitate stopping lifting altogether or stopping the specific exercise that exacerbates it.[24,25]

Exertional Headache in Pheochromocytoma

Episodic headache is a symptom of pheochromocytoma that may be brought on by exertion. The characteristic headache is bilateral, throbbing, and often indistinguishable from classic migraine. It is commonly accompanied by nausea and vomiting. Duration is variable, from a few minutes to rather prolonged. Diagnosis is aided by the fact that these patients are frequently hypertensive without their headache. Their blood pressure during the headache is dramatically elevated, with a series of case reports demonstrating pressure 200-300/120-210.[20] There has been a case report, however, of a patient with exercise-induced headaches caused by a pheochromocytoma without recorded blood pressure elevation.[32] These headaches should be managed by treating the underlying pheochromocytoma.[20]

External Compression Headaches

Athletes can experience headaches due to the constrictions from tight headbands, helmets, and goggles.[5,8,15,26] Typically, the pain is localized to the area under pressure, and it may be relieved by eliminating the pressure.[5,8,26] The etiology has been attributed to local nerve compression,[8,15] and prolonged compression in some athletes has triggered classic migraine headaches.[5,26]

Summary

The exercise-induced headache syndromes are summarized in Table 5. Guides to the evaluation and management of the individual syndromes have been presented, but a repeat word of caution is necessary. Although the incidence of severe underlying organic disease is likely to be less than the 10% in Rooke's study, exercise-induced headaches can mask underlying pathology. They should not be treated as trivial and benign, until they are carefully evaluated and potentially severe organic etiologies have been ruled out.

TABLE 5. Exercise-induced Headaches

Type of Headache	Onset	Symptoms	Duration	Other Characteristics	Prevention	Treatment
Acute effort migraine	Few minutes after extremely intense exercise	Scintillating scotomata Unilateral throbbing retro-orbital headache Nausea and vomiting	Generally few minutes to an hour Occasionally several hours	Less common in highly conditioned athletes	Increase conditioning level Long gradual warm-up Avoid intense exercise when poorly acclimated	Generally not necessary If headache prolonged, treat as classic migraine
Vascular headache with prolonged exercise	After prolonged low-intensity exertion	More gradual onset after exercise Intense throbbing pain Variable location Unilateral or bilateral No scotoma or focal neurologic signs Nausea	One to many hours	Common in poorly conditioned athletes Often associated with dehydration, exercise in heat, hypoglycemia, exercise at high altitude, and alcohol consumption	Increase conditioning level Avoid dehydration, excessive heat loss, hypoglycemia, alcohol, exercise at high altitude when poorly acclimated	Analgesics, especially NSAIDs Treat associated conditions
Benign exertional headache	Precipitated by any level of physical activity however brief or mild	Generally a throbbing headache, but not clearly a vascular pattern Variable location but generally consistent for each patient Increased effort or neck movement may intensify headache	Few minutes to many hours	May have headaches associated with other maneuvers that cause increased intrathoracic pressure	Prophylactic indomethacin or other NSAIDs	Indomethacin and other NSAIDs acutely

Migraine precipitated by minor head trauma ("footballer's migraine)	Few minutes after minor head trauma without unconsciousness	Scintillating scotomata and other visual disturbances Paresthesias & hemiplegic symptoms common Unilateral throbbing retro-orbital headache Photophobia Nausea and vomiting	Few hours to 2 days	Not to be confused with migraine which develops following severe head trauma and which appears weeks to months after trauma	Not enough data available for prophylaxis	Treat as classic or hemiplegic migraine
Weightlifter's headache	Sudden onset while straining to lift weights	Occipital, upper cervical Steady, severe Burning or "boring"	Days to weeks Subsides gradually	Possibly a form of cervical ligament strain	May require stopping lifting	Rest Possible benefit from physical therapy (?)
Exertional headache in pheochromocytoma	Spontaneous or exertion-related	Bilateral throbbing headache often indistinguishable from classic migraine Nausea and vomiting	Variable	Frequent baseline hypertension Blood pressure during headache frequently 200–300/120–210		Treat underlying pheochromocytoma
Exertional compression headache	Variable	Pain under compressed area	Generally abates shortly after relieving pressure	Typically caused by tight headband, helmet or goggles. May trigger classic migraine.	Loosen headband or goggles Refit helmet	Remove offending equipment
Exertional headache related to organic head and neck lesions	Within a few minutes of exertion	Variable	Generally brief—seconds to minutes	Underlying lesions: Arnold-Chiari deformity, platybasia, basilar impression, subdural hematoma, brain tumor		Treat organic lesion

REFERENCES

1. Appenzeller O: Cerebrovascular aspects of headache. Med Clin North Am 62:467–480, 1978.
2. Ashworth B: Migraine, head trauma and sport. Scott Med J 30:240–242, 1985.
3. Atkinson R, Appenzeller O: Headaches in sports. Semin Neurol 1:334–344, 1981.
4. Behrman S: Migraine as a sequelae of blunt head trauma. Injury 9:74–76, 1974.
5. Bennett DR. The athlete with headache. In Mellion MB, Walsh WM, Shelton GL (eds): The Team Physician's handbook. Philadelphia, Hanley & Belfus, 1990, pp 218–225.
6. Bennett DR, Fuenning SI, Sullivan G, Weber J: Migraine precipitated by head trauma in athletes. Am J Sports Med 8:202–205, 1980.
7. Diamond S: Exercise and headaches: When pain hinders athletic gain. Physician Sportsmed 19(8):79–94, 1991.
8. Diamond S: Treating athletes who have posttraumatic headaches. Physician Sportsmed 20(9):167–179, 1992.
9. Diamond S, Medina JL: Prolonged benign exertional headache: Clinical characteristics and response to indomethacin. Adv Neurol 33:145–149, 1982.
10. Dimeff RJ: Headaches in the athlete. Clin Sports Med 11: 339–349, 1992.
11. Espir MLE, Hodge ILD, Matthews PHN: Footballer's migraine. BMJ 2:352, 1972.
12. Haas DC, Pineda GS, Lourie H: Juvenile head trauma syndromes and their relationship to migraine. Arch Neurol 32:727–730, 1975.
13. Headache classification. Committee of the International Headache Society: Classification and criteria for headache disorders, cranial neuralgias, and facial pain. Cephalalgia 8(Suppl 7):12–73, 1988.
14. Indo T, Takahashi A: Swimmer's migraine. Headache 30: 485–487, 1990.
15. Jacobson RI: More "goggle headache": Supraorbital neuralgia. N Engl J Med 308:1363, 1983.
16. Kalenak A, Petro DJ, Brennan RW: Migraine secondary to head trauma in wrestling. Am J Sports Med 6:112–113, 1978.
17. Katchen MS: Exertional headaches with multiple triggers. Aviat Space Environ Med 61:49–51, 1990.
18. Kim JS: Swimming headache followed by exertional and coital headaches. J Korean Med Sci 7:276–279, 1992.
19. Lambert RW, Burnett DL: Prevention of exercise induced migraine by quantitative warm-up. Headache 25:317–319, 1985.
20. Lance JW, Hinterberger H: Symptoms of pheochromocytoma, with particular reference to headache, correlated with catecholamine production. Arch Neurol 33:281–288, 1976.
21. Massey EW: Effort headache in runners. Headache 22:99–100, 1982.
22. Matthews WB: Footballer's migraine. BMJ 2:326–327, 1972.
23. Mizoguchi K, Utsunomiya H, Emoto H, Shimizu T: Benign exertional headaches induced by swimming. Kurume Med J 37:261–263, 1990.
24. Paulson GW: Weightlifter's headache. Headache 23:193–194, 1983.
25. Perry WJ: Exertional headache. Physician Sportsmed 13(10): 95–99, 1985.
26. Pestronk A, Pestronk S: Goggle migraine. N Engl J Med 308:226–227, 1983.
27. Rasmussen BK, Olesen J: Symptomatic and nonsymptomatic headaches in a general population. Neurology 42: 1225–1231, 1992.
28. Rooke ED: Benign exertional headache. Med Clin North Am 52:801–808, 1968.
29. Sands GH, Newman L, Lipton R: Cough, exertional, and other miscellaneous headaches. Med Clin North Am 75: 733–747, 1991.
30. Silbert PL, Edis RH, Stewart-Wynne EG, Gubbay SS: Benign vascular sexual headache and exertional headache: interrelationships and long term prognosis. J Neurol Neurosurg Psychiatr 54:417–421, 1991.
31. Silbert PL, Hankey GJ, Prentice DA, Apsimon HT: Angiographically demonstrated arterial spasm in a case of benign sexual headache and benign exertional headache. Aust NZ J Med 19:466–468, 1989.
32. Swanson RW, Haight KR, Wilson TW, Sher N: Pheochromocytoma: An unusual presentation and sequela. Can J Cardiol 8:47–49, 1992.
33. Vernay D, Deffond D, Fraysse P, Dordain G: Walk headache: An unusual manifestation of ischemic heart disease. Headache 29:350–351, 1989.

16

Common Skin Problems in Athletes

Loren H. Amundson, M.D.
Gene F. Burrish, M.D.

Skin problems are common in athletes and impact upon participation and performance. Given their frequency, it is important that the physician caring for athletes possess skill in diagnosis and treatment of those problems. Important also is an understanding of the many functions the skin performs, including protection against abrasion and mechanical injury, regulation of body temperature within close limits, keeping out chemicals and pathogens while protecting the body's fluid content, and filtering out harmful ultraviolet radiation.[6] It is also necessary that the physician understand skin structure, so as to know how the above tasks are accomplished, and readers are referred for review to one of several excellent dermatologic texts (see list of recommended texts following references).

The physician should likewise be aware of the many environmental factors that affect the skin and in addition the damage that can be caused by inappropriate care. The importance of skin care should be stressed in health classes.[1] Daily skin care should include fresh, clean underclothing and socks, as well as clean clothing and equipment for practice and competition. Equipment is involved in many sports-related skin problems, as the skin is invariably exposed to trauma during athletic training and competition.[9] Preventive techniques are often not adhered to by athletes, especially student-athletes.

Effective management of skin problems in athletes, as with problems of other body systems, follows accurate diagnosis. A trained eye is an important factor in dermatologic diagnosis. Inquiry into the type of sport and level of involvement by the patient is necessary to develop a framework for diagnosis; examples include spatial relationships between a skin eruption and the sport activity, environmental factors such as sunlight, utilization of self-care medication or other therapy; there are also other aggravating factors.

To be an effective dermatotherapist for the athlete, one must understand the principles of skin care, be familiar with the pharmacology of topical and systemic agents, and be acquainted with various physical modes of therapy such as cryotherapy. Glucocorticoids represent the most commonly used topical agents, and it is incumbent upon the sports physician to understand fully the indications and complications of corticosteroid therapy when used topically, intralesionally, or parenterally.[27]

Athletes with bacterial skin infections, viral lesions of herpes simplex and molluscum contagiosum, and infestations should be temporarily disqualified from competition.[12]

INJURY TO THE SKIN

Sun Damage. Sunlight produces both short-term reactions and more serious long-term damage. The athlete and the sports physician both are usually familiar with short-term conditions, including sunburn and miliaria (sweat gland occlusion). However, the long-term effects of sunlight, including solar elastosis, actinic keratoses, and skin cancer, are usually far from the mind of the competitive athlete; the sports physician must be able to counsel the student-athlete on the need to prevent prolonged sun damage to the skin.

Sunburn, which is mainly midrange ultraviolet light (UVB), is usually not a diagnostic problem, nor is the therapy difficult, although it sometimes interferes with competition. First- and second-degree sunburn responds well to analgesics and cool compresses, whereas systematic corticosteroids can be used to combat acute distress of burns that are more extensive. Aspirin taken 1–2 hours prior to sun exposure may reduce sunburn significantly.[9] Taken in high doses for 24 hours, and started immediately after a significant sun exposure, it may reduce the severity of the burn and provide adequate analgesia.[27] Tanning booths that give mainly long-wave ultraviolet light (UVA) are currently popular, and athletes frequently use them to prevent or control the amount of sunburn obtained through sports participation. However, UVA-tanned skin offers little protection against a UVB burn. Also, the long-range effects of UVA are suspected to cause skin damage, and the use of tanning booths can only be decried.

Protective sun agents provide an appropriate preventive option for the athlete. Most sunscreens are labeled for their ability by way of sun protective factors (SPFs) to block the burning UVB rays of the sun. Some UVA rays are also blocked by these products; however, two new specially designed preparations appear to offer extended coverage in the UVA range: Filteray and Photoplex. These newer sunscreens appear to be better (i.e., they retain SPF value) than the older physical blocking agents such as zinc oxide and titanium dioxide. Sunscreens, especially those with an SPF of 15 and above, are effective but must be applied before exposure to the sun and reapplied every few hours after heavy sweating or swimming[21] (Table 1). Oily sunscreens may cause folliculitis.[13] Suntan lotions contain oils that change the optical properties of the skin to speed up the sun's tanning of the skin, and some contain chemicals that stain the stratum corneum to produce an artificial tan that lasts a few days, but these lotions offer little or no protection against sunburn.[4]

Excessive sun exposure frequently leads to a herpes labialis flare-up, necessitating 10–14 days for complete resolution.Similarly distressing for the active athlete are a variety of photosensitive and photoallergic reactions, especially in athletes taking a variety of systemic medications (Table 2). "Sun poisoning" may also occur, especially in those with type 1 and type 2 skin (light complexion, blue eyes, blond or red hair). If the exposure is ex-

TABLE 1. Sunscreens*

PABA sunscreens	Non-PABA sunscreens+
PreSun 15	Bain de Soleil Sport
Sunbrella	Bull Frog Gel
	Piz Buin 15
PABA ester sunscreens	PreSun Active 30
PABAFILM	TiScreen 15 (30)
Sundown	
Sea and Ski	Physical sunscreens
	A-fil
PABA-ester combination sunscreens	Clinique
Bain de Soleil	Covermark
Coppertone Supershade 15	Shadow
Clinique 19	
Estee Lauder 15	
Sundown 15 (sunblock)	

PABA = paraaminobenzoic acid

*Modified from Fitzpatrick TB, Eisen AZ, Wolff A et al (eds): Dermatology in General Medicine, 3rd ed. New York, McGraw-Hill, 1987, pp 1516–1517.

+These sunscreens are PABA free and are formulated to resist sweating and water.

TABLE 2. Photosensitive/Photoallergic Substances and Conditions*

TOPICAL	SYSTEMIC
Acne medications	Antifungals
Vitamin A acid (Retin-A®)	Griseofulvin (Grisactin®)
Isotretinoin (Accutane®)	
	Antihistamines
Coal tar derivatives	Diphenhydramine (Benadryl®)
Acridine	
Anthracene	
Phenanthrene	Diseases
Pyridine	Lupus erythematosus
	Polymorphous light eruptions
Cosmetics	
Indelible lipsticks	Porphyria(s)
Perfumes and aftershave lotions having essential oils	
	Food additives
	Saccharin
	Cyclamates
Plants	
Celery	Furocoumarins
Lemon	Methoxsalen
Lime	(Oxsoralen®)
Soap deodorants	Miscellaneous
(photoallergic)	Birth control agents
Halogenated salicylanilides (tri- and tetrachlor-; brominated)	Chlordiazepoxide HCl (Librium®)
	Furosemide (Lasix®)
Bithionol	
Hexachlorophene	Sulfa drugs and analogues
Dichlorophene	Sulfonamides
Carbanilides	Hypoglycemics
	Sulfonylurea (Dymelor®)
Sunscreens	Tolbutamide
Paraaminobenzoic acid (PABA)	(Orinase®)
Digalloyl trioleate	Chlorpropamide
(Sunstick®)	(Diabinese®)
	Diuretics
	Thiazides (HydroDIURIL®)
	Phenothiazines
	Chlorpromazine (Thorazine®)
	Promethazine (Phenergan®)
	Prochlorperazine (Compazine®)
	Other antibiotics
	Tetracycline
	Doxycycline (Vibramycin®)
	Nalidixic acid (NegGram®)

*Modified from Mellion MD (ed): Office Management of Sports Injuries & Athletic Problems. Philadelphia, Hanley & Belfus, 1988.

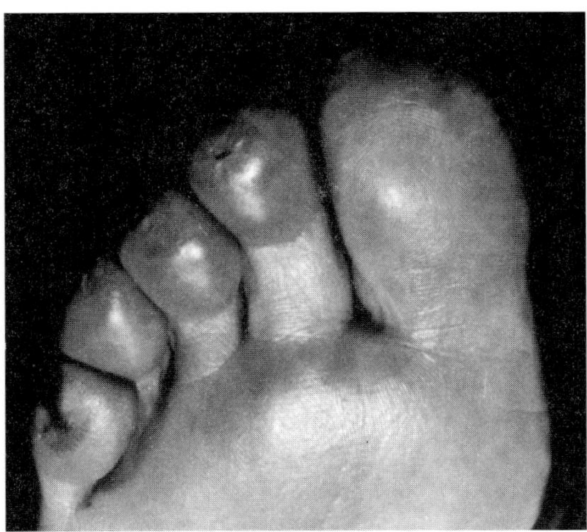

FIGURE 1. Chilblains

treme, the patient may present with a toxic clinical picture characterized by fever, chills, nausea, and prostration, necessitating aggressive supportive care including intravenous fluids.[9] Those with sensitive skin should wear a sunscreen whenever significant sun exposure is anticipated—a lifetime preventive activity.

Hypothermia. The skin is likewise susceptible to the effects of cold. Chilblains (Fig. 1) and frostbite, heralded by discomfort and altered sensation in the affected area (the former causing pruritus, dermatitis, and shallow skin ulcerations; the latter leading to numb, white patches, especially of the nose, earlobes, digits, and male genitalia) are more common in the distance runner, although any sport with skin exposure to a cold environment (e.g., cross-country skiing, winter hiking, ice-skating) may be causal.[22] Therapy includes rapid rewarming and protection from trauma; further damage may be prevented by generous use of friction-reducing emollients. Some resultant numbness and superficial erythema, even blistering, may be noted for a few days. Localized skin damage from inappropriate therapy with dry ice and liquid nitrogen does occur, whereas ice massage only rarely causes frostbite.[28]

Localized Conditions

Abrasions. Abrasions probably constitute the most common dermatologic lesion seen in athletes. A variety of terms apply: turf burn, mat burn, cinder burn, road rash, raspberry, and others. Whatever the cause or location, therapeutic measures must be followed by preventive techniques. Therapy can include initial cleansing with water or hydrogen peroxide, then the application of an antibiotic ointment and dry gauze. Another, more recent approach uses DuoDERM, an occlusive hydrophilic dressing that provides an optimal healing environment for the epithelium, which spreads both from the margins of the abrasion and from the remaining central islands of epithelium in the skin.[29]

Dressings are designed to prevent infection, protect the wound, and reduce pain. After the wound has been washed with soap and water, a DuoDERM dressing is applied to the wound and surrounding area with an overlapping margin of at least 3/4 inch (Fig. 2). As there is usually an accumulation of the tissue fluid that wells up under the dressing initially, it is recommended that the dressing be changed at 24 hours and again if fluid re-collects and extends to within 1/4 inch of the edge of the dressing. At this time, the fluid often has a slightly foul smell, which does *not* indicate infection. If removed, the wound and any dressing materials adhering to it are lavaged gently with water, and another piece of DuoDERM is reapplied. It is left in place until healing is complete: for most abrasions, a week or less. One of the advantages of DuoDERM is that once the dressing is in place there is little or no pain. This process seems to work for all abrasions except the very deepest, which are essentially third-degree burns, in which case initial treatment with Silvadene is indicated.

Other occlusive dressings include Tegaderm, OP-Site, and Bioclusive, which are polyethylene membranes. They are less effective for large abrasions because they lose their adhesive quality when damp and are less absorbent. DuoDerm has a wet-tack property, which provides adherence to wet as well as dry skin. All occlusive dressings must be used with caution in diabetic patients because of the ever-present threat of infection.

Chafing. Intertrigo results from mechanical irritation, regardless of location, and is aggravated by sweating and protective equipment (pads, cups, etc.).[34] Chafing is frequent in runners and bikers, and the nipples, axillae, and groin bear the brunt of insult, even to the point of bleeding. Prevention includes cleanliness, loose clothing, talc or Zeosorb to keep the area dry, and/or lubricating creams such as Cramer's Skin Lube and Eucerin. For females, a sports bra may be indicated. Therapy includes air, cool compresses, heat lamps, and mild corticosteroid creams. Patients should be monitored for secondary infection.

Blisters. Intraepidermal blisters abound in athletes who wear shoes and are also seen in other body areas where friction occurs. Frictional forces are greater if the skin is moist; less if the skin is dry, greasy, or very wet. Some may be prevented by hardening the skin with 10% tannic acid soaks.[12] Other preventive measures include proper shoes and high-bulk acrylic socks, polypropylene liners in shoes, application of Vaseline to skin or sites of

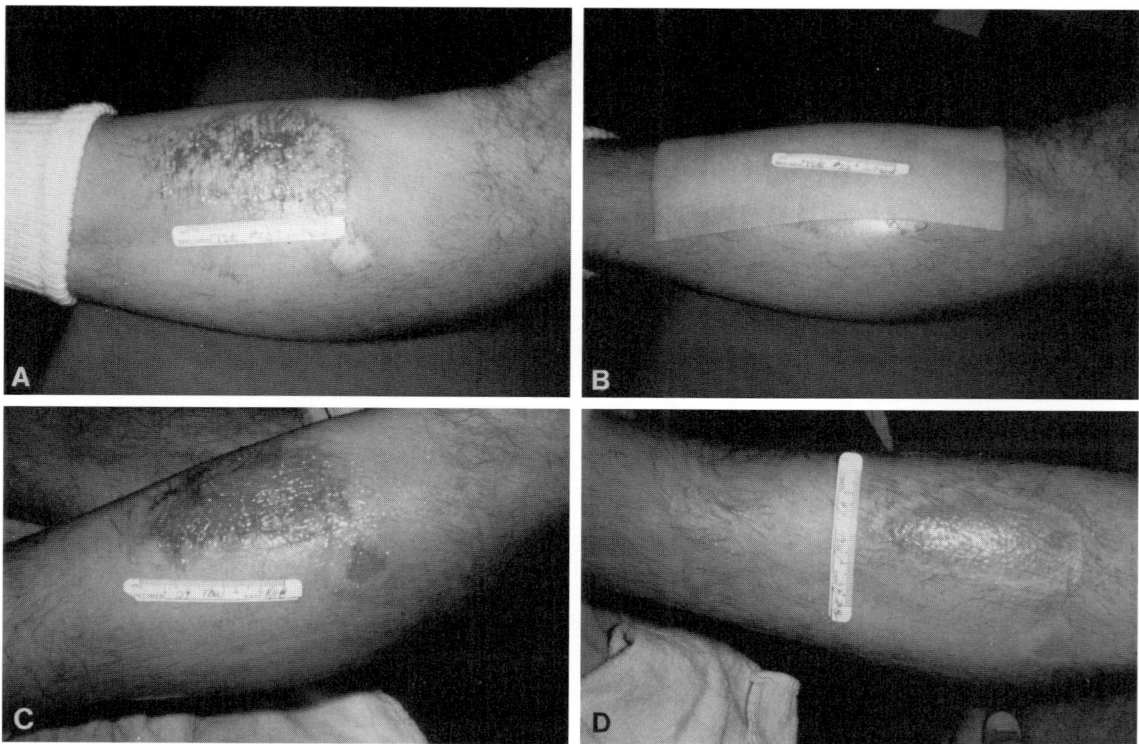

FIGURE 2. *A,* Turf burn, calf, 4.5 by 7.5 cm, day of injury. *B,* DuoDERM dressing applied. *C,* Turf burn, calf, 2 days post-injury; reepithialization under way. *D,* Turf burn, calf, 5 days post-injury; wound clean, dry, and well-healed.

friction in the shoes, talc to reduce moisture, and adhesive tape or moleskin over potential or previous blister sites.

Once a blister has formed, there are management options: Some advocate needle aspiration and adhesive taping, using the epidermal layers as an occlusive dressing.[12] Others prefer to remove the blistered layers of skin and expose the base, believing that this prevents repeat blisters during healing and makes the lesion easier to keep clean and noninfected. Following removal of the blister roof, a tape adherent such as Tuf-Skin is sprayed on, causing some initial discomfort due to its alcohol content. Following that application, a circular or oval piece of moleskin large enough to cover the blister and a 3/4-inch border is applied and left in place until healing is complete. Most failures occur from initial neglect of the lesion, then allowing infection to dictate care.

In patients with recurrent blisters, mild forms of epidermolysis bullosa should be considered.

Calluses and Corns. These lesions, most common on the feet, represent physiological responses to friction or pressure that the skin was not designed to sustain. They are not confined exclusively to the feet, gymnasts and golfers suffering their share of calluses on the hands, and bicyclists occasionally over the ischial rami. Effective therapy depends on the modification of causative factors, such as changing hand grips or a cycle seat, adjustment of footwear, or use of metatarsal inserts. If additional or ongoing therapy is warranted, it is best provided by intermittent paring and trimming, sanding with a pumice stone, and, occasionally, the use of salicylic acid plasters. Plantar corns (clavi) can also be treated with liquid nitrogen.[32] Such physical or chemical debridement can keep the patient comfortable while removing excessive keratinous accumulation. The less surgical the eradication, the better.

Hemorrhage. Several types of soft tissue hemorrhage are seen in the athlete. Subcutaneous ecchymoses occur frequently in the tips of the great and second toes—most often seen in tennis and basketball players and caused by frequent fast starts and stops, in addition to more chronic trauma from long-distance running. Likewise, black heel (talon noir) may be seen on the plantar surface of the heel even in the seasoned athlete (Fig. 3). Prevention rests in thicker socks, moleskin, and emollient creams prior to practice and competition.[16] Diagnosis is sufficient therapy.

Hematomas, seen as blood blisters or contusions in the more superficial intradermal and subcutaneous tissues, and deeper in the muscle with collision/contact sports, may require only limited ther-

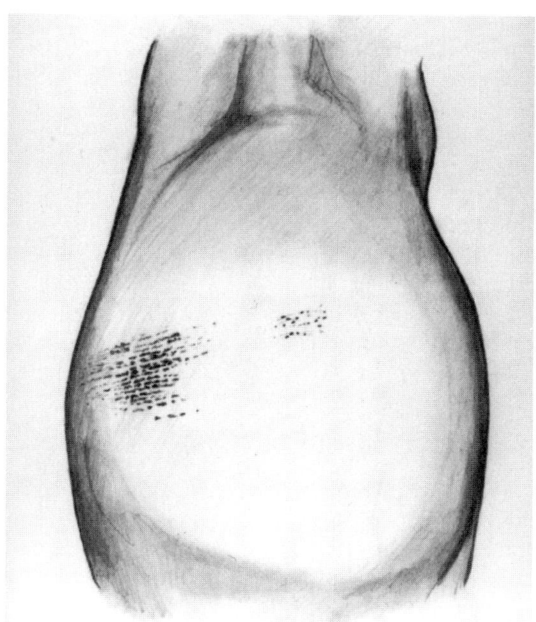

FIGURE 3. Black heel ("talon noir"), a form of ecchymosis.

apy such as rest, ice, compression, and elevation (RICE). More aggressive therapy, especially of deep muscle hematomas, may be indicated to prevent long-term disabilities and complications such as myositis ossificans, more familiar to the athletic trainer and physical therapist than to many physicians.[7]

Nail Hemorrhage. Injuries to the nail may cause it to separate from its underlying bed (onycholysis) or give rise to acute subungual hemorrhage, a more painful condition. Treatment for the former is supportive, whereas evacuating the blood with a hot wire, twirling a needle or a no. 11 blade, or yet other methods offers instantaneous relief for the latter. Loss of the nail will depend on the extent of the injury.

Lacerations. A variety of lacerations occur in the competitive athlete. Assurance of an immune tetanus status is comforting. Appropriate wound care, including surgical repair, ensures the best protection against infection and promotes early healing.[10]

Bites and Stings. For athletes sensitive to a variety of insect bites, common mosquito repellants containing diethyltoluamide (DEET) deter most would-be invaders.[26] Unattended insect bites frequently lead to infection and must be monitored by those responsible for the athlete, especially in environments that combine sweat, dirt, and occlusion. For athletes demonstrating systemic sensitivity to stinging insects (bees, wasps, etc.), the physician must instruct the athlete as to risks and make injectable adrenalin available to those responsible for on-field evaluation and care. Several self-contained bee sting kits are available commercially, and one belongs in the field athletic bag.

Ingrown Nail. Ingrown nails occur frequently, and their causes include trimming the nails too deeply at the corners and the use of tight-fitting footwear, especially in tennis, basketball, and long-distance running. Neglected nails can produce an extreme amount of periungual inflammation, sometimes leading to the development of excessive granulation tissue (pyogenic granuloma), usually next to a great nail, which is also more commonly ingrown.

The treatment of an ingrown nail necessitates appropriate care of the inflammatory periungual tissue (soaks and antibiotics), sometimes nail removal, and stressing the need for appropriate footwear. Cutting the great toe nail straight across without snipping off the protruding corners is the best preventive measure. A pyogenic granuloma, usually presenting as "proud flesh" with a moist, glistening top, may arise anywhere on the skin—usually following trauma—but it most often arises in conjunction with an ingrown nail (Fig. 4). This lesion can be handled by surgical removal of the granulation tissue and adjacent ingrown nail. Hemostatics are sometimes indicated to deal with the vigorous ooze created by cutting into the growth.

Dermatofibroma. Dermatofibroma results from microtrauma to the skin—common in the athlete—and most are seen on the legs (Fig. 5). This small, slightly elevated, firm papule, often brown in color, usually measures less than 1 cm across, it and dimples when pinched (Fig. 6). The lesion is benign and no therapy is indicated.

Nodules. Repetitive friction and skin trauma may lead to the development of firm, flesh-colored nodules in athletes.[17] Most common on the dorsal

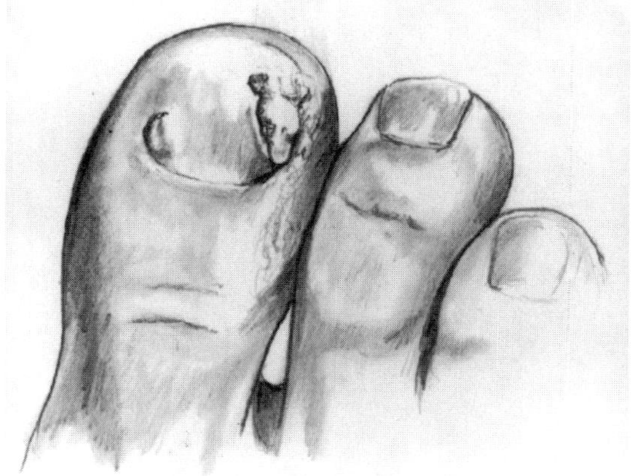

FIGURE 4. Ingrown toenail with excessive granulation tissue (pyogenic granuloma).

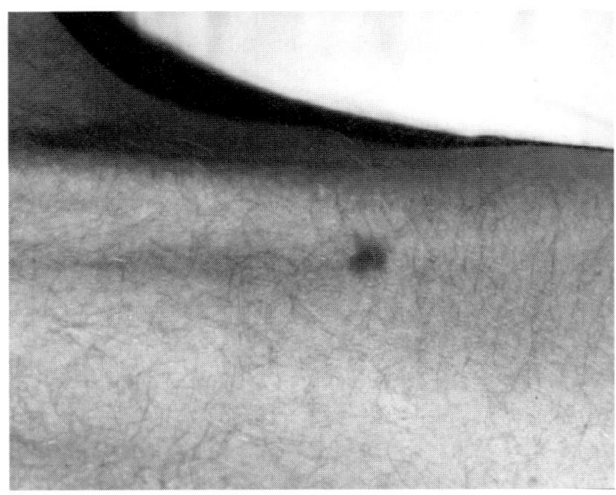

FIGURE 5. Dermatofibroma on the thigh.

aspects of the feet in football players and surfers, these intradermal, connective tissue tumors result from a proliferation of collagen in the dermis. Conservative or surgical treatment may be indicated for such benign lesions.

Striae. Striae result from the loss of dermal collagen and elastic supporting fibers that allows the dermis to pull apart.[12] The lesions are initially red to dusky blue and later change to permanent, pale, atrophic fracture lines.[26] Seen most frequently in athletes who gain considerable weight and/or muscle (weightlifters and gymnasts), these permanent skin changes are also seen in some growing teenagers, females having a higher incidence.[13] Topical and systemic corticosteroids also can cause striae, especially in intertriginous areas following the use of topical fluorinated steroids.[15] Striae are most common over the anterior shoulder, breasts, lower back, abdomen, buttocks, and thighs, running perpendicular to the direction of skin tension. Also to be considered are striae caused by the use of systemic anabolic-androgenic steroids.

Green Hair. Cosmetic discoloration of the hair, most often greenish in tint, may be seen in blond swimmers. Chlorine additives are often considered responsible and may create bleaching effects, with blonding of hair; however, copper deposition in the hair matrix is the reason for the green tint.[9] Shampooing after swimming usually prevents this problem. Therapy with 3% peroxide bleach in a 2- and 3-hour session is helpful, as is local application of a commercially available chelating agent (Metalex).

OTHER PHYSICAL FACTORS

Heat. Erythema ab igne, revealing characteristic hyperpigmentation and reticulated erythema, is sometimes seen after prolonged use of local heat for treatment of persistent painful joints or muscles (Fig. 7).[22] Prevention is the key.

Cold. Erythema pernio (chilblains) sometimes follows exposure to a cold, wet environment, with skin lesions' developing 12–24 hours after the injury. In addition to the symptoms and signs discussed under Hypothermia, red to blue plaques may be seen, most commonly on the feet and lower extremities; they usually disappear in 1–2 weeks[22] (Fig. 8). Therapy is rarely indicated.

Dry skin may occur during prolonged cold exposure in winter sports, secondary to loss of hydration in the keratin layer. The skin appears dry and roughened, and it may crack or chap, leading to eczema, winter itch, asteatotic eczema, or eczema craquelé. Therapy includes limiting use of soap to axilla and groin, moisture (bathing) followed by lubricants (Alpha Keri, Dermol), and application of bland emollients several time daily (Tables 3 and 4). Hu-

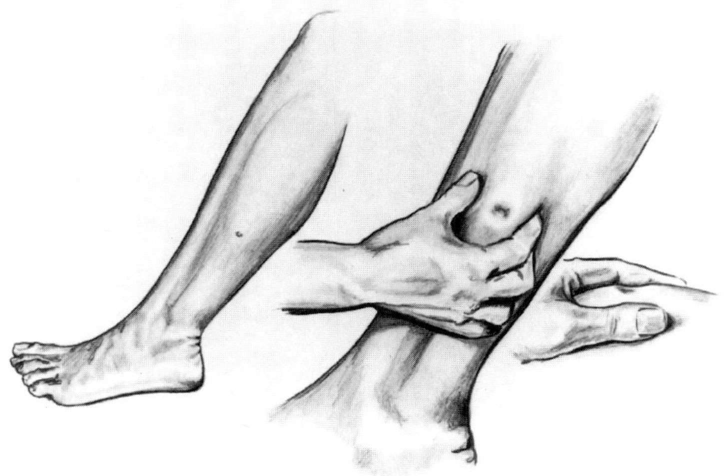

FIGURE 6. Dermatofibroma. This is a benign lesion that "dimples" when pinched.

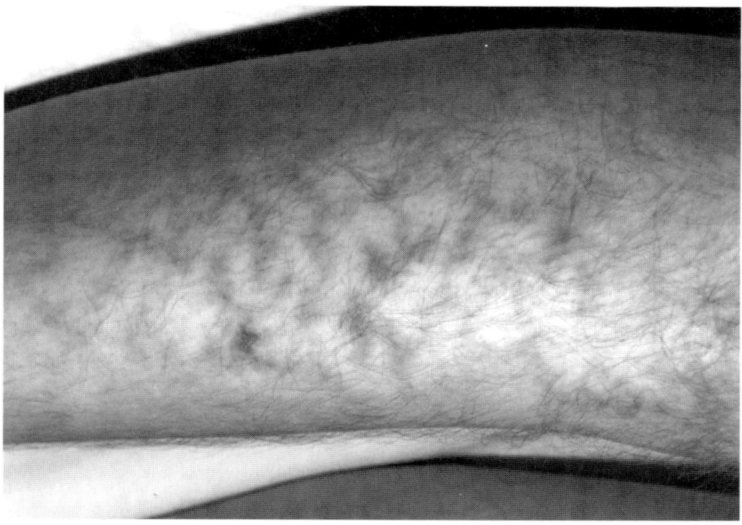

FIGURE 7. Erythema ab igne on the leg caused by chronic use of an electric heating pad.

midification of the home environment and improved general skin care are preventive.

Moisture. Hyperhidrosis is common in many high-energy athletes, and it may adversely affect manual dexterity and aggravate several pedal skin problems.[33] Twenty percent aluminum chloride in anhydrous ethyl alcohol (Drysol) applied to completely dried palms and soles at bedtime may be helpful. Strict attention to produce directions is important.

PHYSICAL URTICARIA

An interesting but distressing group of induced urticarias have a common pathogenesis in histamine. Immunoglobulin E is involved in some, but complement does not appear to play a role.[19] Phys-

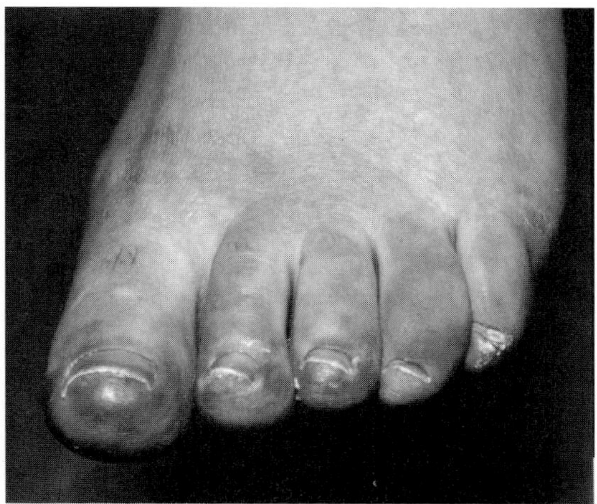

FIGURE 8. Pernio (chilblains) following prolonged cold exposure while wearing tennis shoes.

TABLE 3. **Lubricants and Emollients for Dry Skin***

Ointments/creams	Lotions (suspensions
(water-in-oil	of powder in water)
oil-in-water emulsions)	Cetaphil
Lanolin based	Wondra
Aquaphor	Aloe Vera
Nivea	Esoterica Dry Skin
Eucerin	Eucerin
Keri	Vaseline Intensive
Petroleum based	Care
Lanolor	Wibi
Keri Creme	Alpha Keri
Lubriderm	Lac-Hydrin
Cold cream USP	Ultra Mide
Hydrophilic ointment USP	
Vaseline Dermatology Formula	

*Modified from Mellion MD (ed): Office Management of Sports Injuries & Athletic Problems. Philadelphia, Hanley & Belfus, 1988.

TABLE 4. **Amount of Ointment or Cream Needed for Topical Use***

Area covered	One application (gm)	One application twice daily for 1 week (gm)
Hands, face, head, or anogenital region	2	30
One arm or anterior or posterior trunk	3	40
One leg	4	60
Entire body	30–60	600

*Modified from Mellion MB (ed): Office Management of Sports Injuries & Athletic Problems. Philadelphia, Hanley & Belfus, 1988.

ical exertion, pressure, cold, heat, and solar, aquagenic, and cholinergic factors may lead to exercise-related forms of urticaria, accentuated by rapid changes in body temperature and by emotional stress—all factors common to sports activities (Fig. 9 and 10). Severe reactions can occur.[20]

Prevention is difficult, short of the total avoidance of inciting factors.[9] Gradual exercise may be used to "desensitize" athletes to this form of urticaria; pharmacologic intervention is often not successful. Therapy used in selected cases includes antihistamines such as diphenhydramine (Benadryl), cyproheptadine (Periactin), and hydroxyzine (Atarax, Vistaril); corticosteroids; and sunscreens.[19] Occasionally, two of the aforementioned H_1 antihistamines must be used in combination to obtain an adequate result. Another approach is to use an H_1 antihistamine plus the H_2 antihistamine cimetidine (Tagamet) in combination (Table 5).

Exercise-induced anaphylaxis may be seen in these athletes, with symptoms' occurring within 5 minutes of beginning exercise or with symptoms delayed until exercise has been completed.[19] The patient typically experiences pruritus, usually generalized, followed by urticaria. The severity varies and may progress to include bronchospasm, hypotension, arrhythmias, and gastrointestinal symptoms—true anaphylaxis, which must be treated as such. This exercise-induced syndrome is more common in those with a family history, including related problems such as atopic dermatitis and asthma.

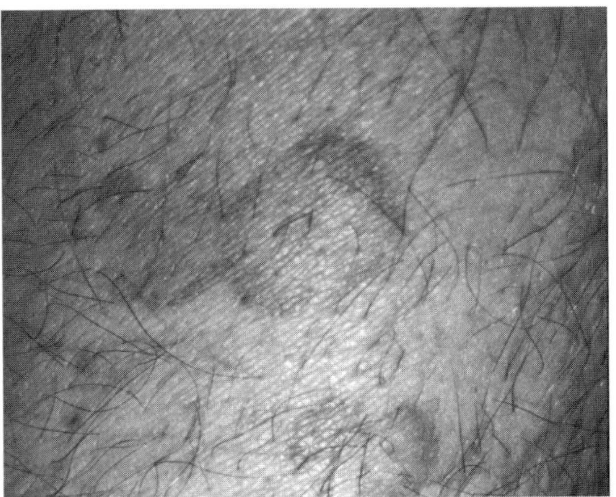

FIGURE 9. Characteristic wheals of acute and chronic urticaria.

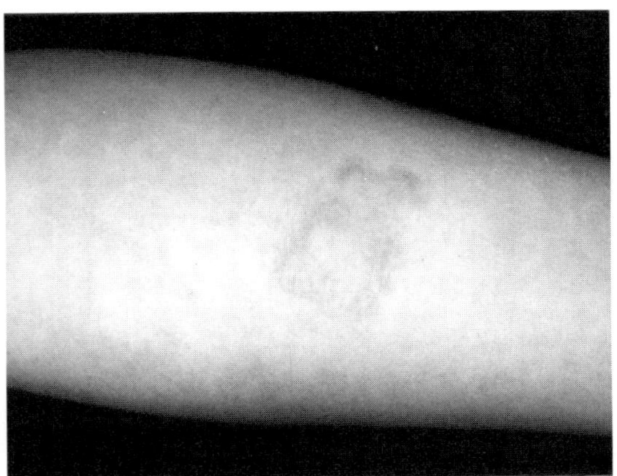

FIGURE 10. Cold urticaria documented by an icecube provocative test.

TABLE 5. **Physical Urticarias***

Inciting Factor	Suggested Therapy†
Solar	Sunscreens, clothing
Cold	Cyproheptadine
Heat	H_1 antihistamines Cyproheptadine
Cholinergic	Hydroxyzine
Exertion, pressure	H_1 antihistamines H_2 antihistamines

*Modified from Mellion MB (ed): Office Management of Sports Injuries & Athletic Problems. Philadelphia, Hanley & Belfus, 1988.

†Combinations of medications sometimes indicated.

CONTACT DERMATITIS

Allergic Dermatitis. Dermatitis is an inflammatory process of the epidermis and upper dermis. Common symptoms and findings include itching that leads to scratching, reddening of the skin, and development of papules and even blisters when the process is acute; more chronic cases reveal thickening and lichenification. Allergic contact dermatitis, the prototype being poison ivy, is common in susceptible athletes, especially those exposed to weedy areas during training or competition; these individuals develop specific T-cell antibodies against the allergen. Other common allergic causes include paraphenylenediamine (blue and black) clothing dyes, nickel-containing metal, all "caine"-containing medicaments and benzoin preparations (tincture of benzoin, Tuf-Skin).[11]

Potent skin sensitizers such as ethylenediamine and neomycin also put the athlete at risk for dermatitis and are best not used at any time. Clear fingernail polish applied to the metal may prevent nickel dermatitis contracted from buttons, shoulder pads, and other equipment.

Irritant Dermatitis. Assessment of irritant contact dermatitis is often not difficult; the condition is usually due to physical and mechanical agents, and the history and location of the lesions are diagnostic. Common irritants include adhesive tape, lime, dry ice, astroturf, poorly fitting gear, cold-pack chemicals from a leak in "liquid ice," a variety of clothing fibers, rubber-containing straps, pads, leather gloves, shoes and chin straps, and a variety of skin products. The hallmark of therapy is to eliminate continued exposure to the irritant. Often one need suggest only symptomatic relief such as cool, wet compresses or the use of antipruritic lotions and creams (no "caines"), including topical corticosteroids, as therapy for less active dermatitis. At times systemic antihistamines are indicated, which may interfere with athletic performance. Rarely, a short course of systemic corticosteroids may be necessary.

INFECTIONS

Bacterial Infections. Temporary cessation of athletic activities is often indicated for common infections, including impetigo and furunculosis (boil).[11] Diagnosis is usually easy; impetigo represents a superficial infection of the skin caused by *Staphylococcus aureus* or group A streptococci or a combination of the two, whereas furunculosis, most commonly a staphylococcal abscess, forms as an infection deep in the hair follicle. Both commonly occur in athletes and are aggravated by sweat, dirt, and occlusion. Athletes who wear heavy, protective padding, as in hockey and football, are susceptible to a type of bacterial folliculitis called acne mechanica. Seventy percent of boils develop after a bruise or break in the skin, most being located on the extremities. Associated causative factors include skin lubricants, elbow and forearm pads, whirlpool baths, and athletic tape.[8] Prevention is important but difficult—finishing the season is curative.

Impetigo can often be cleared by using warm, wet compresses, a 5–10% benzoyl peroxide solution, or a topical antibacterial ointment such as bacitracin, Bactroban, or Polysporin. An oral course of penicillin or erythromycin may be indicated, since untreated steptococcal skin infections can lead to acute glomerulonephritis. Furuncles may develop deeper pockets and become fluctuant, necessitating incision to facilitate rapid drainage. Incision and drainage is sufficient (without a wick).[33] Antibiotics are not ordinarily necessary in the treatment of a furuncle; widespread, recurrent, or resistant furunculosis, however, may best be aided by culture and appropriate systemic antimicrobial therapy. The adhesive tape that is used to secure a gauze dressing can produce enough injury in the adjacent stratum corneum to foster new lesions in the same area, and therefore circumferential dressing is preferred if at all possible. Some sports physicians find that bacitracin or Polysporin ointment applied to an area of furunculosis reduces the development of satellite lesions. When in doubt a course of oral antibiotics should be followed.

A more recent addition to the folliculitis field is hot tub folliculitis, caused by the *Pseudomonas* organism (Fig. 11). The papulovesiculopustular lesions, occasionally heralded by mild systematic symptomatology and located in areas where the skin has been covered by swimwear or other clothing, are usually diagnostic and may be accompanied by external *Pseudomonas* otitis.[30] The course is benign and self-limited, rarely necessitating diagnostic testing or therapeutic measures. Other *Pseudomonas* infections seen in athletes include green lesions of the nails and interdigital webs; the latter are best treated with gentamicin (Garamycin) ointment.

Discrete craters of 1–3 mm are frequently seen on the soles of tennis and basketball players (Fig. 12). The condition, called pitted keratolysis, is precipitated by hyperhidrosis (external or essential), is caused by the *Corynebacterium* species, and is aggravated by occlusive footwear.[23] Therapies include topical and oral erythromycin.

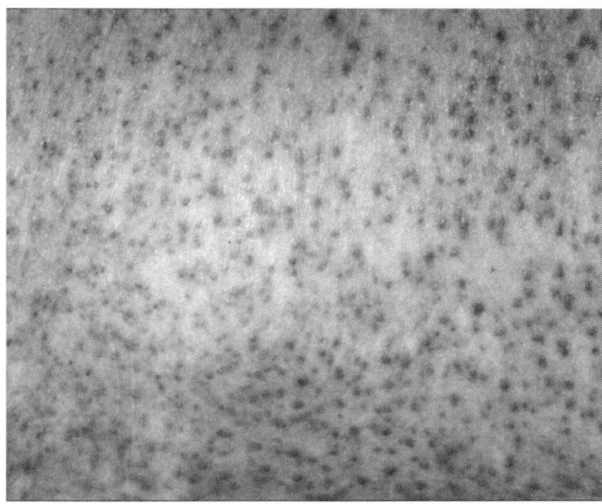

FIGURE 11. Folliculitis on the trunk caused by *Pseudomonas aeruginosa* ("hot tub folliculitis").

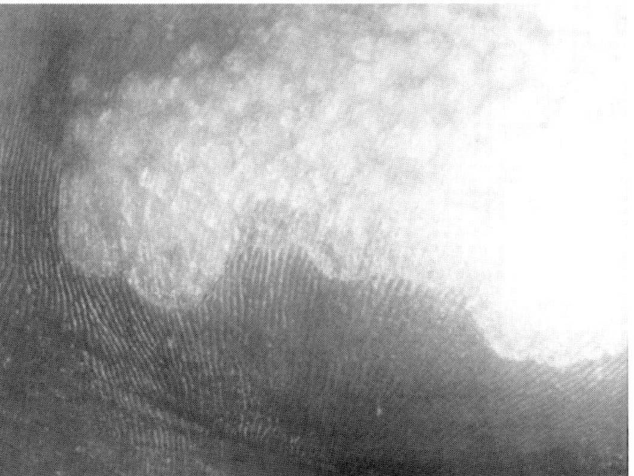

FIGURE 12. Pitted keratolysis. Closeup view demonstrating the characteristic "pits" over the heel due to hyperhidrosis and bacterial colonization.

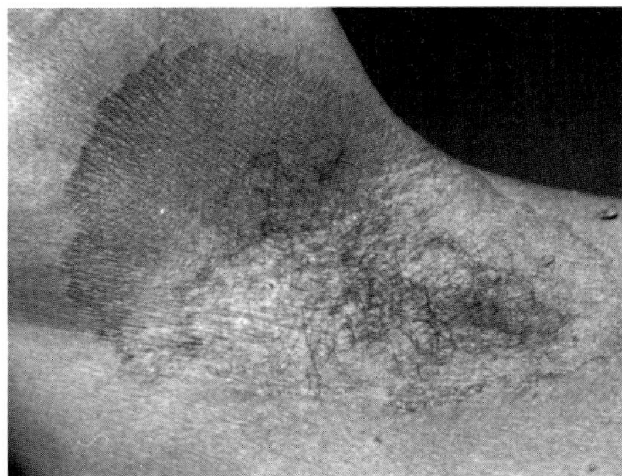

FIGURE 13. Erythrasma of the left axilla caused by the gram-positive bacillus *Corynebacterium minutissimum.* This could easily be mistaken for tinea; however Wood's light and KOH examinations can differentiate the two infections.

A less common bacterial infection in the crural area is erythrasma, caused by *Corynebacterium minutissimum* (Fig. 13). Seen most frequently in long-distance runners in temperate climates, this infection fluoresces coral red under a Wood's light; it also responds to systemic erythromycin.

External otitis (swimmer's ear) is the bane of aquatic participants.[25] Effective therapy includes otic wicks saturated with acid-alcohol or antibiotic-corticosteroid drops followed by measures that promote a more aerobic environment for the external ear, including removal of excess cerumen.[2] Prevention of recurrent otic dermatitis externa in susceptible individuals may include the use of VoSol or Burow's solution (Domeboro), used after swimming and postcompetition showers. A hair dryer may also be helpful.

Fungal Infections. Fungal infection prototypes are dermatophytic tinea pedis (athlete's foot) (Fig. 14) and tinea cruris (jock itch). Diagnosis of most fungal infections can be made from clinical features, those often altered by self-treatment using a variety of over-the-counter preparations.

Fungal infections commonly result from the macerating effects of chronic perspiration, which reduces the natural barrier effects of the stratum corneum. Tinea pedis is a common infection of the lateral intertoe spaces, especially in postpubertal males. Tinea cruris is common in men and rarely seen in women. *Candida albicans,* an opportunistic yeast, can cause much trouble in warm, moist parts of the body. Classic involvement of intertriginous areas and the easily identifiable 1- to 2-mm satellite lesions just beyond the main area of the dermatitis make the diagnosis easily apparent. Tinea versicolor, seen commonly in swimmers and divers, creates more cosmetic than medical concerns for the student-athlete; it usually fluoresces gold to orange under Wood's light.[26]

Preventive measures include daily changes of socks and shorts, use of absorbent foot powder, wearing leather shoes, and daily cleansing of athletic shower and dressing facilities. Therapy may involve modification of the athlete's conditioning or training, allowing a more optimal environment to exist for a period of time. The availability of Monistat-Derm makes therapy for dermatophytic and monilial infections very effective, ably backed up by a variety of other topical antifungal agents. Ongoing use once or twice weekly during a sports season may reduce recurrences. A newer antifungal drug—1% naftifine hydrochloride cream or gel (Naftin)—may be used for more recalcitrant cases. Three percent selenium sulfide shampoo, which is applied, left on for 3–5 minutes after a shower, and repeated daily for 5 days,

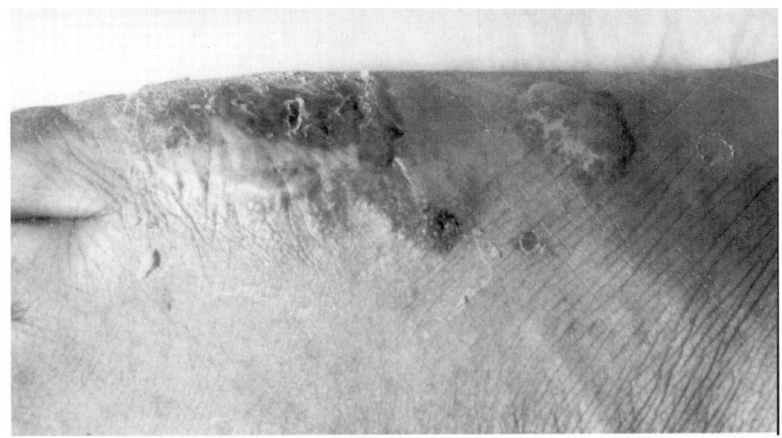

FIGURE 14. Tinea pedis on the lateral foot caused by *T. mentagrophytes.* Note the vesiculopustular eruption in addition to the more common scaling.

usually constitutes a satisfactory course of treatment for tinea versicolor. Topical 2% ketoconazole (Nizoral) cream can be used daily for 2 weeks. In severe cases of tinea versicolor, Nizoral 400 mg orally and repeated in 1 week may be indicated.

Viral Infections. Common warts are usually easy to recognize because of their resemblance to a cauliflower sprig, the surface often including irregular and rough crypts or invaginations accompanied by black dots representing thrombosed capillary tips. They rarely interfere with athletic competition and have a low rate of infectivity. Warts tend to be self-limited, and the athlete who has no symptoms and is willing to wait may be justly rewarded, as most warts resolve spontaneously within a few months—presumably a response to immunologic activity.

These common lesions can be effectively treated by a variety of methods, including liquid nitrogen, intermittent application of strong acids, home therapy with weak acids such as 10% salicylic acid and 10% lactic acid in flexible collodion (Duofilm), gentle electrodesiccation, and curettage under local anesthesia. Other, less common methods are the use of 0.025% Retin-A gel and 2–5% fluorouracil. A greater confluence of warts—called a mosaic, often several centimeters in width, and most common on the sole of the foot—is best handled by the application of a commercial 40% salicylic acid plaster, cut to the shape of the warts and held in place with adhesive tape for 2–3 days. Following removal and foot soaks or a bath, including gentle clearing of the remaining debris, a new plaster can be reapplied for another several days. Continued therapy for 1–2 months often causes the wart to regress. Elliptical excision of warts should be avoided, especially on the plantar surface, and strong acids, liquid nitrogen, and cautery should not be used during the athletic season. For therapy of troublesome, painful plantar warts during the athletic season, weekly injection of 1% xylocaine into the base of the wart until it shells out can be recommended (Fig. 15). The wart usually responds to therapy in 1–3 weeks, occasionally requiring more prolonged therapy.[18] CO_2 laser therapy may be helpful for resistant warts.

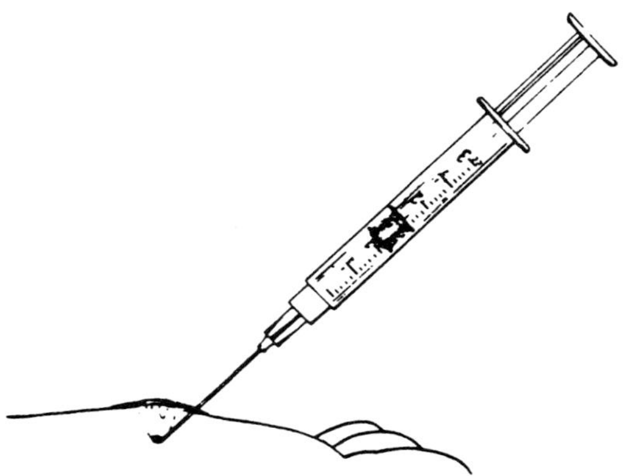

FIGURE 15. Technique for injecting 1-2 cc of lidocaine into the base of a plantar wart.

Another viral infection, molluscum contagiosum, produces small translucent papules (2–4 mm) that may be single, grouped, or inoculated along a scratch (Koebner's lines). Although such lesions may occur almost anywhere on the body, the hands and face are common locations, as are the face and upper body of boxers and wrestlers. The translucent quality and umbilication of this small papule simplifies the diagnosis (Fig. 16). A variety of therapies that evacuate the papular molluscum body include a tiny incision and drainage of the papule with a knife blade, curettage, light spark from an electric needle, application of liquid nitrogen, or continued diligent application of salicylic and lactic acid preparations.[5]

Herpes simplex virus can affect any cutaneous location or adjacent mucosa in the athlete; however, the most frequent locations are the face and hands, often following sun exposure or trauma, respectively. Common in wrestlers, it is known as herpes gladiatorum (Fig. 17). The most effective preventive measure is daily scrubbing of the mats after practice and competition, which is often done by the wrestlers themselves, who know the competitive price of an acute episode. If a trigger factor can be reasonably assumed, the athlete may be able to avoid it—usually a significant saving to conditioning and competition. The lesions are initially small: 1- to 2-mm vesicles grouped together on an erythematous base. An initial attack may be dramatic, with considerable pain, adenopathy, and fever. Acyclovir (Zovirax) is an antiviral agent now available for topical, oral, and systemic use. Cool compresses (Domeboro) and oral acyclovir provide

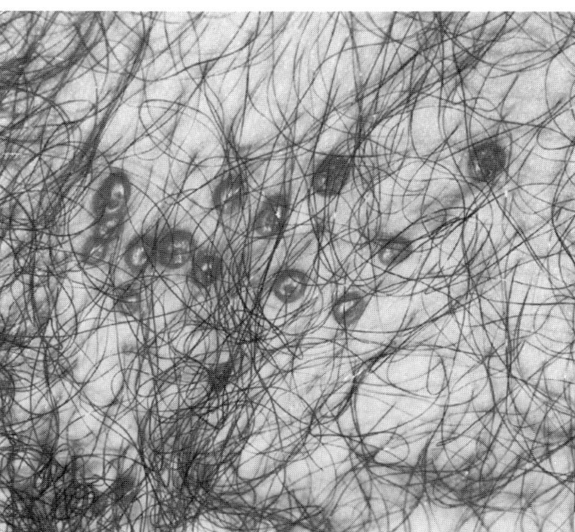

FIGURE 16. Molluscum contagiosum in the groin area.

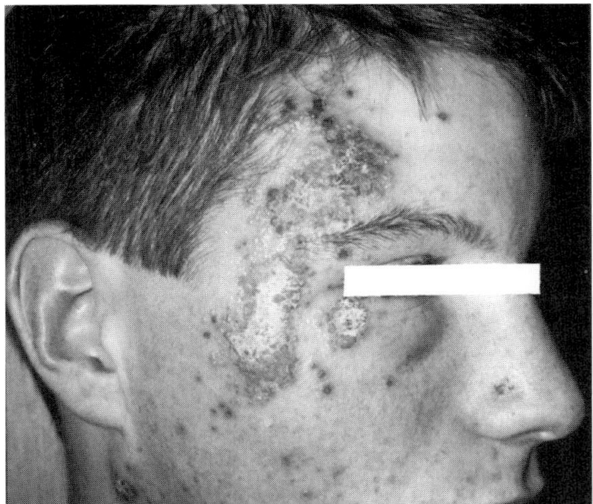

FIGURE 17. Herpes gladiatorum in a wrestler.

rapidly effective therapy; however, infected athletes should be sidelined until freed of lesions in order to prevent spread. Oral acyclovir may also be used both for recurrent episodes and for prophylaxis during an athletic season in situations when recurrent attacks produce an unusual degree of distress or frequent extended periods away from competition.

INFESTATIONS

Pediculosis. Lice, more the bane of the younger classroom student (head lice) than the student-athlete (pubic lice), most commonly occur under circumstances of inadequate hygiene. However, the camaraderie of athletes often puts them in close physical contact, as do athletic endeavors. Public lice (crabs) are therefore not uncommon and affect mature adults of both sexes and all socioeconomic strata. Head and public lice that are spread by close personal contact are easily eradicated by a single application of gamma benzene hexachloride (Kwell) products. Nits on eyelashes—sometimes a secondary area for public lice to inhabit (similar hairshaft diameter)—can be removed by bedtime application of generous amounts of petrolatum to the eyelids until cleared.[31] Head lice, less common in the athlete, may also be treated with a newer product: permethrin 1% cream rinse (Nix), also used as a single application.

Scabies. Still at epidemic levels in this country, scabies should be suspected in athletes complaining of generalized itching that is worse at night and seen especially in those participating in sports leading to close body contact. Because the female mite can survive 1–3 days off the body, scabies can be spread by fomites such as towels, uniforms, and equipment.[15] Although proof of infestation is gratifying (recovering the mite from a burrow), a high index of suspicion and environmental factors often lead to appropriate assumptions and therapy. Itchy papules of the breast areolae or penis are nearly pathognomonic. Therapy is effective with a single application (neck to toes) of Kwell lotion in the evening after a bath. Rebathing the next day completes one treatment cycle, which is usually sufficient. Newer, permethrin 5% cream (Elimite) has also proven to be highly effective. Therapy for scabies is not complete without provision of systemic antipruritics, as it may take 3–4 weeks for the itching to subside, this being completed once the inflammatory skin changes have been replaced with normal epithelium. Judicious use of topical corticosteroids may be helpful. However, widespread skin involvement often makes this therapy impractical and expensive. If multiple cases are seen in the same athlete environment, it behooves the physician to personally supervise the application of a scabicide to all close contacts. All family members and sexual contacts likewise need a course of topical therapy.

EXACERBATION OF PREEXISTING DERMATOSES

Athletes appear in the training room, on the practice field, and in competition with a variety of skin problems common to their age groups. As stated earlier, prevention is key to skin problems, which can affect participation and performance; this applies equally to exacerbation of preexisting skin problems seen in the athlete. Environmental factors play a significant role: the combination of sweat, dirt, and occlusive protective equipment serves to aggravate several preexisting skin conditions, including acne, atopic dermatitis, dyshidrosis, psoriasis, and seborrheic dermatitis. These are discussed further.

Acne. Acne is rarely a diagnostic problem. Much more difficult is the control of this distressingly common skin affliction of youngsters, especially during competitive athletic seasons in many sports. Control of acne is attainable, however, and the objectives are twofold: short-term cosmetic results and long-term prevention of scarring. Preventive and therapeutic measures include the wearing of loose-fitting, dry, clean, absorbent cotton clothing and the avoidance of abrasive skin cleansers and constant picking at acne lesions.[24] In spite of athletic lifestyles and environment, much can be done to improve the lot of the athlete with acne by the judicious use of benzoyl peroxide, retinoic acid derivatives, and antibiotics, the latter two both topical and systemic.[14] Most athletes find sunshine to be helpful, noticing improvement in acne during the summer, with worsening during the winter. A special problem is presented by the athlete with frequent cystic acne who may be psychologically distressed by the slowly evolving cystic lesions. Once a cyst has developed, hot compresses and a small incision to drain its contents when fluctuant are helpful. A more recent innovation—the early intralesional injection of 0.1–0.3 ml of 1/4% triamcinolone acetonide suspension—usually leads to rapid disappearance of the cyst with no surgical trauma to the skin surface.[6] Well-conditioned athletes may be treated with Accutane, a derivative of vitamin A; however, they should not start a new strenuous athletic program during such therapy. Athletes with severe acne may benefit from dermatologic consultation when Accutane is considered for curative systemic use to help prevent recurrences.

Atopic Dermatitis. Athletes with an atopic background are at risk to develop this distressing dermatitis. The chronic thickening and excoriation of flexural areas at the elbows and knees often flare during athletic competition. These athletes are at increased risk to also develop exercise-related urticaria and anaphylaxis, exercise-induced bronchospasm (asthma), and allergic rhinitis (even progressing to nasal polyps). They likewise may develop aspirin sensitivity.

The treatment for a flare-up of atopic eczema is both rewarding and frustrating. Appropriate avoidance of excessive soap during bathing is helpful, as is frequent use of bland emollients such as Vaseline or Eucerin, sometimes used in conjunction with topical corticosteroids. A short course of systemic corticosteroids may offer considerable relief for a flare-up that threatens to interfere with athletic competition.[3] Other measures useful during flare-ups include adequate rest, generous oral hydration, relief from emotional tension, and use of systemic antipruritic agents. Fall and winter sports participants are at greater risk for flare-up of atopic eczema, and many do not learn the need for continuing gentle topical care; for this reason, the sports physician must frequently give a pep talk to ensure patients' compliance with measures that will allow the athletes to be available for optimal participation. Athletes with an atopic background are also more susceptible to viral and bacterial infections.

Dyshidrosis. A common dermatitic condition affecting both the younger and the more mature athlete is dyshidrosis. Deep-seated vesicles affecting the hands and feet, or both, constitute common locations, lying along the sides of the digits and on the palms or soles (Fig. 18). Bullae are occasionally produced, and when they do occur, secondary infection is common, especially in the active athlete. Differential diagnosis includes fungal dermatophytosis, contact dermatitis, and atopic dermatitis. These athletes, uncomfortable during significant flare-ups, usually display ongoing hyperhidrosis. Wet compresses in the acute stage (Domeboro), often followed by topical corticosteroids and oral antibiotics for chronic cases, are the mainstays of therapy. Continuing therapy also is important, as an acute flare-up can cause distressing interference with athletic competition, say, on the hands of a golfer or gymnast or on the feet of a runner, basketball player, or football player.

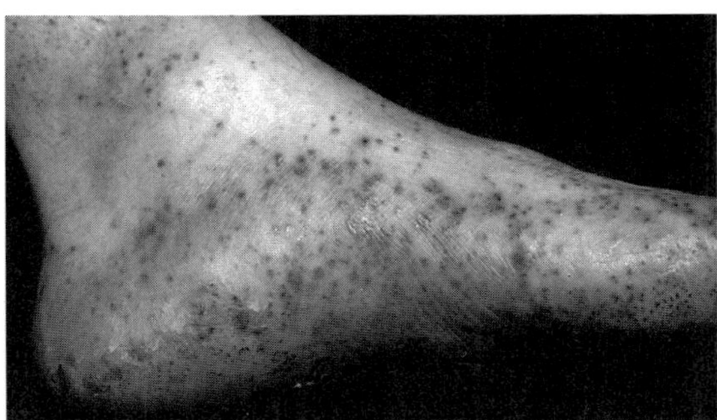

FIGURE 18. Dyshidrotic eczema on the foot.

Psoriasis. Athletes with this common, chronic, relapsing papulosquamous skin disorder are at risk for flare-ups especially on the hands and feet during athletic competition. The diagnosis of psoriasis is usually made by clinical observation alone, and a positive family history is present in about 50% of cases.[4] The main approach to treatment for most patients involves topical corticosteroid preparations, topical tars, and UVA. Improvement is noted with summer sunshine, and many patients benefit from using an artificial ultraviolet (UVB) sunlamp at home, having learned how to administer appropriate amounts. For hand and foot flare-ups, the effectiveness of corticosteroid ointments can be enhanced with occlusive wrapping using saran wrap or other plastic film. One must be cautious, however, about long-term atrophy from excessive use of topical corticosteroids.

Seborrheic Dermatitis. All athletes are acquainted through the media with the ever-expanding variety of dandruff-fighting shampoos and conditioners. When itching is added to dandruff, one can assume an inflammatory process is present, or seborrheic dermatitis. In some cases, the scaliness becomes heavy and the process even exudative. Additional areas of involvement, besides the scalp, may include the central forehead, ear canals, central face, mid-chest, axillae, umbilicus, groin, and intergluteal cleft. Treatment of seborrheic dermatitis, regardless of location, requires frequent scalp shampooing. This therapy alone often makes the dermatitis located elsewhere easier to control. Topical corticosteroid solutions are also used as an adjuvant to scalp care. If other areas of the body require therapy, mild hydrocortisone creams or Cetacort lotion is usually helpful. Flare-ups may be seen during a particularly tense athletic season, and the physician must be ready to intercede.

CONCLUSION

The sports physician can effectively diagnose and treat most skin disorders seen in the athlete. Many are preventable and most respond to therapy without significant side effects. Encouraging athletes' compliance with the treatment regimen of course augments the chance of successful outcome, and clinicians can relate compliance to the athlete's dedication to success. Noncompliance is less likely to be a factor if the physician and athlete have a sound doctor-patient relationship, and the physician dedicated to sports is likely to cultivate this type of contact. Another member of the sports medicine team—the certified athletic trainer—is most helpful in prevention, early diagnosis, and supervision of therapy.

REFERENCES

1. American Academy of Pediatrics Committee on Sports Medicine: The athlete and the skin. In Smith NJ (ed): Sports Medicine: Health Care for Young Athletes. Elk Grove Village, IL, American Academy of Pediatrics, 1983, pp 130–141.
2. Amundson LH: Disorders of the external ear. In Vogt HB (ed): Primary Care: Disorders of the Ears, Nose and Throat. Philadelphia, W.B. Saunders, 1990, pp 213–231.
3. Amundson LH: Managing skin problems in athletes. In Mellion MB, Walsh WM, Shelton GL, (eds): The Team Physician's Handbook. Philadelphia, Hanley & Belfus, 1990, p 249.
4. Amundson LH, Caplan RM: Dermatology I: Home Study Self-Assessment Program. Kansas City, American Academy of Family Physicians, Monograph 108, 1988, pp 21–22.
5. Amundson LH, Caplan RM: Dermatology II. Home Study Self-Assessment Program. Kansas City, American Academy of Family Physicians, Monograph 109, 1988, pp 20–21.
6. Amundson LH, Caplan RM: The skin and subcutaneous tissues. In Taylor RB (ed): Family Medicine: Principles and Practice, 2nd ed. New York, Springer Verlag, 1983, pp 1069–1144.
7. Aronen JG, Chronister RD: Quadriceps contusions. Physician Sportsmed 20:130–136, 1992.
8. Bartlett PC, Martin RJ, Cahill BR: Furunculosis in a high school football team. Am J Sports Med 10:371–374, 1982.
9. Basler RSW: Skin lesions related to sports activity. Prim Care 10:479–494, 1983.
10. Berger A: Traumatic Skin Injuries: Home Study Self-Assessment Program. Kansas City, American Academy of Family Physicians, Monograph 157, 1992, pp 24–29.
11. Bergfeld WF: Dermatologic problems in athletes. Prim Care 10:151–160, 1984.
12. Bergfeld WF: The diagnosis and treatment of dermatologic problems in athletes. In Schneider RC (ed): Sports Injuries: Mechanisms, Prevention, and Treatment. Baltimore, Williams & Wilkins, 1985, pp 636–651.
13. Bergfeld WF, Taylor JS: Trauma, sports and the skin. Am J Ind Med 8:403–413, 1985.
14. Bikowski J: Effectively treating acne vulgaris. Physician Sportsmed 20:100–107, 1992.
15. Birrer RB: Common skin problems in athletes. In Birrer RB (ed): Sports Medicine for the Primary Care Physician. Norwalk, CT, Appleton-Century-Crofts, 1984, pp 239–248.
16. Bodine KG: Black heel. J Am Podiatry Assoc 70:201, 1980.
17. Cohen PR, Eliezri YD, Silvers DN: Athlete's nodules: Sports-related connective tissue nevi of the collagen type (collagenomas). Cutis 50:131–135, 1992.
18. Drez D Jr: Forefoot problems in runners. In Mock RP (ed): Symposium on the Foot and Leg in Running Sports. American Academy of Orthopaedic Surgeons, St. Louis, Mosby, 1982, pp 73–75.
19. Eisenstadt WS, Nicholas SS, Velick G, Enright T: Allergic reactions to exercise. Physician Sportsmed 12:95–104, 1984.
20. Escher S, Tucker A: Preventing, diagnosing and treating cold urticaria. Physician Sportsmed 20:73–84, 1992.
21. Fitzpatrick TB, Eisen AZ, Wolff A, et al (eds): Photomedicine. Dermatology in General Medicine, 3rd ed, New York, McGraw-Hill, 1987, pp 1516–1517.
22. Henderson JM, Hrabal TL, Baumert PW, et al: Sports Medicine II: Home Study Self-Assessment Program. Kansas City, American Academy of Family Physicians, Monograph 161, 1992, pp 25–26.
23. Houston SD, Knox JM: Skin problems related to sports and recreational activities. Cutis 19:487–491, 1977.
24. Hudson A: How I manage acne in athletes. Physician Sportsmed 11:117–120, 1983.
25. Levine N: Dermatologic aspects of sports medicine. J Am Acad Dermatol 3:415–424, 1980.
26. Liteplo MG: Sports-related skin problems. In Vinger PF, Hoerner EF (eds): Sports Injuries: The Unthwarted Epidemic. Boston, John Wright, 1982, pp 188–202.
27. Louis DS, Honkin FM, Eckenrode JF: Cutaneous atrophy after corticosteroid injection. Am Fam Physician 33: 183–186, 1986.
28. McMaster WC: Cryotherapy. Physician Sportsmed 10:112–119, 1982.
29. Mertz PM, Marshall DA, Eaglstein WH: Occlusive dressings to prevent bacterial invasion and wound infection. J Am Acad Dermatol 12:662–668, 1985.
30. Randt GA: Hot tub folliculitis. Physician Sportsmed 11:74–80, 1983.
31. Schamberg IL: Dermatoses of the groin. J Fam Pract 8:825–833, 1979.
32. Sheard C: Simple management of plantar clavi. Cutis 50: 138, 1992.
33. Stauffer LW: Skin disorders in athletes: Identification and management. Physician Sportsmed 11:101–121, 1983.
34. Webster SB: How I manage jock itch. Physician Sportsmed 12:109–113, 1984.

RECOMMENDED DERMATOLOGY TEXTS

Arndt K: Manual of Dermatologic Therapeutics, 4th ed. Boston, Little, Brown and Company, 1989.

Fitzpatrick T, Eisen AZ, Wolff A, et al: Dermatology in General Medicine, 4th ed. New York, McGraw-Hill, 1993.

Moschella S, Hurley H: Dermatology, 3rd ed. Philadelphia, W.B. Saunders, 1992.

Sams WM, Lynch PJ: Principles and Practice of Dermatology. New York, Churchill Livingston, 1990.

Sober AJ, Fitzpatrick TB: Year Book of Dermatology. St. Louis, Mosby, 1992.

17

Principles of Musculoskeletal Rehabilitation

Guy L. Shelton, M.A., R.P.T., A.T.C.

Adequate rehabilitation of the musculoskeletal system is essential for the early, safe return of the athlete to participation. Because every athlete is different in goals, level of skill, level of participation, and degree of competitiveness, the rehabilitation program must be specific to that athlete. The "cookbook" approach, wherein each athlete with a specific problem is handed the same sheet of exercises for that "given" problem, is not suitable. Most athletes will follow an exercise program better if they feel knowledgeable about the program and confident that it is designed for them.

The primary care physician's role is to arrive at an accurate diagnosis, initiate a definitive treatment program, and follow up appropriately to ensure that healing, treatment, and rehabilitation goals are being met. Orthopedic referral is warranted when a specific diagnosis cannot be made, when the definitive treatment might include surgery or specialized immobilization, or when a seemingly minor problem fails to respond to appropriate measures. Physical therapy should be considered a basic component of the treatment program.

The physical therapist or athletic trainer performs a musculoskeletal evaluation to establish a baseline from which progress will be measured; a customized treatment and rehabilitation program is then initiated. The therapist teaches the athlete the components of the program, its rationale, proper exercise techniques, and guidelines for progressing or limiting activities. Appropriate motivation of the athlete should be provided along with the exercise instruction. If an athlete has problems with the rehabilitation program, then the therapist can reevaluate and modify the athlete's program. In short, the therapist serves as the athlete's teacher and coach for the rehabilitation program.

GOALS OF THE REHABILITATION PROGRAM

The overall goal of the treatment and rehabilitation program is to return the athlete to his or her desired level of participation as soon as safely possible. Consideration must be given to the amount of healing time required for the specific injury, length of time away from participation, the athlete's compliance with the treatment and rehabilitation program, and the athlete's motivation to return to play. With many injuries, the athlete may face deadlines to get well and resume participation. These deadlines often conflict with the time required for adequate healing and rehabilitation. While these participation considerations must occasionally be addressed, they should be carefully thought through so as not to jeopardize the long-term ability of the athlete to participate.

In order to decrease recovery time and promote healing, swelling and tissue congestion in the injured area must be controlled and reduced. Further, nutrient supply for rebuilding injured tissue must be facilitated. Morbidity is decreased by minimizing deconditioning through early initiation of the reconditioning program. It is also important to prevent further injury by allowing adequate healing and providing appropriate protection during recovery.

STEPS IN TREATMENT AND REHABILITATION

Prevention

The initial step in treatment of athletic injuries is prevention. The old adage that "an ounce of prevention is worth a pound of cure" is certainly true when dealing with injuries. There are four aspects of prevention: the physical condition of the athlete, proper equipment, a safe playing environment, and the preparticipation physical examination. Even the recreational athlete must be aware of his or her level of fitness and skill. Enhanced flexibility and strength as well as the athletes' recognition of their own skill levels and physical limitations helps to prevent injuries. Appropriate use of both standard and special protective equipment, clothing, and footwear decreases the risk of injury. The playing surface, surrounding environment, and atmospheric conditions are factors in certain injuries. A preparticipation screening examination, particularly in interscholastic athletes, those with previous injuries, those over 35 years old, or those with cardiac risk factors, may help identify certain preexisting conditions that need either further work-up or definitive treatment. This approach may prevent the underlying condition from causing a new injury or a reinjury in a previously afflicted area.

Triage and Initial Management.

Once an injury occurs, the triage process must begin. An evaluation on the field must be done to rule out any life-threatening problem. This must be done within the limitations of your skill level. An "on-the-field diagnosis" or working assessment must be made until a more specific diagnosis can be determined. The initial management of the injury must also be planned. This might include basic first aid measures and simple treatment, stabilization of the more seriously injured patient, rapid transportation to an emergency facility for definitive care, or a combination of the three. Initial management could also mean referral to an orthopedic surgeon or other specialist for further evaluation. It is important to stress that any decision made at this point be a conservative one.

Basic Athletic First Aid

Early implementation of basic athletic first aid helps to minimize pain and swelling, to protect the injury from further injury, and to facilitate an early start with rehabilitation. The steps in basic athletic first aid are best remembered by the mnemonic PRICES, which stands for **P**rotection, **R**est, **I**ce, **C**ompression, **E**levation, and **S**upport.

Protection. This means protecting the injured area from further injury. In cases of lower extremity injuries, crutches (Fig. 1) should be used if ambulation causes *any* pain, swelling, limping, or buckling of the extremity. They should continued to be used until these symptoms are not present and more serious injury is ruled out. Sometimes the use of an immobilizer or splint is warranted, especially if the athlete is in significant pain or if a fracture is suspected. In upper extremity injuries, a sling may be used to provide protection for the injured limb.

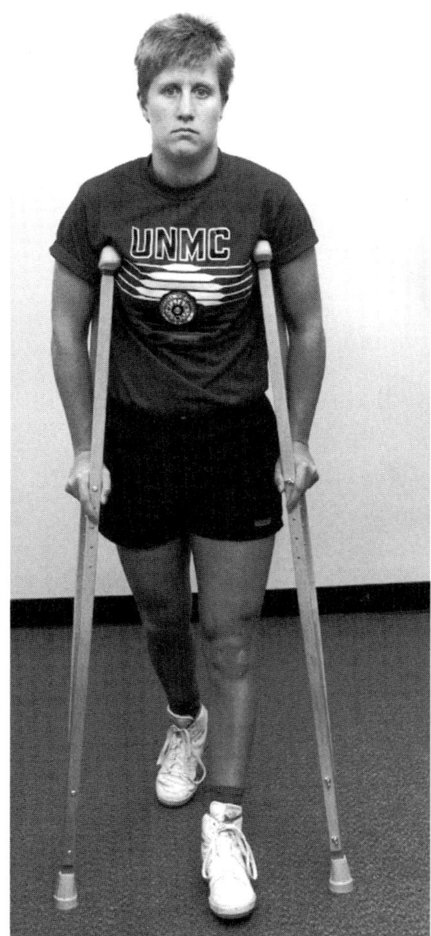

FIGURE 1. Partial weight bearing with axillary crutches to protect injured lower extremity.

Protective positioning instructions to the athlete help the athlete avoid inadvertent motions that could cause additional stress to the injury. In any situation, if the severity of the injury is in question, the use of a stretcher to transport the athlete provides maximum protection and decreases the likelihood of further injury.

Rest. Avoiding use of the injured part also helps to prevent further damage. The need for rest in more severe injuries is apparent. Absolute rest in minor injuries, however, is usually too strict. If one can be sure that an injury is not serious in nature, then *relative rest* may be employed. Relative rest means providing enough protection to keep the athlete asymptomatic. Some lower extremity injuries, for example, may not require crutches but may require abstaining from running or cutting even if the athlete can walk without symptoms.

Ice. Use of ice causes vasoconstriction and thus limits the blood flow to the injured area.[37,48] It further decreases tissue metabolism and so reduces tissue damage.[37,48] Ice also mitigates firing of pain nerve receptors.[37,48] This helps reduce muscle spasm. Many methods of cooling tissue have been used. Chipped ice packs and reusable frozen gel packs have been shown to provide better deep cooling that chemical cold packs and circulating freon gas.[49] Immersion of the injured part in iced water is also effective. Ice massage with a block of ice directly on the skin is useful over a small area. Treatment duration varies with the intensity of the cold and the patient's tolerance. A maximum of 30 minutes of cold followed by at least 30 minutes without cold packs is a general rule to use. Shorter treatment durations must be used if patient tolerance dictates.

Compression. Used in conjunction with ice, compression provides a physical limitation to the space that swelling many occupy. This also helps the edema dissipate so that it can be more readily reabsorbed by the circulatory system. Generally, elastic or double knit compression bandages are wrapped distally to proximally, overlapping about half the width of the bandage. Pneumatic and hydraulic compression devices are also helpful but are somewhat costly.

Elevation. This is a simple matter of using gravity to assist fluid to run downhill. By elevating the injured part above the level of the heart, venous return is enhanced and extravascular fluid is drained away from the injured area. Elevation is especially effective when combined with ice and compression.

Support. Although a form of protection, support implies a more functional type of protection. This would be appropriate for minor injuries without any significant symptoms where the athlete is going to return to play right away. An example of this would be supportive taping of the ankle for a minor ankle sprain.

Definitive Diagnosis and Treatment

Because a problem must be adequately defined before it can be properly solved, one must reach a specific and definitive diagnosis. Often this is the point at which the primary care physician first encounters an athlete. A detailed history and physical examination will provide sufficient information to make the diagnosis in many cases. Sometimes radiographs or other tests will be necessary. Referral to orthopedic, sports medicine, or other consultation is appropriate whenever the diagnosis or treatment approach is not clear.

The treatment program generally takes one of three forms. Treatment with **immobilization** should be used with some fractures and certain types of severe sprains. Immobilization, however, can have detrimental effects on muscle function, fitness, and articular cartilage nutrition. While immobilization may be the only proper way to treat certain injuries, a functional or rehabilitative treatment program must also be included following immobilization to help the athlete return to participation as soon as safely possible.

Second, **surgical treatment** should be undertaken in unstable fractures, certain severe sprains and strains, and as final definitive therapy for those problems for which more conservative treatment has failed. As with immobilization, functional or rehabilitative treatment should always be included in the follow-up postoperative care. In many surgical cases, some form of gentle rehabilitative exercises and other treatments may be initiated immediately after surgery.

Third, **functional treatment** involves progressive stages of exercise and activity. It should be initiated as soon as possible following injury, immobilization, or surgery. This minimizes deconditioning, the detrimental effects of immobilization, and recovery time. The remainder of this chapter is devoted to various aspects of the functional or rehabilitative treatment program.

Treatment with Physical Agents

Cold, heat, water, sound, electricity, and air have long been used in treating musculoskeletal injuries. Treatment with these various physical agents, however, does not constitute the primary, long-term treatment in any situation. If they are used to control acute symptoms or those occurring during rehabilitation, they may allow certain therapeutic exercises to be initiated sooner and progressed more rapidly. Diathermy, electrical stimulation, infrared light, and ultrasound should be applied only by individuals licensed or certified to do so because of the possible dangers inherent with these methods.

The use of **cold** has already been discussed in the section on the acute management of injuries. Ice can also be used to control flareups of inflammation during rehabilitation. Ice massage can provide local analgesia to painful areas prior to exercise or deep friction massage.

Therapeutic **heat** is used to facilitate circulation in an injured area. Warmer tissues are also easier to stretch.[54] Heat can be applied through moist heat packs, hot water bottles, electric heating pads, warm compresses, short- and microwave diathermies, infrared light, ultrasound, and whirlpool baths.

A good compromise that is sometimes used is **contrast treatment**. The injured part is warmed for 1–4 minutes and then cooled for 1–2 minutes. The ratio of heating to cooling time is adjusted based on the likelihood for creating swelling. Shorter heating times and longer cooling times are used in more acute situations.

Swelling should always be monitored when any form of heat is used. Any increase in swelling or other signs of inflammation as a result of any applied heat indicates a need to remove the heat and apply cold immediately.

Electrical stimulation has several potentially useful benefits. It can be used to facilitate muscle contraction as the initial part of a strengthening or reeducation program.[3] Transcutaneous electrical nerve stimulation (TENS) may be used to assist in pain control in acute injuries.[40] Iontophoresis, the use of a continuous direct current to infiltrate therapeutic medications into tissues, can be helpful in treating local inflammation and scar tissue.[10,25]

Ultrasound has several useful therapeutic effects.[25] It can be used to create heating deep in tissues. Phonophoresis uses the mechanical effects of ultrasound to drive medications, mixed into creams and applied topically, into tissues. This is most commonly used with hydrocortisone for an anti-inflammatory effect. The mechanical effects of ultrasound help decrease tightness in collagen tissue.

EMG biofeedback measures the muscle contraction being performed and allows the athlete to monitor muscle activity during contraction. Additional feedback to the athlete helps the athlete maximize muscle contraction and control during rehabilitation. Several authors have advocated EMG biofeedback to facilitate selective vastus medialis oblique control to enhance patellofemoral stability.[26,44,45,57]

Again, these physical agents are used only as an adjunct to therapeutic exercise in the rehabilitation program. With the exception of basic heat and cold, the treatments discussed should be done only by professionals trained in such application.

Therapeutic Exercise

The most important physical modality used in the rehabilitation of the athlete is therapeutic exercise. No matter what the athlete's level—recreational, fitness, or competitive—anyone trying to resume an active, vigorous activity must, at some point, undergo some active, vigorous retraining. Several points must be considered in designing and implementing a program of therapeutic exercise.

First, and probably most important, the program must be accomplished without persistent symptoms.[30] Increased pain, swelling, limping, instability, or alteration of mechanics signal that the injured part is not able to handle the stresses being applied to it. Using symptoms and functional milestones rather than a timetable as a barometer for progress allows the athlete to be advanced when ready and held back when not ready for more stressful activities. Table 1 illustrates a functional "timetable" for ankle sprain rehabilitation.

TABLE 1. **Sample Rehabilitation Program for Ankle Sprains Based on Symptoms and Functional Milestones**

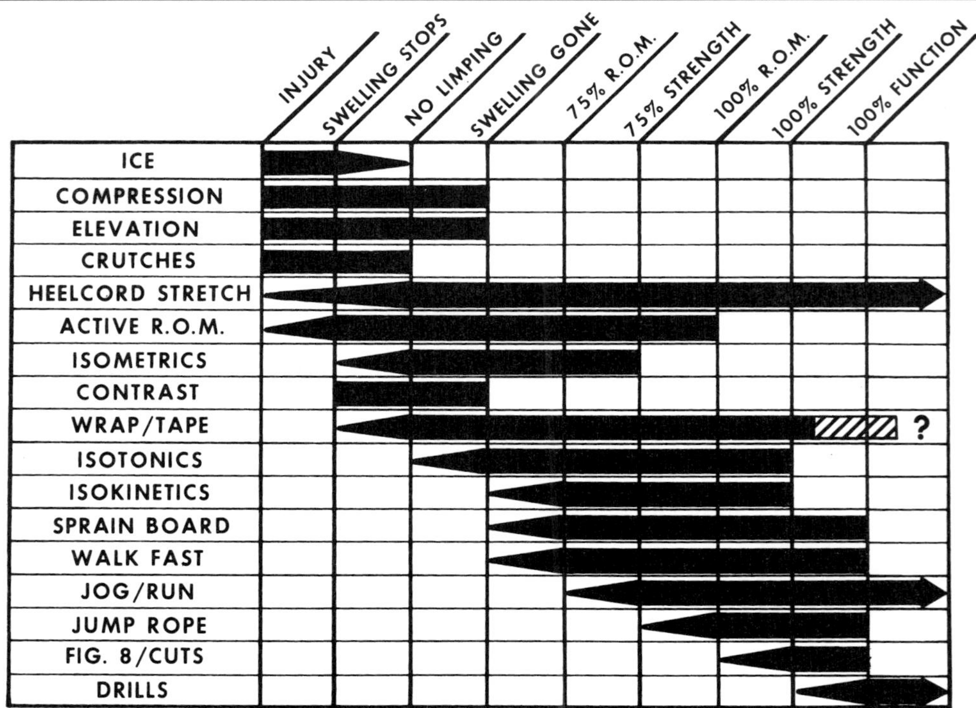

Adapted from Garrick (23).

Second, no "cookbook" program is going to work well for each athlete.[61] Although general treatment goals may be similar for a given injury type, the specific program is based on the goals of the individual athlete. Healing constraints, levels of irritation, progress, and the athlete's tolerance to the exercise program inform the currently appropriate exercise program and readiness of the athlete to be progressed. Knowledge of existing exercise techniques, creativity in modifying old exercises and developing new ones, and knowledge of injury pathology, biomechanics, and kinesiology help the practitioner create a customized exercise program for the athlete.

Third, the exercise program must be realistic but adequate. Very few other than the seriously competitive athlete will devote several hours a day to rehabilitation. All phases of rehabilitation must be addressed, however, or the program will be incomplete and less effective.

Fourth, all components of the exercise program must be goal oriented. Each activity in the program should have a specific reason for inclusion. Extraneous exercises increase the time required to complete the program daily and thus also increase the rate of noncompliance.

Fifth, time must be spent maintaining and improving conditioning in the uninjured areas and the overall fitness of the athlete. A prolonged period of relative inactivity during healing and rehabilitation can cause a significant decline in the athlete's physical condition. Neglecting these components will only increase the time needed to get back to performance levels once healing and injury rehabilitation are complete.

Finally, the athlete must be educated about the various rehabilitation activities. He or she must understand not only the exercise techniques and protocols, but also the rationale for doing the program a certain way. The athlete must be an active participant in the rehabilitation process. If the athlete knows how to monitor progress and problems, then he or she can make some modifications in the program without total dependence on the supervising medical or allied health professional.[46]

Strengthening exercises include isometric, isotonic, and isokinetic techniques. Isometric exercises are muscle contractions against a resistance so that there is no effective joint movement. Resistance can be readily adjusted by altering the effort of the muscle being contracted. These exercises are therefore suitable for strengthening muscles during acute and subacute stages of recovery because additional stress to the injured tissues can be comfortably adjusted by the athlete. Gentle, repetitive isometric contractions around the joint also facilitate the hemodynamic effect around the injury and thus decrease swelling. Isometric strengthening extends about 20° around the specific joint position.[32] A technique known as "multiple angle isometrics," in which isometric exercises are done at about every 20° through the available range of motion, can be used to work on isometric strength through the range while minimizing irritation.[16]

Isotonic exercises[24] are muscle contractions performed against a constant resistance. Resistance is applied with ankle weights, weight machines, free weights, elastic bands, or the athlete's body weight. The speed of the contraction can be varied by the athlete. Variable resistance isotonic exercise is a hybrid of isotonic exercise using exercise machines such as Eagle (Cybex, Ronkonkoma, NY), Body-Masters (Rayne, LA), Nautilus (Nautilus, DeLand, FL), and Universal (Universal Gym Equipment, Cedar Rapids, IA) equipment. The speed of contraction is still varied by the patient, the machine resistance is fixed, but the load experienced by the limb is varied by the use of cams or variable length lever arms. In all modes of isotonic exercise, there is a concentric (or shortening contraction) phase and an eccentric (or lengthening contraction) phase. Eccentric contractions require more muscle energy expenditure, put more stress on the muscle,[21] and are the most important contraction mode for many athletic activities. Various strategies for weight training have been used.[17,33,64]

Isokinetic exercises[24] are muscle contractions against a fixed speed of movement in which the resistance not only varies but accommodates through the range of motion according to the input ability of the musculoskeletal lever system. Examples include Cybex and Orthotron (Cybex, Ronkonkoma, NY), Biodex (Biodex Medical Systems, Shirley, NY), Kin-Com (Chattanooga Group Inc., Chattanooga, TN), and Lido (Loredan Biomedical Inc., West Sacramento, CA). Isokinetics have several advantages over isotonics and isometrics. Isokinetics load the musculoskeletal lever system maximally through the range of motion according to the length-tension relationship of the muscle. Isokinetic resistance also accommodates to pain, fatigue, and other factors that affect muscle force output, and is therefore relatively safe to use after injury. The controlled, faster speeds of movement allow individual muscle training at more functional limb speeds. Equipment cost and availability are two drawbacks to isokinetic exercise.

In any strengthening mode, the muscle must be overloaded in order to strengthen. Overload can be accomplished by increasing the intensity or resistance, increasing the number of repetitions, increasing the frequency of the workouts, increasing the speed of movement, changing the mode of exercise, or a combination of the above.[53] With a healing injury, however, the intensity of the exercise is probably the most critical parameter to control. Too much intensity (resistance) too soon in the healing process is more likely to cause increased symptoms.[36] Therefore, a high-repetition, low-resistance approach is generally used initially.[36,61] Progression to a more traditional low-repetition, high-resistance program is done as symptoms allow.

Additionally, the mode and technique of the exercise may create inappropriate stresses on the healing injury. Modified standard exercise techniques must be made with certain injuries to avoid these stresses or provide appropriate stimulus.[2,20,27,29,61] Careful consideration to and understanding of the specific injury and the associated biomechanics is essential for a safe and tolerable strengthening program. Selected strengthening exercises are illustrated in Figures 2 through 26.

Flexibility exercises are essential to any rehabilitation program. Adequate joint range of motion allows normal kinesiological relationships to occur between limb segments during activity. Good tissue extensibility, especially after surgery, is essential for pain-free tissue excursion during movement. Appropriate musculotendinous flexibility allows more efficient muscle action at extremes, decreases joint compression forces, and decreases musculotendinous overstress.[1,59]

Joint range of motion decreases when injury causes inflammation. Pain causes inhibition of normal muscle function. Swelling increases the pressure within the joint and decreases the ability of the joint to move. Prolonged limitation of motion causes the joint capsule, muscle, and tendon to adaptively shorten and thus further restrict motion. Gentle active range of motion exercises can be started as soon as swelling is under control.[23] Assisted or passive range of motion exercises help to increase range of motion beyond active limits or where active exercises are too uncomfortable. In situations where adaptive shortening has occurred, passive joint mobilization exercises performed by the physical therapist can be helpful.[55] Some of these exercises can be taught to the athlete. In all situations, emphasis must be placed on increasing range of motion gradually without increasing symptoms. In cases of severely restricted range of motion due to adaptive shortening, more vigorous assisted and passive exercises can be done by the physical therapist with appropriate modalities to control symptoms.

Inadequate musculotendinous flexibility is a contributing or causative factor in certain injuries.[1,13,21,44,59,61] Inflexibility increases the force against which antagonistic muscles must contract, thus increasing fatigue and decreasing efficiency of these muscles.[56] Forces in joints, tendons, and other associated structures are also increased by inflexibility, increasing risk of overstress and injury.

Following injury, musculotendinous flexibility decreases due to muscle spasm around the injury, which occur in an effort to protect and guard the injured area. When inflammation or immobilization limits joint range of motion, normal extensibility of the musculotendinous unit cannot be maintained. Gentle stretching exercises are begun as soon as comfortable following an injury. Emphasis is placed on smooth, static stretching technique.[1,4,54] Ballistic or bouncing stretches stimulate the stretch reflex,[21] and the resulting muscle contraction prevents the muscle from elongating. Ballistic stretches may also create undue force on the injured area and increase inflammation. As range of motion increases and inflammation decreases, additional stretching techniques are included for associated and uninjured areas.

The athlete must be taught to stretch properly. Adequate time must be allowed so that the repetitions can be held long enough for the muscles to adapt to a more flexible, elongated position. Although tension must be felt in the intended area, pain should not be experienced. Repetitions must be performed frequently enough to allow lengthening adaptations to develop over time and thus improve flexibility. The specific exercise prescription must be tailored to the individual athlete's own initial level of tightness, specific injury, and tolerance. Anderson[1] illustrates many stretching techniques from which others for the exercise prescription can be modified. This book is an excellent reference for physicians, therapists, and athletes. Figures 27 through 45 illustrate selected flexibility exercises.

Endurance activities should be included in the rehabilitation program as soon as possible following injury.[30] The relative inactivity that occurs during healing and recovery creates significant detraining effects that can decrease performance.[21] Any activity designed to maintain or increase cardiovascular endurance following injury must also avoid any undue stress that might cause reinjury. Bike riding (Fig. 46), single-leg stationary bike riding, upper extremity ergometer training (Fig. 47), swimming, nonweightbearing running in a pool or cross-country skiing may all provide adequate cardiovascular stimulus while altering stresses on an injured lower extremity. Running or riding a stationary bike can provide a similar effect in upper extremity injuries. Again, no symptoms should be created.

Individual muscle endurance also deteriorates following injury. Muscle enzymes decrease with detraining.[21] This inhibits the muscle's ability to use oxygen and to sustain force of contraction. Rehabilitation programs that include a larger number of repetitions at appropriate intensity levels help maintain and regain muscular endurance.

Coordination and agility training is necessary for the athlete to transform the strength, flexibility, and endurance gained into full speed performance

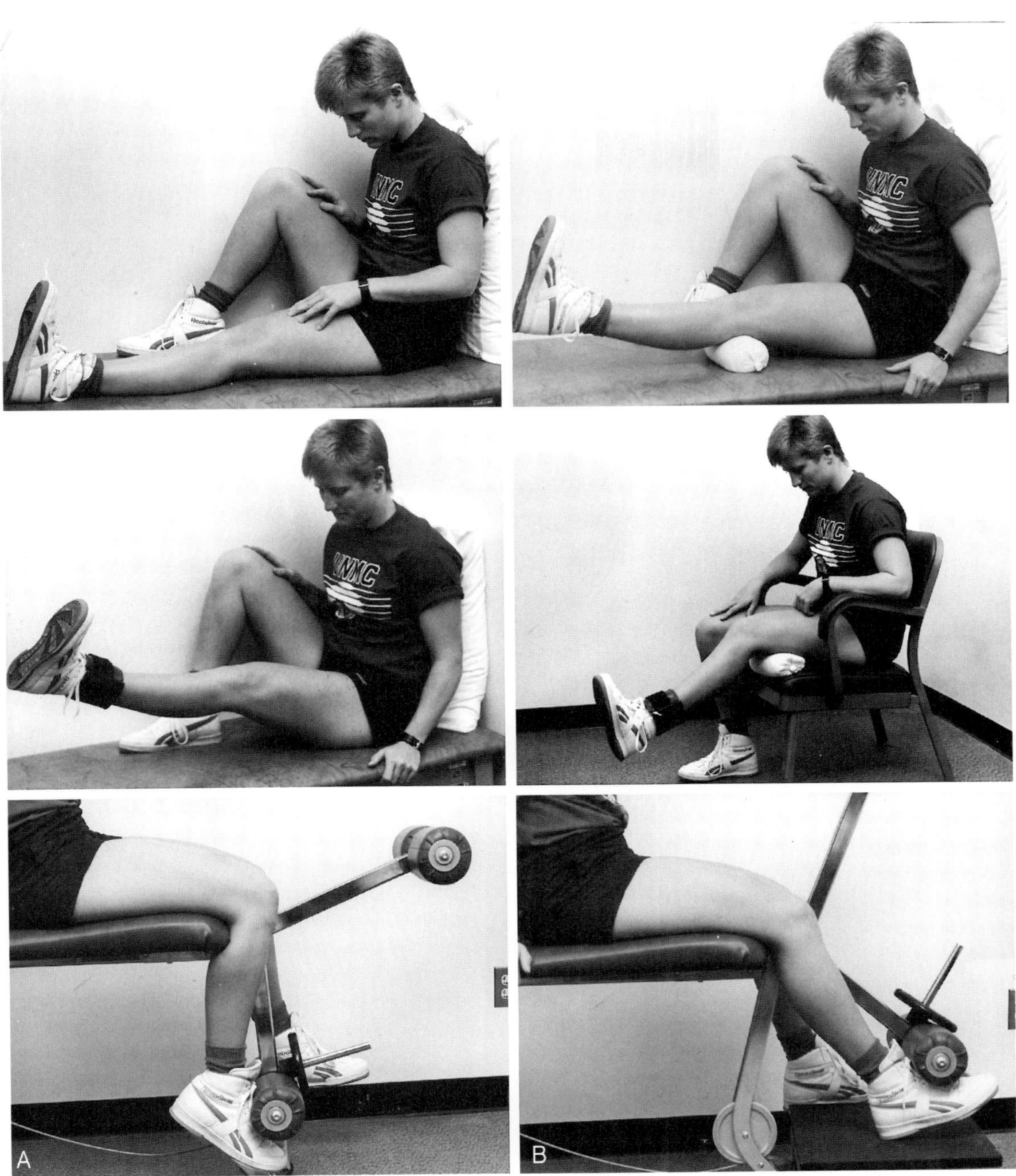

FIGURE 2 (top left). Isometric quadriceps setting. Used in early stage after injury to decrease swelling.

FIGURE 3 (top right). Terminal knee extension. Used in regaining full active knee extension and early quadriceps strengthening. May be done as the initial phase of leg raise.

FIGURE 4 (center left). Straight leg raise with external rotation. Used for quadriceps strengthening. External rotation component used in athletes with patellofemoral problems biases strength toward vastus medialis obliquus (VMO).[61]

FIGURE 5 (center right). Knee extensions with ankle weights. Relatively low intensity exercise but still can cause irritation with patellofemoral problems or acute injuries. Used mostly during intermediate rehabilitation.

Figure 6A (bottom left). Knee extensions on weight machine. Used in advanced rehabilitation. Not a physiologic method of quadriceps strengthening.

FIGURE 6B (bottom right). Knee extensions—45° starting position. Used for quadriceps strengthening. Less pressure on patellofemoral joint than full knee extention techniques in Figures 5 and 6.

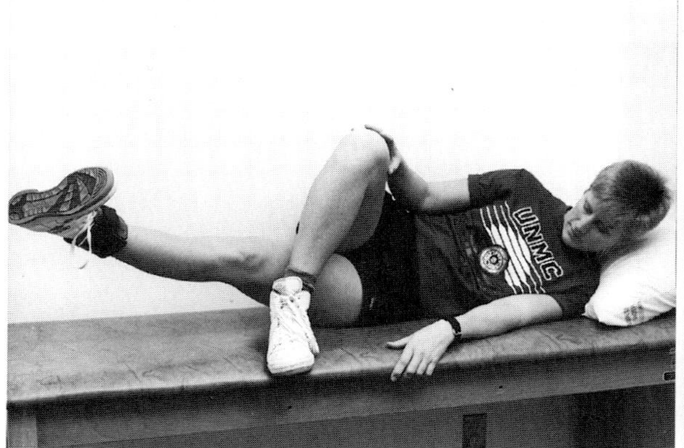

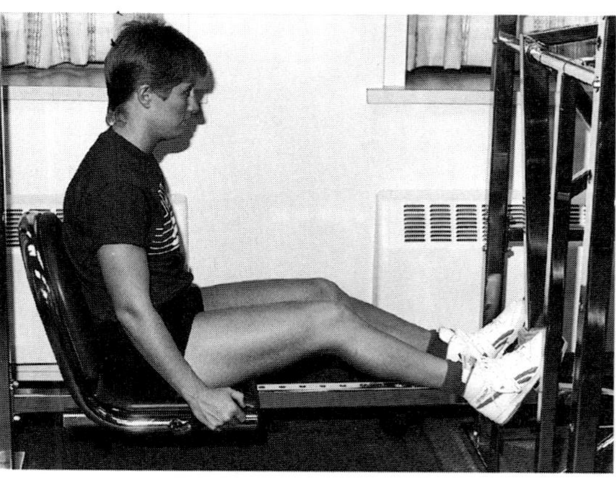

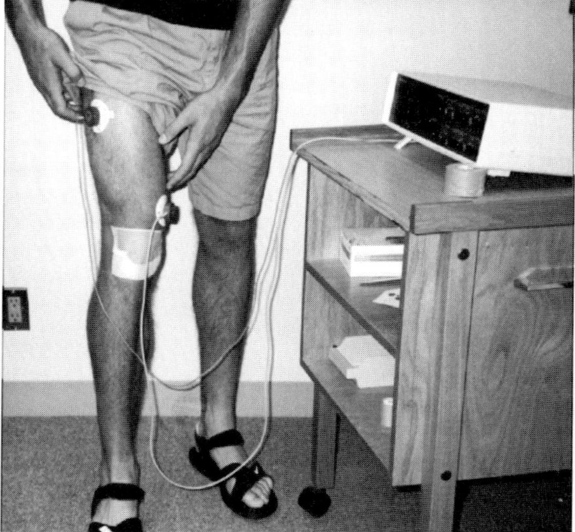

FIGURE 7 (top left). Hip adduction sidelying. With quadriceps set at onset, this can provide additional stimulus to the VMO to improve patellofemoral stability.

FIGURE 8 (top right). Leg press. Closed kinetic chain strengthening for quadriceps and hip extensors. More physiologic method than knee extensions.

FIGURE 9 (left). Mini-lunge or walk-stance with EMG biofeedback for vastus medialis oblique facilitation and patellofemoral taping for stabilizing patellofemoral joint during exercise and functional activity. After McConnell[43–45]

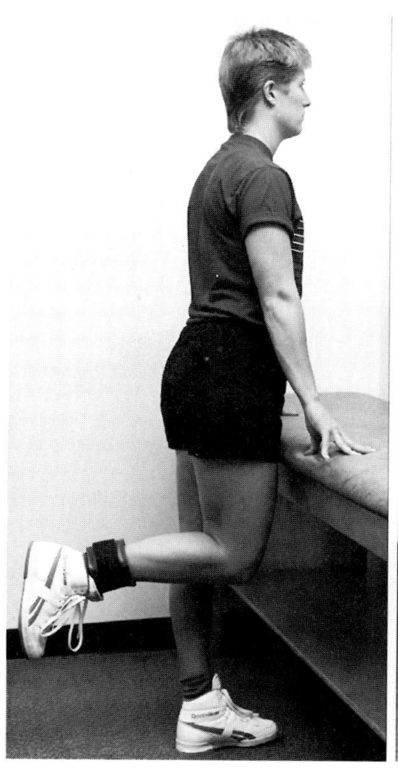

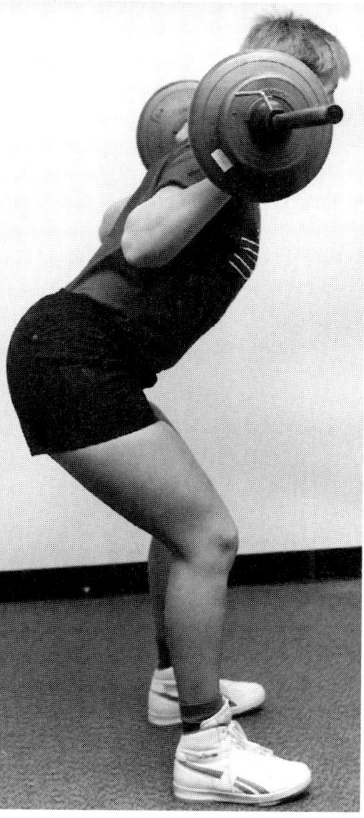

FIGURE 10 (left). Knee curls standing. For hamstring strengthening. May also be done prone on knee curl machine.

FIGURE 11 (right). Mini-squat. Partial depth is preferred over the traditional parallel squat. Keeping shins vertical lessens shear forces at knee. Used in intermediate and advanced phases.[50]

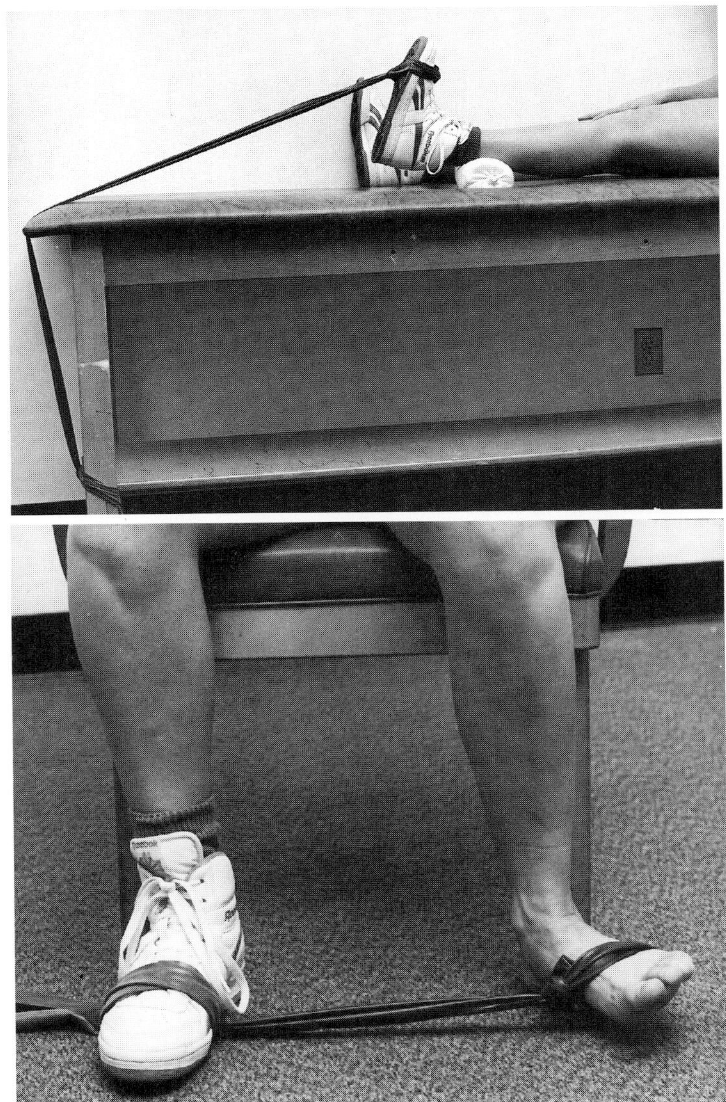

FIGURE 12 (top). Ankle dorsiflexion. Used for ankle rehabilitation. Also helpful for patellar tendinitis when eccentric phase is emphasized.[6]

FIGURE 13 (bottom). Ankle eversion. Used to strengthen dynamic stabilizers with inversion ankle injuries.

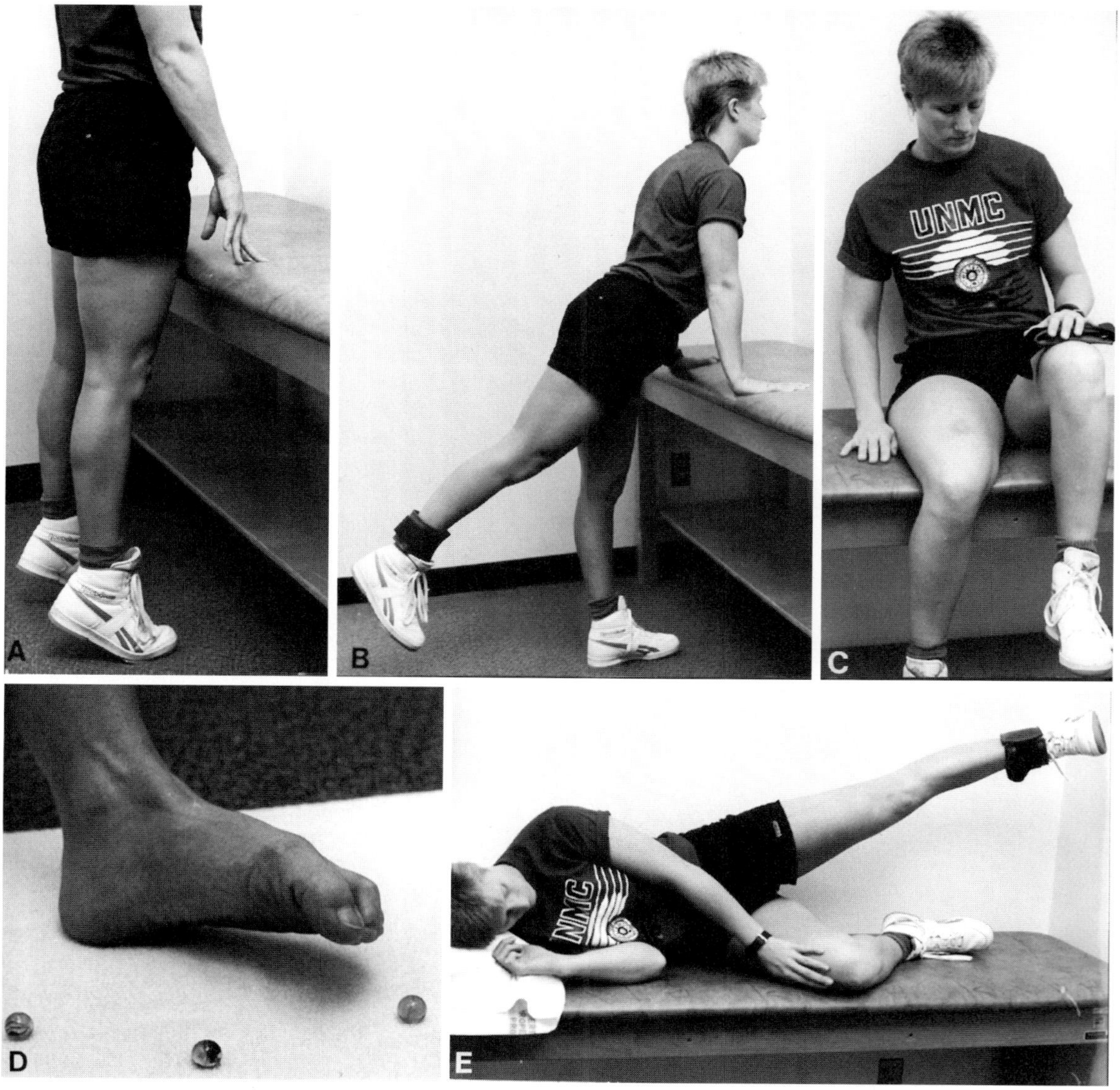

FIGURE 14. *A,* Toe raises. Used to strengthen calf. Start on both legs, progress to only one leg. *B,* Standing hip extension. *C,* Sitting hip flexion. *D,* Toe curls. Marbles or small, smooth stones are grasped by the toes. Used to strengthen foot intrinsic muscles. *E,* Sidelying hip abduction.

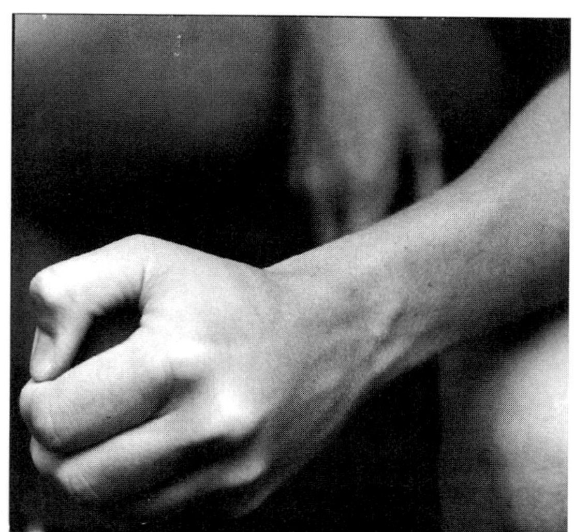

FIGURE 15. Grip strengthening. Used for generalized forearm and hand strengthening. Also helps circulation in upper extremity following injury.

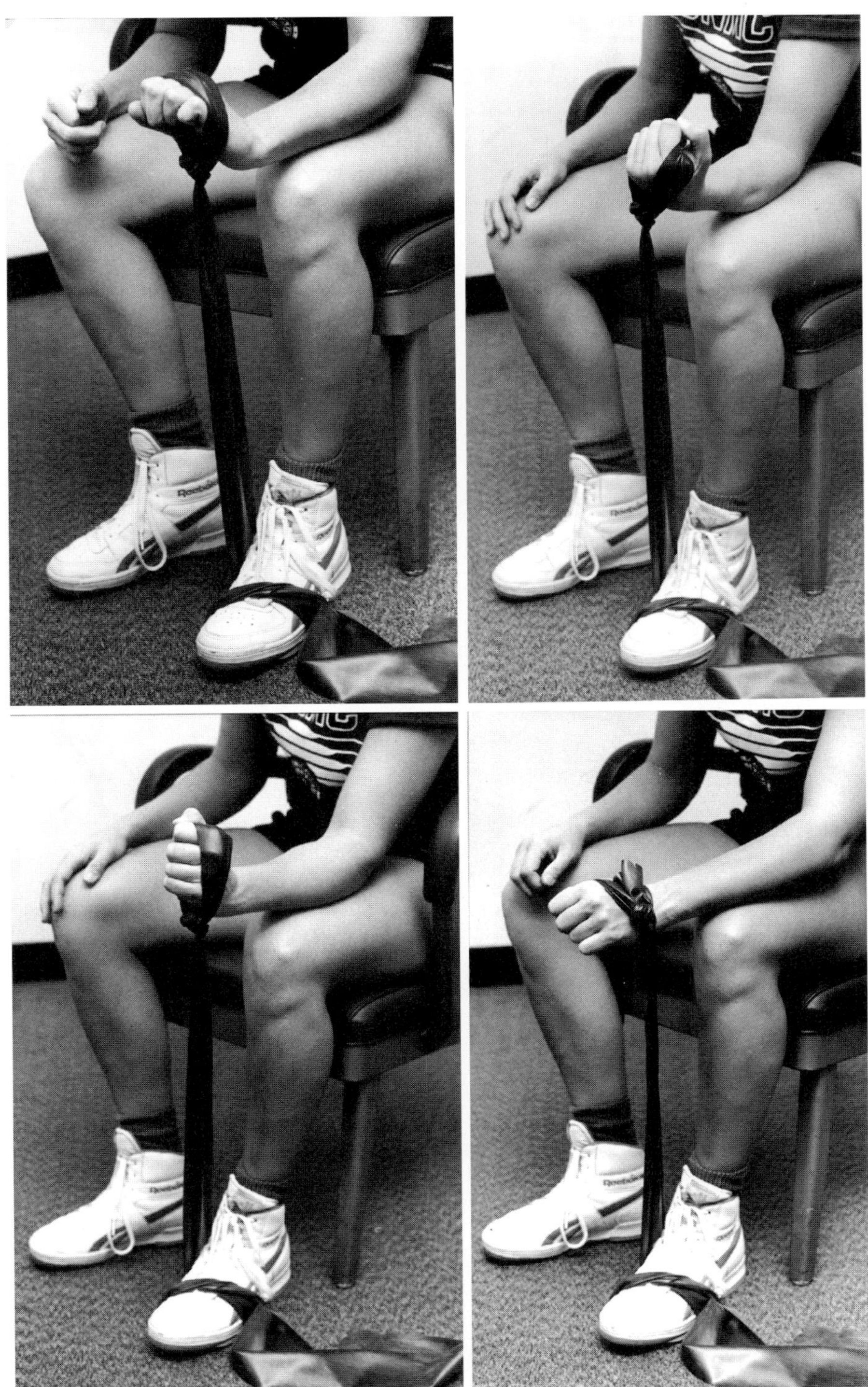

FIGURE 16. Wrist extension ***(top left)*** and flexion ***(top right)*** using elastic band.

FIGURE 17 (bottom left). Wrist radial deviation using elastic band.

FIGURE 18 (bottom right). Forearm pronation using elastic band.

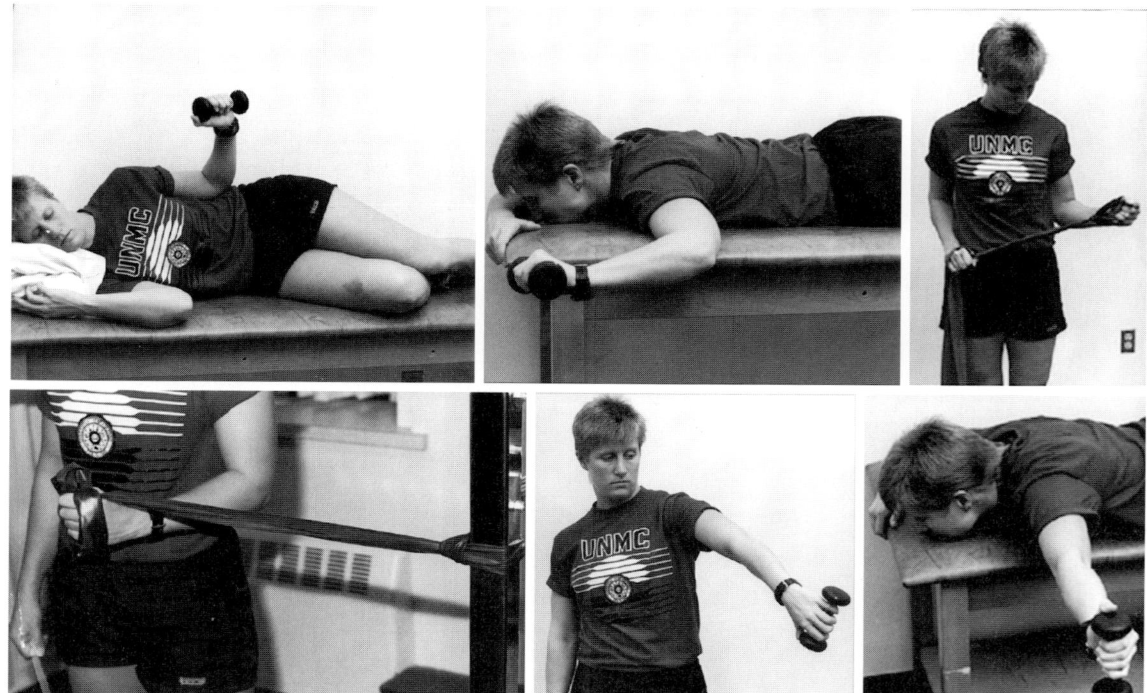

FIGURE 19 (top left). Shoulder external rotation sidelying as suggested by Jobe and Moynes.[27]

FIGURE 20 (top center). Shoulder external rotation prone as suggested by Blackburn.[8]

FIGURE 21 (top right). Standing external rotation using elastic band.

FIGURE 22 (bottom left). Standing internal rotation using elastic band.

FIGURE 23 (bottom center). Isolated strengthening for the supraspinatus as suggested by Jobe and Moynes.[27]

FIGURE 24 (bottom right). Horizontal abduction prone with arm externally rotated for rotator cuff strengthening as suggested by Blackburn.[9]

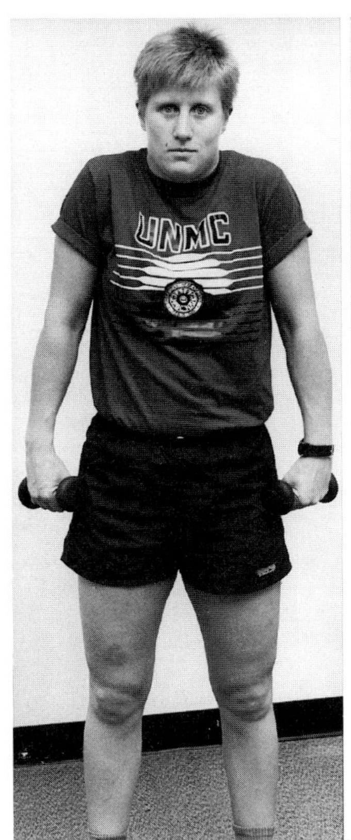

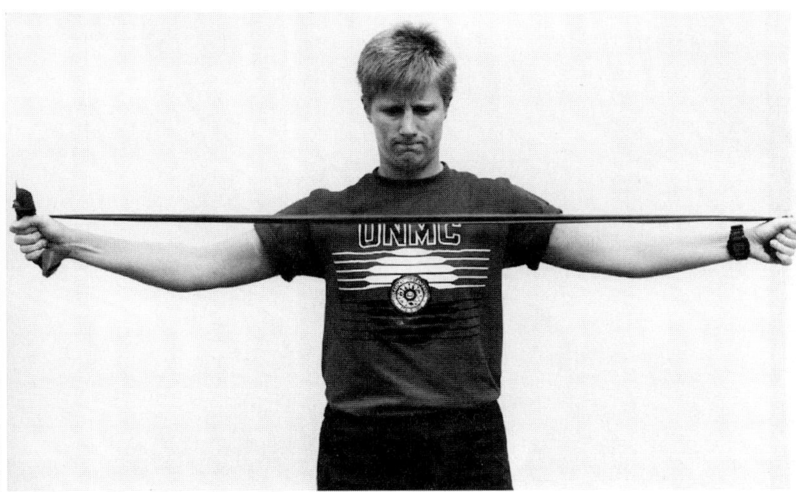

FIGURE 25 (left). Shoulder shrug/scapular adduction for scapulothoracic stability.

FIGURE 26 (right). Scapular adduction with elastic band for scapulothoracic stability.

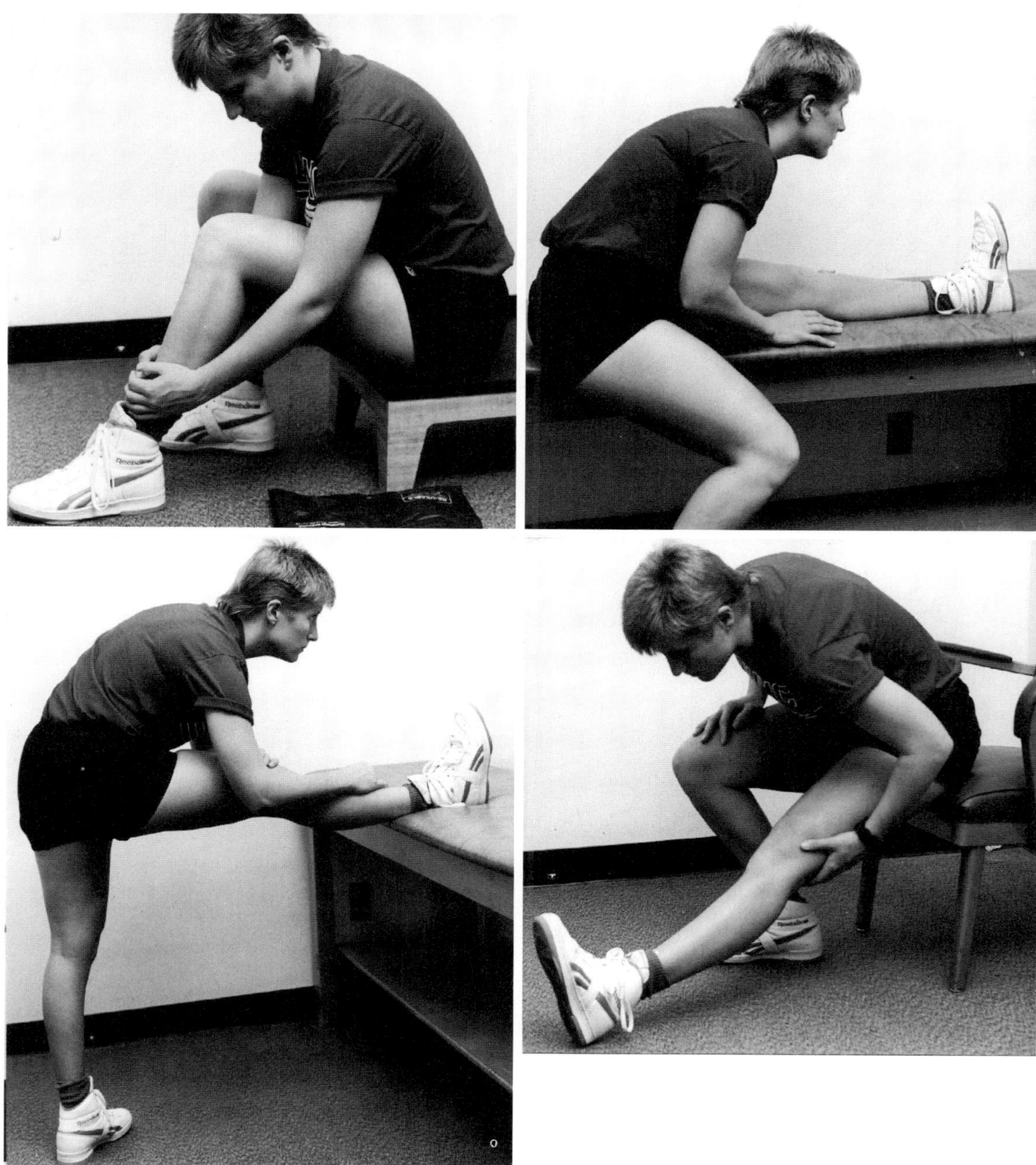

FIGURE 27 (top left). Assisted knee flexion from a low seat. Low seat keeps hip lower than knee and minimizes substitute movement of lifting hip instead of flexing knee.

FIGURE 28 (top right). Hamstring stretching—long sitting at edge of table or couch.

FIGURE 29 (bottom left). Hamstring stretching standing.

FIGURE 30 (bottom right). Hamstring stretching from chair with foot on floor.

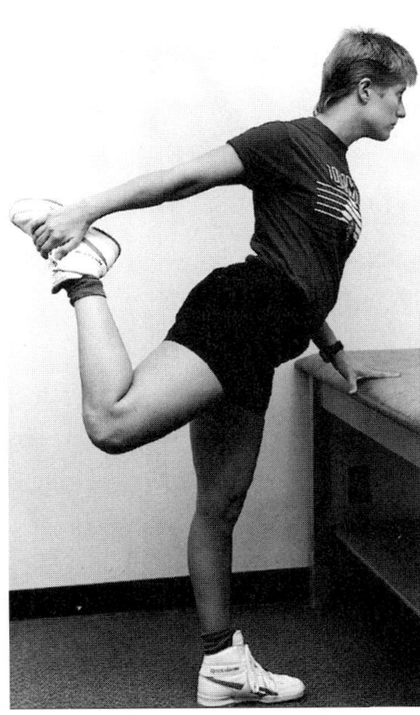

FIGURE 31. Quadriceps stretching. Care should be taken not to acutely flex the knee in athletes with patellofemoral problems.

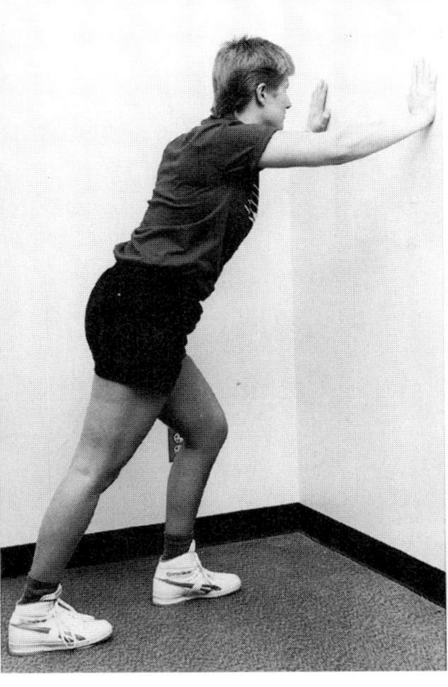

FIGURE 32. Heelcord stretching—knee straight. Used to stretch the gastrocnemius muscle.

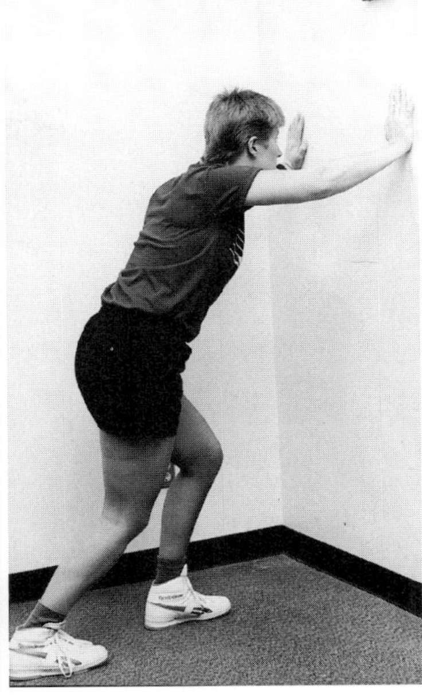

FIGURE 33. Heelcord stretching—knee bent. Used to stretch the soleus muscle and Achilles tendon.

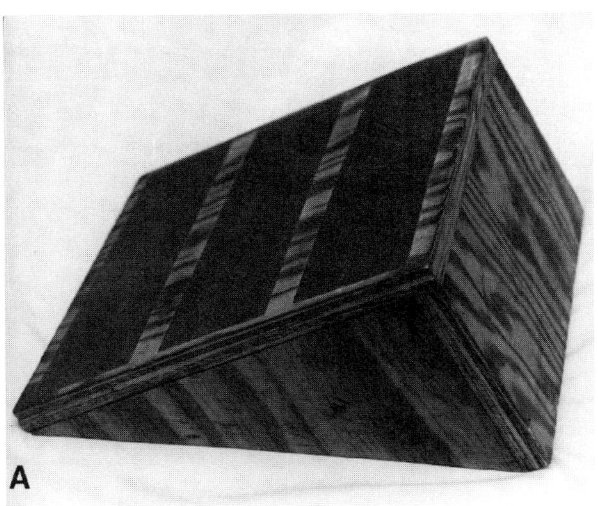

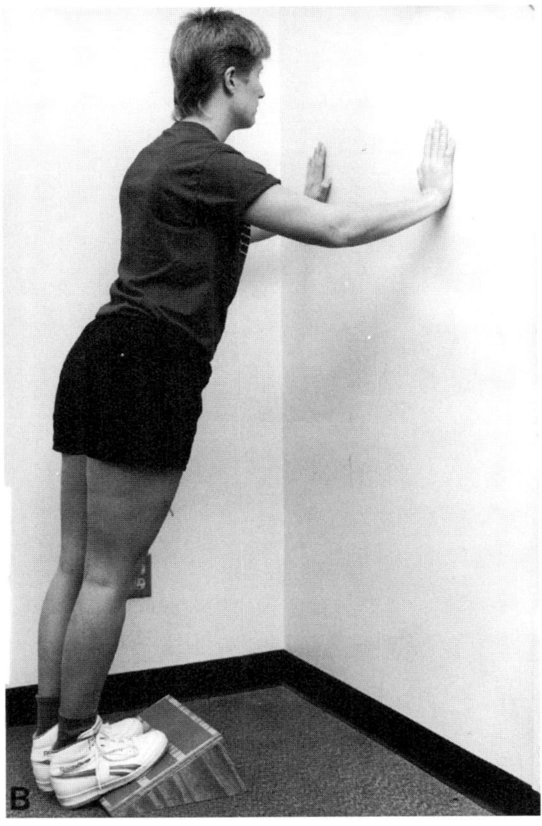

FIGURE 34. *A,* Slant board (12″x12″x6″ high) to increase stretch on calf.[41,42] *B,* Heelcord stretching using slant board.

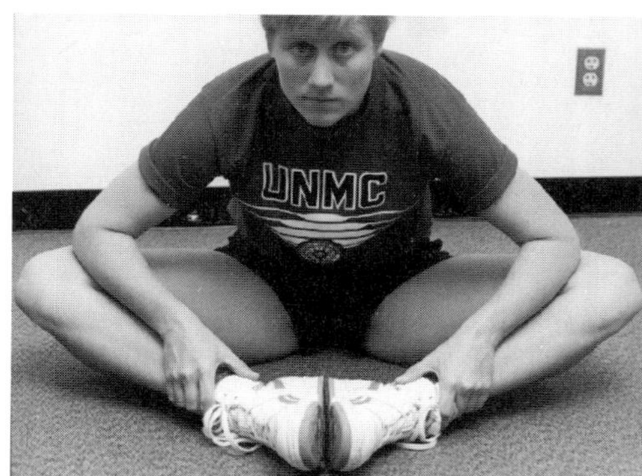

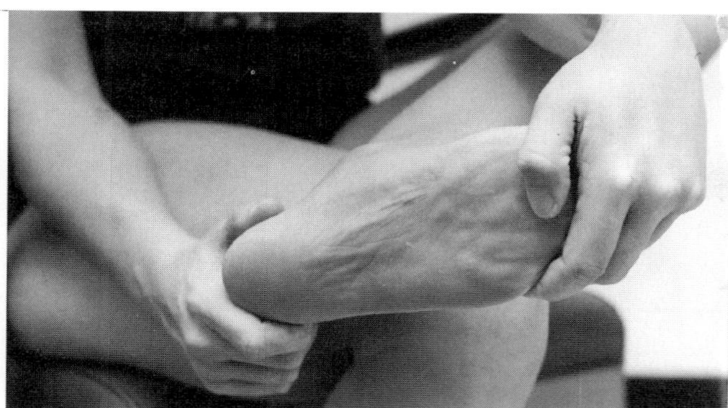

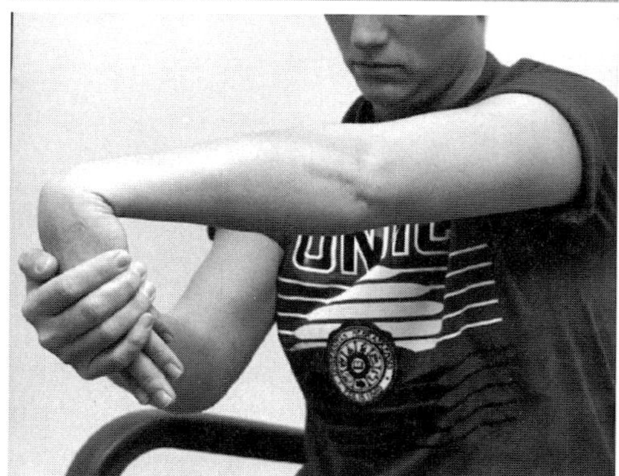

FIGURE 35 (top left). Adductor stretch.

FIGURE 36 (top right). Plantar fascia stretch. Done manually to increase flexibility as a treatment for plantar fascitis.

FIGURE 37 (bottom left). Wrist extensor stretch. Used for lateral epicondylitis.

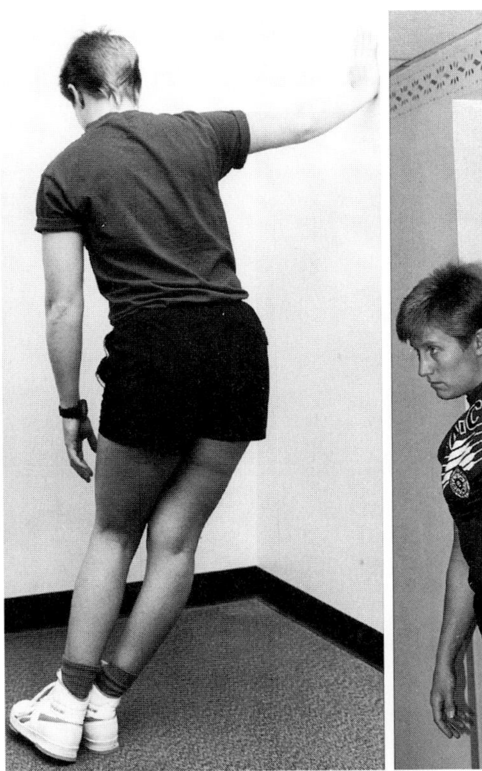

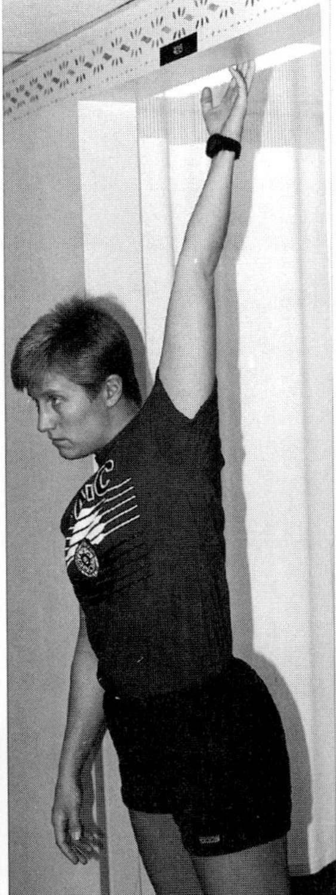

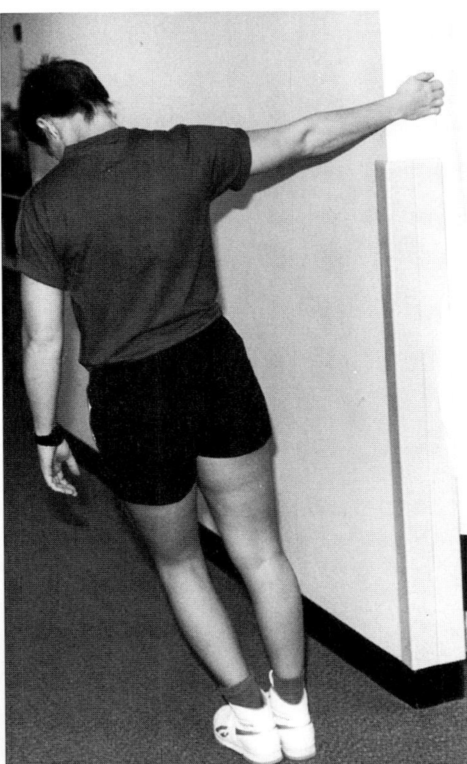

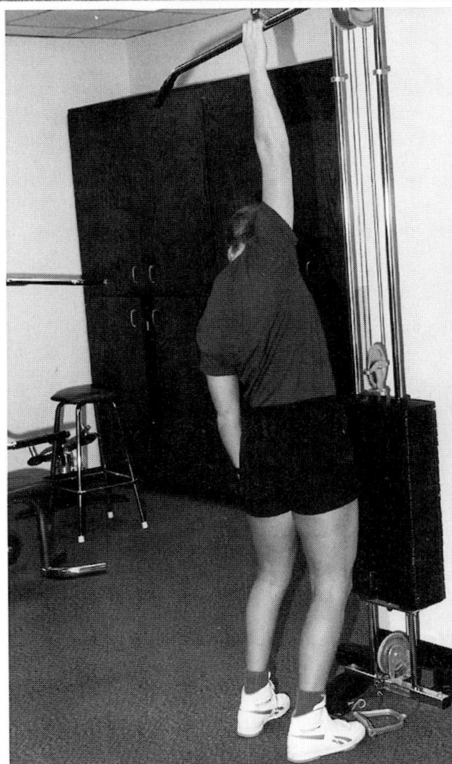

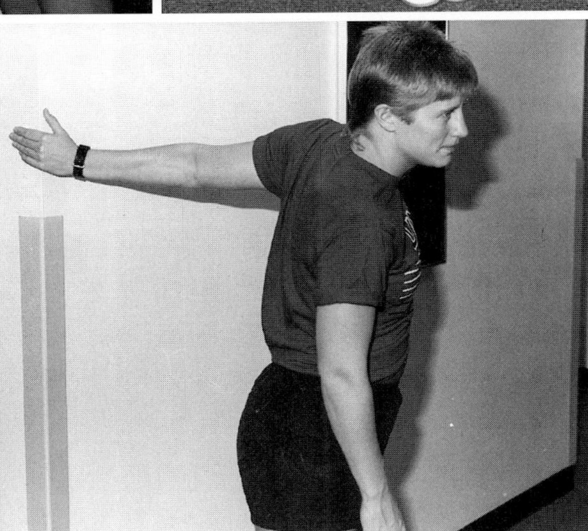

FIGURE 38 (top left). Iliotibial band stretch. Used for iliotibial band friction syndrome.

FIGURE 39 (top center). Shoulder flexion stretch using doorway to anchor hand.

FIGURE 40 (top right). Distraction stretch for glenohumeral joint. Useful as early stretching exercise in impingement syndrome and rotator cuff problems

FIGURE 41 (bottom left). Overhead version of exercise in Fig. 40. This is more advanced technique and should be achieved gradually.

FIGURE 42 (bottom right). Horizontal abduction stretch.

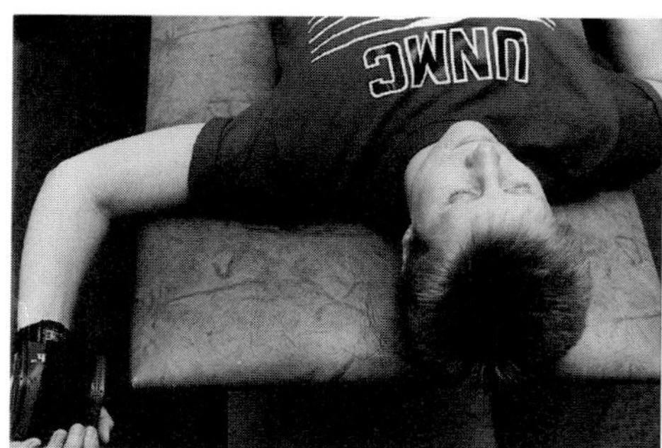

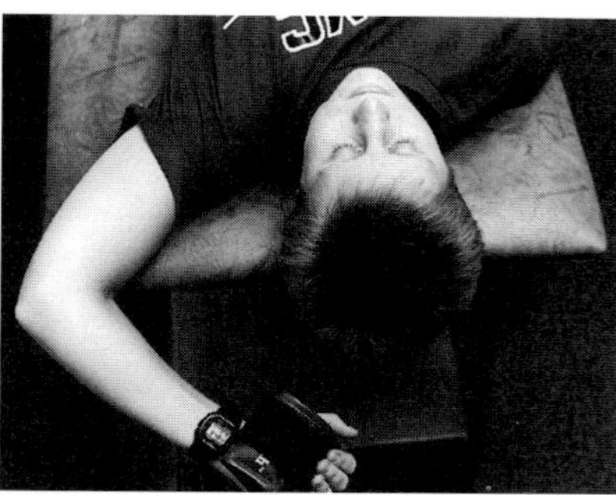

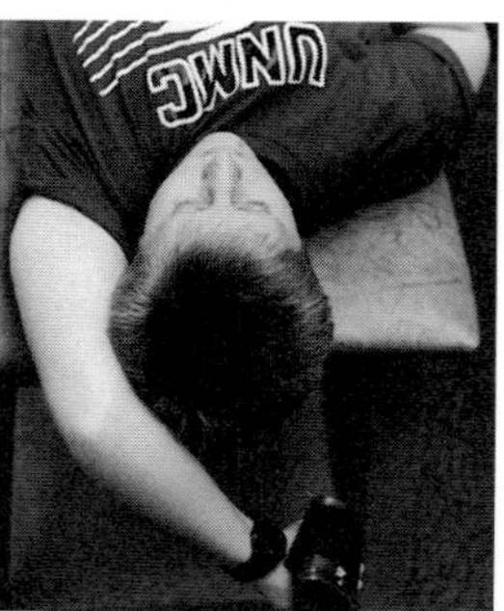

FIGURE 43 (left). Supine external rotation stretch in 90° abduction as suggested by Jobe.[27]

FIGURE 44 (center). Supine external rotation stretch in 135° abduction as suggested by Jobe.[27] Progression of stretch in Fig. 43.

FIGURE 45 (right). Supine external rotation stretch in 180° abduction as suggested by Jobe.[27] Progression of stretch in Fig. 44. Very helpful with shoulder problems in throwing athletes.

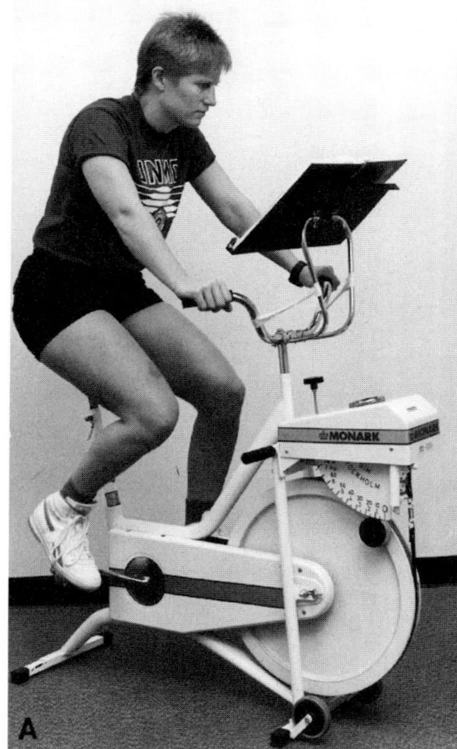

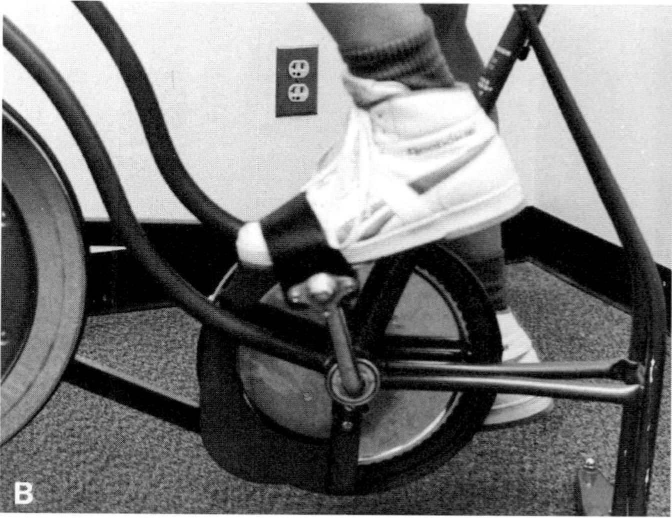

FIGURE 46. *A,* Stationary bicycle riding. Seat height, pedalling resistance, pedalling speed and pedalling phase effort can be adjusted for treatment of various injuries. *B,* Use of toe straps on stationary bicycle to stabilize foot on pedal and facilitate upward pull during the upstroke phase.

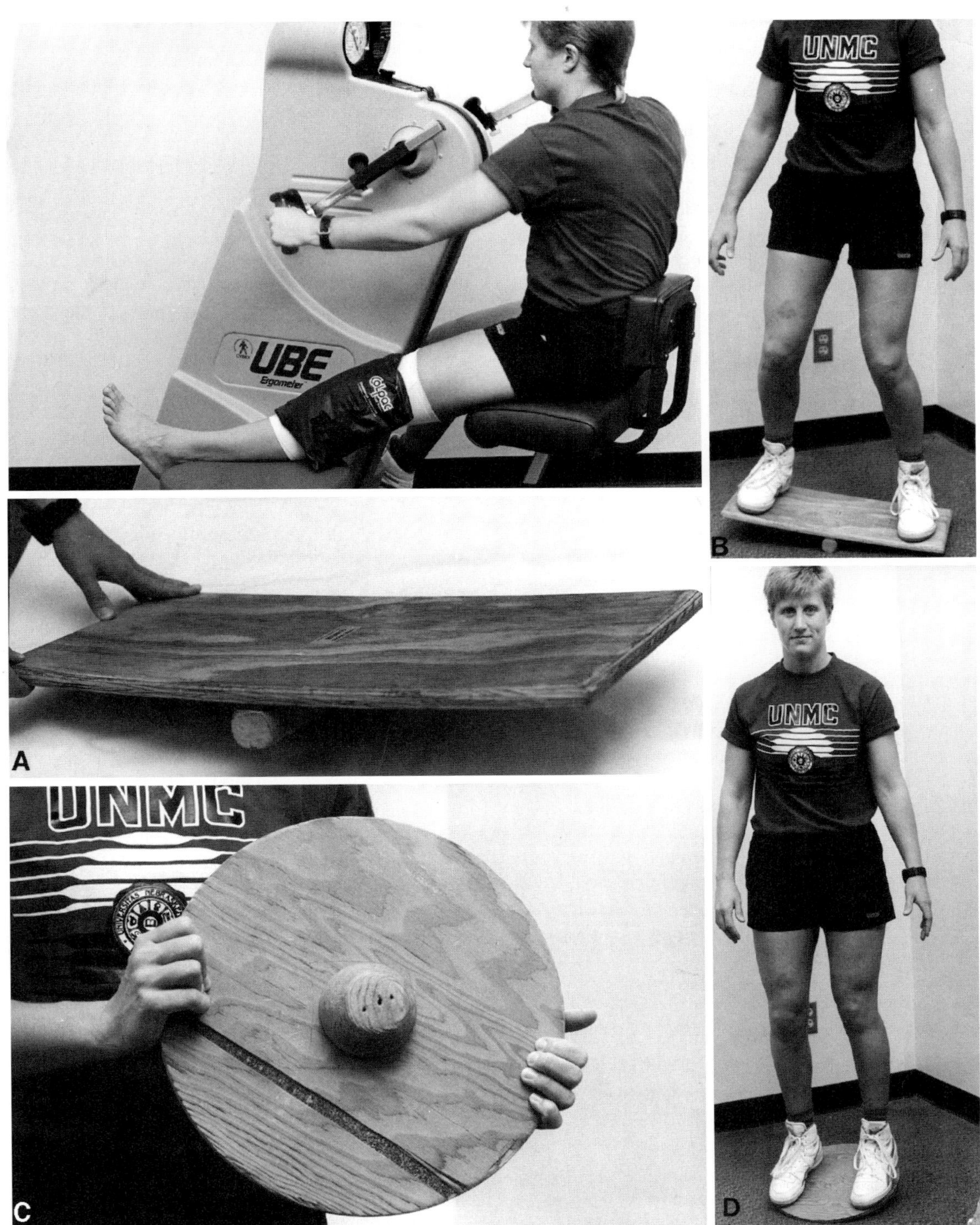

FIGURE 47 (top left). Upper Body Exercise (UBE) Ergometer (Cybex, Ronkonkoma, NY). Used for maintenance of aerobic capacity during rehabilitation and upper extremity endurance training.

FIGURE 48. *A,* Uniaxial balance board (12″x24″ with 2″ tall pivot on bottom). *B,* Uniaxial balance board in use. Foot position can be varied to balance side to side or front to back. *C,* Multiaxial balanace board (15″ diameter with 2″ semi-sphere on bottom). *D,* Multiaxial balance board in use. As balance ability is achieved, the athlete's attention is diverted by playing catch in order to make the reactions more automatic.

skills. Magill[35] states that practice is essential for one to learn skills. Practice variability helps the athlete learn a variety of motor patterns necessary to match the variety of responses a given performance may require.[35] A similar process of skill acquisition is required during rehabilitation as the athlete relearns the skill following injury and detraining.

Tissues that have not been subjected to performance-level stresses for a period of time will be unable to adapt to a sudden resumption of such stresses without risking further injury. Magill[35] states that tasks high in complexity should be practiced in parts rather that as a whole. A gradual progression through increasingly more complex functional activities is advocated by most authors.[7,8,11,12,18,24,28,31,36,40,42–44,52,57,62] Emphasis is placed on proper performance of the skill, no increase in symptoms, and demonstration of confidence with the skill.

Proprioception activities form the basis of coordination and agility activities.[22,39] For lower extremity injuries, bicycling,[47] weight shifting, single leg standing, uniaxial (Fig. 48A and B) and multiaxial (Fig. 48C and D) balance board activities,[22,30,42] and mini-trampoline drills[61] facilitate proprioceptive responses in the rehabilitating limb. For upper extremity injuries, weight bearing through the arms in various positions (sitting pushups, wall pushups, and weighted ball or weighted implement activities are used.[58]

All progressive functional exercise sessions begin with a thorough warm-up program. Warming up consists of getting the blood flowing and stretching all key areas used in the planned activity. Exercise sessions are always concluded with a cool-down session consisting of stretching as above and applying ice to the recovering area to minimize symptoms. The athlete begins with the most basic step in the program, works until achieving the performance criteria, and progresses to the next step *only* in the absence of symptoms. Tables 2 and 3 provide suggested steps of progression for lower and upper extremity injuries respectively.

Protective Equipment

Protective equipment has long been used to prevent injury, and is also essential to help prevent reinjury. Standard protective equipment for a given sport must be adjusted for proper fit. For many recreational sports, the main item of protective equipment is appropriate footwear.

Modified protective equipment may be needed for certain injuries. Additional padding secured inside standard football shoulder pads may provide additional protection for a contusion or acromioclavicular sprain. An oversized football thigh pad may be taped to the thigh to protect a thigh contusion from reinjury in any contact sport.

Special protective equipment includes special padding, taping, and bracing. Virtually any area of the body may be protected from direct contact using either prefabricated or custom-made padding. Taping and bracing are sometimes helpful in limiting extreme motion in an unstable joint. Several authors have advocated taping the patellofemoral joint to promote stability and control pain while progressing with functional rehabilitation.[5,18,43–45,51,57,63] *Taping and bracing should complement the rehabilitation program, however, not substitute for it.*[36,60] There should be a definite need for the supporting device. The specific taping procedure or brace applied should

TABLE 2. Progressive Running Program

Step	Progression Criteria
Bicycle	30 to 45 minutes
Walk	2 miles in 30 minutes or less
Jog	Jog 50 yards, walk 50 yards up to 1/4 mile, increase total distance to 1 mile, then increase jogging and decrease walking until jogging 1 mile straight through.
Run	Increase jogging to 2–4 miles, then increase pace to pre-injury level.
Sprint	Take 10–15 yards to build up to half speed, spring at half speed for 40 yards, take 15–20 yards to slow down and stop. Gradually work from one-half to two-thirds to three-fourths to full speed. Do 10–20 sprints per session.
Figure eight	Gently jog a large (20–30 yard) figure eight. Gradually run the figure eight faster. Then decrease the size of the figure eight by 2–3 yards at a time so that the cutting is progressively sharper. Work down to a 4–5 yard eight. Do 10–20 figure eights in a session.
Basic drills	Work into jumping rope, power jumping activities, stairs, backward running, side-step running, side crossover running, quick starts and stops, cutting, and other basic drill activities important to the athlete's specific sport.
Sports drills	Target these fine-tuning drills to the specific activity the athlete wants to resume.

TABLE 3. Progressive Pitching Program

Step	Progression Criteria
Short toss	Toss ball 10–15 feet for accuracy using good throwing mechanics.
Long toss	Stand in short center field. Throw ball so that it rolls to second base. Then throw so that ball reaches second base in four bounces, then three bounces, then two, and finally one. Use good mechanics and throw for accuracy.
Mound toss	From the mound throw at half speed toward the plate. Emphasize accuracy and mechanics.
Straight throws	Throw straight pitches progressively faster up to three-quarter speed.
Breaking throws	Throw curve and slider pitches progressively faster up to three-quarter speed.
Speed	Increase speed on all pitches toward full speed while maintaining good mechanics and accuracy.
Special pitches	Add any specialty pitches to the program.
Fielding	Work on fielding ground balls and throwing them to various bases from gradually more awkward positions.

provide the desired support[36] and not be just a placebo. Even the simplest wrap or sleeve, however, may provide cutaneous proprioceptive feedback and thus facilitate dynamic stability of the joint.[30]

EVALUATION FOR RETURN TO PARTICIPATION

At some point during the rehabilitation process a decision must be made as to whether the athlete may return to participation. In the situation of the team athlete, various individuals have specific roles in this decision. The physician who provided definitive treatment must make the judgment that adequate healing has taken place. There should be no swelling, pain, or limping.

The team physician, athletic trainer, coach, or the three in some combination must be sure that the athlete is functionally ready to return. Full rehabilitation is the main criterion. Strength is documented through manual[15,38] is isokinetic[16] muscle testing. Flexibility testing and goniometry reveal recovery of mobility. Return of endurance, coordination, and agility is documented by comparing functional and agility tests to preinjury levels. The athlete must then demonstrate full speed performance[18,42] of necessary specific sports skills under the watchful eye of these individuals.

The coach's responsibility is to support the athlete as the athlete works through the rehabilitation process. At no time should the coach try to have the athlete force himself or herself to do an activity beyond what the injury permits.

Finally, the athlete must take an active role in the decision to return to play. The athlete is best aware of how the injured area feels, and should be encouraged to be honest in judging whether the injury is ready. There must not be any lack of confidence on the athlete's part in the performance of his or her skills nor any increase in symptoms after the performance.

Such a team of individuals may not be available to provide guidance to the recreational athlete in deciding when to return to participation. The primary physician and the physical therapist must educate the athlete in the parameters to monitor and guidelines to follow. The recreational athlete must heed this advice and strive to be aware of any symptoms that occur and to be personally honest in dealing with these symptoms.

If there is every *any* doubt as to whether the athlete is ready for participation, then clearance to resume must be withheld until all such doubt is cleared.

GENERAL REHABILITATION PRINCIPLES FOR SPECIFIC INJURY TYPES

Fractures

Early rehabilitation of fractures should always be designed with respect to the type of fracture and method of immobilization or protection. Muscles near the fracture may be exercised only if the risk of disrupting healing is minimal. Fitness of uninjured limbs and the cardiovascular system should be maintained as much as safely possible. Once healing has occurred and immobilization and protection have been discontinued, then specific rehabilitation of the injured limb may be initiated with emphasis on regaining full range of motion and strength lost during healing.

Sprains

Ligament injuries present a challenge to those involved with their rehabilitation. If surgery or immobilization is required, early rehabilitation guidelines used for fractures should be followed. The range of motion and strengthening program should be designed to avoid undue stress on the healing static stabilizers and to not create new symptoms. Strengthening should be maximized in muscles responsible for providing dynamic stability. Coordination and agility activities should focus on helping the entire limb regain synergistic function with the dynamic stabilizers being retrained to help support the joint. Taping or bracing may at times provide additional support, but through rehabilitation provides the quickest and safest return to activity.

Strains and Contusions

Muscle injuries also require thorough rehabilitation before return to play with the least likely risk of reinjury. Stretching exercises should be started gently as soon as possible following injury. Full flexibility must be eventually regained so that the muscle is able to adapt to the extremes of activity. Muscle injuries cause some loss of strength, as does decreased function during healing. Therefore, rehabilitation of the muscle to full strength is essential for full return to activity. With deep contusions, the risk of developing myositis ossificans is always present. Strict adherence to the PRICES principle, cautious use of passive stretching, and conservative progression are the keys to preventing this disabling complication of deep muscle contusions.

Overuse Injuries

Repetitive tissue stress can lead to chronic inflammation and inability to participate in sports. Treatment and rehabilitation seem most effective when multifaceted. Relative rest is essential to control inflammation. Alternate activities provide partial participation to help maintain fitness while decreasing irritating stress. Deep friction massage mechanically increases circulation locally and breaks up scar tissue.[14] Ice helps decrease inflammation. It also provides some analgesia prior to deep friction massage. Anti-inflammatory medication may also be helpful. Injections are rarely used; when they are, they are never given into major load-bearing tendons.

Inflexibility can contribute to musculoskeletal overstress. Therefore, a well-rounded stretching program is an essential part of rehabilitation. Appropriate strengthening helps recondition the total limb and sometimes also helps to correct contributing mechanical faults. Eccentric loading has been reported to be useful in treating tendinitis.[13]

Errors in training and biomechanical faults in performance can contribute to additional stress.[30] These mistakes can be magnified with the high repetition of competitive endurance activities and thus must be identified and corrected. Often a coach or other individual knowledgeable in a particular sports skill is employed to help identify and correct these faults.

SUMMARY

Musculoskeletal injuries are serious in that they can keep the competitive, recreational, or fitness athlete from normal participation. This can have detrimental effects on the athlete's physical and emotional well-being. Therefore, timely and complete rehabilitation is necessary to minimize these detrimental effects.

The PRICES principle is used as first aid in all musculoskeletal injuries. Once a definitive diagnosis is made, a specific course of treatment is initiated. In all forms of treatment, rehabilitative exercises should be started as soon as feasible. As the athlete progresses, presence or absence of symptoms determines the athlete's rate of progress and readiness to return to participation.

REFERENCES

1. Anderson B: Stretching, Bolinas, CA, Shelter Publications, 1980.
2. Antich TJ and Brewster CE: Modification of quadriceps femoris muscle exercises during knee rehabilitation. Phys Ther 66:1246, 1986.
3. Baker LL: Neuromuscular electrical stimulation in the restoration of purposeful limb movements. In Wolf SL (ed): Electrotherapy, New York, Churchill Livingstone, 1981.
4. Beaulieu JE: Developing a stretching program. Physician Sportsmed 9(11):59, 1981.
5. Beckman M, Craig R, Lehman RC: Rehabilitation of patellofemoral dysfunction in the athlete. Clin Sports Med 8:841, 1989.
6. Black JE, Alten SR: How I manage infrapatellar tendinitis. Phys Sportsmed 12(10):86, 1984.
7. Blackburn TA: Rehabilitation of anterior cruciate ligament injuries. Orthop Clin North Am 16:241, 1985.
8. Blackburn TA: The off-season program for the throwing arm. In Zarins B, Andrews JA, Carson WG (eds): Injuries to the Throwing Arm, Philadelphia, W. B. Saunders, 1985.
9. Blackburn TA: Treatment of throwing injuries. Presented at the Cybex Isokinetic Seminar, Las Vegas, NV, October, 1985.
10. Boone DC: Applications of iontophoresis. In Wolf SL (ed): Electrotherapy, New York, Churchill Livingstone, 1981.
11. Brewster CE, Moynes DR, Jobe FW: Rehabilitation for anterior cruciate reconstruction. J Orthop Sports Phys Ther 5(3):121, 1983.
12. Curl WW, Markey KL, and Mitchell WA: Agility training following anterior cruciate ligament reconstruction. Clin Orthop 172:133, 1983.
13. Curwin S, Stanish WD: Tendinitis: Its Etiology and Treatment. Lexington, MA D.C. Heath, 1984.
14. Cyriax J: Textbook of Orthopaedic Medicine. Vol. 1, 8th ed, London, Baillière Tindall, 1982.
15. Daniels L, Worthingham C: Muscle Testing: Techniques of Manual Examination. Philadelphia, W.B. Saunders, 1972.
16. Davies GJ: A Compendium of Isokinetics in Clinical Usage, 2nd ed. La Crosse, WI, S & S Publishers, 1984.

17. DeLorme TL: Restoration of muscle power by heavy resistance exercise. J Bone Joint Surg Am 27A:645, 1945.
18. Doucette SA, Goble EM: The effect of exercise on patellar tracking in lateral patellar compression syndrome. Am J Sports Med 20:434, 1992.
19. Donley PB: Standards of fitness to return to activities for knee injuries. Bull Sports Med, Am Phys Ther Assoc, 4:9, 1974.
20. Einhorn AR: Shoulder rehabilitation: equipment modifications. J Orthop Sports Phys Ther 6:247, 1985.
21. Fox EL, Mathews DK: The Physiologic Basis of Physical Education and Athletics. Philadelphia, Saunders College Publishing, 1981.
22. Freeman MAR, Dean MRE, Hanham IWF.: The etiology and prevention of functional instability of the foot. J Bone Joint Surg 47B:678, 1965.
23. Garrick JG: A practical approach to rehabilitation. Am J Sports Med 9:67, 1981.
24. Gould JA, Davies GJ: Orthopaedic and sports rehabilitation concepts. In Gould JA, Davies GJ (eds): Orthopaedic and Sports Physical Therapy, St. Louis, C. V. Mosby, 1985.
25. Griffen JE, Karselis TC: Physical Agents for Physical Therapists, Springfield, IL, Charles C Thomas, 1982.
26. Jobe FW, Moynes DR: Delineation of diagnostic criteria and a rehabilitation program for rotator cuff injuries. Am J Sports Med 10:336, 1982.
27. Ingersoll CD, Knight KL: Patellar location changes following EMG biofeedback or progressive resistive exercises. Med Sci Sports Exerc 23:1122, 1991.
28. Jones AL: Rehabilitation for anterior instability of the knee: Preliminary report. J Orthop Sports Phys Ther 3:121, 1982.
29. Jurist KA, Otis JC: Anterioposterior tibiofemoral displacements during isometric extension efforts. Am J Sports Med 13(4):254, 1985.
30. Kellett J: Acute soft tissue injuries—a review of the literature. Med Sci Sports Exerc 18:489, 1986.
31. Kerlan R: My bag of tricks for treatment of common throwing shoulder problems. Paper presented at Injuries to the Throwing Arm Meeting, Atlanta, Georgia, February 11, 1983.
32. Knapik JJ, Ramos MV, Wright JE: Non-specific effects of isometric and isokinetic strength training at a particular joint angle. Med Sci Sports Exerc 12:120, 1980.
33. Knight KL: Knee rehabilitation by the daily adjustable progressive resistive exercise technique. Am J Sports Med 7:336, 1980.
34. Lehmann JF, DeLateur BJ: Cryotherapy. In Lehmann JF: Therapeutic Heat and Cold. Baltimore, Williams and Wilkins, 1982.
35. Magill RA: Motor Learning: Concepts & Applications, Dubuque, W. C. Brown, 1980.
36. Malone T, Blackburn TA, Wallace LA: Knee rehabilitation. Phys Ther 60:54 (reprint), 1980.
37. Mannheimer JS, Lampe GN: Clinical Transcutaneous Electrical Nerve Stimulation. Philadelphia, F. A. Davis, 1984.
38. Marino M, Nicholas JA, Gleim GW, et al: The efficacy of manual assessment of muscle strength using a new device. Am J Sports Med 10:360, 1982.
39. Marino M: Current concepts on rehabilitation in sports medicine: Research and clinical interrelationships. In Nicholas JA, Hershman EB (eds): The Lower Extremity and Spine in Sports Medicine, Vol. 1. St. Louis, Mosby, 1986.
40. Markey KL: Rehabilitation of the anterior cruciate deficient knee. Clin Sports Med 4:513, 1985.
41. McCluskey GM, Blackburn TA, Lewis T: Prevention of ankle sprains. Am J Sports Med 4:151, 1976.
42. McCluskey GM, Blackburn TA, Lewis T: A treatment for ankle sprains. Am J Sports Med 4(4):158, 1976.
43. McConnell J: Advanced McConnell Patellofemoral Treatment Plan: Jenny McConnell, Course Notes, Lidcombe NSW, Australia, 1991.
44. McConnell J: The management of chondromalacia: A long-term solution. Aust J Physiother 32:215, 1986.
45. McConnell J: Training the vastus medialis oblique in the management of patellofemoral pain. In Proceedings of the Tenth International Congress of the World Congress of Physical Therapy. Sydney, Australia, May 1987.
46. McKenzie RA: The Lumbar Spine: Mechanical Diagnosis and Therapy. Waikanae, New Zealand, Spinal Publications 1981.
47. McLeod WD, Blackburn TA: Biomechanics of knee rehabilitation with cycling. Am J Sports Med 8:175, 1980.
48. McMaster WC: A literary review on ice therapy in injuries. Am J Sports Med 5:124, 1977.
49. McMaster WC, Liddle S, Waugh TR: Laboratory evaluation of various cold therapy modalities. Am J Sports Med 6:291, 1978.
50. Miller BG: Prophylactic care of the knee. Presented at the Total Care of the Knee Before and After Injury Meeting. Overland Park, Kansas, May 17, 1985.
51. Molnar TJ, Fox JM: Overuse injuries of the knee in basketball. Clin Sports Med 12:349, 1993.
52. Paulos L, Noyes FR, Grood E, Butler DL: Knee rehabilitation after anterior cruciate ligament reconstruction and repair. Am J Sports Med 9:140, 1981.
53. Sanders M, Sanders B: Mobility: active-resistive training. In Gould JA, Davies GJ: Orthopaedic and Sports Physical Therapy. St. Louis, Mosby, 1985.
54. Sapega AA, Quedenfeld TC, Moyer RA, Butler RA: Biophysical factors in range-of-motion exercise. Physician Sportsmed 9(12):57, 1981.
55. Saunders HD: Orthopaedic Physical Therapy: Evaluation and Treatment of Musculoskeletal Disorders, Minneapolis, MN, published by the author, 1982.
56. Sealey DG: Practical considerations in flexibility exercises for knee and lower extremity. In Hunter LY, Funk FJ (eds): Rehabilitation of the injured knee. St. Louis, Mosby, 1984.
57. Shelton GL: Conservative management of patellofemoral dysfunction. Prim Care 19(2):331, 1992.
58. Shelton GL: Rehabilitation of selected shoulder injuries. Presented at the Cybex Isokinetic Seminar, Las Vegas, NV, October 1985.
59. Stone WJ, Kroll WA: Sports Conditioning and Weight Training. Boston, Allyn and Bacon, 1986.
60. Walsh WM, Blackburn TA: Prevention of ankle sprains. Am J Sports Med 5(6):243, 1977.
61. Walsh WM, Huurman WW, Shelton GL: Overuse injuries of the knee and spine in girls' gymnastics. Clin Sports Med 3(4):829, 1984.
62. Yamamoto SK, Hartman CW, Feagin JA, Kimball G: Functional rehabilitation of the knee: A preliminary study. J Sports Med 3(6):288, 1976.
63. Zappala FG, Taffel CB, Scuderi GR: Rehabilitation of patellofemoral joint disorders. Orthop Clin North Am 23:555, 1992.
64. Zinovieff AN: Heavy resistance exercise: The Oxford technique. Br J Phys Med 14:29, 1951.

18

Injuries to the Shoulder and Elbow: Office Evaluation and Treatment

Brian Halpern, M.D.
Brian Incremona, M.D.

Shoulder and elbow injuries are common in athletics today. Although such injuries are not as prevalent as knee injuries, the diagnosis of the problem often leaves the examiner more perplexed. In an examination of a patient who complains of "generalized shoulder pain," the first step toward making a diagnosis is to determine, by history, whether the injury was of the contact or noncontact type. Following this determination, the key to the diagnosis usually lies in the physical examination.

Most complaints are categorized as bursitis or tendinitis and treated as such; yet, the true anatomy and cause of the problem may not be known to the examiner. For this reason, many cases often become recalcitrant or recurrent. Most injuries to the shoulder are soft tissue injuries; therefore, that kind is emphasized in this discussion. Soft tissue injuries occur in the musculotendinous units of the shoulder and elbow. Many times these injuries occur from overuse and poor biomechanics, especially in the case of the throwing athlete. Although professional baseball players, swimmers, and golfers can be afflicted with these syndromes, the recreational athlete is the patient more often encountered. Such patients complain of soreness, mostly from the inflammatory response to repeated microtrauma to the musculotendinous units.

Injuries diagnosed early usually respond well to rest, antiinflammatory medications, stretching and strengthening exercises, and other therapeutic modalities. As an injury becomes chronic, however, weakness and progressive loss of function may be detected. Making an early, accurate diagnosis and initiating treatment based on biomechanics is imperative.

SHOULDER INJURIES

History and Physical Examination

As always, the examiner must begin with the history. Has the patient suffered a traumatic injury that precipitated with pain? The pain pattern, character, duration, and eliciting factors of the injury need to be assessed. A dull, aching discomfort, often felt at night, corresponds with rotator cuff tears, whereas a stabbing, burning pain is more typical of bursitis or tendinitis.

Location of the pain can be helpful in making the diagnosis. Pain over the acromioclavicular joint might suggest degenerative disease, or, if associated with trauma, an acromioclavicular joint sprain may be suspected. Pain deep in the shoulder may come from rotator cuff involvement, synovitis, or a glenoid labrum tear.

A popping or catching noise inside the joint often indicates a glenoid labrum tear.[3] A history of the shoulder's "giving way" or "going out" suggests subluxation or dislocation of the joint. Disclocation is more commonly caused by a contact injury, but subluxation anteriorly or posteriorly can be caused by contact or noncontact injuries. If the stability of the shoulder is affected by either trauma or fatigue, then intraarticular structures such as the labrum may have been torn by traction of the biceps tendon or impingement between the humeral head and glenoid cavity. These types of injuries often result from a combination of acceleration and deceleration forces and internal and external rotation velocities of the humerus.[22] Therefore, it is essential to question the patient as to the phase of the throwing motion (windup, cocking, acceleration, release and deceleration, or follow-through) during which the symptoms occur.

Although the history is often helpful, a definitive diagnosis usually results from the physical examination. Begin with an anterior inspection of both clavicles and the acromioclavicular joints. The uninjured shoulder must always be examined as a "normal" comparison. Look by asymmetry, ecchymosis, swelling, and atrophy.

Palpate over the acromioclavicular joint for pain, crepitus, and instability. Test the stability of the clavicle by pushing down on its distal one-third. Dislocation of this joint can occur in the anterior, posterior, or superior direction. Perform a crossover test by having the patient place the hand of the involved shoulder onto the opposite, uninjured shoulder (Fig. 1). If the patient can perform this maneuver with minimal or no pain, a grade I sprain is probably indicated. If the motion is painful but the patient can resist pressure when the examiner pushes the elbow toward the torso from this flexed position, a grade II sprain is probably indicated. If the patient cannot resist pressure on the elbow at all, a grade III sprain is indicated.[13] Next, inspect and palpate the three posterior rotator cuff muscles (supraspinatus, infraspinatus, and teres minor). Note also the trapezius and latissimus dorsi, which accentuate the rotator cuff. Have the patient push against a wall, and note any winging of the scapula, which signifies possible injury to the long thoracic nerve or scapular stabilizing muscles.

Assess the patient's range of motion beginning with abduction. This motion occurs with glenohumeral and scapulothoracic movement in a 2:1 ratio. For every 3 degrees of shoulder abduction that occur, 2 degrees occur at the glenohumeral joint and 1 degree occurs at the scapulothoracic joint.[17] Check internal and external rotation in the sitting and supine positions with varying degrees of abduction. Also assess the shoulder in adduction, flexion, and extension.

The lateral slide measurement test may be used to assess the functional integrity of the scapular stabilizing musculature. Dysfunction of these muscles has been implicated in the pathophysiologic mechanism of shoulder pain in the throwing athlete. Measurements are taken from the spine to the medial border of the scapula, bilaterally, with the arms in three positions. The first is taken with the arms in neutral rotation, resting at the sides. The second is taken with the hands on the hips, thumbs posteriorly. In the third position, the arms are abducted to 90 degrees with maximal internal rotation. A difference of greater than 1 cm is often found in the second and third positions in athletes with shoulder pain or dysfunction.[21]

To test for anterior instability of the shoulder, perform the apprehension test. With the patient's elbow in 90 degrees of flexion and the humerus in 5 degrees of extension, externally rotate the humerous at 45 degrees, 90 degrees, and 135 degrees of abduction while simultaneously applying downward and forward pressure on the humeral head (Fig. 2).[12] This test stresses the subscapularis, coracohumeral ligament, middle glenohumeral ligament, and inferior glenohumeral ligament.[10] Pain and apprehension constitute a positive test. Relief of this discomfort by application of a direct posterior force on the humeral head is known as the relocation test.[20] A positive test correlates with anterior instability, suggesting subluxation or prior dislocation.

Additional instability testing is done with the patient supine and performance of the anterior drawer test. To test the left shoulder, the patient's left hand

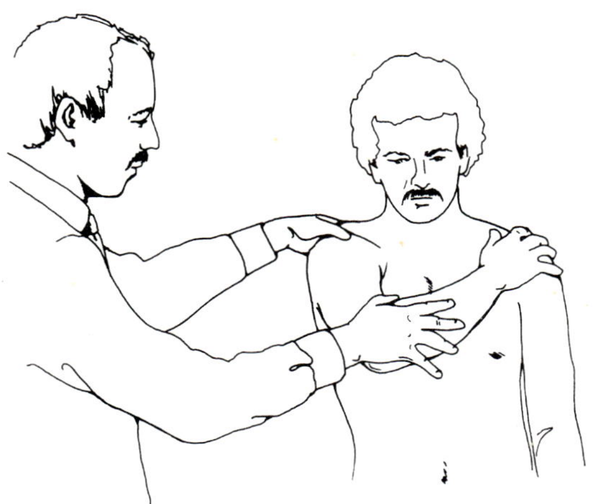

FIGURE 1. Crossover test. Testing for a sprain of the acromioclavicular joint.

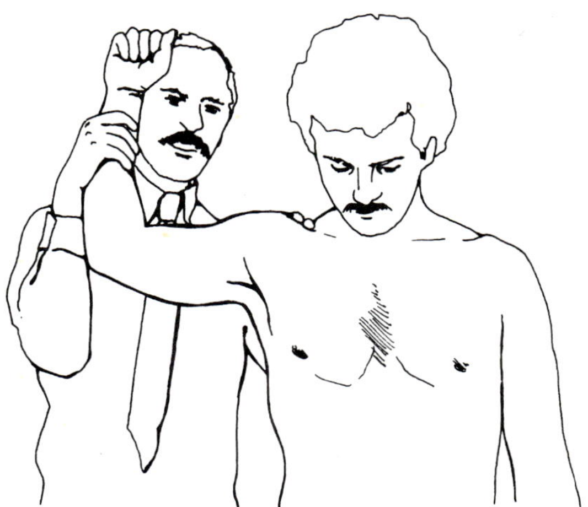

FIGURE 2. Apprehension test. Testing for anterior stability.

is secured under the examiner's right axilla. The examiner's left hand grasps the patient's scapula, pressing the scapular spine forward with the fingers while exerting counterpressure with the thumb over the coracoid process. The shoulder is held in 80–120 degrees of abduction, 0–20 degrees of forward flexion, and 0–30 degrees of external rotation. With the right hand, the examiner grasps the patient's humerus below the humeral head and draws it anteriorly. The anterior displacement of the humerus over the fixed scapula is noted and compared with the opposite shoulder. An occasional audible click may be elicited by this maneuver, usually indicating labral abnormality. In posttraumatic cases, abduction to greater than 120 degrees may be necessary to appreciate a positive sign.

Gerber and Ganz found the anterior apprehension test to be more sensitive in this situation.[12] Laxity may be graded from 1+ to 3+. Anterior and posterior translation of the humeral head further than the opposite shoulder but not beyond the glenoid rim constitute a 1+ instability. In 2+ instability, the examiner is able to pass the humeral head over the glenoid rim. In 3+ instability, the humeral head can be locked over the glenoid rim.[2]

Another variation of instability testing is the load and shift test. With the patient in the supine position, a gentle load is applied to the humeral head to ensure concentric reduction in the glenoid fossa. The head is then stressed anteriorly and posteriorly from a neutral position. Additional load can be applied with varying degrees of internal and external rotation (Fig. 3).[1]

The posterior apprehension test is performed by positioning the affected shoulder in 90 degrees of forward flexion and 90 degrees of internal rotation with the elbow flexed to 90 degrees. A posterior force is applied from the elbow down the shaft of the humerus. As in the anterior apprehension test, pain and apprehension constitute a positive test. This test is probably not as consistent in diagnosis of posterior instability as the posterior drawer test is.[9]

To perform the posterior drawer test, have the patient lie supine. To test the left shoulder, the proximal forearm of the patient is grasped in the examiner's left hand. The elbow is flexed to 120 degrees. The shoulder is held in 80–120 degrees of abduction and 20–30 degrees of forward flexion. With the right hand, the examiner grasps the scapula, placing the fingers over the spine and the thumb just lateral to the coracoid process. The humerus is rotated medially from 60 degrees to 80 degrees of flexion. Posterior displacement of the humerus causes the humeral head to contact the fingers of the examiner's right hand while the thumb glides past the coracoid process. A positive test is frequently accompanied by apprehension.[12] Posterior laxity is often a normal finding in a throwing athlete's shoulder.[3]

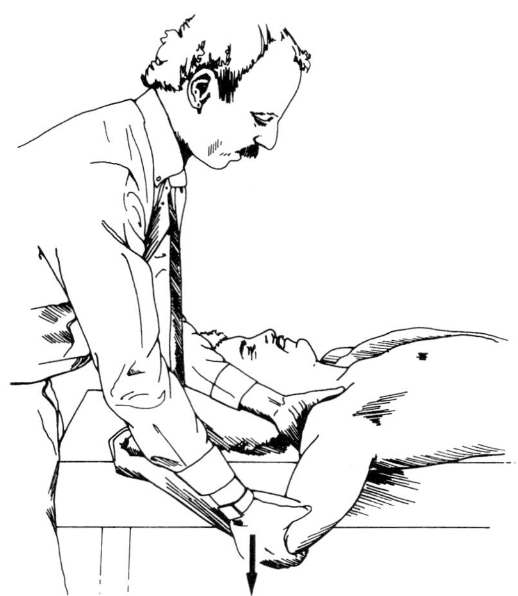

FIGURE 3. Testing for anterior subluxation.

Inferior instability is tested by applying gentle traction to the relaxed upper arm with the patient seated and the shoulder in the neutral and adducted position. Inferior displacement of the humeral head produces the appearance of a sulcus sign in the subacromial region, which can be graded as follows: grade I, less than 5 mm of inferior translation of the humeral head; grade II, 5–10 mm of inferior translation of the humeral head; grade III, greater than 10 mm of inferior translation of the humeral head. It is most commonly present in multidirectional instability.[12,24] The test stresses primarily the superior glenohumeral ligament; however, it is important to realize that with shoulder abduction beyond 45 degrees, the inferior glenohumeral ligament becomes the primary stabilizer.[40]

Injuries to the rotator cuff are best assessed by applying a downward force to the shoulder at 90 degrees of abduction, 30 degrees of forward flexion, and full internal rotation (Fig. 4). Weakness or pain can indicate injury to the supraspinatus muscle or the suprascapular nerve.[3] Test for strength of the subscapularis muscle by having the patient resist internal rotation with maximum adduction of the arm (Fig. 5). Having the patient resist external rotation with maximum adduction of the arm tests the strength of the infraspinatus and teres minor muscle (Fig. 6).

An impingement test is positive when pain is elicited by internal rotation of the humerus in the forward-flexed position (Fig. 7).[14,24] This maneuver tends to drive the greater tuberosity under the coracoacromial arch. Test for "painful arc" of abduction by having the patient slowly abduct the arm

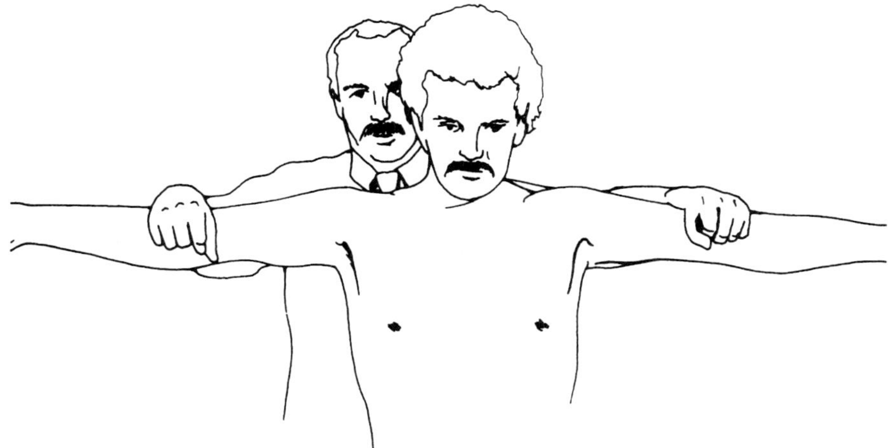

FIGURE 4. Supraspinatus test. Testing for strength of the supraspinatus and deltoid muscles.

from 70 degrees to 120 degrees of abduction. Discomfort during the action suggests rotator cuff inflammation. Slight resistance against this motion may augment the discomfort. Occasionally, the arm may give way or drop at midrange. This is known as the drop arm test.[27] As this syndrome progresses, refractory tendinitis, wearing the supraspinatus and biceps tendon, and partial- or complete-thickness rotator cuff tears can occur.[15]

Thrower's shoulder is also prone to glenoid labrum tears, specifically the anterosuperior portion of the labrum. This lesion is diagnosed by the clunk test, or labral grind test.[3] The examiner places one hand posterior to the humeral head while the other hand rotates the humerus. The arm is brought into full overhead abduction while providing an anterior force to the humeral head. The clunk test is positive when a clunk or grind is felt at the shoulder as the humerus comes into contact with the labral tear (Fig. 8).[3]

The long head of the biceps can be palpated in the bicipital groove. It is best appreciated with the arm in adduction and 15 degrees of external rotation. Tenderness over this area may indicate the presence of inflammation, whether from isolated tenosynovitis or in association with impingement. Resisted forward flexion of the humerus with the elbow extended is known as a straight arm–raising test. Pain elicited with this maneuver, as well as with resisted supination, is suggestive of bicipital tendinitis.[14] Patients with chronic symptoms of subacromial impingement and bicipital tendinitis are susceptible to rupture of the long head of the biceps.[24] By external rotation of the humerus in the adducted position, the subscapularis tendon can be palpated. Similarly, by internal rotation of the humerus, the supraspinatus tendon can be palpated for tenderness.

A radiographic examination of the shoulder should include an anteroposterior (AP) view in internal and external rotation and an axillary or transthoracic view. The AP internal rotation view allows the best visualization of a Hill-Sachs compression fracture of the posterolateral humeral head, seen after anterior dislocation.[27,29] The AP external rotation view is best in order to appreciate cystic or sclerotic changes of the humeral head, as well as osteopenia.[27] These AP views may also reveal (1) ectopic calcifications adjacent to the humeral head, indicating the presence of calcific tendinitis, or (2) a decrease in the acromiohumeral space, indicating the presence of a rotator cuff tear or impingement.

Magnetic resonance imaging is a more sensitive means of detecting tendinitis and tears. It is also useful in detecting bursal fluid and defects in the labral cartilage. For evaluation of impingement, the Neer view will help to detect a hooked acromion or a subacromial spur not visualized on routine AP

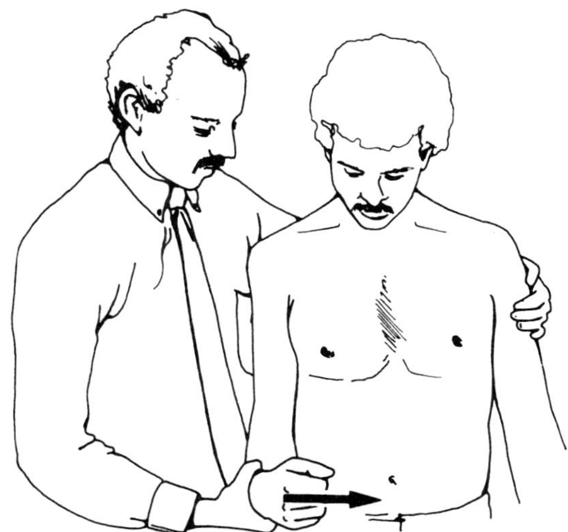

FIGURE 5. Testing for strength of the subscapularis muscle.

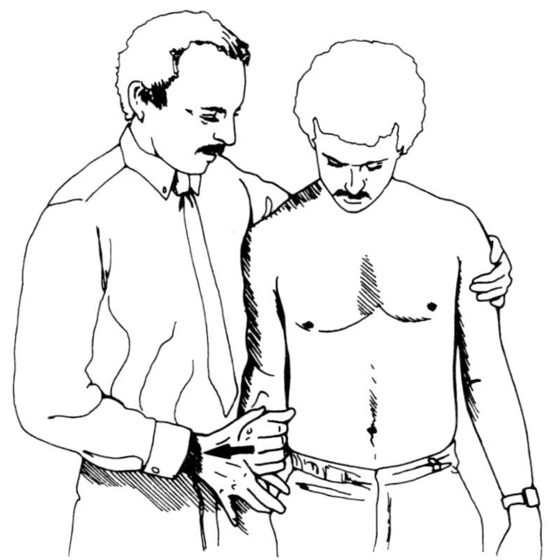

FIGURE 6. Testing for strength of the infraspinatus and teres minor muscles.

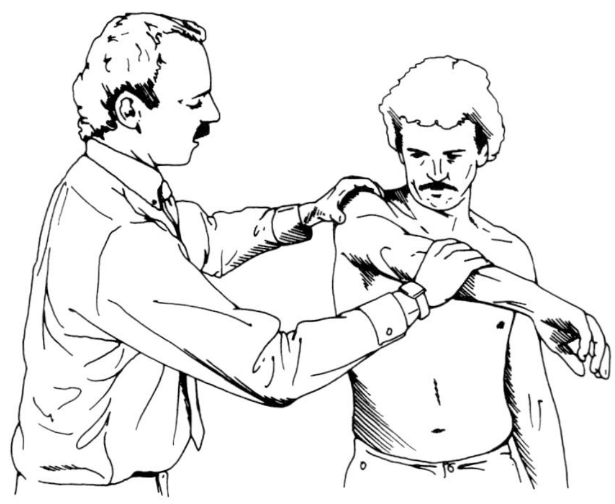

FIGURE 7. Impingement test. Testing for impingement against the coracoacromial arch.

studies.[29] The scapular Y view helps in evaluation of scapular and humeral head fractures and distinguishes anterior from posterior dislocations. The West Point view is also used in evaluation of anterior dislocation to identify an osseous fracture in the glenoid rim. Evaluation of acromioclavicular sprains may be done using routine AP films; however, the Zanca view, which provides 10 degrees of cephalad angulation and 50 percent attenuation of beam intensity, provides the optimal image.[5] The Alexander view may reveal a posterior clavicular dislocation missed on routine AP films.[38] Although stress views using weights strapped to the wrists bilaterally may help in differentiation between grade II and grade III acromioclavicular sprains, the results are seldom clinically relevant.

Injury Patterns

One of the more commonly seen contact injuries is an injury to the acromioclavicular joint. The mechanism usually is direct force onto the point of the shoulder, resulting in a sprain and sometimes a fracture of the distal clavicle. A grade I sprain involves capsular and ligamentous stretching without frank disruption. In grade II sprains, the capsule and acromioclavicular ligament are ruptured. Radiographs of grade II injuries reveal slight elevation of the clavicle when compared with the un-

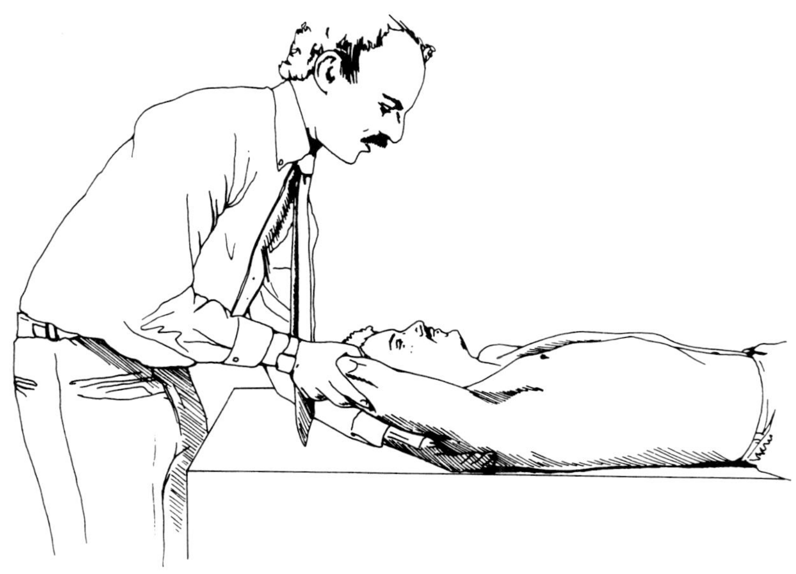

FIGURE 8. Clunk test. Testing for an anterior labral tear.

involved side. Disruption of both the acromioclavicular and coracoclavicular ligaments constitutes a grade III sprain and is accompanied by tenderness and swelling along the ligaments (Fig. 9).

On radiographs, a coracoclavicular distance of greater than 1.3 cm or a coracoclavicular interval greater than 25% that of the uninvolved shoulder suggests a grade III sprain. In an expanded grading system proposed by Rockwood and Young, types I, II, and III acromioclavicular injuries correlate with grades, I, II, and III acromioclavicular injuries correlate with grades I, II, and III sprains, respectively.[31] In a type IV acromioclavicular injury, the displaced clavicle penetrates posteriorly into the trapezius muscle and is seen best using an Alexander view. In type V dislocations, the coracoacromial interval exceeds 100% compared with the uninvolved shoulder. In type VI injuries, the clavicle is displaced inferiorly beneath the coracoid process.[5]

Treatment

Treatment of these injuries is controversial. Grade I and II acromioclavicular sprains usually respond well to ice, immobilization in a sling, and early rehabilitation once some of the pain has resolved. For treatment of grade III sprains, satisfactory results are seen with both closed measures and open surgical reduction, but most grade III sprains can be treated nonoperatively. In their study on shoulder strength after acromioclavicular injury, Walsh et al. demonstrated, from the standpoint of objective strength, that nonsurgical treatment of grade III acromioclavicular joint injuries was as effective as surgical treatment.[39] These findings have been reaffirmed in at least eight other studies.[5] The choice remains with the patient and the treating physician. Types IV, V, and VI acromioclavicular injuries often require surgical repair.

Shoulder subluxation or dislocation is another common contact injury to the shoulder. Subluxation occurs when the humeral head slips over the glenoid rim and then relocates spontaneously, whereas with a dislocation, the humeral head loses contact with the glenoid and lodges along the side of the joint. Subluxation can be so transient that the athlete feels only a sudden pain and the arm "goes dead."[35] Subluxation may occur without contact, particularly in the throwing athlete.

On physical examination, the patient with the more common anterior dislocation is unable to internally rotate the arm and cannot touch the opposite shoulder with the hand of the involved arm. In the case of the less common, posterior dislocation, the arm is locked in internal rotation, and the patient is unable to externally rotate the arm.[34]

Treatment consists of closed reduction, using one of many methods.[32] Following a reduction, three

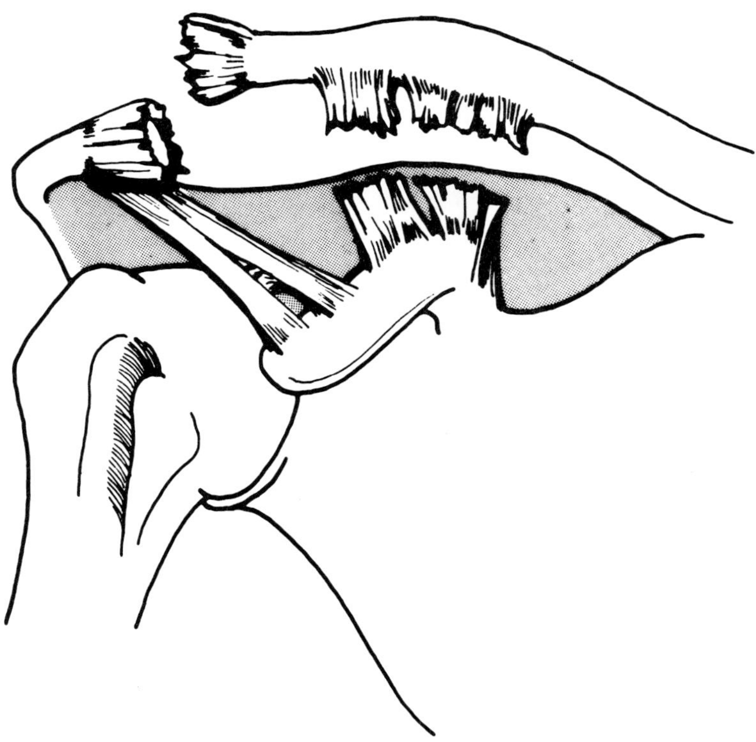

FIGURE 9. Grade III acromioclavicular joint sprain.

weeks of immobilization in a sling succeeded by an intensive rehabilitation program of muscular strengthening exercises emphasizing internal rotation and adduction are recommended. Some authors recommend operative stabilization for first-time dislocations, but long-term follow-up is still limited. Most physicians would agree that one should stabilize the shoulder that has already had three anterior dislocations.

The most common complaint with subluxation of the shoulder is a sudden paralyzing pain during forceful external rotation in the abducted overhead position. The most reliable physical sign is a positive apprehension test. Exercises similar to those used in rehabilitation of a dislocated shoulder are used for subluxation for at least six weeks, with early mobilization of the shoulder.

Most glenoid labrum tears are the result of shoulder instability, the mechanism being forceful subluxation of the humeral head over the fibrocartilaginous labrum.[2] Weakness of the scapular stabilizing muscle (the trapezius, the rhomboid muscles, and the serratus muscles) allows lateral sliding of the scapula and anteversion of the glenoid, resulting in increased anterior motion of the humeral head during abduction and external rotation. Diminished internal rotation caused by a tight posterior capsule and ligamentous structures is often encountered in the throwing athlete and inhibits free rotation of the glenohumeral joint during the acceleration and follow-through phases. The combination of these factors has been demonstrated to contribute to glenohumeral subluxation and dislocation as well as injury to the anterosuperior glenoid and anteroinferior glenoid labrum.[21]

Arthroscopic evaluation of athletes with recurrent anterior instability has revealed a high correlation (94%) with anterior and anteroinferior glenoid labrum tears.[19] The most specific test for this lesion is the positive clunk or labral grind test described previously. Treatment centers on exercises to increase flexibility and muscular strength, specifically the strength of the scapular stabilizers and posterior rotator cuff muscles (Fig. 10, A–L). Often, these injuries do not resolve without definitive treatment. Since simple labral debridement has been shown to afford only temporary relief, repair of the lesion is probably indicated, whether through arthroscopic or open techniques.[2]

In contrast to many labral tears, partial tears of the rotator cuff usually respond to physical therapy. These tears are frequently seen in the thrower's shoulder and are usually the result of repeated microtrauma to the supraspinatus tendon. The biomechanical fault is in the deceleration stage, when weak posterior rotator cuff muscles attempt to restrain the forward movement of the humerus. Occult recurrent anterior instability with secondary impingement also plays a role in rotator cuff injury, particularly in the young athlete, whereas falling on an outstretched arm is often the cause of a rotator cuff tear in the middle-aged.[8]

A partial rotator cuff tear causes pain in the shoulder and is indicated by a positive supraspinatus test. Weakness of the infraspinatus and teres minor may also be demonstrated by physical examination. A complete tear usually results in loss of active abduction beyond the first 30 degrees, whereas passive abduction remains full.[8] Although arthrograms are valuable in the diagnosis of complete tears, partial tears are often missed by an arthrogram. Magnetic resonance imaging is currently the most sensitive noninvasive tool for evaluation of rotator cuff damage.

The rotator cuff muscles are also involved in the impingement syndrome. This chronic inflammatory process of the rotator cuff and, secondarily, the subdeltoid bursa occurs as the muscles impinge against the coracoacromial ligament and the anterior part of the acromion process.[22] The syndrome is more often seen in sports requiring overhead use of the arms such as tennis, swimming, and baseball. Primary impingement syndrome is more common in the older recreational athlete. Posterior capsular tightness—manifested by decreased active and passive internal rotation and cross-chest adduction—and relative weakness of the external rotators of the shoulder are commonly responsible for mechanical impingement and degeneration. In younger athletes, impingement syndrome occurs frequently in association with anterior instability of the glenohumeral joint. A commonly associated physical finding is excessive external rotation of the shoulder. As a result of repeated high-velocity overhead throwing motions, it is believed that microtrauma to the anterior stabilizing structures of the shoulder leads to repeated minimal anterior glenohumeral subluxation, causing secondary impingement.[40]

Arthroscopic evaluation of athletes believed to have impingement syndrome commonly reveals tears of the superior labrum, partial tears of the rotator cuff, or lesions of the biceps tendon.[19] Loss of acromial elevation in the cocking phase of throwing as a result of weakness of the trapezius and serratus muscles increases the likelihood of rotator cuff impingement.[21] A positive impingement test may be elicited by physical examination and is accompanied by complaints of pain and, sometimes, weakness. Testing for both lateral scapular slide and instability of the shoulder is essential for diagnosis.

Treatment for rotator cuff injuries should begin conservatively, except in the instance of an obvious, new, complete tear. Antiinflammatory medications, rest, and strengthening and flexibility exercises with emphasis on the scapular stabilizing muscle groups are the most important elements of conservative treatment (Fig. 10, A–L). Complete

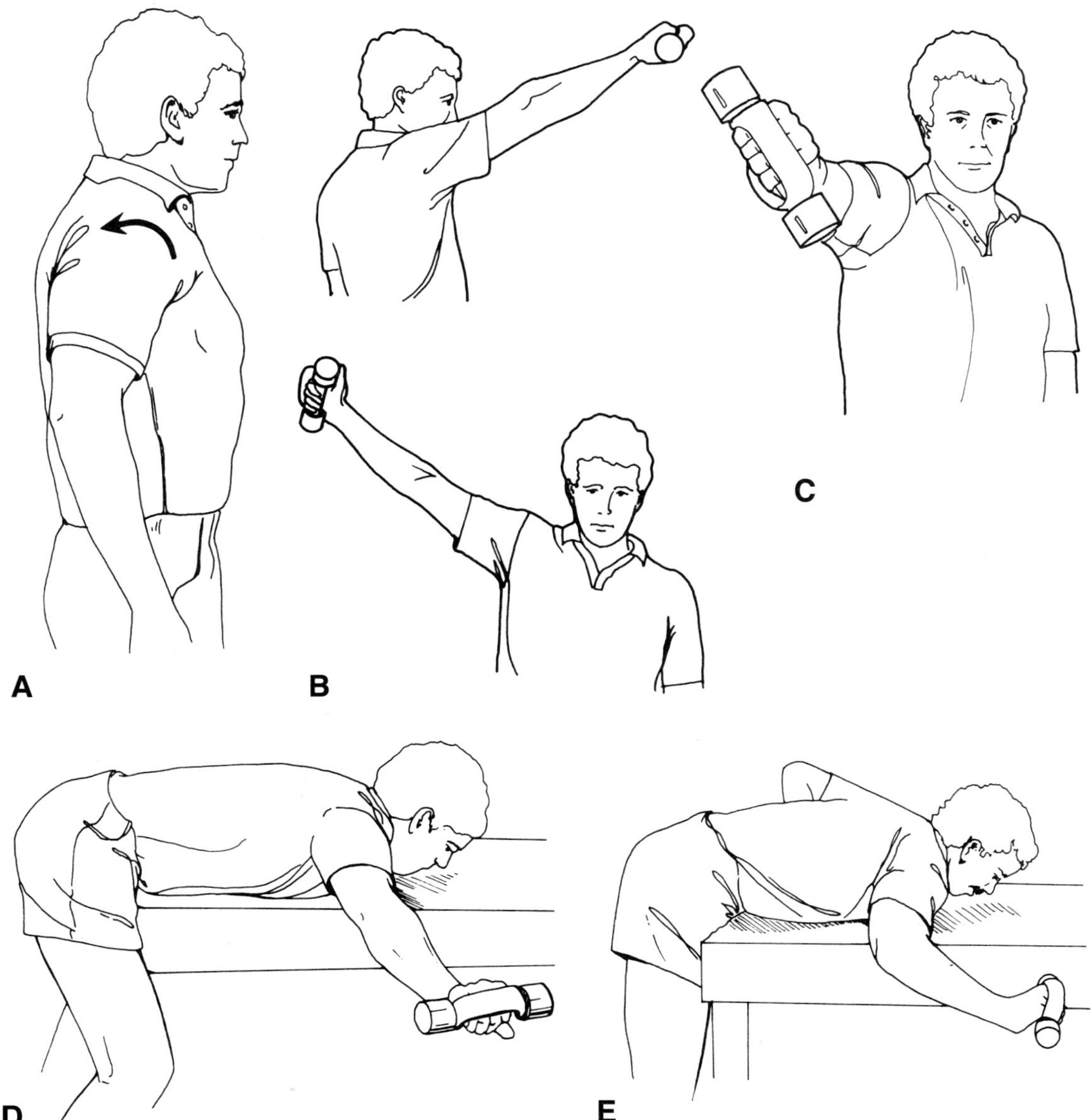

FIGURE 10. *A,* Shoulder shrug with scapular abduction. *B,* The anterior portion of the deltoid muscle is strengthened by forward-flexion exercises. The middle portion of the deltoid muscle is strengthened by abduction exercises. *C,* The supraspinatus muscle may be strengthened by internally rotating and abducting the humerus, keeping the arm below horizontal; but be careful as this may reproduce symptoms. *D,* Shoulder position for strengthening the external rotators. *E,* Strengthening exercise for the posterior portion of the deltoid muscle and the rotator cuff.

rest in a sling often induces adhesive capsulitis, adding another complicating factor to the diagnosis and treatment of the shoulder pain. Adhesive capsulitis (frozen shoulder) causes a chronic, persisting pain and decreased range of motion at the shoulder, especially in active abduction and external rotation.

Shoulder movement and exercises are the key to early recovery after rotator cuff injuries. Strengthening is achieved through a high-repetition, low-weight program.[4] Occasionally, steroid injections may be used in rotator cuff injuries, but such treatment should be reserved for the middle-aged person instead of the young athlete. Arthroscopic subacromial decompression with debridement of partial rotator cuff tears has been proven successful and should be considered if six months of conservative management produces no improvement.

Calcium deposits represent another rotator cuff problem. When calcification in the tendon becomes painful, it causes a reaction in the overlying bursa, which may itself become inflamed.[36] Common symptoms include severe shoulder pain that occurs suddenly and inhibits any movement of the shoulder. In those cases, steroid and anesthetic injections into

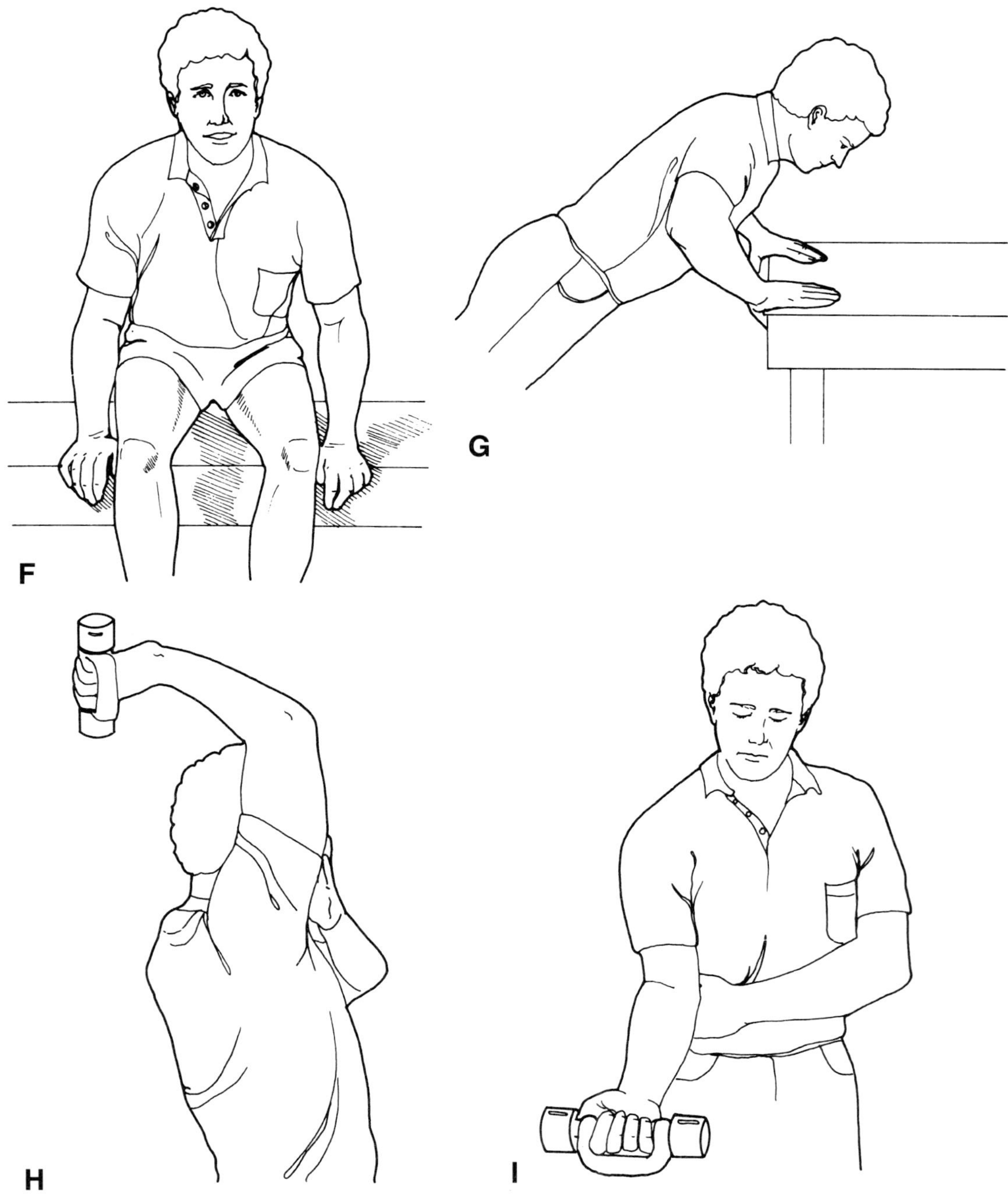

***FIGURE 10** (Continued).* *F,* Strengthening the shoulder depressor, horizontal adductor, and internal rotator muscles. *G,* Modified push-up. *H,* French-curl exercise for strengthening the triceps muscle. *I,* Biceps or elbow curl for strengthening the biceps muscle.

the calcium deposit are indicated to decrease the inflammatory response.[36] Once the acute symptoms have been relieved, the patient can progress to range-of-motion, flexibility, and strengthening exercises.

Closely associated with the rotator cuff tendons and the glenoid labrum is the biceps tendon. Anatomically, the tendon has an intimate attachment to the labrum, riding over the top of the humerus close to the capsule and rotator cuff.[36] The long head of the biceps tendon has an important stabilizing function, especially in the throwing shoulder. If other structures, such as the posterior cuff muscles, are weak, the long head carries more of the load and is susceptible to increasing microtrauma, which results in inflammation.[7] Clinical presentation includes persistent pain in the proximal area of the shoulder with palpable tenderness in the bicipital groove. Treatment often revolves around strengthening the poste-

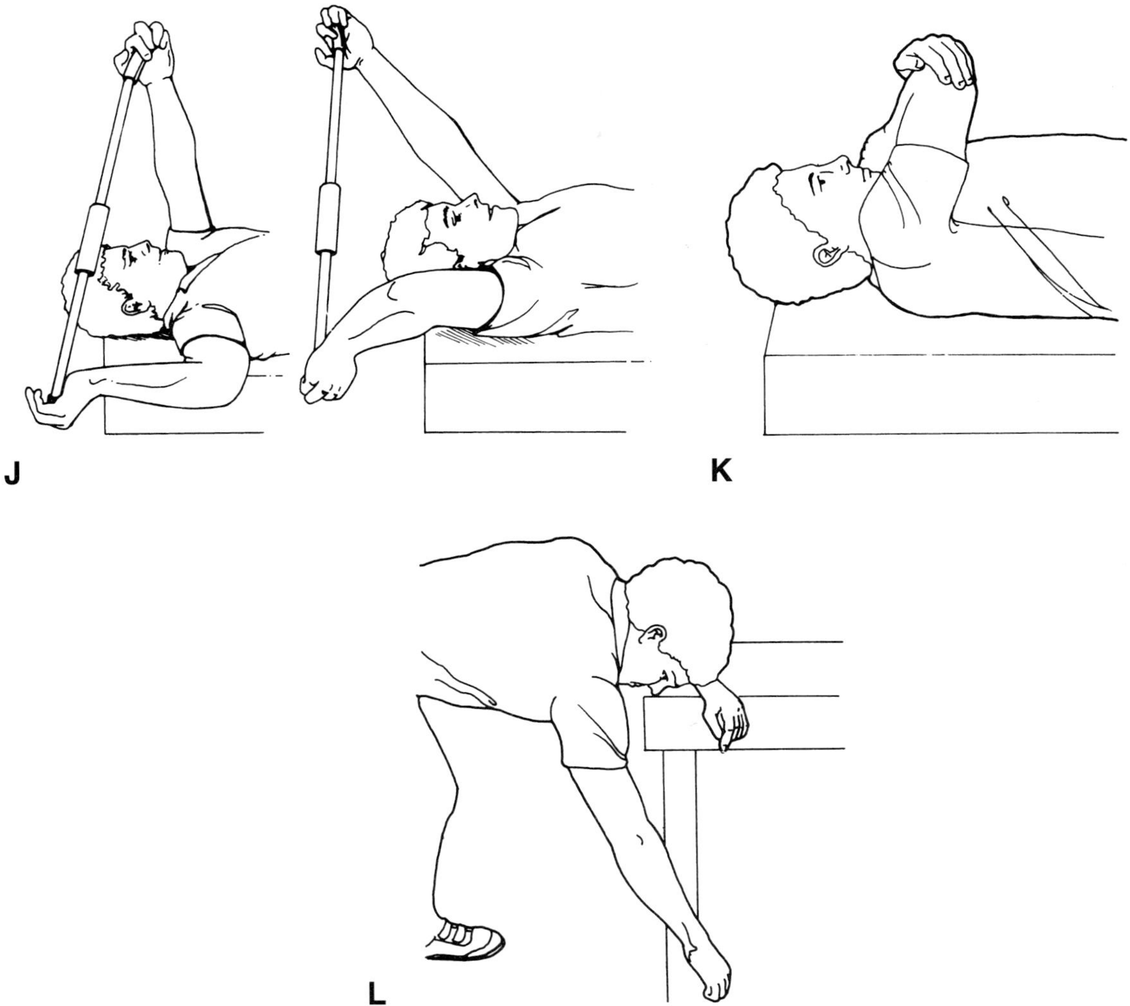

***FIGURE 10** (Continued)* *J,* External rotation flexibility exercises performed with the shoulder abducted from 90 degrees to full abduction. *K,* Stretching exercise for the posterior shoulder structures. L, Pendulum exercises.

rior cuff muscles and the use of antiinflammatory medications. Some authors recommend a steroid injection into the bicipital groove, but this usually affords only temporary relief.[36]

Subacromial bursitis occurs from a blunt injury, usually during a contact sport such as football, when the humerus is driven against the acromion. Blood can often be aspirated from the bursa; an injection of lidocaine relieves the symptoms. Conservative treatment is recommended, including rest, heat, and flexibility and strengthening exercises. Recovery is usually complete by 3–6 weeks.[24]

Sternoclavicular dislocation is an uncommon injury to the shoulder, and anterior dislocation occurs three times as frequently as posterior dislocation. In athletes 22 years of age or younger, epiphyseal separation of the medial clavicle must be considered. Posterior dislocations may cause trauma to the underlying structure of the mediastinum and therefore may require immediate closed reduction with the aid of a towel clip fastened to the clavicle. Anterior dislocations tend to be less stable and may require either the use of a spica cast, with the shoulder in forward flexion, or the use of a sling and swathe.[24]

Finally, vascular compromise should be suspected in any athlete complaining of early fatigue and poor ball control during repetitious overhead activities. During the cocking phase of pitching, for instance, hyperabduction and extension in extreme rotation of the humerus produce excessive pressure on the subclavian and axillary arteries at the anterior scalene and pectoralis minor muscles, respectively. Branch artery compression, subclavian artery aneurysm, and cervical ribs have also been reported. Examination reveals occurrence of the symptoms in the abducted, externally rotated position, along with a diminished radial pulse and proximal bruit. Evidence of finger ischemia may be detected in the presence of a subclavian aneurysm. Doppler examination in the functional position reveals arterial compression at the axillary-subclavian level, which can be confirmed by an arteriogram. Treatment consists of decompression by resection of a portion of the scalene or pectoralis minor muscle or a cervical rib.[28]

ELBOW INJURIES

The elbow is a hinged joint responsible primarily for flexion and extension. Its intimate relationship with pronation and supination of the forearm, as well as rotation of the shoulder, affords it a crucial role in the complex function of the upper extremity in sports. Therefore, it is also subject to a complex array of biomechanical stresses that can lead to injury.

History and Physical Examination

A careful history should include the nature and location of the problem, onset and duration of the symptoms, circumstances surrounding the injury, and exacerbating and relieving factors. The patient's level of athletic participation may offer insight into the type and mechanism of injury.

Begin the examination with inspection for ecchymosis, effusion, erythema, muscular development and symmetry, and gross bony abnormality. Examine for evidence of possible flexion contracture. Normal flexion should be approximately 135 degrees, with extension to 0 degrees. Note the carrying angle as well as the degree of supination and pronation. By applying valgus stress to the elbow in full extension and in 30 degrees of flexion, assess the integrity of the medial collateral ligament (particularly the anterior oblique portion). This ligament is one of the basic stabilizers of the humeroulnar articulation, and it works in conjunction with the anterior capsule and the bony contact of the humerous and ulna. Applying varus stress in a similar fashion, assess the stability of the lateral collateral ligament, although it should be noted that the capsule and bony structures provide proportionately more stability in this direction.[30]

Palpate posteriorly for pain and swelling in the area of the triceps insertion and the olecranon and its bursa. Tenderness is present in these areas with triceps tendinitis and avulsion injuries of the olecranon, whereas a large fluid collection indicates bursitis. Tenderness on palpation anteriorly indicates anterior capsulitis as well as strain or avulsion of the biceps tendon at the area of insertion. Tenderness to palpation over the lateral humeral epicondyle is often demonstrated in tennis elbow. Resisted extension is often demonstrated in tennis elbow. Resisted extension at the wrist (Fig. 11) that produces discomfort at the lateral epicondyle is indicative of irritation of the extensor carpi radialis brevis tendon (the major extensor tendon involved in tennis elbow) and its insertion into the lateral humeral epicondyle. Painful resisted extension of the third and fourth digits suggests involvement of the extensor digitorum communis tendons as well.[30]

Palpate over the medial epicondyle and have the patient resist flexion at the wrist (Fig. 12). Discomfort indicates inflammation in the flexors of the forearm, originating from the medial epicondyle. Finally, perform a neurovascular examination including tapping over the sulcus between the medial epicondyle and the olecranon process. Hypersensitivity with this maneuver (Tinel's sign) may indicate irritation of the ulnar nerve, whether from trauma, traction, or compression. Radiologic evaluation should begin with an AP view in extension, a lateral view in 90 degrees of flexion, and bilateral oblique films.[42]

Injury Patterns

The common patterns of force overload to the throwing elbow include tension overload of the me-

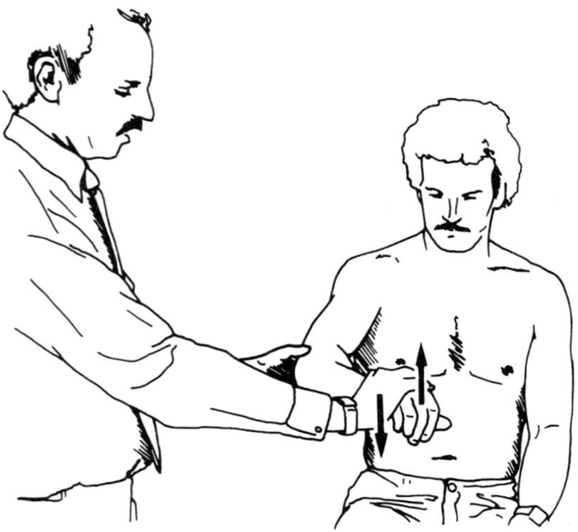

FIGURE 11. Testing for lateral epicondylitis.

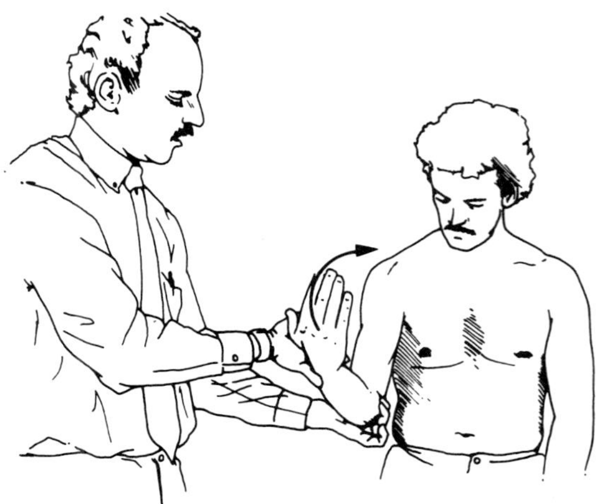

FIGURE 12. Testing for medial epicondylitis.

dial aspect and compression overload of the lateral aspect.[23] Whereas the stress of repetitive overuse is the usual cause of injury in the student-athlete and the professional athlete, the recreational athlete is more likely to sustain injury from intermittent overloading of the muscle-tendon units, compounded by poor conditioning and inadequate warm-up.[42] Although certain disorders are restricted to the child-athlete and the adolescent athlete, most of the pathologic entities classified under the general diagnosis of Little Leaguer's elbow are common to the young and older athlete alike.

During the late cocking phase, distraction forces on the medial elbow result in traction forces that are applied to the medial epicondyle and the wrist flexor musculotendinous units. These forces may cause a sprain of the medial collateral ligament, traction spurs of the coracoid process, or ulnar nerve traction with resultant neuritis.[30]

During the acceleration phase, rapid forward motion of the humerous places a valgus force on the elbow, with resultant medial traction and lateral compression. Medial collateral ligament sprains, ulnar traction neuritis, wrist flexor strains with medial epicondylitis, ulnar coracoid spurs, and calcification of the ulnar collateral ligament all may develop as a result of this medial traction.[30] In 9- to 12-year-old children, bony overgrowth of the medial epicondyle and apophysitis with subsequent avulsion fracture may develop as well.[42] Lateral compression may result in articulocartilage damage in the radiocapitellar joint, and osteochondritis may lead to loose body formation.[30,42] Lateral epicondylitis may occur secondary to extreme pronation of the wrist.[18] The young athlete in particular is prone to avulsion fractures of the lateral epicondyle in addition to osteochondritis dissecans.[42]

During the follow-through phase, the olecranon comes into forceful contact with the fossa while the triceps contracts to decelerate the arm. Triceps tendinitis and strain and olecranon fractures may ensue.[30,42] Although the follow-through phase has been implicated in posterior compartment impingement, it is more likely that the extreme valgus stress during the late cocking and acceleration phases is responsible, with resultant spurring of the posterior medial aspect of the olecranon.[42] In a young athlete, one must entertain the possibility of traction apophysitis of the olecranon.[42]

The patient with Little Leaguer's elbow and related elbow conditions may present with pain, stiffness, or swelling with prolonged activity, which may progress to an inability to throw. Tenderness may be present on palpation over the olecranon, the radial head, and the medial and lateral epicondyles.[25] A positive Tinel's sign and sensory motor deficits in the C7, 8 nerve root distribution indicate ulnar nerve involvement. Radiographs may reveal soft tissue swelling, osteophytosis, osteochondritis with loose body formation of the radiocapitellar joint, or hyperostosis of the medial compartment with fragmentation or separation of the medial epicondylar epiphysis.[18]

Treatment

The cornerstone of therapy for conditions of the elbow is rest combined with a carefully supervised rehabilitation program designed to restore range of motion and strength (Fig. 13 A–F). Antiinflammatory medication, ice, and other therapeutic modalities are useful adjuncts. Splinting of flexion may be necessary for severe sprains of the ulnar collateral ligament; such splinting should be followed by early mobilization. Surgical intervention may be required for conditions that do not respond to conservative measures. Examples of conditions that require surgical treatment include ulnar traction neuritis, which is treated by subcutaneous transposition; recalcitrant epicondylitis, which requires debridement; and displaced medial epicondylar epiphysis, which requires anatomic reduction. Foreign body removal and debridement of osteophytes over the posterior medial olecranon are best achieved using the arthroscopic technique. After restoration of flexibility and strength, the athlete may progress through functional activities with increasing intensity. A full return to activities can usually be achieved by 6–12 weeks.[25]

Olecranon bursitis is caused by acute or repetitive trauma to the tissue over the olecranon. It often appears as a dramatic bulging over the olecranon that is usually painful only to direct palpation. When a preexisting olecranon bursa problem becomes painful or red, aspiration of the contents for analysis by Gram's stain and culture is indicated. Compression, antiinflammatory medication, and avoidance of trauma usually constitute sufficient treatment; however, in recalcitrant cases, aspiration and injection with corticosteroid are occasionally required.

Tendinosis is an overuse syndrome that occurs in throwing and racquet sports as well as in occupational settings. It is a degenerative process described histologically as angiofibroblastic tendinosis (remarkable for lack of an inflammatory component). The tendon of the extensor carpi radialis brevis is involved on the lateral aspect, whereas the tendons of the pronator teres, flexor carpi radialis, and palmaris longus are predominantly involved on the medial aspect. Associated fibrosis, epicondylar osteophytosis, and ectopic calcification of the tendon (in up to 20% of cases) may occur secondarily.[26] Treatment includes rest from the offending activity; antiinflammatory medications; physical modalities, including ice, electric stimulation, and iontophoresis; and a flexibility program.

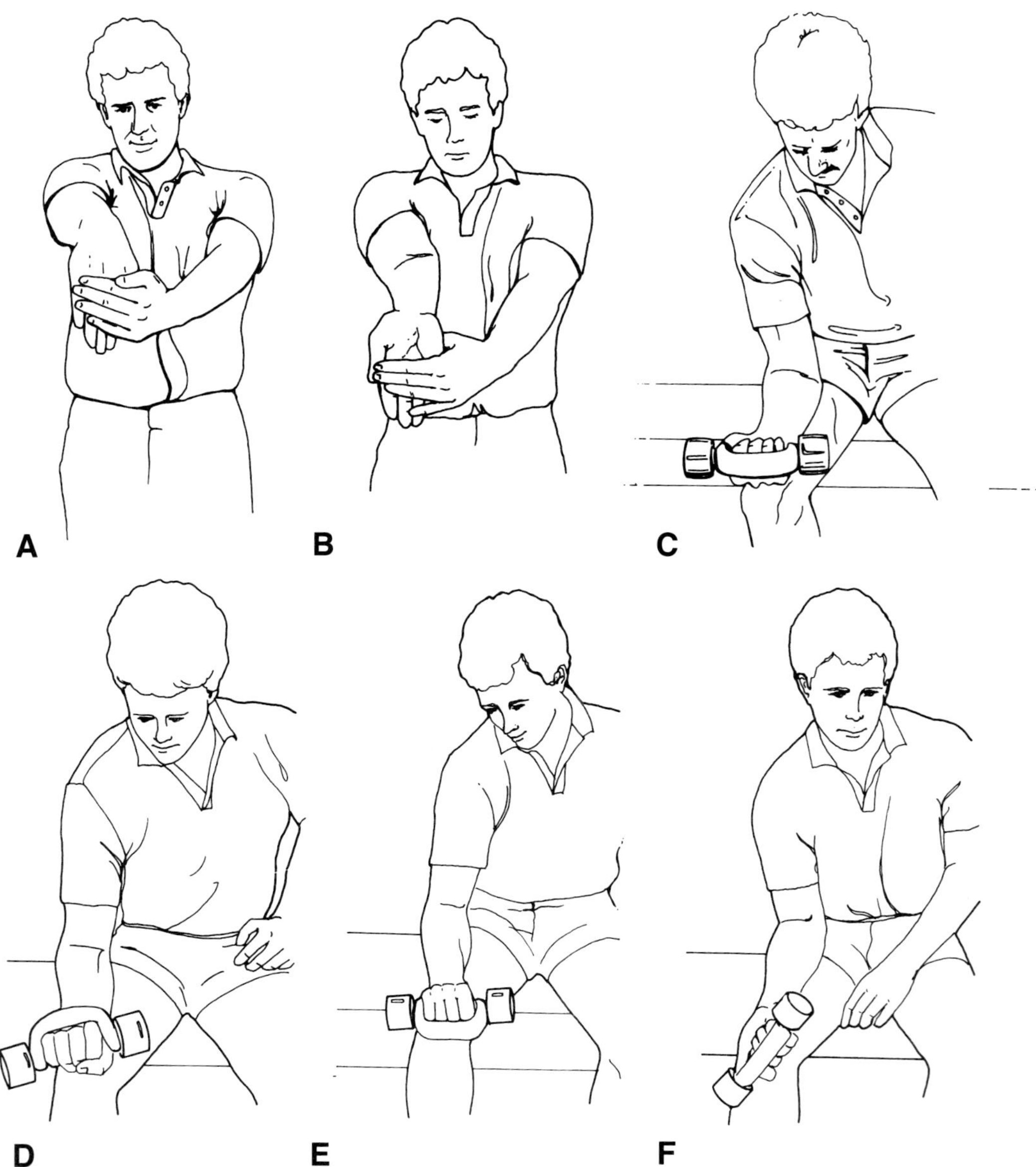

FIGURE 13. *A,* Stretching exercise for wrist extensor muscles. *B,* Stretching exercise for wrist flexor muscles. *C,* Strengthening exercise for wrist flexor muscle. *D,* Strengthening exercises for wrist extensors. *E,* Strengthening exercises for forearm pronator muscle. *F,* Strengthening exercises for forearm supinator muscles.

This is followed by a rehabilitative program made up of strengthening exercises for the flexors, extensors, pronators, and supinators of the wrist (Fig. 13 A–F). Counterforce bracing to reduce overload of the tendons together with an injection of carticosteroids and a local anesthetic is often required in more severe cases. Attention to proper technique, control of intensity and duration of activity, and use of equipment that minimizes force load (i.e., a lightweight racquet with low-range string tension) are essential to reduce the incidence of recurrence. Surgical debridement and resection of exostoses is indicated only rarely, such as when these conditions fail to respond to an aggressive, conservative program after 1 year.[26]

Acknowledgment

The authors give special thanks to the Hughston Foundation.

BIBLIOGRAPHY

1. Abrams JS: Special shoulder problems in the throwing athlete: Pathology, diagnosis, and nonoperative management. Clin Sports Med 10:839–861, 1991.
2. Altchek DW, Warren RF, Wickiewicz TL, Ortiz G; Arthroscopic labral debridement. Am J Sports Med 20:702–706, 1992.

3. Andrews JR, Gillogly S: Physical examination of the shoulder in throwing athletes. In Zarins B, Andrews JR, Carson WG (eds): Injuries to the Throwing Arm. Philadelphia, W.B. Saunders, 1985, pp 51–65.
4. Aronen JG, Regan K: Decreasing the incidence of recurrence of first time anterior shoulder dislocations with rehabilitation. Am J Sports Med 12:283–291, 1984.
5. Bach BR, VanFleet TA, Novak PJ: Acromioclavicular injuries. Controversies in treatment. Physician Sportsmed 20(12):87–101, 1992.
6. Bearden JM, Hughston JC, Whatley GS: Acromioclavicular dislocation: Method of treatment. J Sports Med 1:5–17, 1973.
7. Blackburn TA: The off-season program for the throwing arm. In Zarins B, Andrews JR, Carson WG (eds): Injuries to the Throwing Arm. Philadelphia, W.B. Saunders, 1985.
8. Booth RE Jr, Marvel JP Jr: Differential diagnosis of shoulder pain. Orthop Clin North Am 6:353–379, 1975.
9. Brown DE: Shoulder injuries. Prim Care 19:265–281, 1992.
10. Ferrari DA: Capsular ligaments of the shoulder. Anatomical and functional study of the anterior superior capsule. Am J Sports Med 18:20–24, 1990.
11. Fronek J, Warren RF, Bowen M: Posterior subluxation of the glenohumeral joint. J Bone Joint Surg 71A:205–216, 1989.
12. Gerber C, Ganz R: Clinical assessment of instability of the shoulder. With special reference to anterior and posterior drawer tests. J Bone Joint Surg 66B:551–556, 1984.
13. Halpern BC: Diagnosis and treatment of sprains and strains. GA Acad Fam Physicians (GAFP) 7:3, 1985.
14. Hawkins RJ, Hobeika PE: Impingement syndrome in the athletic shoulder. Clin Sports Med 2:391–405, 1983.
15. Hawkins RJ, Kennedy JC: Impingement syndrome in athletes. Am J Sports Med 8:151–158, 1980.
16. Heppenstall RB: Fractures and dislocations of the distal clavicle. Orthop Clin North Am 6:477–486, 1975.
17. Hughston JC: Functional anatomy of the shoulder. In Zarins B, Andrews JR, Carson WG (eds): Injuries to the Throwing Arm. Philadelphia, W.B. Saunders, 1985, pp 43–50.
18. Hunter SC: Little Leaguer's elbow. In Zarins, Andrews JR, Carson WG (eds): Injuries to the Throwing Arm. Philadelphia, W.B. Saunders, 1985, pp 228–231.
19. Hurley JA, Anderson TE: Shoulder arthroscopy: Its role in evaluating shoulder disorders in the athlete. Am J Sports Med 18:480–483, 1990.
20. Jobe FW, Kvitne RS: Shoulder pain in the overhand or throwing athlete: The relationship of anterior instability and rotation cuff impingement. Orthop Rev 18:963–975, 1989.
21. Kibler WB: Role of the scapula in overhead throwing motion. Contemp Orthop 22(5):525–532, 1991.
22. Leach RE: The impingement syndrome. In Zarins B, Andrews JR, Carson WG (eds): Injuries to the Throwing Arm. Philadelphia, W.B. Saunders, 1985, pp 121–127.
23. McLeod WD: The pitching mechanism. In Zarins B, Andrews JR, Carson WG (eds): Injuries to the Throwing Arm. Philadelphia, W.B. Saunders, 1985, pp 121–127.
24. Neer CS, Welsh RP: The shoulder in sports. Orthop Clin North Am 8:583–591, 1977.
25. Nicola T: Elbow injuries in athletes. Prim Care 19:283–302, 1992.
26. Nirschl RP: Elbow tendinosis/tennis elbow. Clin Sports Med 11:851–870, 1992.
27. Norris TR: History and physical examination of the shoulder. In Nichols JA, Hershman EB (eds): The Upper Extremity in Sports Medicine. St. Louis, Mosby, 1990, pp 41–90.
28. Nuber GW, McCarthy WJ, Yao JS, et al: Arterial abnormalities of the shoulder in athletes. Am J Sports Med 18:514–519, 1990.
29. Pope TL, Chen MY: Imaging the acutely painful shoulder. Emergency Medicine September 15, 1992, pp 122–139.
30. Reid DC: Sports Injury Assessment and Rehabilitation. New York, Churchill Livingstone, 1992, pp 999–1052.
31. Rockwood CA Jr, Young DL: Disorders of the acromioclavicular joint. In Rockwood CA Jr, Matsen FA III (eds): The Shoulder, Vol. 1. Philadelphia, W.B. Saunders, 1990, pp 413–476.
32. Rowe CR: Acute and recurrent anterior dislocations of the shoulder. Orthop Clin North Am 11:253, 1980.
33. Rowe CR: Anterior subluxation of the throwing shoulder. In Zarins B, Andrews JR, Carson WG (eds): Injuries to the Throwing Arm. Philadelphia, W.B. Saunders, 1985, pp 144–151.
34. Rowe CR, Zarins B: Chronic unreduced dislocations of the shoulder. J Bone Joint Surg 64A:494–505, 1982.
35. Rowe CR, Zarins B: Recurrent transient subluxation of the shoulder. J Bone Joint Surg 63A:863–872, 1981.
36. Simon WH: Soft tissue disorders of the shoulder. Orthop Clin North Am 6:521, 1975.
37. Simonet WT, Cofield RH: Prognosis in anterior shoulder dislocation. Am J Sports Med 12:19, 1984.
38. Waldrop JI, Norwood LA, Alverez RG: Lateral roentgenographic pojections of the acromioclavicular joint. Am J Sports Med 9:337, 1981.
39. Walsh WM, Peterson DA, Shelton G, Neumann RD: Shoulder strength following acromioclavicular injury. Am J Sports Med 13:153, 1985.
40. Warner JJ, Deng X, Warren RF, et al: Static capsuloligamentous restraints to superior-inferior translation of the glenohumeral joint. Am J Sports Med 20:675–685, 1992.
41. Warner JJ, Micheli LJ, Arslanian LE, et al: Patterns of flexibility, laxity and strength in normal shoulders and shoulders with instability and impingement. Am J Sports Med 18:366–375, 1990.
42. Whiteside JA, Andrews JR: Common elbow problems in the recreational athlete. J Musculoskel Med 6(2):17–34, 1989.
43. Zanca P: Shoulder pain involvement of the acromioclavicular joint: Analysis of 1000 cases. Am J Roentgenol Rad Ther Nucl Med 112:493–506, 1971.

19

Hand, Wrist, Elbow, and Forearm Injuries

David E. Brown, M.D.
Michael J. Whalen, PA-C

HAND INJURIES

Hand injuries are exceedingly common in athletes. Most tend to be traumatic, unlike elbow injuries, which usually are due to overuse. It is important to question the athlete about the mechanism of injury and to pay careful attention to the actual mechanics and stresses that occurred. The injury mechanism in most cases allows one to "predict" the injury even prior to x-ray examination.

Query the patient on the ability to use the hand after the injury. Were they able to continue to participate? Was or is there an obvious deformity in the hand? If there was a deformity, was it corrected either by the patient or a medical professional prior to your evaluation?

If the injury is nontraumatic, ascertain how long symptoms have been present, where they are located, and what the offending and relieving activities are. What sports does the individual play? How do the symptoms affect the ability to play his or her sport? Are there any neurologic symptoms?

Examination

Observe the hand for deformity, swelling, and resting posture. The tenodesis effect of the flexor tendons can provide useful information about their integrity. Have the patient relax the hand and passively flex the wrist. Note that the fingers are nearly extended. Passively extend the wrist and note that the fingers assume a more flexed position. This indicates intact flexor tendons. If a flexor tendon is injured, that digit will remain relatively extended as you passively extend the patient's wrist. Note skin color and integrity. Document active and passive range of motion (ROM). Palpate for point of maximum tenderness. Is there crepitation present at the point of maximum tenderness? If there is a specific tender point, radiographic evaluation is usually indicated. AP and lateral views are the minimum required. Stress views may be helpful if there is a potential ligament injury. Evaluate motor and sensory neurologic function.

Fractures

Metacarpals. Fractures can occur at the base, shaft, neck, or head. Note any angular, rotational, or intra-articular deformity. Rotational deformities are not well tolerated, although rotational deformity in the ring and small finger metacarpals is functionally better tolerated than in the index and long metacarpals. Remember that malrotation is more apparent in flexion than in extension. Metacarpal neck fractures angulated greater than 30 degrees require closed reduction (Fig. 1). Stable metacarpal fractures can be splinted or casted. Fractures of the base of the fifth metacarpal that are intra-articular and subluxed are unstable and therefore require closed reduction and percutaneous pinning.

Phalanges. Stable, well-aligned phalangeal fractures can be treated with buddy taping or splinting. Phalangeal fractures are prone to rotational as well as angular deformity owing to deforming forces from the flexor and extensor tendons. If unstable, treat with reduction and percutaneous pinning. Intra-articular condyle fractures require anatomic reduction and internal fixation so that early ROM may be instituted to avoid the complication of joint stiffness.

Thumb. Fracture of the base of the thumb metacarpal (Bennett's fracture) is unstable owing to the deforming force of the abductor pollicis longus (Fig. 2). This fracture requires closed or open reduction and pinning to restore and maintain its anatomic position.

Extensor Tendon Avulsion Fractures. A fracture of the dorsal, proximal base of the distal phalanx represents a disruption of the long extensor ten-

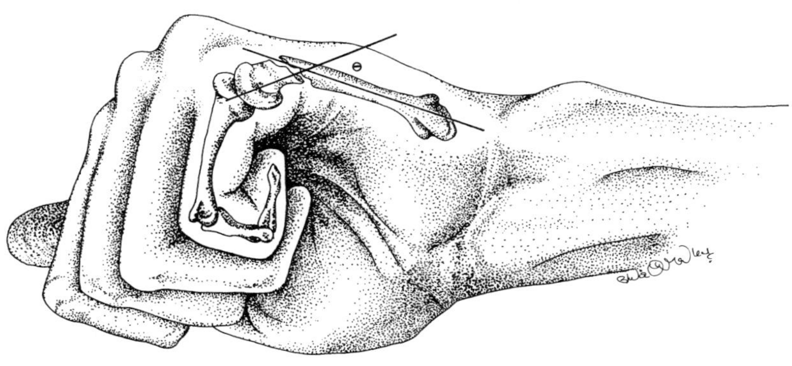

FIGURE 1. Metacarpal fracture with greater than 30 degrees of fracture angulation should be reduced.

don (Fig. 3). The mechanism of injury is similar to that of a simple mallet finger. It is generally caused by a direct blow to the tip of the finger by a ball or an opponent. Small fractures are treated with extension splinting for 4–6 weeks. If greater than 50% of the articular surface of the distal phalanx is involved or if there is distal interphalangeal joint subluxation, open reduction and internal fixation are indicated.

Dislocations

Metacarpophalangeal (MCP) joint dislocations most often occur following hyperextension injuries. These dislocations may be simple or complex. A complex dislocation is irreducible owing to the interposition of the volar plate within the joint. A characteristic dimple is noted at the palmar surface of the MP joint. Open reduction is required for complex dislocations.

Proximal interphalangeal (PIP) joint dislocation occurs with axial loading and hyperextension. This results in dorsal or dorsolateral dislocation. Treatment involves closed reduction and splinting or buddy taping depending on degree of pain, swelling, and range of motion. Volar plate avulsion fracture may occur. Splint in slight flexion for 2–3 weeks followed by early ROM to prevent development of pseudo-boutonniere deformity. If the joint is subluxed because of a large fracture fragment, open repair and fixation are necessary.

Distal interphalangeal (DIP) joint dislocations are less common than are PIP joint disloca-

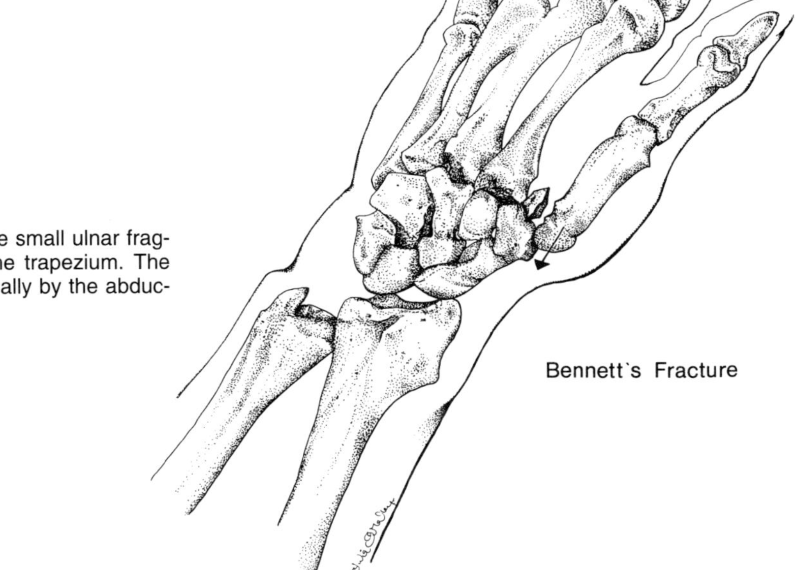

FIGURE 2. Bennett's fracture. The small ulnar fragment remains firmly attached to the trapezium. The larger fragment is displaced proximally by the abductor pollicis longus.

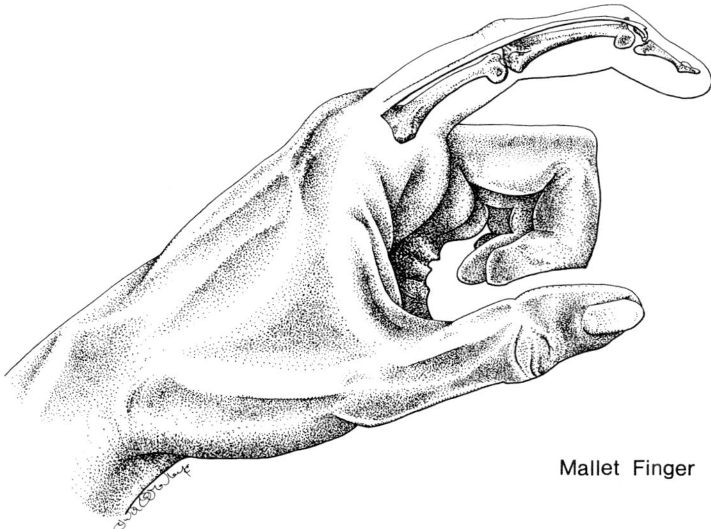

FIGURE 3. Mallet finger. The extensor tendon is usually torn near its insertion. Occasionally a small fragment of the distal phalanx is avulsed by the tendon. The DIP joint cannot be actively extended.

tions. When they do occur they are often open injuries. Following reduction, immobilization should be brief and ROM instituted as symptoms allow. Associated nailbed injuries should be repaired.

Ligament Injuries

Extensor hood rupture at the MP joint most often occurs from a direct blow. The lesion is the result of tearing of the sagittal band of the extensor hood. Rupture of the sagittal band usually occurs on the radial side of the extensor hood. This results in extensor tendon subluxation into the valley between the metacarpal heads. Repair of the defect is indicated when conservative treatment with splinting in extension fails.

Ulnar collateral ligament (UCL) rupture at the MP joint of the thumb occurs from hyperextension and abduction stress (Fig. 4). This injury is known as gamekeeper's or skier's thumb. Laxity is demonstrated by placing radial stress on the slightly flexed thumb. Chronic laxity of the UCL can lead to significant functional disability. Primary repair of complete UCL injuries is indicated.

Collateral ligament injuries of the IP joints are common. Partial tears with minimal laxity can be treated conservatively. Protective splinting or buddy taping should be used until symptoms subside. Complete ruptures of the radial collateral ligament of the index finger can lead to chronic instability and are best treated with primary repair.

Tendon Injuries

Mallet finger deformity is the result of disruption of the extensor tendon at its insertion on the distal phalanx. This injury usually occurs when the fingertip is impacted by a ball or other object. The

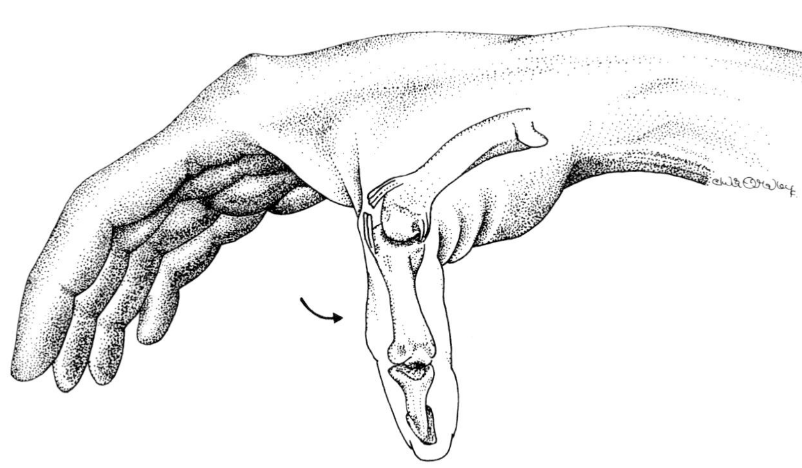

FIGURE 4. Skier's thumb. The ulnar collateral ligament to the metacarpophalangeal joint is disrupted by an abduction force.

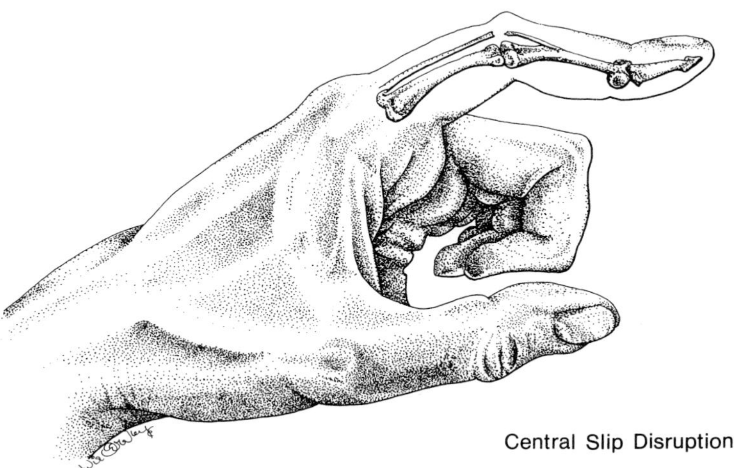

FIGURE 5. Central slip disruption. The central slip of the extensor tendon is disrupted over the PIP joint. This injury is easily missed acutely because the boutonniere deformity develops slowly.

patient cannot actively extend the DIP joint. Passive extension is possible and is usually painless. A lateral radiograph is necessary to rule out a fracture or subluxation. Splint the DIP joint in extension for 6 to 8 weeks. This allows the conjoined extensor tendon to heal in a normal position. If the DIP joint is allowed to flex, the tendon will either fail to heal or will heal in a lengthened position, which is inadequate to produce active extension at the DIP joint.

Central slip disruptions (Fig. 5) at the PIP joint are the result of either direct trauma to the dorsum of the joint or a flexion force while the joint is actively extending. This can result in a boutonniere deformity if not diagnosed and treated acutely. Initially, the injured digit will be swollen and flexed to approximately 30 degrees. Further active extension is impossible. The DIP joint should be normal. Splint the PIP joint in extension and allow active DIP joint flexion for an acute injury. This maintains the lateral bands in their proper position. If the finger remains in flexion, lateral bands sublux volar. This results in a relative extension or hyperextension at the DIP joint. Thus, a late deformity is a fixed flexion contracture at the PIP joint and an extension contracture at the DIP joint.

If an individual with a PIP joint injury presents with a PIP flexion deformity and absent PIP joint extension, it is safest to splint the joint in extension for several weeks. Be aware that ligament sprain may present in a similar fashion. Pain and swelling from the ligament injury may inhibit active PIP extension. After a week of splinting and rest, the patient should be able to demonstrate active PIP extension. The joint may then be mobilized as tolerated.

Rupture of the flexor profundus tendon at its insertion on the distal phalanx results in the inability to flex the distal phalanx (Fig. 6). This is the "jersey finger," commonly seen when an athlete attempts to grasp his opponent's jersey. The finger is forcefully extended during active finger flexion, leading to tendon avulsion. The ring finger is most commonly involved. Primary surgical repair is indicated.

WRIST INJURIES

History

The wrist is subject to a variety of traumatic and overuse injuries. If there is a traumatic onset of pain, the time and mechanism of injury, the onset of swelling, and localization of pain are important to ascertain. The degree of disability that the injury caused to the wrist and upper extremity are important. Patients with moderate or severe pain and disability or restriction of range of motion should have radiographic evaluation. Many wrist fractures are

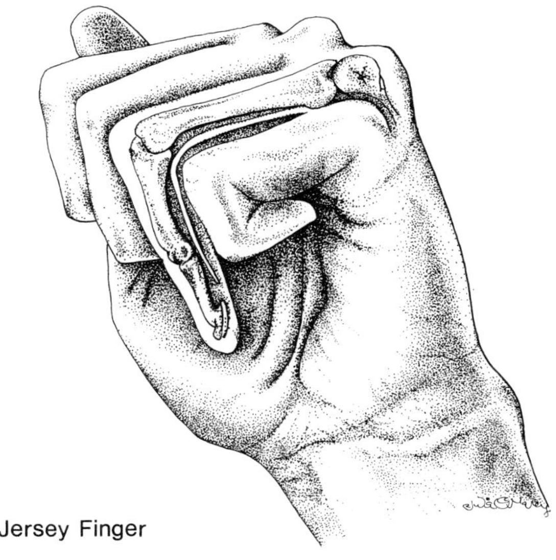

FIGURE 6. Jersey finger. The flexor profundus tendon is detached by a forced hyperextension of the DIP joint. This commonly occurs when an athlete is attempting to tackle an opponent by grasping and pulling on the jersey.

occult in that the initial x-rays may be normal. It is often necessary to splint these injuries and repeat x-rays again in 10–14 days, when the fracture line may be more evident. Wrist ligament injuries may present similarly to wrist fractures with substantial disability and swelling. It is important to repeatedly evaluate patients with persistent functional disability and pain following a traumatic wrist injury.

In patients with chronic overuse injuries, it is important to determine the inciting and relieving factors, location and duration of symptoms, presence or absence of swelling, and response to any previous splinting or medications. Nocturnal symptoms are common in neurologic wrist disorders.

Examination

Carefully evaluate for swelling, deformity, ecchymosis, or masses. Compare to the contralateral side. Assess both active and passive range of motion. Feel for clicks, masses, deformity, and crepitus. It is extremely important to know the topographic anatomy of the wrist in order to determine which structure is maximally tender. The multiple bones, ligaments, and tendon structures that make up or cross the wrist make accurate anatomic understanding important in formulating an accurate diagnosis. Neurovascular status evaluation should include sensibility, motor strength, and sympathetic function (sweating). The two-point discrimination test for sensibility is an easily performed evaluation of nerve integrity.

Phalen's test evaluates nerve compression at the wrist. Determine whether neurologic symptoms begin or worsen with the wrist maximally volarflexed. In a positive test, the symptoms occur or worsen within two minutes. **Tinel's sign** is elicited by tapping over the course of a nerve. When percussing over an abnormal nerve, distal propagation of pain or paresthesia occurs. **Finkelstein's test** detects de Quervain's tenosynovitis. Adduct the thumb into the palm. The examiner should gently ulnar-deviate the wrist while maintaining the thumb in the adducted position. In a positive test, there is exacerbation of pain over the first dorsal compartment.

Fractures

Fractures of the wrist may involve the distal radius, ulna, or carpal bones. Not all wrist fractures present with deformity. Torus fractures in children and nondisplaced distal radius fractures in adults may present with minimal deformity and swelling.

Radius Fractures. Nondisplaced radius fractures can be managed with cast immobilization for 4–6 weeks. Repeat x-rays at 1 week should be obtained to document maintenance of anatomic position. Angulated or displaced fractures require reduction and casting. If unstable, internal fixation may be necessary. Intraarticular fractures usually require reduction and percutaneous pinning or open reduction and internal fixation.

Scaphoid Fractures. Scaphoid fractures are commonly caused by a fall on the outstretched arm. Football linemen seem to sustain these through repeated hyperextension injuries during blocking. These athletes present with pain, swelling, and tenderness over the anatomic snuff box at the wrist. If initial x-rays are negative and there is a clinical suspicion of a scaphoid fracture, the patient should be immobilized in a thumb spica splint or cast. The wrist should be examined and repeat x-rays obtained in 2 weeks.

The majority of these fractures occur through the waist of the scaphoid (Fig. 7). Immobilization in a thumb spica cast is required for at least 6 weeks and commonly for as long as 4 months. Five to 10% still go on to nonunion. Proximal one-third fractures (Fig. 8) have a higher incidence of nonunion. Scaphoid tuberosity (distal one-third) fractures usually unite with 4–6 weeks of immobilization (Fig. 9). Displaced fractures require open reduction and internal fixation because of the high incidence of nonunion.

Hamate Fractures. Direct trauma to the hypothenar eminence can result in fracture of the hook of the hamate. This occurs when a bat, racquet, or golf club forcefully strikes the unprotected hand. Nonunion is common and may result in neuritis of

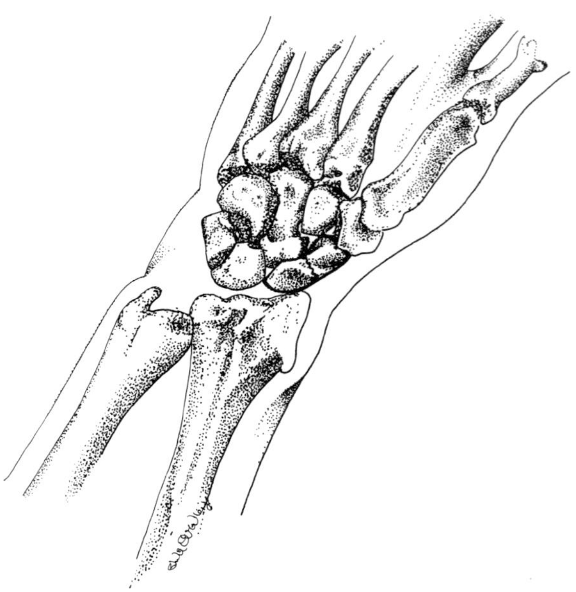

Fracture of the Scaphoid's Waist

FIGURE 7. Scaphoid waist fracture. The fracture through the middle one third of the scaphoid is the most common location.

the ulnar nerve, since the hamate hook forms the radial border of Guyon's canal (through which the ulnar nerve passes). Nondisplaced fractures can be immobilized in a short arm cast with the wrist in slight flexion. The fourth and fifth fingers are immobilized with the MP joints in flexion. Displaced fractures or nonunions are treated with excision of the fracture fragment.

Triquetrum. Dorsal avulsion fractures can be treated with 3–6 weeks of immobilization. Volar fractures are more commonly associated with perilunate dislocation and usually require surgical reduction and repair of soft tissue injuries.

Dislocations

Fortunately, disclocations and fracture-dislocations of the wrist are uncommon athletic injuries. These are devastating injuries and require expedient reduction. Open reduction of the associated fractures with repair of soft tissues is necessary.

Ligament Injuries

Injuries to the ligaments of the wrist most often occur from a single traumatic event. Partial or complete tears can result in intercarpal instabilities. The abnormal wrist mechanics lead to secondary post-traumatic degeneration.

Scapholunate Ligament. The scapholunate is the most commonly injured ligament. This injury classically results from a fall on an outstretched arm with dorsiflexion and axial loading forces across the wrist. Complete rupture leads to scapholunate dissociation. This can be noted on posteroanterior radiographs when the scapholunate interval is greater than 3 mm (Fig. 10). Initial treatment involves immobilization for 4–6 weeks. If static or dynamic instability patterns develop, than a ligament reconstruction procedure or intercarpal fusion may be necessary. It is difficult to return to athletics after these injuries.

Triangular Fibrocartilage Complex (TFCC). TFCC injuries can occur from a fall on an outstretched hyperpronated arm. Ulnar wrist pain is the most common presenting complaint. Ulnar wrist pain that does not respond to conservative treatment should be evaluated with arthrography or MR scan. TFCC tears may benefit from arthroscopic excision.

Tendinopathies

deQuervain's Disease. The abductor pollicis longus (APL) and extensor pollicis brevis (EPB) tendons are located in the first dorsal compartment overlying the radial styloid. They are contained at this level by a thickened segment of the extensor retinaculum. Activities that require repetitive forceful grasping or ulnar deviation can lead to irritation of these tendons at this location. Inflammation of the tenosynovium results in pain and sometimes crepitation. Finkelstein's test causes increased pain, as the APL and EPB are placed in maximum

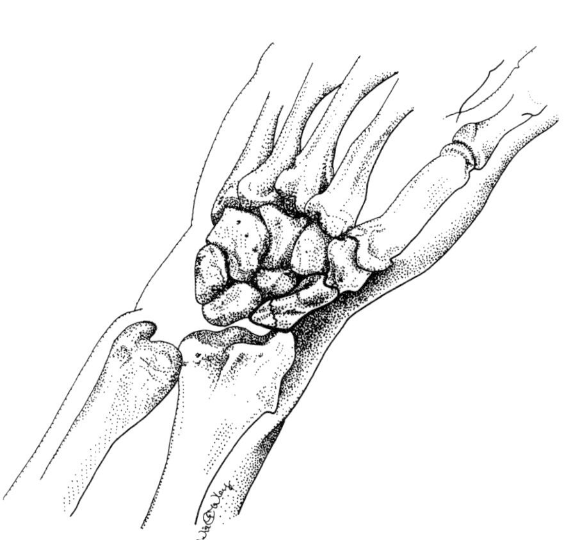

Fracture of the Scaphoid's Proximal Pole

FIGURE 8. Proximal one third scaphoid fractures are notorious fractures that frequently fail to unite.

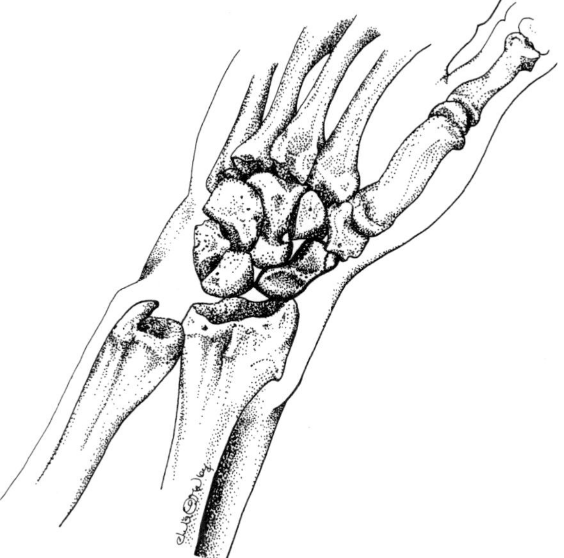

Distal Fracture of the Scaphoid

FIGURE 9. The scaphoid tuberosity fracture unites readily. It is rarely displaced and has good vascular supply.

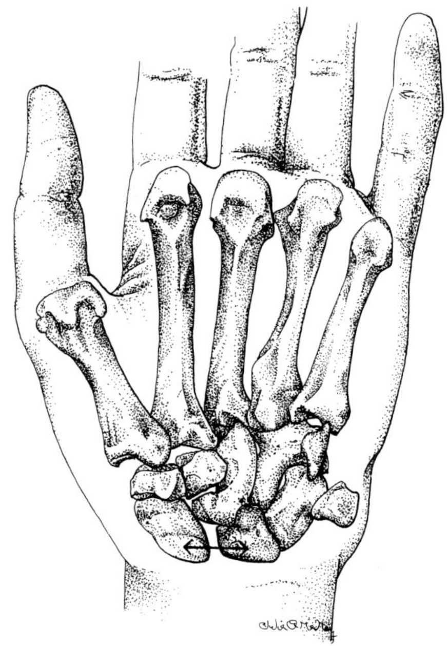

FIGURE 10. Scapholunate dissociation results from a tear of the scapholunate interosseous ligament. There is greater than 3 mm of separation between the scaphoid and lunate.

excursion. Conservative treatment includes splinting and tendon sheath injection. Recalcitrant cases respond to surgical release.

Intersection Syndrome. This is an inflammatory condition located where the first dorsal compartment muscles cross the extensor carpi radialis longus and brevis. Pain, swelling, and crepitation may be present at the dorsal radial wrist. Treatment consists of splinting and antiinflammatory medications.

Neurovascular Injuries

Carpal Tunnel Syndrome (CTS). The median nerve leaves the forearm and enters the hand through the carpal tunnel. It travels through the tunnel with the four FDP, four FDS, and FPL tendons. Acute CTS can occur with trauma but most often is associated with overuse. Tenosynovitis of the flexor tendons is the most common cause. Initial treatment consists of splinting the wrist in slight dorsiflexion and oral antiinflammatory therapy. Injection of the carpal tunnel (but not the median nerve) may provide temporary and occasionally permanent relief. EMG and nerve conduction studies will demonstrate changes consistent with CTS in 85% of cases. Persistent CTS requires decompression to prevent permanent nerve injury.

Ulnar Nerve. The ulna can be compressed within Guyon's canal. This is seen in cyclists owing to prolonged external pressure from the handlebars on the hypothenar eminence. Most commonly the deep terminal branch is involved. It supplies motor fibers to the hand intrinsics but spares the hypothenar muscles. If the main trunk is involved more proximally, ulnar sensory involvement will be noted. Appropriate cycling gloves usually relieve symptoms. A knowledgeable examiner or technician should check the bicycle fit for appropriate size. Additional handlebar padding may be required. Persistent symptoms require temporary cessation of cycling.

Miscellaneous

Ganglions. Ganglions are benign cysts arising from joints or tendon sheaths. They present as painful masses on either the dorsal or volar aspect of the wrist. Conservative treatment with splinting, antiinflammatory drugs, or aspiration may be helpful. Aspiration of the ganglion is performed with an 18-gauge needle and small syringe. A nearly clear jelly-like fluid is obtained. Following aspiration, you may want to puncture the cyst walls several times. The goal is to decompress this cyst and have the cyst walls scar together. Surgical excision is indicated for the painful recurrent ganglion.

Dorsal Impaction Syndrome. Dorsal wrist pain following hyperextension weight-bearing activities is seen in gymnasts and weightlifters. Other causes of dorsal wrist pain, such as occult ganglia, de Quervain's syndrome, and fractures must be ruled out. Treatment consists of relative rest, ice, anti-inflammatory drugs, and technique modification to avoid the hyperextended position. Braces are available that dampen shock and limit the extremes of extension.

ELBOW AND FOREARM INJURIES

History

Evaluation of the painful or injured elbow begins with a thorough history. Date of onset and mechanism of injury are noted. Aggravating activities may provide useful information and point toward specific diagnosis. The location of the pain narrows the differential diagnosis considerably. In acute injury, the mechanism of injury is very important. For example, acute medial elbow pain in a young throwing athlete may be due to a medial epicondylar avulsion fracture or a tear of the flexor muscles or of the ulnar collateral ligament. A fall onto the elbow or arm that results in lateral elbow pain is likely due to a radial head fracture.

Examination

Examination of the elbow begins with inspection and comparison with the contralateral side to note any swelling or deformity. Palpate to localize tenderness or crepitation. Both active and passive range of motion is assessed. Stability to varus-valgus and anterior-posterior stress and strength are tested.

Fractures

Radial Head. A fall on an outstretched pronated forearm is a frequent cause of radial head fractures (Fig. 11). The distal radius and distal radioulnar joint should be evaluated, as there may be associated distal injury. Undisplaced and minimally displaced fractures are treated with brief immobilization followed by range of motion as soon as tolerated. Displaced or comminuted fractures may require open reduction and internal fixation or excision.

Olecranon. Olecranon fractures occur from a direct blow to the olecranon or from the avulsion force of the triceps extending the elbow against resistance. Stress fractures from repetitive extension activities (e.g., pitching) may also occur. Undisplaced fractures may be treated conservatively. Displaced fractures will require open reduction and internal fixation followed by early range of motion.

Medial Epicondyle. Medial epicondylar fractures can occur in skeletally immature persons (Fig. 12). Although these can be secondary to repetitive valgus stresses, they more commonly are seen in the throwing athlete during a significant valgus stress or violent flexor contraction. If the fragment is displaced, it should be reduced and pinned to restore stability. On occasion, the avulsed medial epicondylar fragment is trapped in the joint.

Dislocations. Posterior elbow dislocations account for 90% of all elbow dislocations. These dislocations are termed complex if there is an associated fracture. Radial head and neck fractures and medial epicondyle avulsion fractures are most common. The most frequent mechanism of injury is a fall on an outstretched, extended arm. Careful assessment of the neurovascular status prior to reduction is essential. Treat simple dislocations with gentle closed reduction. Reduction is accomplished by longitudinal traction in full extension. As soon as the palpable and audible reduction is accomplished, flex the elbow to maintain the reduction. Immobilize in a sling or posterior splint but start range of motion as soon as it is tolerated by patient comfort.

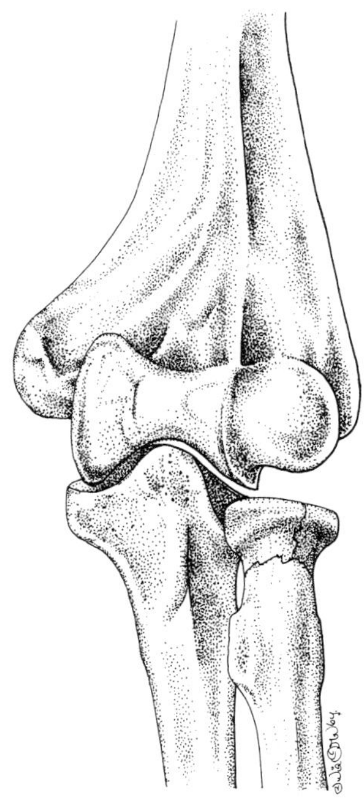

Radial Head Fracture

FIGURE 11. Radial head fractures result from axial compression injuries. Nondisplaced or minimally displaced fractures should be mobilized early.

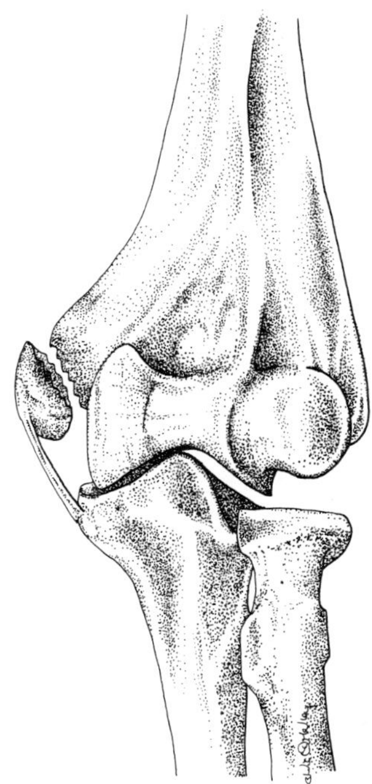

Medial Epicondyle Fracture

FIGURE 12. Medial epicondyle fractures occur in late adolescence from a valgus stress to the elbow. The ulnar collateral ligament is attached to the fracture fragment.

Complex dislocations may require surgical intervention for fracture reduction and soft tissue repair. Patients should be counseled at time of injury that loss of terminal extension is common.

Ligament Injuries

Ulnar collateral ligament injuries (Fig. 13) occur from valgus stress at the elbow. This injury may present as an acute event or as a chronic overuse syndrome. In the acute setting, the patient may report a "pop" over the medial elbow during a throw. Valgus instability may be hard to detect clinically owing to muscle spasm and guarding. Stress radiographs are helpful in demonstrating medial joint opening. Primary repair or reconstruction is indicated.

Chronic injuries present with medial elbow pain. Ulnar nerve symptoms may result from stretching of the nerve. Conservative treatment, including ice, NSAIDs, and rest should continue until the elbow is no longer tender. Resumption of throwing activities should be gradual, using a progressive throwing program.

Anterior capsular strain may occur with a hyperextension injury. Diffuse anterior elbow pain is usually the presenting symptom. Conservative treatment includes ice, NSAID, and early active range of motion. Aggressive-passive range of motion to gain terminal extension should be avoided, as this may lead to myositis ossificans.

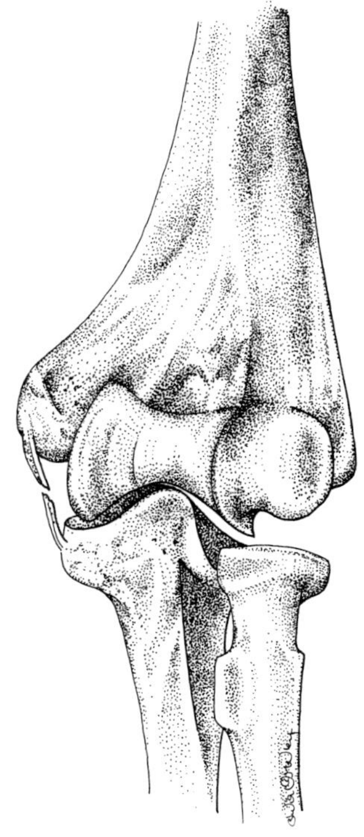

UCL Rupture

FIGURE 13. Adults injure the ulnar collateral ligament from hyperabduction injuries and during elbow dislocations. Throwing athletes usually need surgical repair. Most other athletes may be treated with protected early motion.

Tendinitis

Medial and lateral epicondylitis occur frequently with activities that require repetitive forceful forearm use (racquet sports, golf, throwing sports). Patients present with pain localized to either the medial or lateral elbow. The pain may occur with or after forceful activity or it may be constant.

Pain localized to the medial epicondyle that is exacerbated by resisted wrist flexion and forearm pronation is indicative of medial epicondylitis. Not uncommonly, patients with medial epicondylitis have associated ulnar nerve symptoms. These are primarily sensory and mild. Pain at the lateral epicondyle that is exacerbated by resisted wrist and or finger extension is indicative of lateral epicondylitis. Passive forearm pronation and wrist flexion may provoke pain. Neurogenic or intra-articular causes of medial or lateral elbow pain need to be considered.

Treatment of medial or lateral epicondylitis includes rest, ice, avoidance of aggravating activity, and oral anti-inflammatory agents. If symptoms are more acute or do not respond to the above measures, add phonophoresis and splint the wrist. Splint lateral epicondylitis in mild wrist dorsiflexion. This places the common wrist extensors at rest, reducing tensile forces at the lateral epicondyle. Splint medial epicondyle injuries in neutral wrist position, which places the flexor pronator mass at rest, reducing tensile forces at the medial epicondyle. Do not splint medial injuries in wrist flexion, as this may cause pressure in the carpal tunnel.

When the symptoms of medial or lateral epicondylitis are caused by a specific sport, the patient's equipment and mechanics should be assessed. For example, lateral epicondylitis is a frequent cause of lateral elbow pain in tennis players who may need a change in grip size, string tension, or racquet size. Enlist the help of a professional instructor in this type of evaluation. When symptoms subside, rehabilitation for flexibility and conditioning is imperative. Some patients will not respond to these treatment methods. A corticosteroid injection may provide relief and allow initiation of rehabilitation. Patients who fail to progress with conservative measures may require surgical intervention for debridement and release of the degenerative tendon.

Anterior or posterior elbow pain due to distal biceps or triceps tendinitis occurs less frequently than medial or lateral tennis elbow. These conditions present with pain localized to the affected tendon. Again, treatment includes rest, ice, and oral anti-inflammatory medications.

Neurovascular

Cubital tunnel syndrome involves the ulnar nerve as it crosses the medial aspect of the elbow through the cubital tunnel. There is posteromedial elbow pain with paresthesias and numbness on the ulnar side of the arm and hand. Motor involvement is uncommon. Tinel's sign is frequently positive over the cubital tunnel. Nerve conduction studies may demonstrate slowing of conduction velocity across the elbow. Initial treatment consists of relative rest, ice application, and oral anti-inflammatory medications. If motor weakness is present, or if conservative therapy fails to provide relief, surgical decompression or anterior transposition of the ulnar nerve may be necessary.

Pronator teres syndrome involves the median nerve. There is compression of the nerve in the proximal forearm by the pronator teres and an aching sensation in the volar forearm with distal radiation of pain. Unlike carpal tunnel syndrome, nocturnal exacerbation is uncommon. Conservative treatment includes avoidance of forceful repetitive pronation, rest, and oral anti-inflammatory medications. Failure of conservative treatment requires surgical exploration and decompression.

Posterior interosseous syndrome involves the radial nerve. The usual lateral elbow pain may mimic lateral epicondylitis. Pain is the predominant symptom and there is no loss of sensation. There may be weakness of the wrist or finger extensors. The posterior interosseous nerve passes through the supinator and may be compressed at the proximal edge or the middle or distal end of the muscle.There will be tenderness at the site of entrapment, which is usually four fingerbreadths distal to the lateral epicondyle. EMG studies may be positive. Surgical decompression is indicated for recalcitrant symptoms.

Miscellaneous

Olecranon Bursitis. Olecranon bursitis may be seen following a single traumatic event, with repetitive stress, or with systemic illnesses such as gout and rheumatoid arthritis. Most often, this is relatively painless. Painful bursal effusions associated with parabursal edema and erythema should be aspirated for Gram stain, culture, and crystal analysis. Septic bursitis requires drainage either by aspiration or open debridement and antibiotic therapy. Treatment of aseptic bursitis consists of application of cold, protective padding and avoiding trauma and compression. Recalcitrant painful olecranon bursitis occasionally requires surgical excision.

REFERENCES

1. Burkholter WE: Closed treatment of hand fractures. J Hand Surg 14A:390, 1989.
2. Gunther, SF: Dorsal wrist pain and the occult scapholunate ganglion. J Hand Surg 10A:697, 1985.
3. Lichtman DM (ed): The Wrist and Its Disorders. Philadelphia, W.B. Saunders, 1988.
4. Linscheid RL: Athletic injuries of the wrist. Clin Orthop 198: 141, 1985.
5. Petrone FA (ed): AAOS: Symposium on upper extremity injuries in athletes. St. Louis, Mosby, 1988.
6. Strickland JW, Rettig AC: Hand Injuries in Athletes. Philadelphia, W.B. Saunders, 1992.
7. Taleisnik J: Pain on the ulnar side of the wrist. Hand Clin 3: 51, 1987.

20

The Spine in Sports

Walter W. Huurman, M.D.

In today's world of increasing physical activity and athletic endeavors on the part of the general population, the spine has joined the knee, ankle, elbow, shoulders, and other anatomic areas as a site for maladies related to athletics. The athlete who presents with a spine problem needs a physician who understands spinal anatomy and biomechanics as well as other pathologic conditions specific to the vertebral column. Owing to the age group of this patient population (young) and general physical profile (more fit), an athlete who develops spine-related symptoms requires a careful search for specific pathology. Because, in the recreational athlete, response to treatment or eventual recovery is not influenced by compensation considerations, results of appropriate treatment can frequently be gratifying to both athlete and physician.

As athletic injuries continue to increase in our very active population, injuries related to the spine increase proportionately. Many treating physicians feel quite uncomfortable dealing with problems of the central nervous system and its protective bony enclosures, the cranium and the spine. Dealing with the athlete's physical problems requires a systematic approach. This is particularly true when anatomical relationships are complex and a variety of possible pathological conditions occur—a situation common to the spine.[14,28] If one approaches the problem with a firm grasp of normal anatomy and biomechanics, the confusion regarding specific diagnoses tends to disappear.

For purposes of direct clinical application, spinal problems related to athletic activity are best managed in a symptom-oriented, differential diagnostic approach. After potential diagnoses are narrowed by taking an accurate history, the physical examination (Table 1), combined with appropriate laboratory and radiographic testing (Table 2), further clarifies the problem and allows the primary care physician to make the all important decision of whether to proceed with treatment or to make a referral to an appropriate specialist.

Neither infallible nor all-inclusive, an anatomic approach will simplify treatment of the patient with perplexing spine-related complaints.

ANATOMY AND FUNCTION

Composed of 24 articulating segments anchored at one end by the skull and at the other by the sacrum, the spinal column provides support for the trunk and extremities and, of equal importance, protects the delicate and unforgiving components of the axial nervous system. Unique anatomic characteristics within each region (cervical, thoracic, and lumbar) supply appropriate amounts of support while providing a varying contribution to the total motion requirements of the body. In its broadest anatomic sense, the spine includes the bony vertebral column, its associated musculoligamentous structures, and the neural components—the spinal cord as well as the intra- and extradural nerve roots.

Each vertebral element comprises an anterior body and a posterior complex of lamina/spinous process. The two are connected by laterally placed "posts" or pedicles. The space created between the posterior aspect of the body, anterior aspect of the lamina and, laterally, the inner margin of the pedicles constitutes the spinal canal, through which the fragile spinal cord and nerve roots pass (Fig. 1).

Anatomically, the differences among cervical, thoracic, and lumbar elements are found primarily in the orientation of the facet joints, which posteriorly provide articulation from one vertebral segment to the next, and in the size of the anteriorly located vertebral bodies.

Cervical Vertebrae

The seven cervical vertebrae provide more motion than found in any other spinal region.[28,38] The facets are located somewhat laterally and are ori-

TABLE 1. Elements to Observe in the Spinal Physical Examination

Stance
Erect? Liting to the side? Bent forward?
Gait
Rate (normal, slow, guarded)
Position (normal, flexed, listing)
Palpation
Tenderness to palpation (generalized, localized)
Muscle spasm (unilateral, bilateral)
Range of Motion
Active (patient standing)
Forward flexion
Lateral bending
Truck rotation
Extension
Single stance extension
Passive (performed supine)
Straight leg raise
Lasegue's maneuver
Hip flexion, abduction, external rotation (FABER)
Muscle Strength
Patient standing
Trendelenburg test (hip abductors)
Tip-toe walking (gastrocsoleus)
Heel walking (tibialis anterior)
Toe extension (extensor hallucis)
Patient sitting
Hip flexion (iliopsoas)
Knee extension (quadriceps)
Elbow flexion (biceps)
Elbow extension (triceps)
Wrist flexion (flexor carpi)
Wrist extension (extensor carpi)
Index finger abduction (first dorsal interosseous)
Tendon Reflexes
Patellar
Tendoachilles
Biceps
Triceps
Wrist extensors
Sensation
Dermatomal distribution

ented parallel to the frontal plane. With respect to the transverse plane, the cervical facet is tilted in a relatively shallow angle from anterosuperior to posteroinferior. A proportionately large lateral mass is positioned between the lamina and the short, narrow pedicle. On either side, the small transverse process contains a foramen, through which the vertebral artery passes in its route from a subclavian origin to the cranial vault via the foramen magnum. The volume of the cervical canal, bounded by the relatively small vertebral body anteriorly, the pedicle and lateral masses laterally, and the lamina posteriorly, is sufficient to allow a slight (3 mm) amount of anterior-posterior gliding of one segment upon another without damaging the spinal cord.[38]

TABLE 2. Radiographic Studies for Assessing Spinal Symptoms

Laboratory
Complete blood count with differential
Urine analysis
Sedimentation rate
C-reactive protein
HLA B_{27}
Electromyography
Radiography
Routine plano views
Anteroposterior
Standing lateral
Oblique
Special Studies
Computed tomography
Myelography
Nuclear imaging
Magnetic resonance imaging

The volume of the cervical spinal cord does not fill the vertebral canal to the degree that the thoracic cord does. Injury to the cervical cord, however, can be more devastating than other neural injuries because sensory and motor innervation to both upper and lower extremities pass through this segment.

Anteriorly the intervertebral body spaces in all three regions consist of a semifluid nucleus pulposus and its restraining envelope, the annulus fibrosus. The avascular nucleus acts as an effective shock absorber between bony segments. The enveloping annulus solidly unites the vertebral bodies and consists primarily of fibrous bands arranged in lamellar fashion, much like rings on a tree. Within the spinal canal, on the dorsal aspect of the vertebral body, the continuous posterior longitudinal ligament provides an anterior wall for the canal and blends with the annulus fibrosis at each level. Its ventral companion, the anterior longitudinal ligament, in like fashion continuously joins the anterior margin of each vertebral body.

Flexion, extension, lateral bending, and rotation greater than that found in either of the other two regions predispose the articulations of the cervical spine to degenerative change. The relatively small muscular attachments here are less effective in absorbing forces of direct trauma than in the lumbar spine: the lack of supporting bony attachments makes the cervical spine more vulnerable than its ribbed thoracic counterpart.

Thoracic Spine

The thoracic vertebral complex differs from the cervical in that at each level a rib joins the vertebral

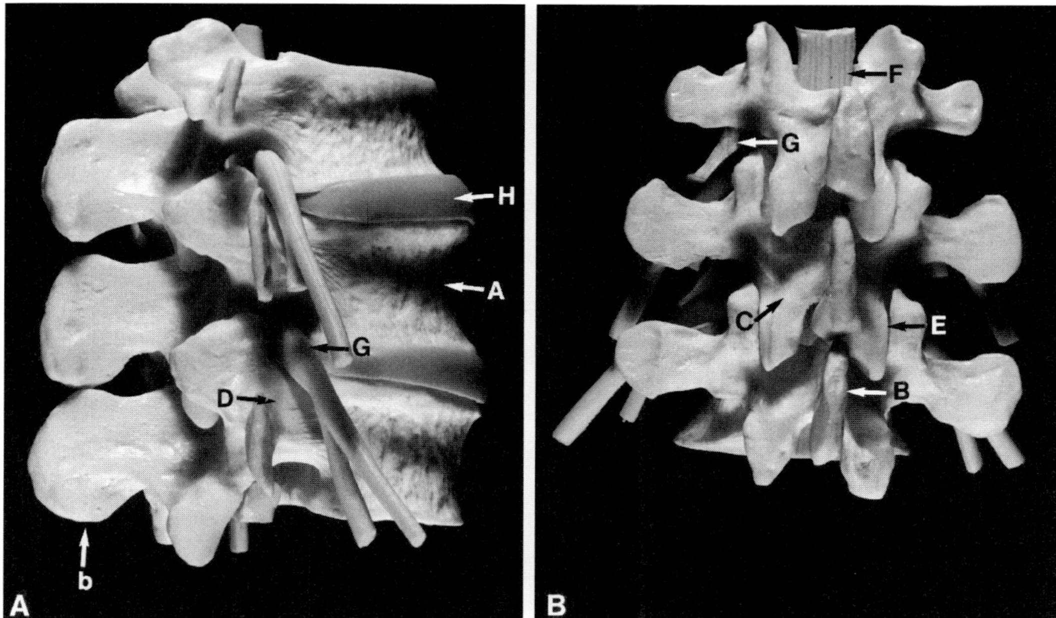

FIGURE 1. *A,* Lateral anatomic view of vertebral elements: **A,** vertebral body; **b,** spinous process; **D,** pedicle; **G,** nerve root exiting from foramen; **H,** intervertebral disc. *B,* Posterior anatomic view of vertebral elements: **B,** spinous process; **C,** lamina; **E,** facet joint, **F,** spinal cord; **G,** nerve root exiting from foramen.

column just anterior to its transverse process. The vertebral bodies are somewhat larger than their cervical counterparts. The facet joints are re-oriented parallel with the frontal plane but at a more significant angle from the horizontal seen in the transverse plane. The spinous processes angle inferiorly, actually overlapping to some extent and thus covering the interlaminar space.

The spinal canal through most of the thoracic spine is proportionately smaller in relation to the spinal cord than it is in the cervical spine. There is, consequently, less margin for intervertebral instability. Unlike the cervical and lumbar spine, the bony elements of the thoracic are not left to "fend for themselves" when it comes to providing structural support for the axial skeleton; the rib cage provides needed additional stability to protect the thoracic neural elements. The rib pairs provide skeletal protection for the heart, great vessels, and lungs, while significantly adding cylindrical stability to the vertebral column, joining anteriorly through the sternum. Although direct muscular support is again limited, the large posterior thoracic muscle masses (trapezius, rhomboids) significantly absorb forces applied to the thoracic spine.

Lumbar Spine

The lumbar bony elements are larger than those at the cervical and thoracic levels. Broad, thick vertebral bodies combine with large facet joints, transverse processes, lamina, and spinous processes to form a secure base for attachment of larger supportive muscles and ligaments. These soft tissues act as "guy wires" to maintain alignment and provide for the strong, coordinated torso movement necessary in most athletic endeavors. Lumbar facet joints are aligned more or less parallel to the sagittal plane, so as to permit flexion and extension while resisting rotation. As one approaches the inferior segments of the lumbar spine, gradually increasing height of the vertebral bodies anteriorly serves to create a lordotic curve. Although a certain amount of lordosis is necessary for normal, painless function, an increase in this curve predisposes the individual to acute and chronic injuries as will be described later in this chapter. [4,15,27,29,38]

PATHOLOGY AND TREATMENT

Unlike other areas of the athlete's anatomy, physical complaints related to the spine are not those of instability, giving way, or loss of strength, but primarily pain. Among the many characteristics of spinal pain, the most clinically important finding is whether the discomfort is radicular or nonradicular. Continuing in anatomical fashion, one may look at each segment of the spine in relation to the radicular or nonradicular nature of the pain and there begin formulation of an accurate diagnosis.

Posture and Its Effects

As the only support for the head and trunk, alignment of the spinal elements in normal anatomical relationship is key to maintaining mobility and decreasing "wear and tear." A spine held in malalignment because of poor posture will transfer increased stress to the soft tissue structures leading to muscle/ligamentous fatigue, pain, and ultimately, degeneration in the bony structures themselves.

In the cervical spine a gentle lordotic curve placing the atlas (C1) only slightly forward of the midsagittal line should result in optimal positioning for head support and maximum pain-free motion. A normal 20 to 40° thoracic kyphosis serves to balance cervical and lumbar-lordotic curves, placing the body's center of gravity just anterior to the fifth lumbar vertebrae.[31] A spine in balance results in a head that is not thrust too far forward or a lumbar spine in excessive swayback. The supporting muscular elements, as noted earlier, may be envisioned as "guy wires" that maintain the upright stance. A balanced spine distributes forces generated by the erect stance throughout the bony elements in proportion to the ability of each segment to withstand the generated stress. If the "guy wires" are not balanced, excessive flexion (i.e., the anterior muscle groups overpowering posterior) or extension (i.e., dominant posterior musculature) will ultimately result in symptoms of pain and fatigue.

Regardless of specific anatomic pathology, a normal response to spinal pain is tightening of the "guy wires" to position the bony elements in such a relationship to one another to produce the least pain. Unfortunately, this subconscious response often creates spinal imbalance and the original problem is then compounded. Restoration of stability to neutrality is necessary; physical therapy to restore such balance is beneficial.[29]

The Athlete's Cervical Spine

Athletic injuries to the cervical spine are relatively few and, with the exception of thankfully rare but well-publicized trauma resulting in cervical spinal cord compromise,[34,35] are usually transient and treatable. Those injuries that present to the primary care physician, for the most part, include ligamentous sprain and strain or minor bony injury.

Nonradicular Cervical Pain

Soft Tissue Injuries

Forward or lateral flexion of the neck resulting in stretch of posterior or contralateral ligamentous and muscular elements may result in fiber disruption. There will be local tenderness to palpation with pain aggravated by motion. Little or no swelling is evident, muscle strength in the upper and lower extremities normal, and neurologic testing unremarkable. Routine anteroposterior, lateral, and oblique radiographs should be augmented by flexion-extension lateral views to rule out segmental instability. When findings are locally limited and radiographs negative, treatment with analgesics, a soft supportive collar and physical therapy with heat, ice, and ultrasound should suffice to allow complete healing and a return to physical activity in 2–3 weeks.[32,33]

When radiographs do reveal sufficient soft tissue damage to allow for abnormal increase in motion between segments, however, the duration of treatment becomes more prolonged, requiring 8–12 weeks of more rigid immobilization.[12] Occasionally, if pain persists after a course of nonoperative care, surgical stabilization may be necessary. It is beyond the scope of this discussion to address these problems in detail, and any treatment should be made by a surgeon well schooled not only in cervical spine injury but also in the demands of the athlete's particular sport.

Bone Injuries

Bony injuries of the cervical spine are usually caused by violent application of vertical or shear loading, for example, the athlete's spearing an opponent in football, diving into shallow water, or landing inappropriately in a gymnastic maneuver.[1,34,35,36] If fortunate, the individual may sustain only a minor injury to the osseous structures that does not result in significant neural compromise. Much like minor cervical soft tissue injury, such limited bony injury results in localized tenderness pinpointed by palpation and aggravated by motion; muscular weakness or other neurologic abnormalities are absent. A minor compression fracture of the vertebral bony does not visibly compromise stability on a radiograph, but rather appears as slight wedging on the lateral view. It needs to be treated much as if a soft tissue injury—with 3 weeks of collar immobilization. Similarly, a radiographically visualized but nondisplaced fracture of the spinous process with sparing of ligamentous soft tissues can result from overaggressive neck flexion. In such cases, when an avulsion fracture exists and stability has not been compromised, prognosis for successful nonoperative treatment is greater than when complete ligamentous disruption exists. Three to six weeks of immobilization with a firm collar will allow bony union and restoration of stability. When the fracture is accompanied by instability, as documented on the lateral flexion/extension radiographs, treatment is more complex, requiring halo stabilization and/or surgical intervention.[16]

If the patient presents on physical examination with an obvious rotational deformity of the neck accompanied by limited motion, facet subluxation is likely. Unilateral subluxation shows a greater rotational deformity than bilateral. In either case, pain is only moderate and neurologic findings are absent, but both rotational and flexion/extension movements are limited. Oblique radiographs are required to make the diagnosis; occasionally computed or plain tomography will be necessary as well to visualize the pathology.[26,28] The importance of adequate radiologic studies cannot be overemphasized. Before clearing an individual for return to competition, the treating physician must assure that adequate films have failed to demonstrate any evidence of bony abnormality. The films obtained must include clear visualization of the C7–T1 relationship. This may require a "swimmer's view" in individuals whose cervicothoracic soft tissues interfere with a clear radiographic study. Accepting less than optimal radiographic visualization is inconsistent with appropriate care. Treatment of individuals with instability or malalignment frequently includes surgical intervention, so therapy from an appropriate specialist should be sought.

Radicular Cervical Pain

Indicative of neural compromise, radicular pain most often requires a more aggressive investigational approach and treatment is more involved. One must always assume that the athlete with cervical radiculitis has sustained a potentially devastating injury. Symptoms involving more than one extremity point to spinal cord compromise, whereas single extremity involvement represents trauma to a nerve root. Before resuming activity, an accurate diagnosis must be made and any identified pathology sufficiently documented and treated.[14,22]

Soft Tissue Injuries

Recurrent radicular pain aggravated by cervical motion indicates neurologic compromise involving soft tissue or bony damage. Further athletic participation may result in permanent injury to the spinal cord and nerve roots; therefore withdrawal from participation is mandatory. In addition to symptoms of extremity pain and paresthesias, the physical examination may show decreased (if the injury is to the nerve root or peripheral nerve) or increased (if the damage is to the spinal cord) deep tendon reflexes. Specific muscle weakness or distribution of sensory disturbances may aid in identifying the vertebral level of the injury. Standard anteroposterior, lateral and oblique radiographs should be augmented by lateral flexion-extension and odontoid images. If these are negative, CT or MRI may be required to identify fragments of displaced disc material.[17,20,26] Electromyography is additionally helpful in delineating the level and degree of injury and may, when repeated, aid in measuring recovery[14] (See Table 2).

In the absence of radiographically documented instability, bony injury, or soft tissue lesion, such as a herniated nucleus pulposus, treatment with a soft collar and analgesics should resolve symptoms over a few weeks. Radiculitis in such instances may well be secondary to direct root contusion and, with resolution of edema, symptoms will resolve.[33] Failure of this regimen indicates necessity for referral.

Bone Injuries

Any fracture that results in mild instability and/or neural compression will often cause radicular symptoms. Compression fracture of the vertebral body, laminar fracture, facet subluxation-dislocation, or lateral mass disruption should be suspected when the force of injury is particularly violent. When not evident on routine radiographs and tomographs,[99m] technetium bone scanning helps identify the site of injury.

When an acute fracture is identified and significant instability (greater than 3–4 mm of subluxation in lateral flexion-extension views) is ruled out, treatment in a firm collar for 6 weeks, if the immobilization promptly relieves radicular symptoms may be sufficient.[12] If (1) such a therapeutic approach does not relieve symptoms, (2) symptoms resume after an adequate period of immobilization, (3) the radiculitis is caused by osseous foramenal narrowing, or (4) the level of injury is to the lower (C_6,C_7) cervical elements, the assistance of a neurosurgeon or orthopaedic surgeon should be sought.

In addition to acute fracture, degenerative disease of the cervical spine caused by repeated trauma may result in osteophyte formation and partial obstruction of the vertebral foramen with resultant nerve root compression (see Fig. 2). A common problem in athletes who have participated in collision sports, degenerative cervical disease may respond to conservative measures such as immobilization and intermittent cervical traction. However, when motor dysfunction or persistent symptoms exist, surgery is recommended.

Cervical Radiculitis Secondary to Neural Injury

On occasion an athlete will sustain a temporary injury to the neural structures lasting from a few seconds to several minutes or hours. The individual may present on the sideline with complaints of paresthesias, burning or stinging in the upper extremities, or tingling throughout the body. When temporary, such symptoms are usually the result of vertical or shear stresses, which cause compression of the cord or

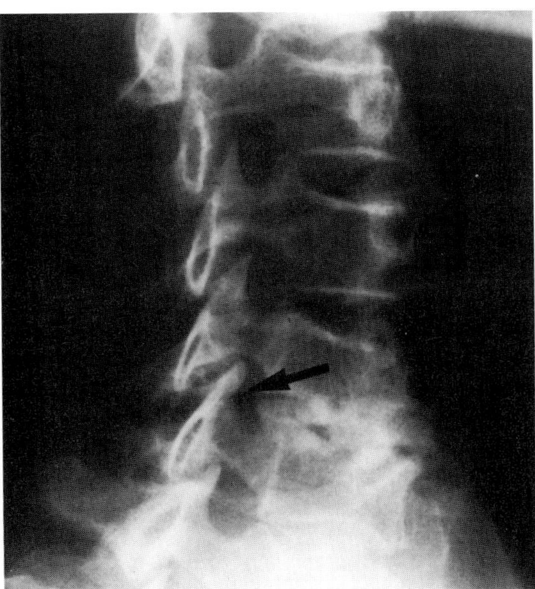

FIGURE 2. Degenerative changes in C5-C6 with foraminal encroachment are seen best on this oblique x-ray.

nerve root by osseous or ligamentous structures that have not been rendered unstable but only briefly distorted enough to transmit force to the neural element. Such events, when isolated, are usually inconsequential, but in the presence of continuing symptoms (pain, limited motion, or radicular symptoms lasting more than 10 minutes), significant pathology must be ruled out before allowing the individual to resume play. Initially, the individual's neck should be placed in a cervical collar until flexion-extension lateral and oblique radiographs are obtained.

A recently identified pathology that may cause temporary paresis is congenital narrowing of the spinal canal. This has resulted in temporary quadriplegia, an extremely frightening experience. In 39,377 exposed participants, the rate of transient paralysis or paresthesia in one football season was 7.3 per 10,000.[36]

The presence of repeated radicular symptoms ("stingers," "burners") or temporary quadriparesis demands an in-depth evaluation and search for etiology.[13] Tables 3A and 3B outline a recommended approach toward resumption of collision sports in instances of resolved neural compromise. Torg has developed guidelines that may be followed if the spinal canal be found to be abnormally narrow.[36,37] In his review of 117 permanent quadriplegics injured between 1971 and 1984, none had experienced prodromal symptoms of temporary paresthesias. Conversely, none of the players who experienced an episode of temporary neurologic symptoms sustained further neurologic injury after returning to play. In such instances, however, I believe rather strongly that until further evidence is compiled with regard to the natural history of such an anomaly, individuals with documented cervical canal narrowing, especially those with suspected instability, should not be allowed to participate in activities in which they are at potential risk. The Torg ration, which compares width of the spinal canal to width of the cervical vertebral body, has not proved infallible in identifying cervical spinal canal stenosis. Many athletes have enlarged veterbral bodies that make the ratio of canal to body width less than 0.8—the plain x-ray diagnostic parameter for stenosis.[37] Therefore, when spinal stenosis is suspected by a decreased canal-body ratio, an MRI study is necessary to confirm the diagnosis. Any individual with recurrent neurologic symptoms merits an MRI study of the spinal canal.[2,10]

Injuries to the Thoracic Spine

Soft tissue or bony injury of the thoracic spine as a result of athletic trauma is unusual; more often the forces are transmitted along this sturdy midline axis to injure the more vulnerable cervical or lumbar elements. Additionally, as a result of more rigidity between its segments, the thoracic spine is protected from degenerative processes to a greater degree. However, inflammatory or neoplastic invasion in

TABLE 3A. Investigation of Recurrent Cervical Radiculitis

X-ray studies:
- AP, Lateral, Oblique
- Lateral Flexion/Extension Views
- Pillar Views

Computed tomography
Magnetic resonance imaging

If all studies are negative, treat the symptoms and return to sport activity when asymptomatic.

TABLE 3B. Treatment of Proven Instability

IMMOBILIZE

SOMI Brace × 8 weeks

+

Philadelphia Collar × 4 weeks

↓

Stress lateral flexion/extension x-ray

No instability	<3.5mm instability	>3.5mm instability
↓	↓	↓
Return to Activity	Probably OK	Probably fusion candidate

this region is not uncommon in the general population. Although we do not often associate inflammatory and neoplastic problems with athletes, such problems must not be forgotten when formulating the differential diagnosis of a spinal complaint.[18,32]

Nonradicular Thoracic Pain

Soft Tissue Injury

More commonly associated with work stress and tension than athletics, thoracic symptoms of non-radicular pain most frequently represent muscle spasm or fatigue caused by overuse. Physical findings on examination include point tenderness and soft tissue firmness over the involved muscle fibers. Motion, particularly truncal rotation, increases the pain; massage temporarily alleviates it. For those symptoms that persist over several weeks, anteroposterior and lateral radiographs as well as basic laboratory testing (complete blood count, sedimentation rate or C-reactive protein as shown in Table 2) should be obtained to rule out the existence of metastatic disease, occult fracture, infection, or noninfectious inflammatory disease.

Treatment of nonradicular soft tissue discomfort should be directed toward the symptoms and consist of analgesics, muscle relaxants, and when pain is persistent, physical therapy. Occasionally an inciting activity can be identified in taking the history and an alteration made in frequency or method of performance of that activity.

Bone Injury

On occasion, progressive bone deformity may be the source of nonradicular thoracic discomfort. Most commonly seen in older adolescents, both the symptomatic flexible roundback condition as well as Scheuermann's disease present with localized interscapular or lower thoracic pain aggravated by prolonged standing, sitting, and bending activities.[7,39] Findings on physical examination generally are limited to an increase in roundback deformity, either in the form of a long graceful curve representing flexible adolescent-type postural roundback or a more sharply angulated, rigid kyphosis, as frequently seen in Scheuermann's deformity (Fig. 3). The diagnosis is based on the findings shown in the standing lateral radiograph; and when the kyphosis as measured between T12 and an upper thoracic vertebra exceeds 40°, the diagnosis of roundback is confirmed (Fig. 4). In the case of Sheuermann's disease, three successive thoracic vertebral bodies must each be anteriorly wedged more than 5° and, on occasion, the vertebral end plate may be slightly irregular (Fig. 5).

In the case of the former, i.e., flexible roundback, treatment consists primarily of postural exercise.

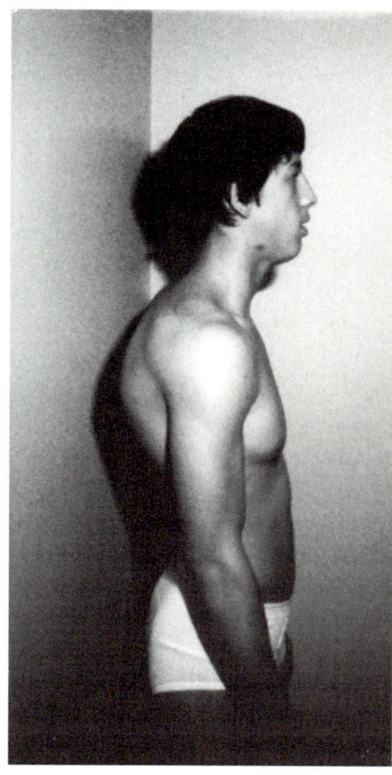

FIGURE 3. Relatively sharply angled dorsal kyphosis in a 16-year-old male typical of Scheuermann's disease.

When severe, treatment similar to that offered for Scheuermann's kyphosis may be carried out.

In Scheuermann's disease, where structural deformity exists, successful, permanently corrective brace treatment is possible (Fig. 6).[21] Such treatment should be directed by a physician well versed in the fundamentals of spinal deformity care.

Radicular Thoracic Pain

Radicular thoracic pain—that radiating laterally toward the anterior axillary line or distally accompanied by gluteal or lower extremity paresthesias—whether due to soft tissue, bone, or a primary neural etiology, should be subjected to in-depth investigation upon first presentation. When physical findings include (1) hypesthesia or hyperesthesia, (2) alterations in deep tendon reflexes, (3) pathologic reflexes (Babinski, clonus), (4) muscle atrophy and weakness, or (5) a change in foot posturing (progressive varus, cavus, or cavovarus deformities), neural function is presumed to be compromised.

MRI has shortened evaluation nearly to that of a single test. Although osseous abnormalities are less well identified, spinal cord compromise by tumor, abscess, or a herniated thoracic disc is readily identifiable on such images; a follow-up CT scan will confirm bone pathology.[17,20] The athlete with such a problem should be referred to a spinal surgeon without delay.

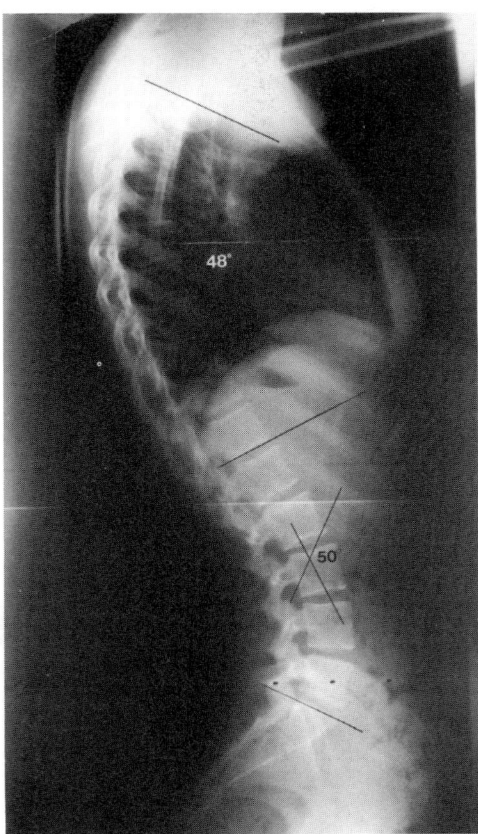

FIGURE 4. Flexible adolescent roundback deformity. Note that there are no structural abnormalities or wedging of the vertebral bodies.

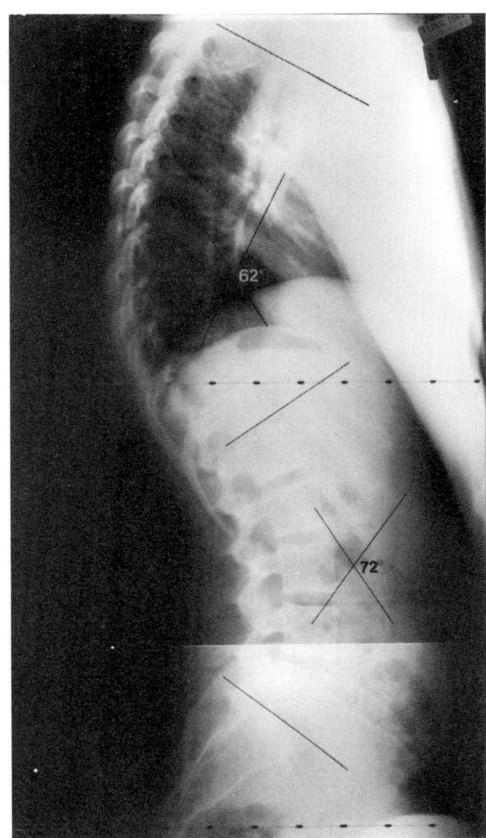

FIGURE 5. Standing lateral x-ray shows slight wedging of the vertebral bodies typical of Scheuermann's disease.

The Lumbar Spine

The athlete has not been spared the curse of pain in the lumbar area, which is the site of most complaints. The usual degenerative disease of middle age is accelerated in sport participants and, in addition, overuse syndromes are common. Physical activities easily and safely performed by the young adult can cause painful, career-shortening or career-ending injuries in two other groups of individuals, those who have either not yet reached bony maturity or those who are approaching middle age. A true appreciation of such predisposition by the physician will keep both the younger and older athletes actively participating.

Nonradicular Lumbar Pain

Soft Tissue Injury

Sudden, violent movement may tear muscle/ligamentosus fibers and cause localized pain, spasm, and postural deformity. Such an event is easily recalled by the individual, and physical examination demonstrates limited motion in flexion, lateral bending, or rotation and palpable localized tenderness. Prompt treatment with analgesics, physical therapy (ice massage, heat or ultrasound), and modified activities will limit disability to a few days. Return to activity must be gradual and preceded by strengthening and stretching exercises to decrease risk of reinjury.[32,33] Emergence of the "back school" concept of stabilizing the spine through strengthening the "guy wire" supporting soft tissues has clarified the nonoperative approach.[29] The key to success is an individualized approach to sound exercises applied to the large variety of pathologic conditions[27] (Table 4).

Bone Injury

Acute failure of the lumbar bony elements is rare. Conversely, overuse compromise of the lumbar skeleton is all too common and increasing in frequency. No age group is spared but the adolescent, skeletally immature athlete seems to be particularly prone to these problems. Vulnerability of the immature vertebral endplate and pedicle is unfortunately too often ignored by those overseeing junior and senior high school athletes. A training regimen designed for the mature individual too often results in a function-impairing overuse injury to the youth's spine

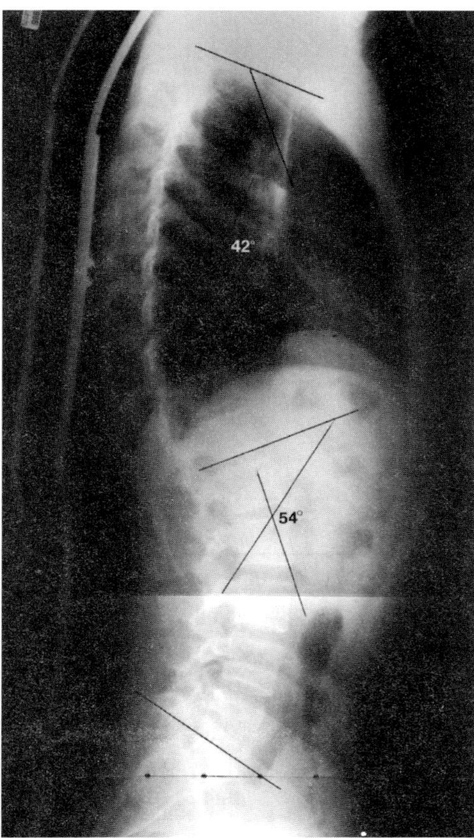

FIGURE 6. The same adolescent patient in Figure 5 but with a Milwaukee brace. Note significant passive correcton of the deformity.

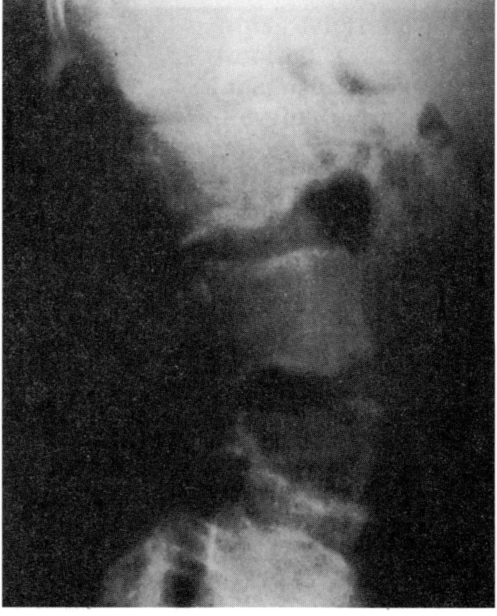

FIGURE 7. Radiographic appearance of lumbar vertebral bodies in a teenage gyrnnast reveals evidence of repeated end-plate fracture and growth plate irregularities.

TABLE 4. **Muscles Requiring Optimal Flexibility for Postural Alignment and Spine-safe Maneuvers**[27]

Upper Extremity
Pectoralis major and minor
Subscapularis
Teres major
Latissimus dorsi
Levator scapula
Trapezius
Lower Extremity
Hamstrings
Quadriceps
Psoas major and minor
Iloacis
Quadratus lumborum
Gluteus maximus, medius, minimus
Piriformis
Iliotibial band
Gastrocnemius
Soleus

(Fig. 7). The physician needs to be aware of these probabilities and to be able to recognize and treat such injury. Adequate treatment necessitates communication with coaches, trainers, and the athletes themselves regarding appropriate alteration in activity.

Anatomically, the pedicle (see Fig. 1) of the lower lumbar vertebra is prone to overuse failure by virtue of both its size and orientation. Roughly cylindrical, it is best suited to resist stresses directed along its long axis. Unfortunately, the variable degree of lordosis present in the lower lumbar spine area orients the pedicle obliquely, placing it in an inopportune position to resist vertical loading.[15,38] Such shear loading is encountered specifically in gymnasts during dismounts or in any athlete working out with weights during upright lifting activities, such as military presses, squats, or dead lifts. In addition, torsional stress, as is delivered to the pedicle during activities such as a tennis serve, also predisposes the area to injury. Repeated stress results in development of a "stress fracture" across the delicate, oblique pedicle. [3,4,11]

Poorly localized pain begins insidiously and gradually increases in intensity and frequency as long as physical activity continues. The discomfort is activity related, begins during or shortly after exercise, and lasts for a variable period. Physical examination reveals normal neurologic testing (deep tendon reflexes, muscle strength and sensation), a negative straight leg-raising test and only mild limitation of lumbar motion. The athlete has small restriction of forward flexion; however, extension, particularly when standing on one leg (Fig. 8), elicits discomfort, and the individual is able to localize pain to the region and side of pathology.

Seen best on oblique radiograph (Fig. 9), the stress fracture or spondylolysis may often also be visualized

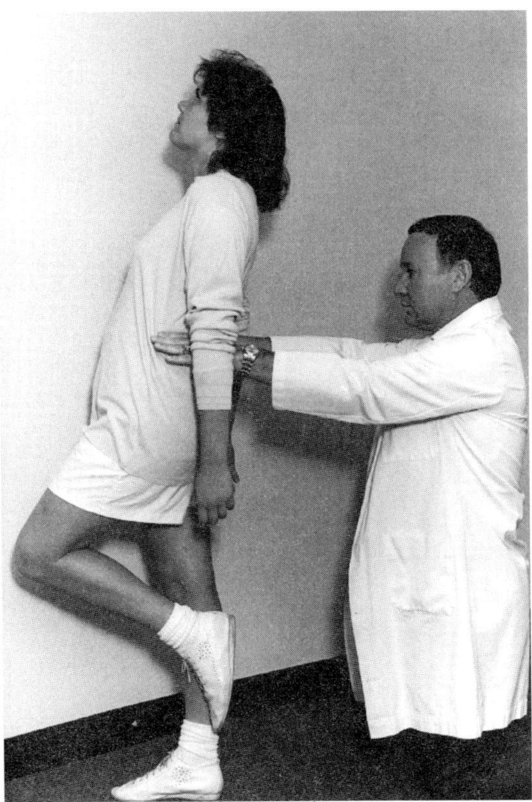

FIGURE 8. Single leg hyperextension test aggravates discomfort in the presence of spondylolysis.

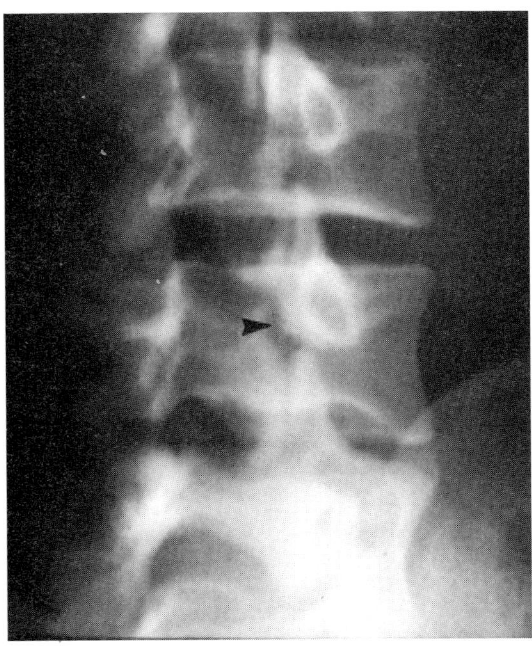

FIGURE 9. Oblique x-ray of the lumbosacral spine demonstrates spondylolytic defect in the L4 pars interarticularis (arrow).

on the lateral view. Anatomic proximity to the nerve root occasionally results in radicular symptoms, especially when the deficit is of long standing and a mass of callus has developed in an attempt at healing. When single leg-stance hyperextension aggravates the symptoms, but plain x-rays are not diagnostic, ^{99m}technetium bone scanning can be extraordinarily helpful in localizing early pathology.[5,25] A three-phase imaging sequence and computerized reproduction of the images further enhances anatomic localization of the problem (Fig. 10A). Computerized and plain tomographic imaging are additional,[8] and usually unnecessary, methods of further radiologic evaluation (Fig. 10B). When bilateral spondylolysis is present, potential exists for spinal instability because the anterior structure (veterbral body) is no longer connected to the posterior elements. Under such circumstances, only the anterior and posterior longitudinal ligaments along with the annulus fibrosus secure the vertebral column at the level of the lesion. If these soft tissue structures are stretched, the superior vertebral body may displace anteriorly on the one below, creating a spondylolisthesis. In the adult, spondylolisthesis is frequently stable and nonprogressive. In the adolescent, however, not only may the slippage be progressive, but in the supine position it may be partially or completely reduced. It is therefore imperative that at least one of the lateral radiographs views be taken in the standing position (Fig. 11).

Treatment of the all-too-frequent spondylolysis is staged. As in any fracture, the spondylolytic defect will heal if reasonably acute, and if nonunion or pseudarthrosis is not yet established. The bone scan is helpful in determining the age of the defect—one in which there is an active attempt at healing will have increased nucleotide uptake; an established pseudarthrosis in which attempted healing has ceased will appear "cold" on the scan.

If the defect is very acute, simple cessation of all aggravating activity for 6 weeks may result in sufficient bone repair to allow gradual return to sport. Over the ensuing 6 weeks the individual should very slowly work back into conditioning, flexibility, and finally full activity. Instituting an aerobic exercise program will improve muscular endurance and stability of the bony elements, thus preventing reinjury.[23] If, on resumption of athletic endeavors, symptoms recur, institution of more complete immobilization, as in any fracture, may allow for healing. Restoring balance and decreasing shear will occasionally be successful in treating spondylolytic or muscular lumbar pain. Use of a Boston or other antiflexion system may suffice.[19] Unfortunately, in order to immobilize the lower lumbar spine fully, the pelvis-sacrum area much also be stabilized. In some persistent cases, this may be accomplished with a single leg, pantaloon, body cast (Fig. 12) or similar brace, which is worn 24 hours per day. When

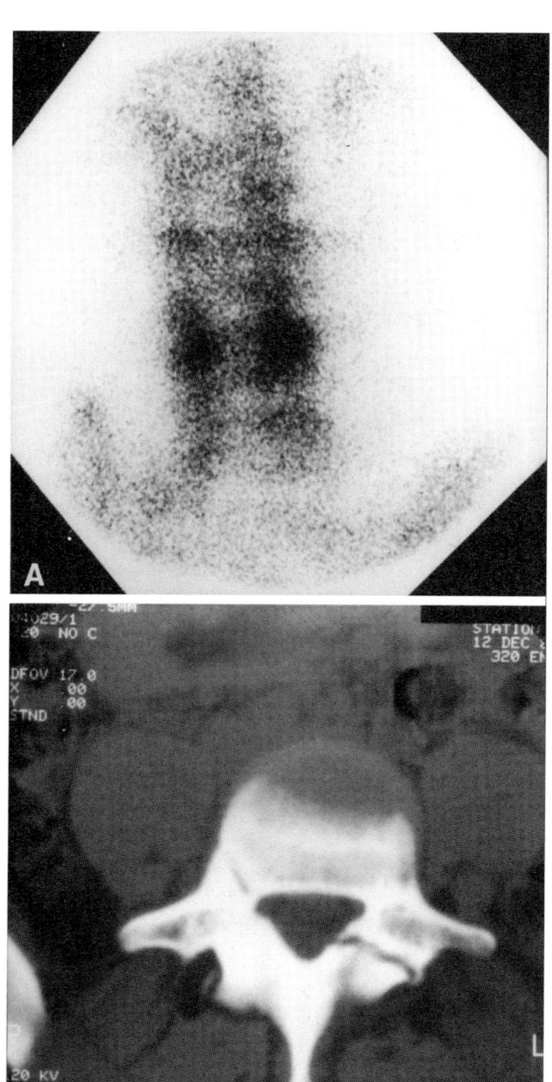

FIGURE 10. *A*, Technetium-99 bone scan demonstrates increased uptake bilaterally in the pars interarticularis region of L4 (same patient as in Figure 9). *B*, CT scan of L4 demonstrates spondylolytic defect on the left and fracture at the base of the pedicle on the right.

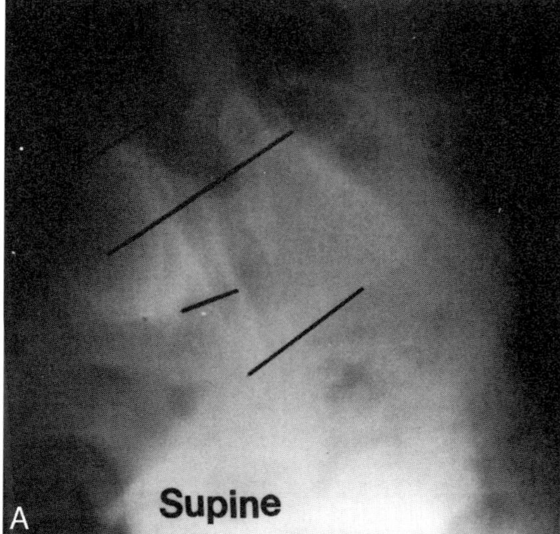

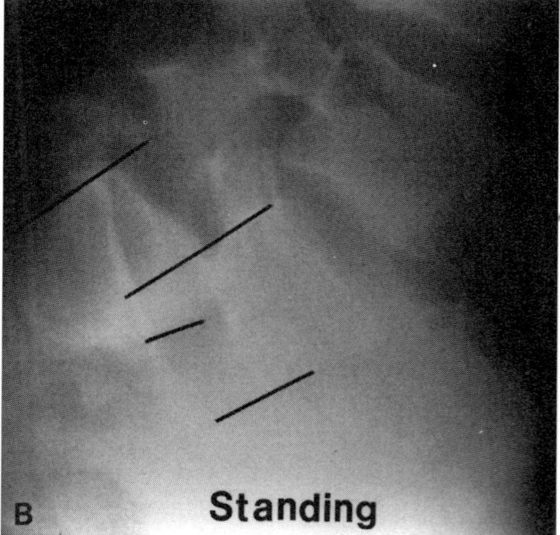

FIGURE 11. L5 on S1 spondylolisthesis increases from Grade II (50%) to Grade III (75%) when the x-ray is taken in the standing position.

the lesion is unilateral, the ipsilateral leg is immobilized; if bilateral, either leg may be selected. The athlete is allowed to be ambulatory in the cast or brace, which is worn for 8–12 weeks. On removal of the cast or brace, activity resumes very slowly. When immobilization is required, a total of at least 6 months of rehabilitation is necessary to return the individual to full athletic activities. The bone scan remains positive for up to 18 months as remodeling continues and the pedicle increases in size and strength in order to resist the forces to which it is subjected. Consequently, ^{99m}technetium scan is not a good yardstick by which to measure success of the healing process; nonrecurrence of symptoms after resumption of activity is the best indicator.

When nonunion is established or symptoms do recur, surgical fusion of the pseudarthrosis is required, and referral to an orthopedic surgeon experienced in spinal surgery is recommended.

The spondylolisthetic deformity, if stable, does not necessarily require treatment beyond that of a good spinal-stabilization exercise program.[27,29] Certainly, with progressive or continually bothersome symptoms, surgical consultation is required. Again, a spinal surgeon familiar with the psychic and physical demands of the athlete's particular sport is best suited to treat such a problem.

The modern-day practice of exposing youths to occult spinal injury by subjecting developing, growing veterbral structures to repeated physical impact and stress may create longer lasting, less treatable pathology. The vertebral endplate is physiologically constructed much like the physeal plate of the long bones, similarly contributing to growth and development of the part. Microfractures of this "growth plate" may recur with ongoing trauma of vertical loading, and subsequent growth may be impaired or deformity created. Although symptoms are intermittent and usually last only a few days, subsequent radiographs (see Fig. 7) reveal the abnormal development and irregular form of the vertebral body portion adjacent to the intervertebral disc. Cessation of the inciting activity may prevent formation of new lesions, but residual deformity will persist. The long-term effect of this irregularity in middle or late adulthood is unclear. It would seem most reasonable, however, that the activity be modified when such a problem is first recognized.

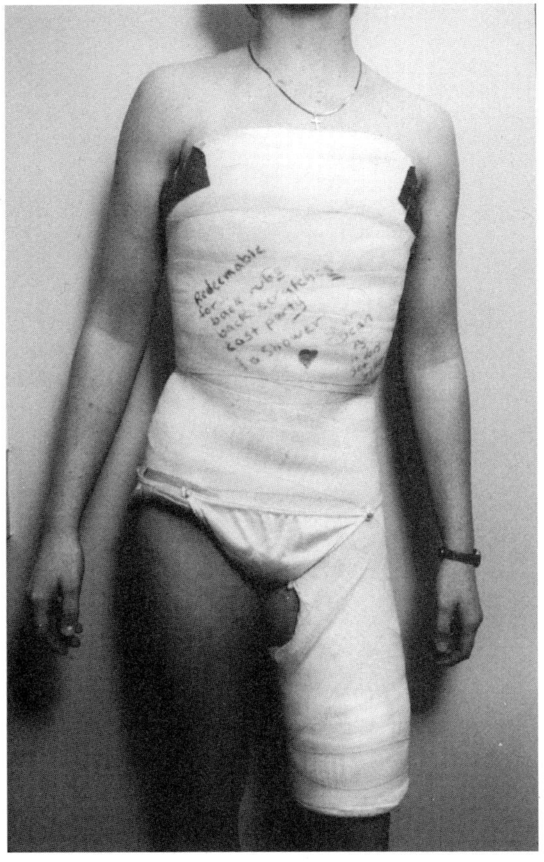

FIGURE 12. Single leg pantaloon cast extending from mid-chest to waist on the right and to the suprapatellar region on the left. Although the patient is ambulatory, the lumbosacral region is immobilized well.

Lumbar Radicular Pain

As the athlete gets older, the usual nerve root compromise seen in the nonathlete likewise become more frequent.[14] Pain radiating into the lower extremity is increased by activity and reduced by rest. Symptoms are similarly aggravated by Valsalva maneuvers (coughing, sneezing, and straining at stool). Physical findings may include protective muscle spasm and limited lumbar spinal motion, but surprisingly often the individual displays a normal degree of flexion, extension, and rotation of the trunk. Straight-leg raise is positive as is Lasegue's maneuver (passive dorsiflexion of the foot with the extremity just short of the painful position in passive straight-leg raising). Altered deep tendon reflexes combined with sensory and muscle strength testing will often define the level of nerve root compromise.

Radiographic evaluation, particularly CT or MRI, is particularly helpful in identifying the offended nerve root and source of its compromise (herniated disc, stenotic spinal canal, or foraminal narrowing by callus).

Initial treatment should be decreased activity, with progress to rehabilitation as the acute symptoms subside. Restoring spinal stability is necessary to protect the lumbar spine from additional microtrauma and any progression of root compromise. A high percentage of success is claimed by some using a nonoperative approach.[30] If such an approach, i.e., rest combined with aggressive physical therapy, analgesics, and muscle relaxants, fails to relieve the symptoms, the patient may well require appropriate surgical intervention. Return to athletic activity in the individual whose symptoms resolve may be permissible, but such a decision should be made on an individual basis. A wise course would be to modify excessively vigorous endeavors.[33]

Other Sources of Spinal Symptomatology

On rare occasion problems not previously mentioned will be the source of symptoms related to the athlete's spine. Unrelated to athletic activity, the individual's risk of developing a disc space infection, benign tumor such as osteoid osteoma, or noninfectious inflammatory process is no lower than in the general population. When the history, physical, laboratory, or radiographic findings suggest one of the more uncommon sport-unrelated diagnoses (e.g., decrease in disc space height, night pain reduced by salicylates, morning stiffness, increased sedimentation rate) treatment is no different than in the nonathlete. Other sources listed in the bibliography are recommended for specific diagnosis and therapeutic approaches to these entities.[33]

Scoliosis

Scoliosis, a condition present to a lesser degree in up to 8% of the population and to a more significant one in 0.3%, has received a great deal of attention over the past 2 decades due to school screening programs. When it is discovered, questions arise regarding what is permissible athletic activity. Athletic endeavors have neither a positive or negative proven effect on idiopathic scoliosis of mild to moderate degree (up to 45°). Additionally no benefit has ever been documented relative to a positive impact on the scoliotic curve itself as a result of an exercise program.

When the adolescent's minor curve becomes progressive, it is usually necessary to begin nonoperative treatment. If such treatment includes some form of bracing, the treating physician must decide the advisability of continued athletic activity. Frequently the treatment regimen will safely allow enough time out of the brace daily for the individual to participate, but each case must be individualized and the final decision made by the scoliosis specialist.

REFERENCES

1. Bundens DA, Rechtine GR, Bohlman HH: Upper cervical spine injuries. Orthop Rev 13:556–564, 1984.
2. Cantu RC: Cervical spine stenosis: Challenging an established protection method. Physician Sports Med 21(8): 57–63, 1993.
3. Ciullo JV, Jackson DW: Pars interarticularis stress reaction, spondylolysis, and spondylolisthesis in gymnasts. Clin Sports Med 4:95–110, 1985.
4. Dietrich M, Kurowski P: The importance of mechanical factors in the etiology of spondylolysis: A model analysis of loads and stresses in human lumbar spine. Spine 10:532–542, 1985.
5. Gelfand MJ, Strife JL, Kereiakes JG: Radionuclide bone imaging in spondylolysis of the lumbar spine in children. Radiology 140:191–195, 1981.
6. Godfrey CM, Morgan PP, Schatzket J: A randomized trial of manipulation for low-back pain in a medical setting. Spine 9:301–304, 1984.
7. Greene TL, Hensinger RN, Hunter LY: Back pain and vertebral changes simulating Scheuermann's disease. J Pediatr Orthop 5:1–7, 1985.
8. Grogan JP, Hemminghytt S, Williams AL, et al: Spondylolysis studies with computed tomography. Radiology 145:737–742, 1982.
9. Gutowsici WT, Renshaw TS: Orthotic results in adolescent kyphosis. Spine 13:485–489, 1988.
10. Herzog RJ, Wiens JJ, Dillingham MI, et al: Normal cervical spine morphometry and cervical spinal stenosis in asymptomatic professional football players: Plain film radiography, multiplanal computed tomography and magnetic resonance imaging. Spine 16(Suppl 6):5176–5186, 1991.
11. Jackson DW, Wiltse LL, Dingeman RD, Hayes M: Stress reactions involving the pars interarticularis in young athletes. Am J Sports Med 9:304–312, 1981.
12. Johnson RM, Owen JR, Hart DL, Callahan RA: Cervical orthoses: A guide to their selection and use. Clin Orthop 154:34–44, 1981.
13. Jordan BD, Warren RF, Tsairis P, Ghllman B: How to evaluate transient quadriparesis. Physician Sports Med 20:(2):83–90,1992.
14. Kikuchi S, Hasue M, Nishiyama K, I to T: Anatomic and clinical studies of radicular symptoms. Spine 9:23–30, 1984.
15. Letts M, Smallman T, Afanasiev R, Gouw G: Fracture of the pars interarticularis in adolescent athletes: A clinical-biomechanical analysis. J Pediatr Orthop 5:40–46, 1986.
16. Mazur JM, Stauffer ES: Unrecognized spinal instability associated with seemingly "simple" cervical compression fractures. Spine 8:687–692, 1983.
17. McAfee PC, Bohlman HH, Han JS, Salvagno RT: Comparison of nuclear magnetic resonance imaging and computed tomography in the diagnosis of upper cervical spinal cord compression. Spine 11:295–304, 1986.
18. Micheli LH: Back injuries in gymnastics. Clin Sports Med 4:85–93, 1985.
19. Micheli LJ, Hall JE, Miller ME: Use of modified Boston brace for back injuries in athletics. Sports Med 8(5):351–356, 1980.
20. Modic MT, Weinstein MA, Pavlicek W, et al: Nuclear magnetic resonances imaging of the spine. Radiology 148: 757–762, 1983.
21. Montgomery SP, Erwin WE: Scheuermann's kyphosis—long term results of Milwaukee brace treatment. Spine 6: 5–8, 1981.
22. Munnings F: Should athletes return to play after transient quadriplegia? Physician Sportsmed 19(10):127–134, 1991.
23. Nutter P: Aerobic exercise in the treatment and prevention of low back pain. Spine: State Art Rev 4(2):137–145,1990.
24. Paris SV: Spinal manipulative therapy. Clin Orthop 179:55–61, 1983.
25. Pennell RG, Maurer AH, Bonakdarpour A: Stress injuries of the par interarticularis: Radiologic classification and indications for scintigraphy. Am J Radiol 145:763–766, 1985.
26. Post MJD, Green BA, Quencer RM, et al: The value of computed tomography in spinal trauma. Spine 7:417–431, 1982.
27. Robison R: The new back school prescription: Stabilization training, part I. Spine: State Art Rev 5(3):341–355, 1991.
28. Rothman RH, Simone FA: The Spine, 2nd ed. Philadelphia, W.B. Saunders, 1982.
29. Saal, JA: The new back school prescription: Stabilization training, part II, Spine: State Art Rev 5(3):357–368, 1991.
30. Saal JA, Saal JS: Later stage management of lumbar spine problems. Phys Med Rehabi Clin North Am 2(1):205–219, 1991.
31. Seireg A, Arvikar R: Biomechanical analysis of the musculoskeletal structure for medicine and sports. New York, Hemisphere, 1989.
32. Spencer CW, Jackson D: Back injuries in the athlete. Clin Sports Med 2:191–215, 1983.
33. Teitz CC, Cook DM: Rehabilitation of neck and low back injuries. Clin Sports Med 4:455–476, 1985.
34. Torg JS: Epidemiology, pathomechanics, and prevention of athletic injuries to the cervical spine. Med Sci Sports Exerc 17:295–303, 1985.
35. Torg JS, Das M: Trampoline and mini-trampoline injuries to the cervical spine. Clin Sports Med 4:45–59, 1985.
36. Torg JS, Gennario SE, Pavlov H, Torg E: Cervical spinal stenosis with cord neurapraxia and transient quadriplegia. Exhibit, American Academy Orthopaedic Surgeons Annual Meeting, Jan. 1987.
37. Torg JS, Pavlov H, Genuarin AT, et al: Neurapraxia of the cervical spinal cord with transient quadriplegia. J Bone Joint Surg 68A:1354–1370, 1986.
38. White AA, Panjabi MM: Clinical Biomechanics of the Spine. Philadelphia, J.B. Lippincott, 1978.
39. Wilson FD, Lindseth RE: The adolescent "swimmer's back". Am J Sports Med 10:174–176, 1982.

21

Office Management of Knee Injuries

W. Michael Walsh, M.D.
Michele J. Helzer-Julin, PA-C, M.S.

For most primary care physicians, orthopedic problems make up a significant percentage of their practice. Many of these orthopedic disorders may be related to sport, especially if the patient population is young and athletic. The knee continues to present the most nettlesome problems for primary care physicians, and indeed for orthopedic surgeons as well.

The purpose of this first of two chapters is to present a logical approach to the injured knee that the physician can undertake in the office. Emphasis is on the evaluation of the acute knee, since this situation usually presents some time constraints. Along the way, reference will be made to significant differences in evaluation of the patient with chronic complaints. The second chapter discusses the group of disorders that account for the greatest percentage of overuse injuries of the knee: tracking problems of the patella.

TAKING A HISTORY

Much important information can be gathered before one even begins a physical examination of the knee. The prime question to be answered is, "How did this knee problem begin?" If the patient indicates that the problem started without any single specific trauma to the knee, then we are immediately guided toward overuse injury. Here we will almost invariably be dealing with a certain well-defined group of inflammatory syndromes, most of which involve the extensor mechanism of the knee—that is, the quadriceps, the patella, the patellar tendon, and other related soft tissues such as the synovial plica and the infrapatellar fat pad. More will be said about these entities in the next chapter.

In the youngster with insidious, nontraumatic onset of knee pain, other more unusual explanations must be at least considered, such as osteochondritis dissecans and neoplasm. In older age groups, too, apparent overuse may imply somewhat different pathology. Symptoms of a degenerative meniscus tear, for example, may occur from trauma that is trivial or unremembered. Osteoarthritis or the inflammatory arthritides also may occur without specific trauma. Across all age groups, the vast majority of patients who report knee pain, especially bilateral anterior knee pain that is not related to a specific traumatic episode, will be suffering from one of the extensor mechanism syndromes.

If the knee problem is due to a single definite injury, it is important to have the *athlete* specify precisely what occurred. What was he or she doing at the moment the knee was hurt? Was there a direct force applied to the knee by some other object, such as another player's body? If so, where did the force strike the leg and into what position was the knee forced? Was it a noncontact mechanism of injury? What was the athlete doing at that precise moment? Coming down from a rebound or jump shot? Making a turn?

Next press the patient for specific details as to what he or she *felt* when the injury occurred. Did the patient feel or hear a "pop?" Did he or she feel something actually slip out of place? Did the athlete feel immediate pain? If so, where was the pain located?

Next ask the athlete about immediate disability. This is usually the history of falling to the ground and being unable to get up and continue. This situation implies an injury quite different from one in which the athlete is able to continue playing during the game or practice and develops soreness and disability overnight. If the athlete fell to the ground, in what posture was the knee originally held? If the knee was initially flexed, who straightened it out? Was it the coach, the trainer, a teammate, or the athlete himself? As the knee was straightened, was there a sensation of something "going back into place?" This history suggests an acute patellar dislocation that was reduced by simple knee extension, whereas a knee that could not be straightened out from the moment of injury would suggest a mechanical blockage to knee extension, such as a displaced bucket-handle tear of a meniscus.

Finally, and very importantly, there is the question of swelling. A large swelling within the first two hours after injury is invariably a hemarthrosis. Few injuries create an immediate hemarthrosis. The most common of these is a tear of the anterior cruciate ligament, which accounts for 80% of the athletic knee injuries that produce immediate onset of hemarthrosis. The other injury likely to cause hemarthrosis is an osteochondral fracture of one of the joint surfaces. Remember, though, that swelling may not necessarily accumulate within the joint. If one of the capsular ligaments (that is, the actual joint capsule itself) has been torn, any swelling may not be retained within the knee. Therefore, if the rest of the history sounds serious, but the story of swelling is relatively benign, one should not be misled into minimizing this athlete's injury. The same advice goes for the history of pain. Remember that completely torn knee ligaments are generally less painful than partially torn ligaments. Often, the patient with a complete tear will soon be able to walk without significant pain and without instability. However, if the knee ligaments are completely torn, twisting, pivoting, or cutting activity will usually provoke joint instability symptoms.

If the knee injury is chronic, there are some additional symptoms about which you should ask. First is the symptom of "giving way." What does giving way mean to the patient? Is it a sudden weakness in the leg causing the knee to bend in a direction in which knees normally bend—that is, into flexion or mild hyperextension? If so, this is usually a muscular phenomenon. Any chronically disabled lower extremity may eventually experience this reflex, muscular type of giving way. On the other hand, is the patient using "giving way" to indicate true joint subluxation symptoms, with "bones going out of place?" This is a far more significant problem that may indicate laxity of ligaments or patella. Usually joint subluxation does not occur while simply walking straight ahead but rather with twisting, pivoting, or cutting activity.

What about popping? Popping is so ubiquitous as to be practically useless in terms of specific diagnosis. All sorts of things can create popping in and around knee joints, whether injured or not. However, if either you or the patient can recreate this popping sensation during the physical examination, some usefulness may come from it. Painful popping is likely more significant than nonpainful popping.

Patients may also complain of locking or catching sensations. What is the difference between these two symptoms? We generally use "locking" to mean some mechanical interference with knee motion that is of relatively long duration. Usually this occurs with the knee in flexion, causing inability to fully extend. The patient may eventually learn some maneuver to "unlock" the knee. A history of true locking is typical of meniscus injury or loose bodies within the joint. If a loose body is the trouble, many times patients will also report feeling a small lump arise in a subcutaneous location that they can manipulate around and eventually see disappear into the confines of the knee joint. "Catching" is a much more transient phenomenon. It usually occurs with the knee in extension, causing an inability to flex. It is a sensation for which the patient generally does not perform a specific maneuver to correct. These catching episodes are highly typical of extensor mechanism disorders.

PHYSICAL EXAMINATION

After a carefully taken, detailed history, proceed with the physical examination of the knee. The patient must be adequately exposed. You must be able to see and get to *both* lower extremities, including the feet. Examination gowns are adequate, but gym shorts are ideal. Having a few pair of "loaner" shorts in your office in assorted sizes is very helpful. Simply pulling the pants leg up is *not satisfactory!* You must have better access to the entire limb in order to do an adequate examination.

The patient's situation will determine the way in which you proceed. If it's a chronic problem or one of gradual onset, then do not rush to have the patient assume the supine position on the examination table. Look at the patient in the standing position from both front and side to detect any deformities or asymmetries of the lower extremities. Note any varus, valgus, lack of complete extension, recurvatum, or rotational deformities. See the next chapter on tracking problems of the patella for more complete details on abnormal rotation of the femur and tibia. Remember that foot deformities can have a roll in creating knee problems. Take particular note of any pes planus or pronation. The next chapter on patellar problems gives further details on the foot exam as it pertains to knee pathology. Next, watch the patient walk. Is there a limp? Is there a varus or valgus thrust? Is there some other evidence of abnormal mechanics of gait? If possible, observing the patient walk or even jog over a longer distance, such as down a hallway, will give you a much better idea of lower extremity mechanics.

In chronic or overuse problems, have the patient sit on the side of the examination table with both knees flexed to 90°. Here, a number of observations can be made about the extensor mechanism (discussed in the next chapter). Additionally, the earliest and most subtle sign of swelling in the knee joint may be obliteration of the concavity that almost all

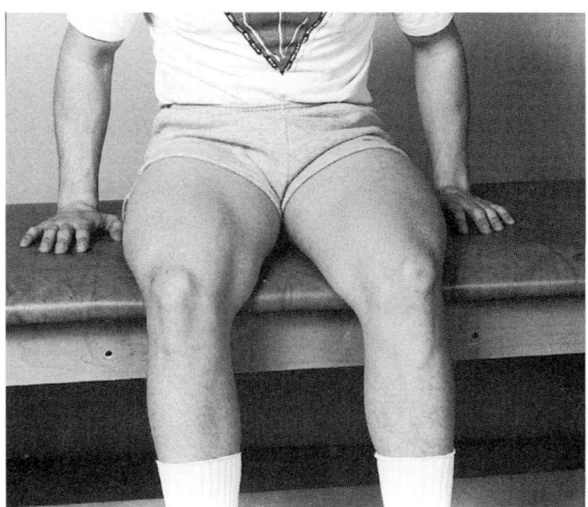

FIGURE 1. **Patient sitting with knees flexed 90°.** Note normal concavity adjacent to anteromedial joint line, just medial to patellar tendon. Obliteration of this concavity by mild puffiness may be the first subtle sign of knee swelling.

of us have over the anteromedial part of the knee joints adjacent to the patellar tendon (Fig. 1).

Now have patients with a chronic knee problem lie flat on their back. In an acute knee injury, the examination is usually started with the patient lying supine. In either case, start with examination of the uninjured knee first! If both knees are symptomatic, start with the less symptomatic knee first. Try to arrange your office examination table so that both knees can be conveniently examined. If this is impossible, have the patient turn around with his head at the opposite end of the table for each knee. To neglect the normal knee is to miss a vast amount of information! There is a wide range of normal findings in knees. Joints may be more or less lax, depending on our normal make-up and collagen composition. One has no idea whether ligament laxity or patellar hypermobility is significant unless one first establishes what is "normal" for *this particular patient*. The other benefit in beginning with the normal knee in the acute setting is that it demonstrates to the patient what to expect when you examine the more painful injured side. By doing a gentle examination with finesse, you set the patient's mind at ease. With a rough examination of the good knee, the response will be, "You're not going to do that to my hurt knee, are you?"

For the sake of brevity, we will not describe the complete examination on the normal side. This will become clear as we discuss the examination of the injured limb.

Observation

Even if you begin the examination with the patient lying supine because it is an acute injury, take a few moments simply to observe the leg. How does the patient hold the extremity? Does the leg lie flat on the table with the knee coming to full extension? Is there some obvious deformity of the leg? Can you visualize swelling that appears to be either inside the joint or in the extraarticular soft tissues? Believe it or not, there are probably some diagnoses that could be made without going any further in the knee examination, just by simple observation. An example would be prepatellar bursitis, in which the prepatellar bursa would be easily visible as a localized "goose egg" sitting superficial to the patella and clearly contained within a bursal structure. The point is to take some time to observe what can be seen.

Initial Palpation

Lay your hands on the patient's knee for a little bit of very gentle palpation. One of the benefits of this approach is to allay fears the patient may have about your manipulation of the knee. Once you make the initial contact in a very gentle fashion, you may often set the patient's mind at ease. About the only thing to really palpate for at this point is effusion within the joint. Use your hand closest to the patient's head to milk any effusion out of the suprapatellar pouch into the subpatellar region where it is most easily felt.

Ligament Examination

The most important question you should ask yourself at this point of examining the acutely injured knee is, "Is this knee stable?" Next, examine the ligaments. If the injury is extremely painful, and if the patient cannot fully extend the knee, place a pillow under the knee to hold it in the flexed position while the patient completely relaxes the thigh musculature (Fig. 2.). As with all these ligament stress tests, patients must keep their head down and be relaxed. If they pick their head up to see what you are about to do, it is impossible to relax the thigh. With the patient in this position, perform the Lachman test, which has been proved to be the most reliable indicator of anterior cruciate ligament injury. This test is done by holding the distal thigh with one hand while applying an anterior drawer type of maneuver to the tibia with the opposite hand (Fig. 3). The test should be done in approximately 15° of flexion, just about the same degree of flexion that is comfortable in most acutely injured knees. Squeezing on sore, injured areas may cause the patient to contract the muscles, invalidating the test. Be careful not to do this. If the test is positive and the subluxation itself is painful, then the patient may allow you only one good chance to perform the Lachman test. One positive response is enough! If the patient is a 280–pound defensive football lineman, and if your hands are relatively small, you may find the Lachman test impossible to perform.

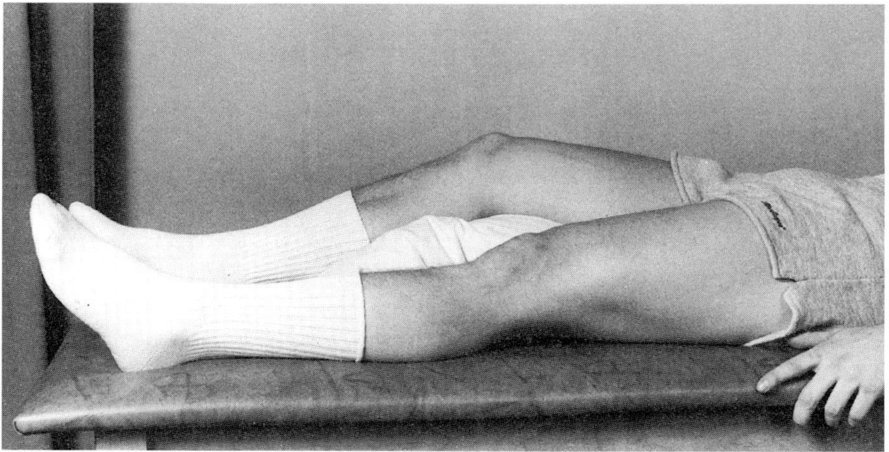

FIGURE 2. **Positioning**. A patient with acute knee injury is comfortably positioned on the examination table with the injured knee in slight flexion on a pillow. The opposite leg and head are flat. All muscles are relaxed.

In this case, have an assistant stabilize the distal thigh with two hands while you apply the anterior force on the proximal tibia with *both* hands (Fig. 4). John Feagin has described a variation of the Lachman test, done with the patient in the prone position. This is done with the foot and ankle held by your upper arm against your body. It allows both hands to be free and uses the force of gravity to help to create the anterior subluxation of the proximal tibia (Fig. 5). My experience, however, has been that getting into this position with an acutely injured knee is not very comfortable, so this variation has been of greatest help in large patients with a chronic problem.

Interpretation of the Lachman test, like all ligament stress tests, is based on comparison with the normal knee. The beauty of the Lachman test is that it may help you decide not only whether the anterior cruciate ligament has been hurt but also to what degree. If there is a mild increase in the Lachman test over the normal side, but it still has a good, firm endpoint, then there is probably a partial tear of the anterior cruciate ligament. If the Lachman test is markedly positive with a "mushy" feel to the endpoint, then most likely the anterior cruciate ligament is completely torn. When the Lachman test is positive, especially when accompanied by a history that is extremely typical, you may wish to stop the examination here. This is an injury that primary care physicians usually do not want to deal with. The athlete should be sent to an orthopaedic consultant as soon as feasible. On the other hand, if you are seeing the patient soon after injury, you may be able to

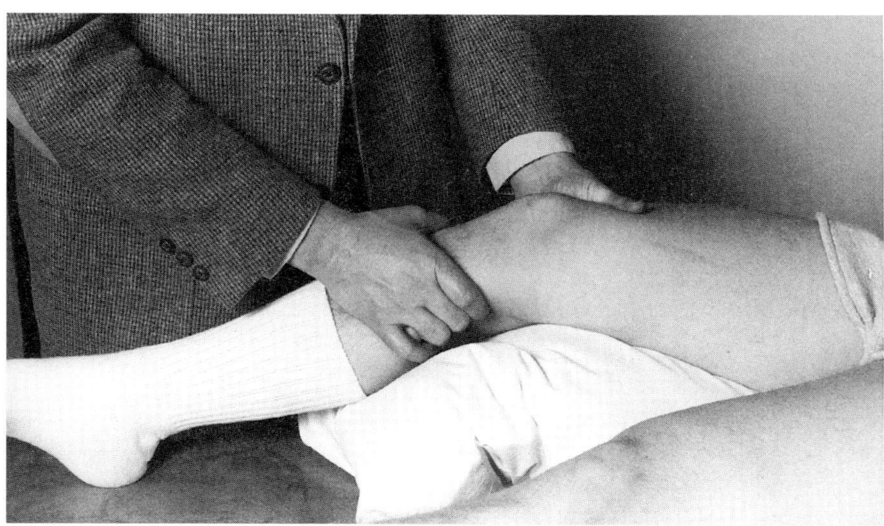

FIGURE 3. **Lachman test.** A Lachman test in a patient with acute knee injury can be done with the leg on a pillow. An attempt is made to sublux the tibia anteriorly while holding the distal thigh with the opposite hand. This test is done in approximately 15° of flexion. Anterior subluxation of the tibia indicates injury to the anterior cruciate ligament.

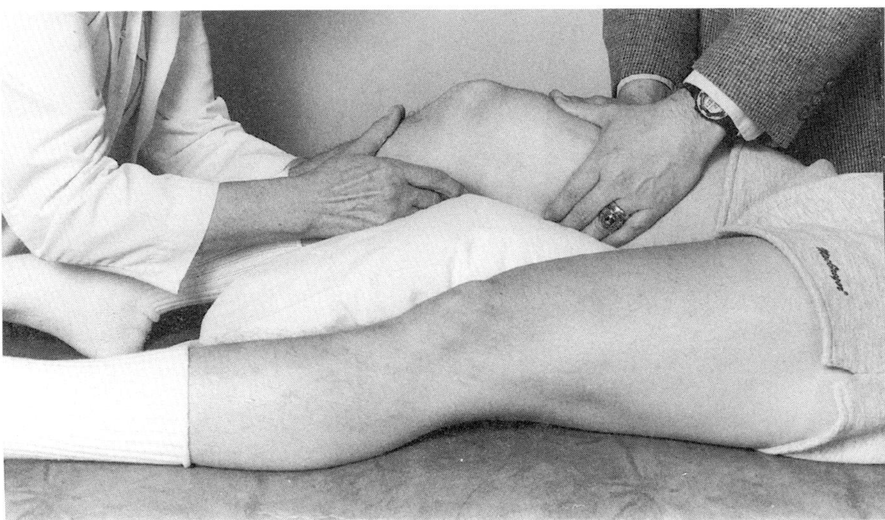

FIGURE 4. **Alternative method for performing Lachman test** in a patient with a large thigh. The distal thigh can be stabilized by an assistant while the examiner uses both hands to apply anterior force to the proximal tibia.

detect findings that later will not be discernible by a consultant. The patient is also more comfortable than he or she will be later, so you should proceed with whatever further examination is possible.

Next, perform the abduction stress test to check the medial collateral ligament. This can be done with the knee on a pillow but is probably better done with the thigh lying flat on the examination table and the foot over the side (Fig. 6). One of the examiner's hands grasps the forefoot while the other hand is placed on the lateral side of the knee. As you get the patient into this position, reassure him or her that you are not going to release the foot suddenly and make the knee bend. The thigh lying flat on the table helps greatly in relaxing the musculature. With the knee at about 30° to 45° of flexion, gently stress the knee into a position of valgus, using the hand on the lateral side of the knee as a fulcrum. What you are feeling and looking for is an opening along the medial joint line, which may actually be visible in a thin, unswollen knee or may be detectable only as a feel. The opening may be only noticeable as a slight clunk when the medial femur and tibia come back to the neutral position. Done with the knee in 30°–45° of flexion, this is a secure, reliable test for integrity of the medial compartment ligaments. Why do this test with the knee flexed? When the knee is fully extended, it is stabilized by the posterior cruciate ligament. Therefore, one can have a complete rupture of the medial compartment ligaments, and, so long as the posterior cruciate ligament remains intact, the knee will be stable to either abduction or adduction stress with the knee in full extension. This stabilizing effect of the posterior cruciate is relaxed by flexing the knee, thereby allowing the instability created by the medial compartment tear to be felt. If the knee can be straightened comfortably, however, the abduction stress test should be tried in progressively straighter positions until the fullest possible extension is reached. A knee that is unstable in flexion but stable in extension demonstrates that the medial ligaments are ruptured and that the posterior cruciate ligament is probably intact. If significant instability exists both in flexion and in extension, the posterior cruciate ligament as well as medial ligaments may be ruptured.

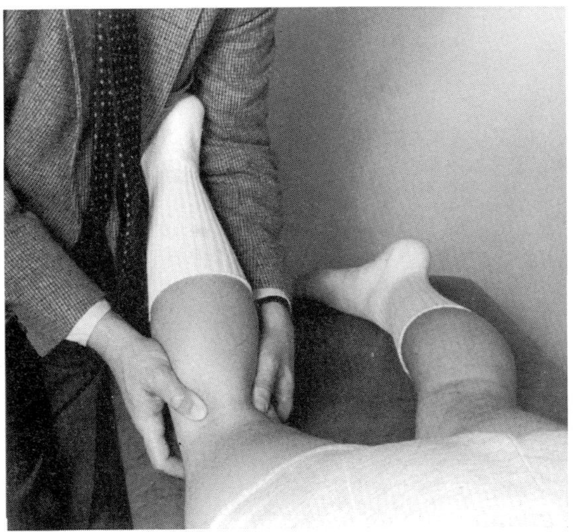

FIGURE 5. **Feagin modification of the Lachman test.** The patient is in prone position. The examiner holds the foot under his arm. Both thumbs are used to sublux the tibia anteriorly beneath the distal femur. Both index fingers are used to palpate anterior tibial subluxation in relation to femoral condyle.

Your hands can now be reversed to perform the adduction stress test in both flexion and extension (Fig. 7). If gross instability is present in comparison to the normal knee, this may be a helpful finding. However, realize that the adduction stress test is

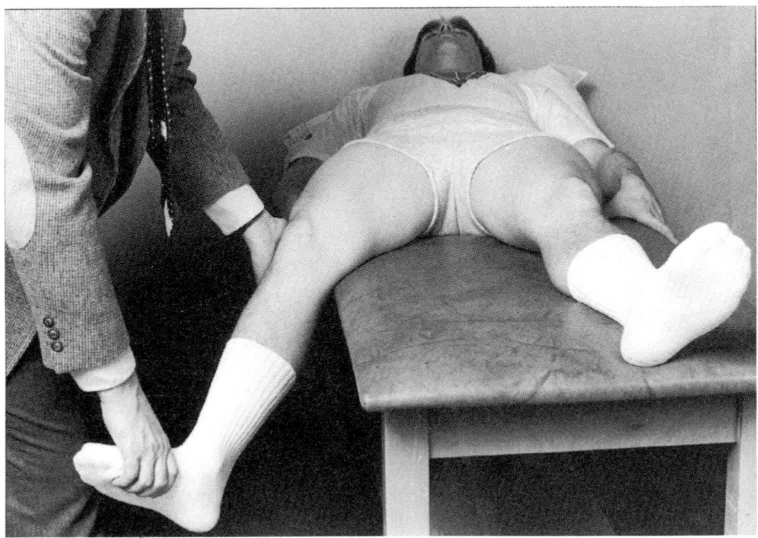

FIGURE 6. **Position for performing the abduction stress test in flexion.** The thigh rests flat on the examination table, with muscles relaxed. The opposite leg and head must also be flat. A hand placed along the lateral aspect of knee is used as fulcrum, while the opposite hand on the patient's foot applies abduction or valgus. See text for details.

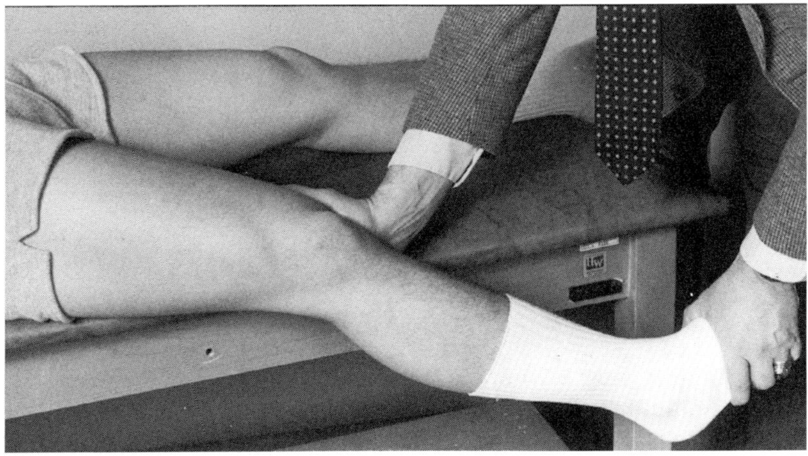

FIGURE 7. **Position for performing adduction stress test in flexion.** Hand position is opposite that shown in Figure 6. Adduction or varus is applied to the knee. See text for interpretation.

much less useful overall than the abduction stress test. First, most knees will demonstrate a mildly positive adduction stress test in 30° of flexion. Second, even with the knee in flexion, there is a great stabilizing influence of the iliotibial band. Consequently, an adduction stress test that is no different from that on the opposite side should not be viewed with any great amount of comfort. Serious lateral compartment injuries to the lateral collateral ligament, popliteus, or arcuate complex may still exist.

Another major point may be raised. The abduction or adduction instability in full extension is a reliable indicator for posterior cruciate injury *only* in the acute setting. It is not reliable in the chronically injured knee, when posterior cruciate injury will be best shown by some of the tests discussed later.

Range of Motion

You have now examined the knee for the two most common ligament ruptures that you will encounter. If these tests are negative, carry on with further tests. Determine whether there is enough comfortable range of motion in the knee to allow other manipulations to be done. Gently assist the patient with the acutely injured leg to see how much extension and flexion is possible in comparison to the opposite side. Lack of full range of motion will not provide a specific diagnosis, but if the knee lacks full extension, and has lacked it since the very moment the injury occurred, then you may be dealing with a displaced meniscal tear. It may be of some benefit, especially in the chronically injured knee, to ascertain whether the lack of full extension is accompanied by the "springy" feeling of hamstring muscle spasm causing "pseudolocking" of the knee versus the more solid feel of meniscal or other mechanical blockage to full extension.

Other Ligamentous Tests

If the knee can easily flex to 90°, then you can proceed with the traditional drawer tests. Do these with the patient supine and relaxed, with the head completely flat. The hip is bent to 45° and the knee to 90° (Fig. 8). The foot is then placed flat on the examining table. The most convenient way to stabilize the foot is to sit on the toes gently, securing the foot to the examination table. Both hands are then free to grasp the proximal tibia, with thumbs along the anterior aspect of both medial and lateral tibial plateau, flanking the patellar tendon. Your index fingers behind the tibia can easily palpate the hamstring tendons, making sure that they are relaxed. The anterior drawer is then a matter of pulling on the proximal tibia, attempting to sublux it anteriorly beneath the distal femur. The posterior drawer is the simple converse of the anterior drawer. The posterior drawer is performed by pushing the proximal tibia posteriorly rather than pulling it forward.

Several words of caution are in order. These drawer tests can be done with the foot and tibia in various degrees of internal or external rotation. The interpretation is technically somewhat different, depending on the degree of rotation. Simply put, internal rotation of the tibia causes tightening of the cruciate ligaments, whereas external rotation causes relaxation. The primary care physician should do the drawer tests routinely with the foot and tibia in neutral rotation—that is, with the toes pointing straight ahead on the examination table.

Carefully define the starting position for the drawer test. If the posterior cruciate ligament has been ruptured, gravity itself may create a posterior sag of the proximal tibia when the knee is first placed in position to perform the drawer test (Fig. 9). Then, when you do the anterior drawer maneuver, you will pull the posteriorly subluxed tibia into neutral position and may interpret this maneuver as a positive anterior drawer test, when, in fact, it is the reduction of a spontaneous posterior drawer test. The only way to avoid this pitfall is by careful comparison with the uninjured knee.

The anterior drawer test is not as reliable as the Lachman test for detecting anterior cruciate ligament injury. There are many structures that influence the anterior drawer test other than the anterior cruciate ligament. We commonly see a normal anterior drawer test when the anterior cruciate ligament has been completely ruptured. Remember, the anterior drawer test alone is *not* a reliable indicator for anterior cruciate injury, even though we continue to use it along with the Lachman test in evaluation of the anterior cruciate.

How do you correlate the posterior drawer test with the instability in full extension discussed earlier? These two tests are both helpful in evaluation of the posterior cruciate ligament, though usually in different settings. Specifically, the positive abduction stress test or adduction stress test in full extension is helpful when the posterior cruciate has been injured along with the medial or lateral compartment ligaments, and the patient is evaluated in the acute period. On the other hand, if the mechanism of injury has been a direct blow to the anterior portion of the flexed knee, as in a dashboard injury, the posterior drawer sign may also be positive immediately following the trauma. The posterior drawer sign, however, is routinely positive in *all* patients with chronic posterior

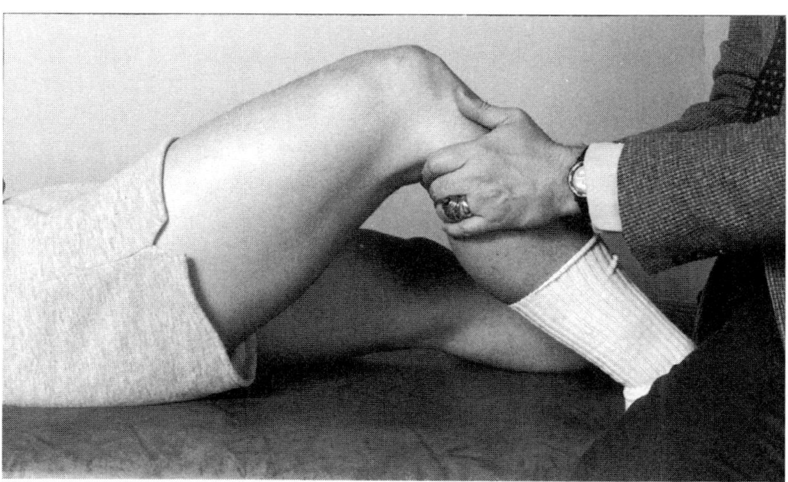

FIGURE 8. **Position for anterior and posterior drawer tests.** Hip is flexed 45°. Knee is flexed 90°. The tibia is in neutral rotation. Anterior pull or posterior push can be applied to the proximal tibia with both hands. See text for interpretation.

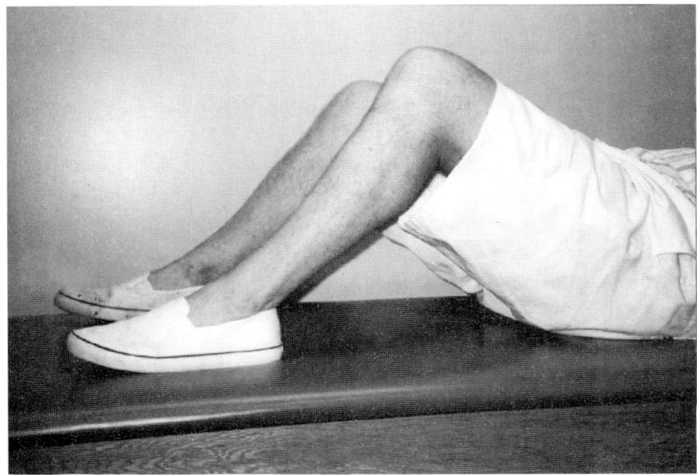

FIGURE 9. Posterior sag of proximal left tibia seen in posterior cruciate ligament tear. Compare with normal position of opposite right knee.

cruciate instability. The best recommendation is to do both the abduction and adduction stress tests as well as the posterior drawer test in all knees you evaluate.

Several other ligament stress tests can be performed on the knee. However, they are rather subtle and more difficult to describe, perform, and interpret. For example, you may be aware that the instability created by an anterior cruciate ligament rupture is really a rotatory type of instability. Usually there is an anterior rotatory subluxation of the lateral tibial condyle in the last 30° or so of extension. This is the phenomenon that produces the symptoms of joint instability that patients report. Tests are available that demonstrate this anterolateral rotatory instability. The two most commonly used are the jerk test and the pivot shift test. Both tests elicit the same phenomenon, but in opposite directions. It is therefore easiest to perform both tests sequentially as the ending position for one test is the starting position for the other test.

Begin the pivot shift with the knee in complete extension (Fig. 10A,B). Next, internally rotate the foot and apply gentle valgus stress. Slowly bring the knee into flexion. In the anterior cruciate deficient knee, the lateral tibial plateau progressively subluxes anteriorly in early flexion. The pivot shift phenomenon occurs with further knee flexion as the anteriorly displaced tibia reduces. Prepare to follow the pivot shift test with the jerk test by keeping the knee in flexion with the thigh adducted and the tibia slightly internally rotated. Hold the foot with one hand while the other hand exerts light pressure anteriorly in the region of the fibular head. Extend the leg slowly. The tibia will sublux anteriorly with a jerk at 50°–30° and reduces as the knee extends fully. To learn the other fine points of the ligament examination, accompany your orthopaedic consultant to the operating room to examine several knees under anesthesia. It is here that you can easily learn the feel of these more subtle tests. In the meantime, the diagnostic maneuvers described above, if carefully and repeatedly done, will allow you to identify the vast majority of athletic knee ligament injuries you encounter.

Patellar Stability

By this stage of the examination, you should have already answered the most important question: whether the knee is stable. If the answer is "yes" but the patient has experienced a significant traumatic episode with obvious disability, the ex-

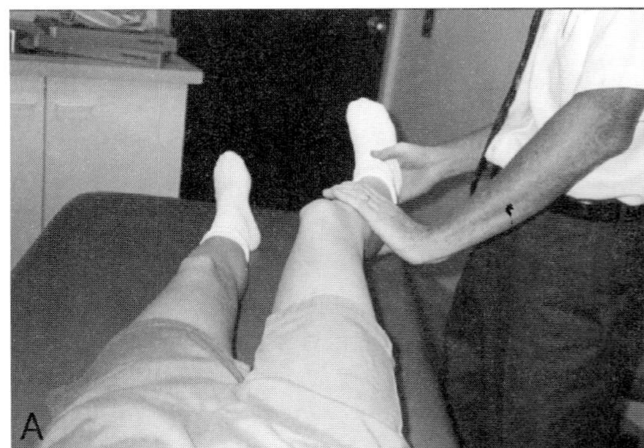

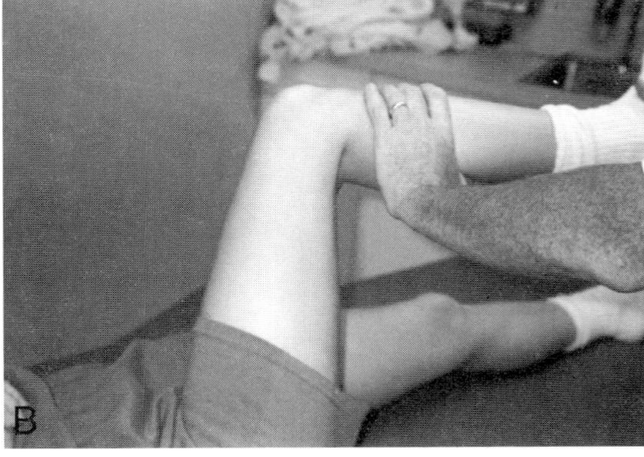

***FIGURE 10.* Pivot shift maneuver and jerk test.** Note that *A* is starting position for pivot shift and ending position for jerk test. Similarly, *B* is starting position for a jerk test and ending position for pivot shift. See text for details.

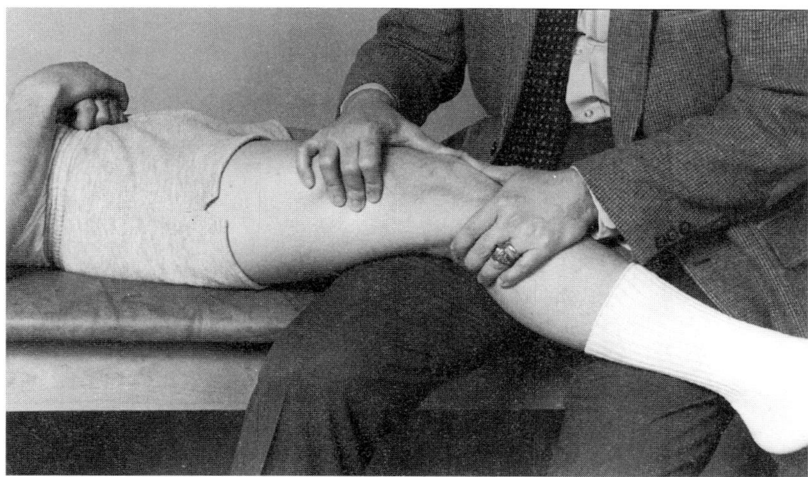

FIGURE 11. **Testing for patellar hypermobility.** The patient is flat on the table and relaxed. The knee is flexed across examiner's thigh, with the patient's foot and ankle on the examiner's other thigh. Thumbs are placed along medial edge of patella and lateral displacement is applied to the patella.

tensor mechanism may have been injured. You might reasonably ask yourself next, "Is this patella stable?" That should be fairly easy to determine. First, look for the predisposing physical findings that are discussed in the next chapter by examining the uninjured knee. You can feel confident that, in the absence of predisposing factors, the patient will not likely have sustained one of the common athletic injuries of the extensor mechanism.[7] On the other hand, the patient certainly could be predisposed and yet the patella may not be the culprit responsible for this acute episode.

After looking for predisposing findings, it is prudent to test for patellar hypermobility. This is best done by sitting on the side of the examination table with the patient's knee flexed across your thigh (Fig. 11). The patient's ankle and foot can then conveniently rest on your other anterior thigh, causing the knee to remain flexed approximately 30–45°. Again, with the patient's head flat and muscles completely relaxed (especially the quadriceps), position your thumbs along the medial edge of the patella and push firmly, trying to displace the patella over the lateral edge of the femoral condyle. With rare exception, patellar dislocations and subluxations will be lateral. Not only are you looking for hypermobility of the patella in comparison to the opposite side, but also in comparison to other knees you have examined. You are also interested in the feeling of apprehension or discomfort the patient may experience. If a patellar dislocation is the source of the acute knee injury, the patient will usually bolt up off the table, grab you by the wrists, and tell you not to displace the patella again (Fig. 12). Also important

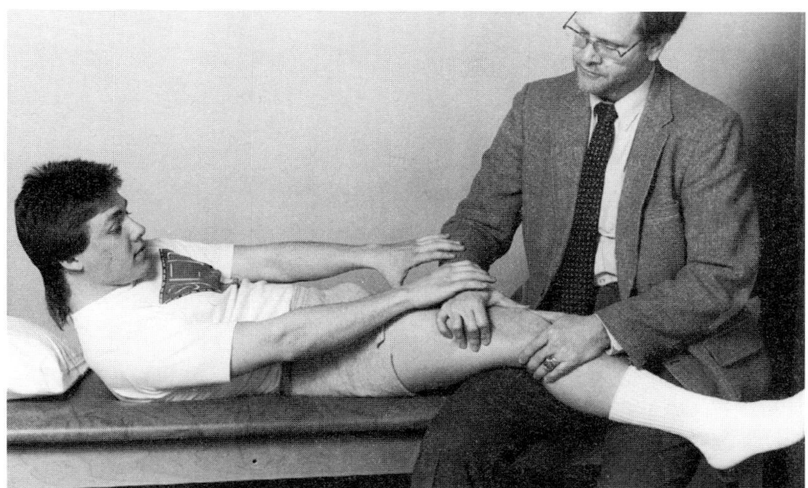

FIGURE 12. **Positive apprehension test**. Lateral displacement of the patella causes the patient to feel that the patella is about to slip out of place.

is the subjective report by the patient that this is the same sensation he or she felt when the knee was twisted and something "went out of place."

Meniscal Examination

If you are now confident that this acutely injured knee has neither ruptured ligaments nor acute patellar instability, then you are dealing with a more benign process. Often, this will be an injury to one or both of the menisci. If the knee is not too painful, two tests can be used to diagnose a torn meniscus. The better known of these is the McMurray test (Fig. 13), done by acutely flexing the knee as far as possible. The foot and tibia are then either externally rotated to test the medial meniscus, or internally rotated to test the lateral meniscus. While holding the tibia in the appropriate rotation, the knee is brought down from a position of acute flexion into extension. The classic finding is a painful pop along the appropriate joint line. In other knees, there may be pain over the appropriate joint line without a real pop being felt. There may be a pop that the patient associates with his or her symptoms that is not particularly painful. There may be a painful pop or clicking sensation that comes and goes, or changes with every repetition of the test.

The other test you should be familiar with is the Apley compression test (Fig. 14). This is performed with the patient prone and the knee flexed to 90°. The examiner pushes downward on the sole of the patient's foot toward the examination table, compressing the menisci between tibia and femur. Then, with the tibia in either external rotation (for medial meniscus) or internal rotation (for lateral meniscus), the knee is taken through a range of motion while maintaining the compression. The most common Apley test response with a torn meniscus is pain over the joint line on that side of the knee.

Other physical examination is less specific for a torn meniscus. There may be tenderness over the joint line, but this may be present from any condition that causes synovitis in that area. It is extremely unlikely to find a knee with a significantly torn meniscus that does not have palpable effusion. While a torn meniscus may be the cause of an acute episode, it is often seen as the reason for chronic knee disability. In the older patient, the meniscus can undergo degenerative change so that even a minor twist can result in a symptomatic tear.

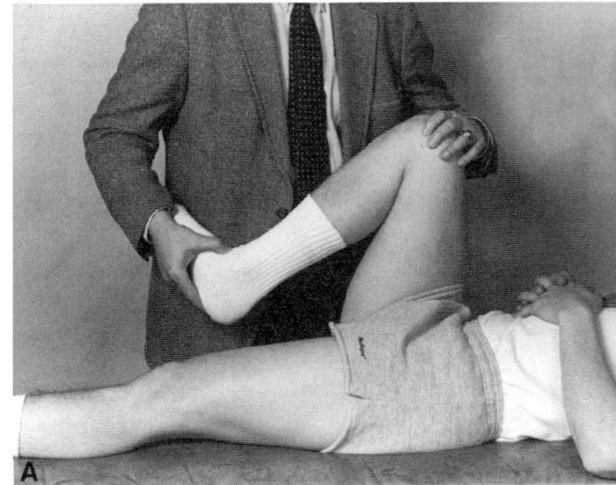

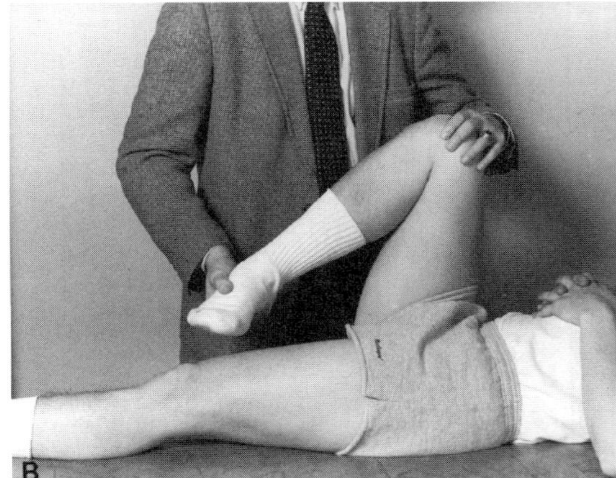

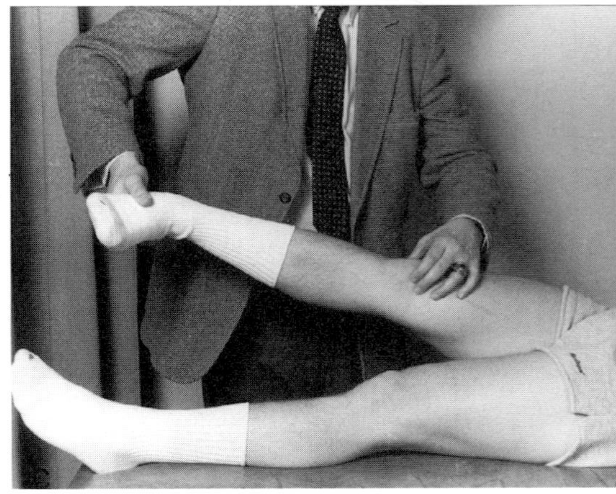

FIGURE 13. **McMurray test.** *A,* Starting position for testing the medial meniscus. The knee is acutely flexed, with the foot and tibia in external rotation. *B,* Starting position for testing the lateral meniscus. The knee is acutely flexed and the foot and tibia are internally rotated. *C,* Ending position for the lateral meniscus. The knee is brought into extension while rotation is maintained. Ending position for medial meniscus would be the same, but with external rotation.

Advanced Palpation

Having gone through this entire routine, try to identify other areas of tenderness or localized puffiness that might be present. There are too many potential sore spots to catalogue. Any particular ligament that is torn may be tender or puffy at one of its attachments or along its course. The various bursal structures about the knee may be swollen or tender, including the semimembranous gastrocnemius bursa, which is best seen when viewing the knee from behind. This is the bursa that, when

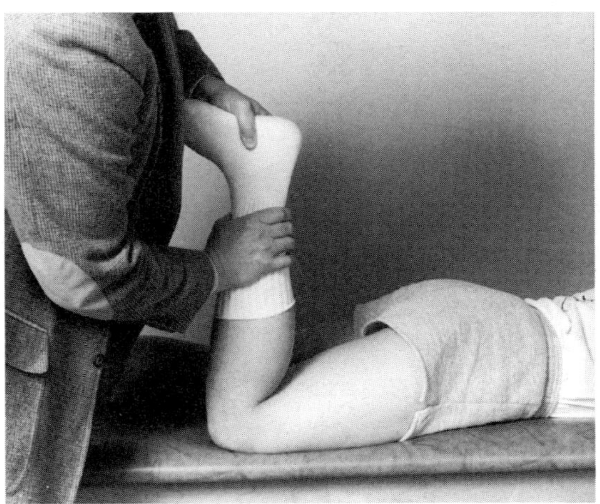

FIGURE 14. **Apley compression test.** Patient is prone. The examiner applies pressure on the sole of the foot toward the examination table. The tibia is rotated externally for the medial meniscus or internally for the lateral meniscus. The knee is then flexed and extended.

fluid-filled, is referred to as a "Baker's cyst" or a "popliteal ganglion." In addition to the bursae, any of the tendinous structures about the knee may be tender from an inflammatory process. It is through a thorough knowledge of knee anatomy that these tender or puffy spots become meaningful. Frequent reference to an anatomy textbook, dissection of the cadaver knee, or watching surgical dissections done by your orthopaedic consultant will facilitate such familiarity.

Other Examinations

Other areas outside the knee joint itself should at least be briefly considered. Muscular findings such as quadriceps atrophy and atonia; weakness of hip flexors and hip abductors; and tightness of hamstrings, heel cords, quadriceps, and iliotibial band are all important. Hip range of motion should be checked, especially in adolescents, where a slipped capital femoral epiphysis may produce referred medial knee pain.

Knee Aspiration

We are often asked about the usefulness of knee aspiration in the evaluation of the acutely injured knee. We aspirate very few knees, believing that through careful history-taking and the thorough but gentle examination described above, we can evaluate most knee injuries. However, many orthopaedic surgeons believe that knee aspiration in the acute setting is helpful, stating that the risk is acceptably small. Consequently, we have no reason to inveigh against knee aspiration, if it helps and if it is done in a precise and careful way. To be completely honest, there are some occasions in dealing with tense, painful hemarthrosis when we aspirate the knee for comfort alone. The only pitfall is that frequently the hemarthrosis reaccumulates, since the cause for hemarthrosis has not been treated through the aspiration.

If you decide to aspirate the knee joint, it is important to prepare the knee thoroughly with an antibacterial soap, just as one would do in the operating room. Simply swabbing the skin with a little alcohol before performing a knee aspiration would leave you open to liability should complications ensue. The superolateral approach is useful for knee aspiration (Fig. 15A and B). The suprapatellar pouch extends several centimeters above the proximal edge of the patella in most knees. The only pitfall in going too far proximal to enter the suprapatellar pouch is that in some knees the pouch itself is congenitally separated from the knee joint proper, so that you may not find the fluid you are anticipating. An approach at about the proximal lateral pole of the patella itself is satisfactory. After anesthetizing the skin and deeper soft tissue with local anesthetic, insert a large bore *spinal* needle into the joint, aiming for the interval between the patella and the femoral trochlea. It is important to use a spinal needle, since using a needle with an open bore will punch out a plug of skin as the needle passes through, and may deposit that patch of contaminated skin within the knee joint. Using the largest bore possible is important because, in the acute situation, the joint is often filled with early blood clot and it is difficult to aspirate the knee. You may need to flush with sterile saline to aspirate a knee that has already begun to form clots. Using the superolateral approach, the last bit of fluid can be obtained by having the patient carefully flex the knee and externally rotate the hip. The needle and syringe can hang over the edge of the table in a dependent position, encouraging fluid to exit the joint (Fig. 15B).

After aspirating the contents with a syringe, squirt any blood into a bowl or basin and look for floating fat droplets on the surface (Fig. 16), which may indicate that there is an obscure bony injury that may not be visible on x-ray. Synovial fluid analysis is beyond the scope of this discussion. It is usually helpful only in the chronic knee problems in which there is some question of an inflammatory process. This is usually not the situation in dealing with an injured athlete. In the acute injury, a bloody or fat-containing aspirate indicates a serious injury and warrants orthopaedic referral.

If you go to the trouble of aspirating a knee, get as much information as possible. Inject 5–10 cc of 1% lidocaine for some local anesthetic effect. This will not give total anesthesia within the joint but may help facilitate some of the examination discussed previously. Be sure to repeat the Lachman test under the analgesia. Lidocaine and aspiration may allow a better evaluation of this test. Again, re-

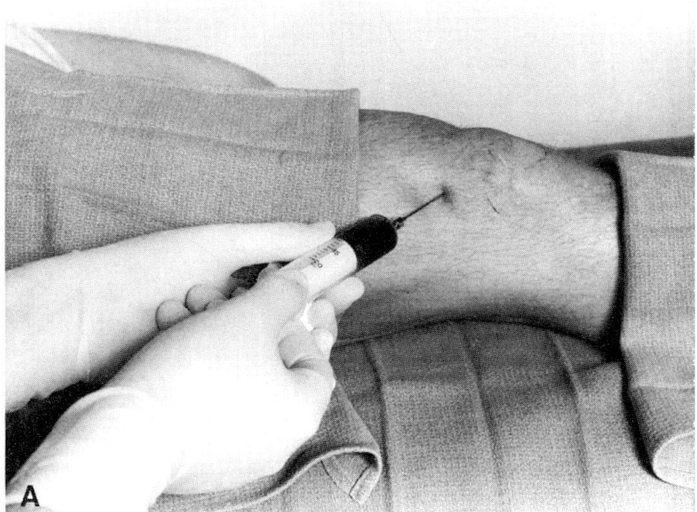

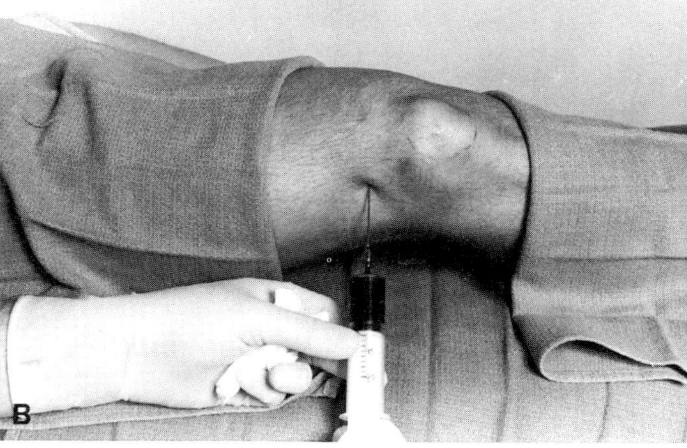

FIGURE 15. **Knee aspiration.** *A,* Large-bore spinal needle is used through superolateral approach to aspirate the knee. *B,* Having the patient gently externally rotate the hip and flex the knee over the side of table can help to aspirate the last bit of fluid.

member that the greatest percentage of acute hemarthroses of the knee will be secondary to rupture of the anterior cruciate ligament.

X-ray Evaluation

X-ray all *acutely* injured knees. Even in chronic knee problems where the diagnosis seems certain through history and physical examination, it is advisable to obtain x-rays. One would hate to miss osteochondritis dissecans or a primary bone tumor in a knee that otherwise seemed to have patellar or meniscal problems. Some patients with typical problems of the extensor mechanism—that is, bilateral knee pain of nontraumatic onset and the presence of predisposing findings—can be treated for a few weeks to see if the problem can be cured. If unsuccessful, one should certainly go ahead with x-rays if they have not been previously obtained.

A routine anteroposterior and lateral view are used in most acutely injured knees. Oblique views are not obtained unless something suspicious is seen. In chronic problems, other views may be helpful. For example, in a situation suggestive of osteochondritis dissecans, be certain to obtain an intercondylar notch view. In the patient with chronic knee complaints whose knee will flex easily to 90°, we prefer to take the lateral x-ray at that position. This gives the best indication of positioning of the patella, as discussed in the next chapter. In patients beyond middle age, obtain the anteroposterior view in the weight-bearing posture. The joint space can then be assessed more accurately and may lend evidence of a degenerative process.

In all knees, it is useful to take some type of infrapatellar x-ray. The traditional "skyline" or "sunrise" view is not adequate, though, because these views are made with the knee flexed greater than 90°. Almost all unstable kneecaps will seat in the trochlea when the knee is flexed. Therefore, the infrapatellar view should be made with the patellofemoral joint in more moderate flexion, approximately 30°–45°. It is also convenient and helpful to obtain x-rays of both

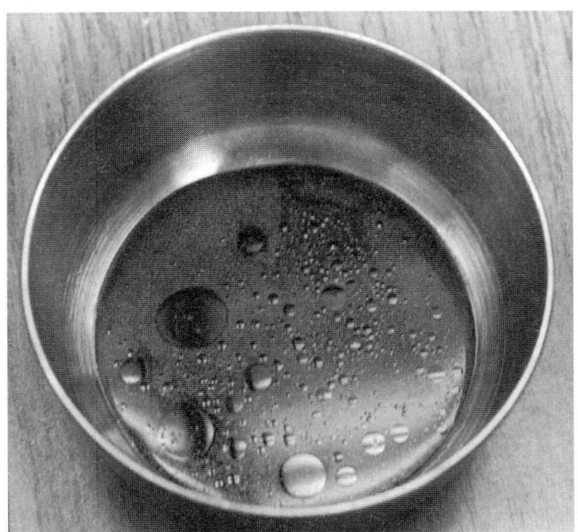

FIGURE 16. Fat droplets in knee aspirate indicate bony injury and communication of marrow cavity with the interior of the joint.

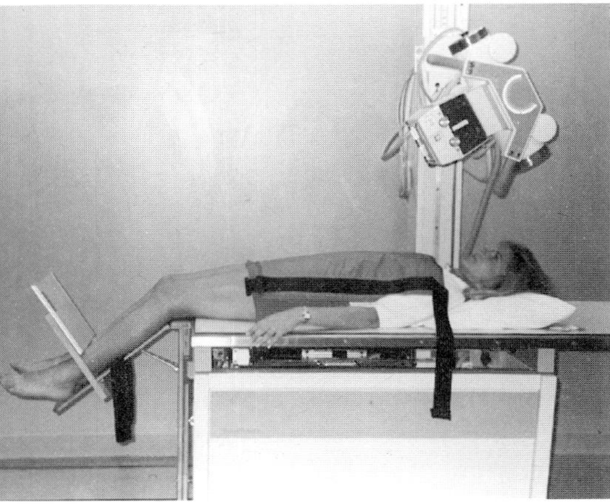

FIGURE 17. Cassette holding jig for modified Merchant view.

patellofemoral joints on the same cassette by holding the knees together as the film is exposed (Fig. 17). Even if the other knee is not involved, this provides a ready comparison for some of the subtle position changes that one may see on this view.

Stress x-rays are not a routine part of x-ray evaluations of every acutely injured knee. However, in the youngster with open epiphyses, the possibility of epiphyseal fracture exists. It is axiomatic that if you feel apparent knee joint instability in a patient with open growth plates, you should proceed with a varus and valgus stress x-ray. In many instances, the stress film will show an opening at the level of the growth plate rather than at the joint (Fig. 18). This confirms an epiphyseal fracture separation, usually of the Salter I or II type, which should be treated by appropriate immobilization.

The vast majority of cases, x-rays of the acutely injured knee will be negative. The most common positive finding in the acute knee is some type of osteochondral fracture. These fractures may occur at any one of the joint surfaces but are especially common in patellar dislocation, in which they originate from either the lateral edge of the femoral trochlea or the medial facet of the patella. If a loose osteochondral fracture is seen within the joint, orthopaedic consultation is indicated, even though not all such loose bodies need surgical removal. Some small osteochondral fractures may not produce future problems.

Two avulsion fractures that occur around the knee can lead to a specific diagnosis. A small avulsed

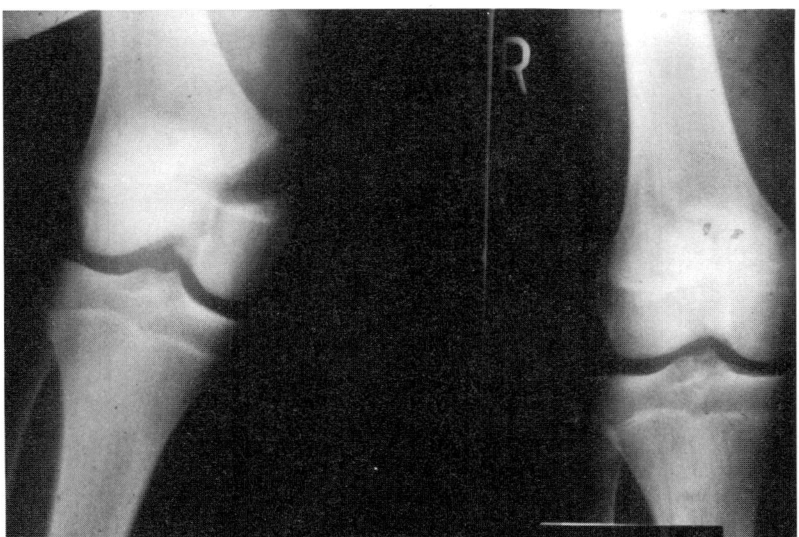

FIGURE 18. Positive stress film in a skeletally immature patient shows opening at growth plate, rather than joint line, when abduction stress is applied.

piece of bone just below the lateral joint margin on the tibia has been called the "lateral capsular sign"[8] (Fig. 19). This bone is pulled off by the lateral capsular ligament and is usually accompanied by an anterior cruciate ligament tear. The lateral capsular sign is considered virtually pathognomonic for anterolateral rotatory instability of the knee. A crescent-shaped piece of bone may be avulsed from the most proximal part of the fibular head (Fig. 20). This has been termed the "arcuate sign" and indicates a significant injury to the posterolateral corner of the knee.[1] The musculotendinous, ligamentous, and meniscal complex in the posterolateral knee is referred to as the arcuate complex. Acute injury to this part of the knee causes a posterolateral rotatory instability. Either of these avulsion fractures indicates significant ligamentous disruption and should be referred for orthopaedic consultation.

Currently, we have abandoned the use of arthrography. It was never a very useful part of the evaluation of the acutely injured knee. In the chronic setting, the lack of diagnostic accuracy proved to be more confusing than helpful.

MRI has truly come of age as the most useful diagnostic imaging technique for evaluating knee injuries. Its advantage over arthrography are many in that it does not use ionizing radiation or dye, does not require an injection, and provides accurate information on menisci, ligaments, and joint surfaces. Disadvantages are few. Its value in detecting loose bodies or providing useful information on the patellofemoral joint is limited. The cost is relatively high and some insurance companies refuse reimbursement for certain preliminary diagnoses. The main disadvantage lies in the patient who suffers from claustrophobia. Some centers have "open air" MRI's for large or claustrophobic patients but the quality and sensitivity of this type of scan is diminished.

MRI has shown a high degree of accuracy for detecting medial meniscus tears. Sensitivity has been reported as high as 94%.[5] Its sensitivity in detecting abnormalities of the lateral meniscus is somewhat less. One study[5] shows this to be 78%. A grading system for meniscus abnormalities has been proposed which provides a useful means for grading the various degrees of meniscal tears. Grade I signal is globular and is localized to the center of the meniscus, and there is a distinct zone of dark, low-intensity meniscal substance separating it from all

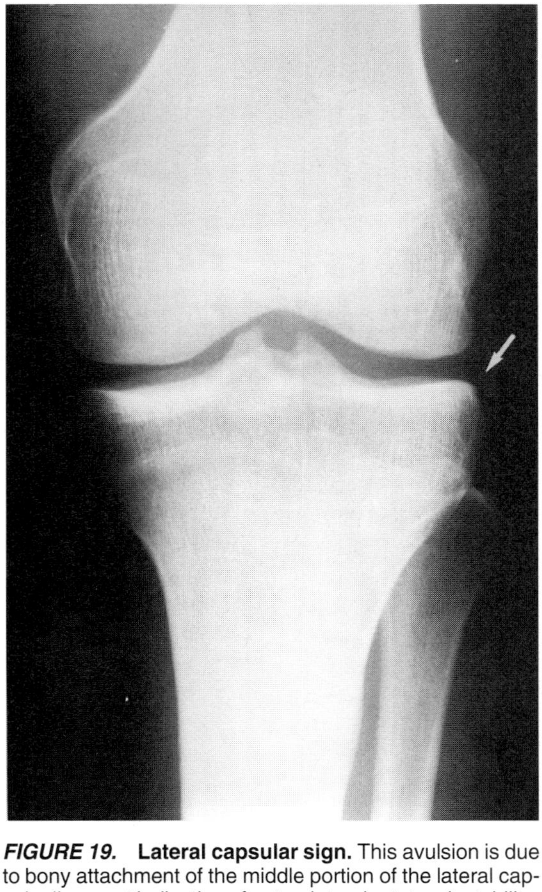

FIGURE 19. **Lateral capsular sign.** This avulsion is due to bony attachment of the middle portion of the lateral capsular ligament indicative of anterolateral rotatory instability.

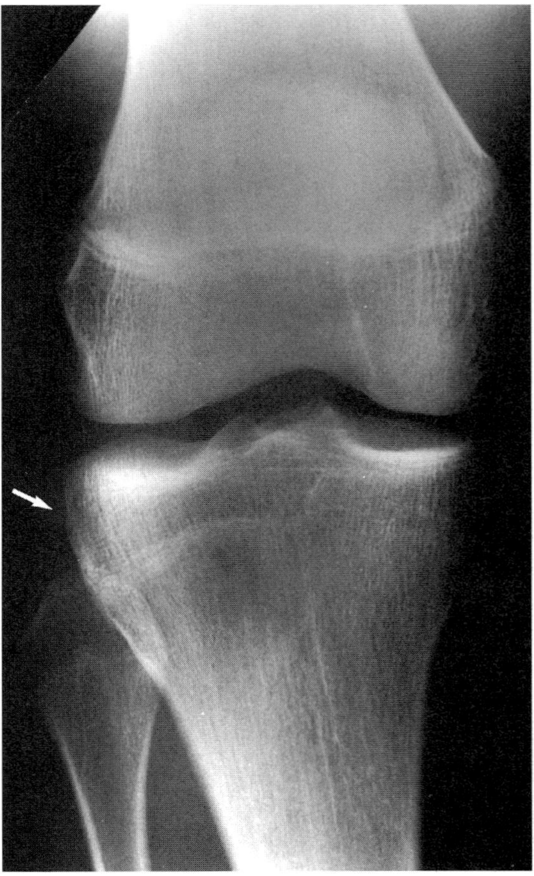

FIGURE 20. **Arcuate sign on knee x-ray.** Avulsion fracture from the proximal fibula indicates injury to the arcuate complex and posterolateral rotatory instability.

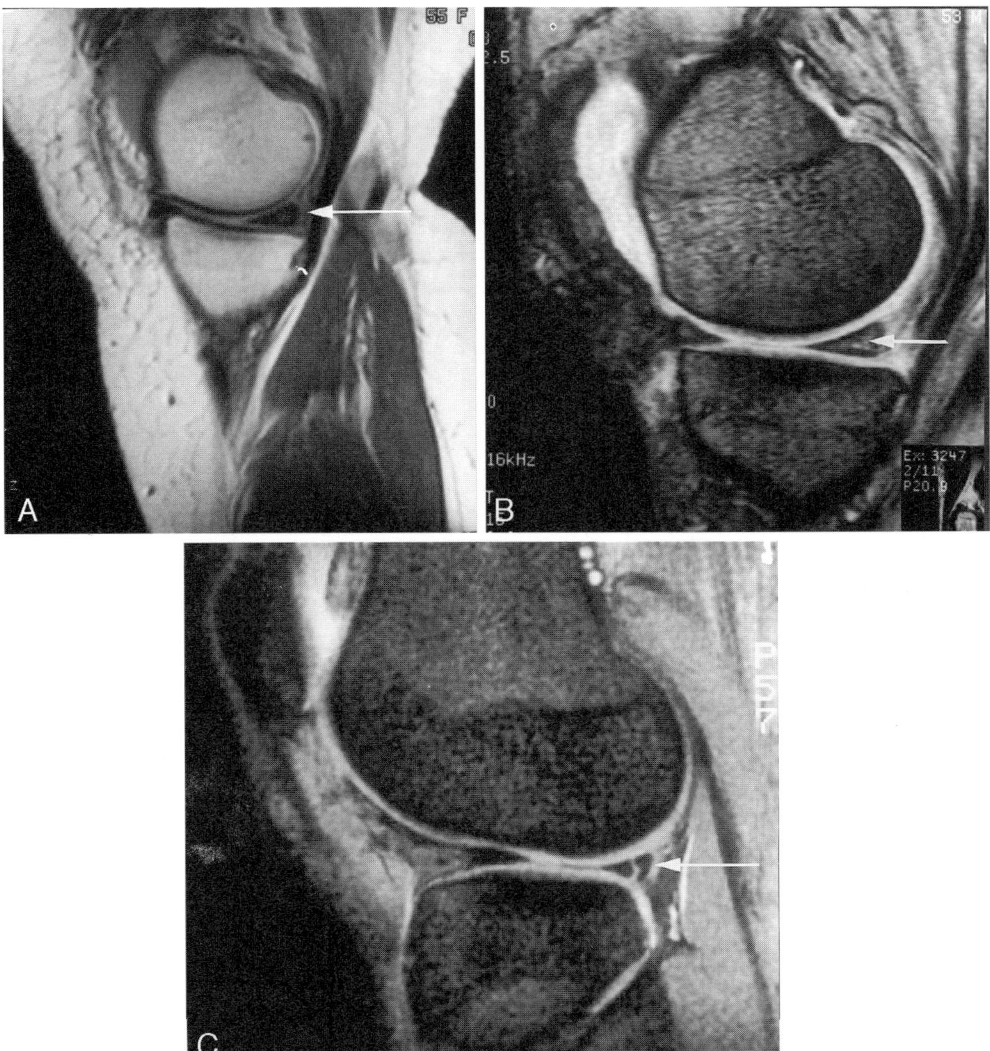

FIGURE 21. **MRI grading of meniscal tears.** *A,* poorly defined "globular" zone of increased signal intensity (arrow) corresponding to grade I change. *B,* linear zone of hyperintensity (arrow), not communicating with the articular surface, corresponding to grade II change. *C,* linear band of hyperintensity (arrow) communication with both articular surfaces corresponding with grade III change; that is, a complete tear.

free meniscal edges (Fig. 21A–C). This abnormality is not visible with arthroscopy. It corresponds to histologically identifiable degeneration in the central substance of the meniscus. A grade II signal is a linear signal that does not connect with the articular surface (Fig. 21B). Histologically, this corresponds to a more advanced stage of the abnormality seen in grade I. A grade III signal is either linear or irregular in appearance and reaches a free meniscal edge (Fig. 21C). This signal closely corresponds with meniscus tears at the time of arthroscopy.

Ligamentous structures including the anterior cruciate ligament, posterior cruciate ligament, medial collateral ligament, and lateral collateral ligament are also easily identified on the MRI (Fig. 22A and 22B). Tears can be identified as to whether they are complete or partial. Accuracy in detecting anterior cruciate ligament tears has been reported as high as 95%.[4]

There are also other abnormalities within the knee joint that are easily identified on MRI that are not apparent on arthrography or plain x-ray. Osteochondritis dissecans lesions can not only be identified but can be further elucidated as to whether the overlying articular cartilage is intact, or whether there is synovial fluid between the fragment and the condyle; osteonecrosis can be identified on MRI even when changes are too subtle to show up on a plain x-ray; any fluid-filled structures such as meniscus cysts, ganglions, or popliteal cysts cannot only be identified but can be accurately measured and noted as to whether or not they make a connection within the joint itself; joint effusions and hemarthroses can be

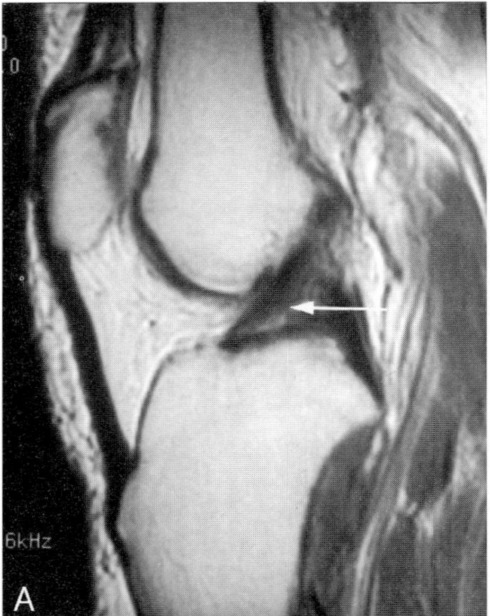

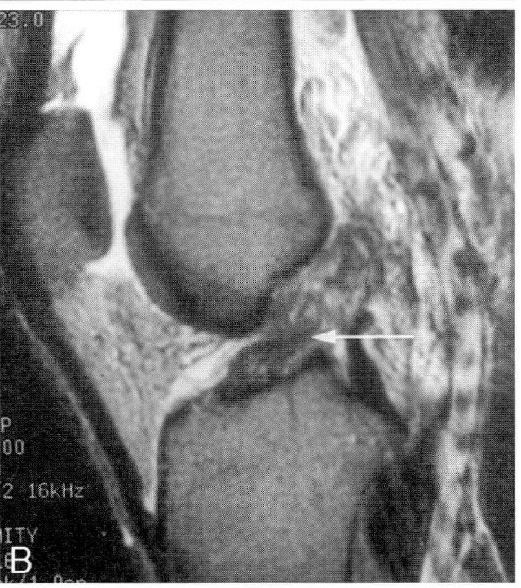

FIGURE 22. **Anterior cruciate ligament.** *A,* MRI image of normal ACL (arrow) consisting of multiple fibers with a straight course. *B,* MRI image of torn ACL (arrow). Note irregularity in the ligament as well as no visible attachment of proximal ACL at the femur.

quantified; arthritic changes and chondromalacia can be quantified and localized.

INITIAL ASSESSMENT AND TREATMENT

To the nonorthopaedist, this detailed evaluation of one peripheral joint may seem somewhat overwhelming. However, with a little practice, you will spend much less time evaluating an injured knee than you would in working up a complicated diabetic or heart patient. One item that maybe helpful in the initial assessment is the use of a special knee examination sheet or checklist. It not only saves time by allowing you to circle and check items, it also helps you remember to ask all the pertinent questions and do all the pertinent tests.

As mentioned earlier, the most significant athletic knee injury that you are likely to encounter is a grade III sprain of the knee ligaments. A grade III sprain is synonymous with a complete tear of the ligament. By definition, a completely torn ligament causes joint instability. This injury is diagnosed, then, by the presence of instability on one of the tests described earlier. If there is obvious instability in the acutely injured knee, prompt orthopaedic consultation is indicated. If you see the patient 24 hours after injury and the knee is swollen and painful, you may not be able to decide whether there is joint laxity or not. That's all right. If x-rays are not helpful and orthopaedic consultation is not immediately available, then the right approach is to place the athlete on crutches, with limited weight-bearing on the injured extremity, as well as to recommend elevation of the extremity, application of ice to the knee, and oral anti-inflammatory medication. The commercially available knee immobilizers are not particularly useful except when the patient is extremely uncomfortable getting around on crutches. In most instances, however, the knee immobilizer will not be terribly comfortable, either, because it forces the knee into full extension. Some sort of compressive wrap may be beneficial. We use only the white elastic bandages that contain far less elastic than the brown bandages. The white bandages may be wrapped snugly around the knee joint with less risk of constricting circulation. A foam rubber or felt pad over the specific area of tissue damage may likewise be helpful. For example, in the common sprain of the medial ligaments from their femoral attachment, there will usually be marked tenderness to palpation over the medial epicondyle of the femur. A foam pad over that area wrapped on with the white elastic bandage may reduce both edema and pain. If you have aspirated fluid from the knee, it is important to place the knee in a bulkier compression dressing, including fluffed sponges, an ABD roll, or perhaps cast padding beneath the white elastic bandage to minimize reaccumulation of fluid.

The athlete must be started on some type of early rehabilitative exercises. The simplest of all knee exercises is the quadriceps setting exercise, in which the patient simply tightens the quadriceps and holds it maximally contracted for a count of 6 seconds, then relaxes it for a count of approximately three seconds. Fifty quadriceps setting exercises should be encouraged each hour the patient is awake. Additionally, while lying with the leg elevated, using ice, the patient should do ankle-pumping exercises almost constantly. Instruct the patient to pull the foot into maximum dorsiflexion and hold it for a count and then push the foot down into maximum plantar flexion and hold it for a count, and do this repeatedly. Both the quadriceps setting exercises and the ankle pumping minimize swelling throughout the limb, which facilitates the repeat examination a day or two later.

The aggressive use of rest, ice, compression, elevation, and simple rehabilitative exercises for a day or two may facilitate the examination. If you are still not convinced that the examination is adequate, you can continue the conservative care for another day or two.

If you are convinced that you have performed an excellent examination of the knee, and there is no joint instability, the injury may be only a mild or moderate ligament sprain (grade I or grade II injury). These two grades are differentiated only by the relative amount of swelling, pain, and disability. In grade I or II injuries, no joint laxity should be evident on performing the stress tests described earlier. Do not immobilize mild to moderate knee ligament sprains in the athlete, as this invites increased atrophy and prolonged disability. Instead, manage them with crutches and the simple athletic first aid described above, followed by a rehabilitative exercise program.

If you are convinced that there is no ligament injury, the next most important issue is whether there is acute injury to the extensor mechanism. The management of acute patellar dislocation is described in the next chapter.

If the ligaments and patella have not been injured, a meniscal tear may be present. Suspected meniscal tears are not surgical urgencies and may be managed with limited weight-bearing and rehabilitative exercise.

One thing you must *not* do with the acutely injured knee is to simply hide the leg inside a knee immobilizer or cast without making a diagnosis. To be certain that there is no ligamentous damage and to decide to manage the patient yourself is quite acceptable, especially if orthopaedic care is not available. However, to let a patient molder in a cast or knee immobilizer for 6 weeks without a diagnosis is not appropriate.

In almost all chronic knee problems, it is reasonable to try conservative care first. Any problem marked by inflammation and swelling can be treated with nonsteroidal anti-inflammatory medication. The most important facet of nonsurgical treatment is an appropriate rehabilitative exercise program. One cannot be "cookbookish" about this advice, because the exercises will be considerably different, depending on the exact diagnosis. For the sake of brevity, the details of individualized rehabilitative exercise routines are not addressed here. Instead, the reader is referred to Chapter 17 for information on general rehabilitation concepts and advice about specific programs.

Certain problems respond better than others to a rehabilitative approach. For example, recurrent locking of the knee caused by a bucket-handle tear of the medial meniscus obviously will not heal through exercise. However, there is really no harm in trying a rehabilitation program for a short period of time. Lack of complete extension and persistent effusion would warrant orthopaedic referral, however. Even if the patient has to resort to surgical treatment later, this early introduction to rehabilitation will make it easier to recover from surgery. If the patient has a degenerative meniscal lesion that is marked more by pain and swelling than by mechanical locking, the entire process may well resolve with anti-inflammatory medication and exercise. If significant symptoms persist, a degenerative meniscal tear is ammenable to arthroscopic debridement.

Bracing of the knee is a consideration. The most successful bracing is done for the extensor mechanism. Even a simple neoprene rubber knee sleeve may give enough patellar support to help. Other more elaborate, yet relatively inexpensive braces for the patellofemoral joint are available (Fig. 23). Meniscal lesions usually are not affected by bracing techniques. Many expensive custom-made braces are now available for ligamentous instabilities, but it is advisable to send the patient for orthopaedic consultation before incurring the expense (several hundred dollars) of one of these custom-made braces. Generally, bracing by itself is not acceptable but may be of benefit when combined with rehabilitative exercise.

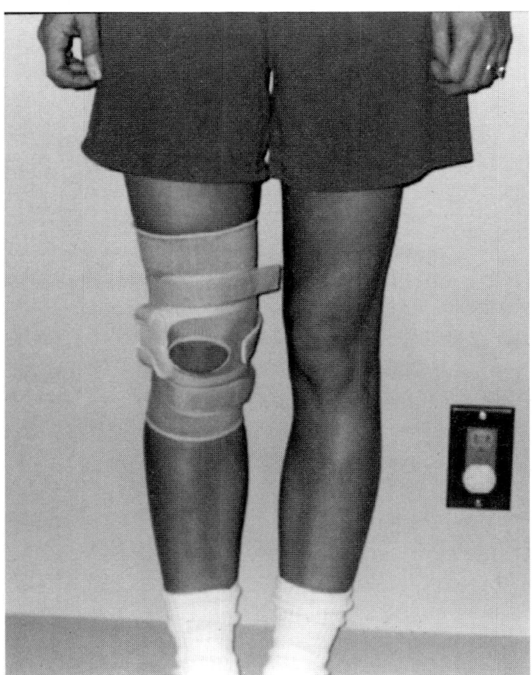

FIGURE 23. **Palumbo patellar stabilizing brace.** Adjustable lateral buttress helps prevent lateral subluxation of patella (DynOrthotics, Dania FL).

SPECIFIC INJURIES

Grade I or II Ligament Sprains

In mild to moderate knee ligament injuries, the athlete eventually should be able to return to sport. These injuries are best managed initially through protection and simple athletic first aid. A very brief period of knee immobilization may help symptoms but should not replace crutch use. The rehabilitation program, started early, should progress through more and more complicated exercise techniques and functional activity. Again, the reader is referred to chapter 17 on rehabilitation.

The only other issue to be addressed is that of confidence. This can probably be determined only by directly questioning the athlete as to whether he or she has total confidence that the knee will hold up the stress of athletics. The length of recovery from Grade I or II sprains of the knee ligaments varies so widely that it is impossible to give the athlete an accurate estimate at the time of the first examination. The physician is well advised to describe briefly the functional goals the patient will have to attain before returning to sport, rather than arbitrarily giving the athlete a specific length of time before he or she may return.

Tears (Grade III Sprains) of the Medial Ligaments

When a complete tear of the medial ligament complex is diagnosed, the athlete should be referred to an orthopaedic surgeon. It is current thinking that not all medial ligament tears require surgical repairs. However, it is necessary to prove that this is an isolated injury of the medial ligaments, with no involvement of the cruciates or meniscal structures. MRI is extremely beneficial here. If the MRI confirms an isolated medial collateral ligament tear, many orthopaedic surgeons currently choose treatment with immobilization only. Studies now exist to substantiate the closed treatment approach.[3] In this instance, the knee is usually immobilized at 30 degrees of flexion for two weeks and then allowed 30 to 90 degrees of flexion in a brace (Fig. 24). Return to sporting activities with nonsurgical treatment is based on regaining full range of motion, muscular strength, and a progression through functional activity program.

Other orthopaedic surgeons, however, believe that direct surgical repair for grade III injuries yields the best prognosis. If the surgical approach is chosen, this is a good opportunity to reexamine the ligaments under anesthesia. In addition, medial collateral ligament repair may be preceded by an arthroscopy if intra-articular pathology is suspected on MRI or physical exam. Following surgical repair, immobilization is generally continued for 6 to 8 weeks. Crutches are continued for an additional several weeks following removal of the immobilization. This is all combined with an extensive rehabilitative exercise program. Running and a progression through functional activities may be resumed approximately six months following surgery. Regardless of whether surgical or nonsurgical treatment is chosen, the prognosis is quite favorable in isolated tears of the medial ligament complex.

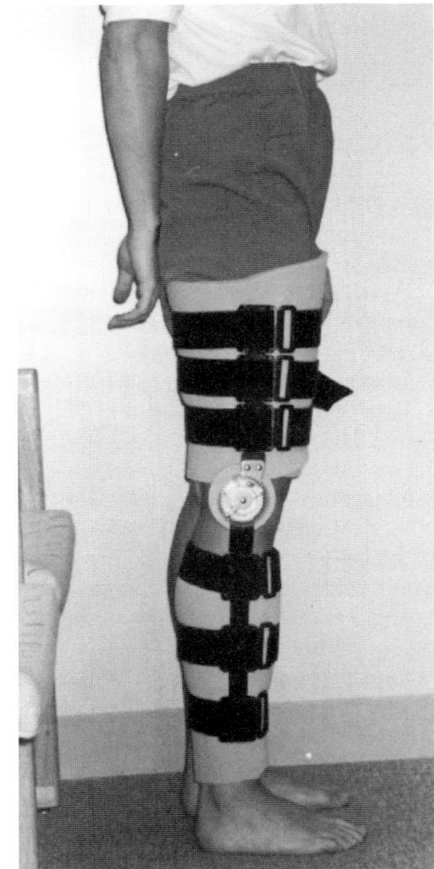

FIGURE 24. **Adjustable brace** provides protection with controllable range of motion (Vantage Orthopaedics, Inc., Cincinnati, OH).

Tears (Grade III Sprains) of the Cruciate Ligaments

Without a doubt, injuries of the anterior cruciate ligament are the most problematic. Factors affecting prognosis include the amount of ligament tissue torn, location of tear, associated meniscal tears, joint surface damage, congenital laxity of the joint, and the athlete's functional goals. All anterior cruciate ligament injuries should be referred to an orthopedic surgeon. The orthopaedist, along with the patient, should make the final decision about the mode of treatment. If the injury to the cruciate ligament is only partial, and laxity is mild, the patient may not require surgical repair or reconstruction.

However, most athletes with an anterior cruciate ligament tear will undergo some sort of surgical treatment, if not for reconstruction of the ligament, then for associated intra-articular pathology. Although MRI has supplanted the need for diagnostic arthroscopy in most instances, some patients will require arthroscopy to treat any associated meniscus or articular surface pathology even if they choose nonsurgical treatment for their anterior cruciate ligament injury.

If surgical reconstruction of the anterior cruciate ligament is chosen, various techniques are popular. Routinely, all reconstructions are accompanied by an exam under anesthesia and arthroscopy. In the young adolescent, if the cruciate has been avulsed directly off either of its bony attachments, a direct repair may be in order. Usually, though, the tear occurs in the middle third of the ligament so that the cruciate's tenuous blood supply is disrupted and no direct repair is possible. In this instance, an augmentation or substitution type of procedure may be chosen. Depending on the orthopaedic surgeon, this could mean an intra-articular procedure in which some tissue such as patellar tendon, hamstring, or allograft is placed back through the center of the knee joint to attempt recreating something resembling a normal anterior cruciate ligament. Less commonly, the orthopaedic surgeon may choose an extra-articular substitution in which lateral joint structures, such as the iliotibial band, are used to substitute for the anterior cruciate.

Previously, it was taught that the "golden period" for treating knee ligament tears extended 7–10 days after injury. It was felt that if knee ligaments were torn and needed to be repaired, they should be fixed during this time period. The current thinking regarding anterior cruciate ligament tears, however, is to let the knee "quiet down" for at least 3 weeks after injury before attempting any surgical intervention.[2,6] The goals during this 3-week delay are to regain full motion and eliminate effusion and soft tissue swelling. Studies have shown lower incidence of postoperative complications, such as knee stiffness, with this technique. This 3-week delay is not appropriate for direct repair of the avulsed anterior cruciate ligament.

Any of these surgical repairs or reconstructions is followed by immobilization for some period of time, crutches for an additional length of time, and extensive rehabilitation. The current thinking allows an athlete with an anterior cruciate injury to return to sports 6–9 months postoperatively, but this time frame varies. Some residual laxity may persist. Long-term bracing may be necessary as well as modification of life-style. Overall, the prognosis for anterior cruciate reconstruction is quite good as it allows for satisfactory return to pre-injury activity levels in most individuals.

Acute ruptures of the posterior cruciate ligament are encountered much less frequently. Isolated posterior cruciate ligament tears are routinely treated nonsurgically with bracing and rehabilitative exercises. This is, however, a complicated problem and does warrant orthopaedic consultation. Surgical reconstruction of the posterior cruciate ligament is not as satisfactory or predictable as anterior cruciate ligament reconstruction. Many patients are left with some residual laxity. The length of time to return to sports following posterior cruciate ligament reconstruction is approximately 9–12 months.

Tears (Grade III Sprains) of the Lateral Ligaments

Isolated injuries to the lateral compartment ligaments are not very common in sports. The lateral collateral ligament (or fibular collateral ligament) is in itself not a very important stabilizing structure. Most injuries to this extracapsular ligament alone can be treated nonsurgically. Injuries to the middle portion of the lateral capsular ligament are usually found in combination with tears of the anterior cruciate ligament. When the lateral capsular sign is seen on an x-ray of an acutely injured knee, the problem should be referred to an orthopaedic surgeon as if it were an anterior cruciate rupture. Complete tears of the arcuate complex in the posterolateral corner of the knee, though less frequent, certainly occur. If an arcuate sign is encountered on x-ray, these injuries too should be referred for orthopaedic evaluation. Direct suture repair may be warranted, and it carries a good ultimate prognosis. Massive injuries of the lateral ligament complex, though not common in sports, may be associated with damage to the peroneal nerve, which may severely worsen the outcome.

Acute Patellar Dislocation The treatment of acute patellar dislocation is described in the next chapter.

Meniscal Injury

Though tears of the menisci are not emergencies, competitive athletes may feel a sense of urgency in having the problem resolved. If so, orthopaedic consultation should be obtained, with the thought of proceeding with MRI or arthroscopic evaluation of the knee joint. If a meniscal tear is encountered, a decision must be made as to whether repair or removal is the best treatment. Meniscus repair is a growing trend in orthopedics. MRI is, at times, able to identify whether a meniscal tear is peripheral (in other words repairable) or not. Realistically, whether a meniscal tear is repairable or not is determined by direct arthroscopy. If the tear is vertical at or near the periphery, then it is amenable to suture repair. Most orthopaedic surgeons currently recommend reattachment of a peripheral tear of either meniscus. Though the sutures are placed arthroscopically, a skin incision is commonly used to retrieve the sutures and to tie them beneath the skin. Meniscus repair is routinely performed as outpatient surgery. Immobilization is often used following meniscus repair. If the procedure proves successful, recovery is expected in about six months. On hearing this time frame, athletes often shy away from meniscal repair, choosing to ignore the potential long-term benefits in favor of a quicker return to sport. Part of the orthopaedic surgeon's job is to counsel the individual athlete regarding the pros and cons of repair versus removal.

The majority of meniscal tears still require removal of the torn portion of the meniscus, for which arthroscopy clearly has been shown to be the most effective method. The orthopaedist can actually visualize the joint better with the aid of the arthroscope than with an open surgical procedure—certainly with less trauma to the patient. An arthroscopic procedure is outpatient surgery, with a short period of postoperative disability and often a rapid return to activity.

Osteochondral Fractures

The treatment and prognosis for osteochondral fractures depend on their size and location. Osteochondral fractures detected by the primary care physician should be referred for orthopaedic evaluation. A rehabilitative approach may be undertaken if the fragment is quite small. Some osteochondral fragments never produce symptoms sufficient to warrant even arthroscopic surgical treatment. The majority, however, are treated by some surgical means. Arthroscopic removal is most common. If the fragment is massive, some attempt may be necessary to replace and internally fix it. If the fragment has come from a non–weight-bearing area such as one of the joint margins, no real treatment may be necessary other than removal. However, if it has come from a weight-bearing area, then removal must often be followed by a period of prolonged protection. One never likes to see an osteochondral fracture, especially in a young athlete, because it has been well documented that hyaline articular cartilage does not heal to a normal state. Instead, it is replaced by fibrocartilage, which does not stand up well to the stresses of weight-bearing. In fact, such injury may be a harbinger of degenerative changes to come. Protection on crutches following the osteochondral fracture may need to extend for eight weeks or more. However, immobilization is usually not indicated, since joint motion may actually help to stimulate the healing effect.

SUMMARY

Office management of athletic knee injuries requires a thorough, thoughtful approach. The role of the primary care physician includes detailed history-taking, thorough examination, institution of a rehabilitation program, and orthopaedic consultation when indicated. Simple athletic first aid and early rehabilitation should always be applied to any knee injury. If orthopaedic evaluation does not become necessary, the athlete's return to sport can be facilitated through a thorough, progressive program of knee rehabilitation and functional retraining.

REFERENCES

1. DeLee JC, Riley MB, Rockwood CA: Acute posterolateral rotatory instability of the knee. Am J Sports Med 11: 199–207, 1983.
2. Harner CD, Irrgang JJ, Paul J, et al.: Loss of motion after anterior cruciate ligament reconstruction. Am J Sports Med 20:499–506.
3. Linton RC, Indelicato PA: Medial ligament injuries. In DeLee JC, Drez D (eds): Orthopaedic Sports Medicine: Principles and Practice. Philadelphia, W.B. Saunders, 1994, pp 1261–1274.
4. Mink JH, Levy T, Crues JH: Tears of the anterior cruciate ligament and menisci of the knee: MR evaluation. Radiology 167:769–774, 1988.
5. Raunest J, Oberle K, Loehnert J, Hoetzinger H: The clinical value of magnetic resonance imaging in the evaluation of meniscal disorders. J Bone Joint Surg 73:11–16, 1991.
6. Shelbourne KD, Wilckens JH, Mollabashy A, DeCarlo M: Arthrofibrosis in acute anterior cruciate ligament reconstruction: The effect of timing of reconstruction and rehabilitation. Am J Sports Med 19:332–336, 1991.
7. Walsh WM: Patellofemoral joint. In DeLee JC, Drez D (eds): Orthopaedic Sports Medicine: Principles and Practice. Philadelphia, WB Saunders, 1994, pp 1163–1248.
8. Woods GW, Stanley RF, Tullos HS: Lateral capsular sign: X-ray clue to a significant knee instability. Am J Sports Med 7:27–33, 1979.

22

Tracking Problems of the Patella

W. Michael Walsh, M.D.
Michele Helzer-Julin, PA-C, M.S.

Of all knee problems presenting to the typical physician's office, the most common are disorders of the extensor mechanism. The term "extensor mechanism" encompasses several anatomical structures: the various parts of the quadriceps musculature; the quadriceps tendon and attachment into the patella; the patella and its articular surface as well as the corresponding trochlear surface of the femur; the patellar tendon and its attachments to both patella and tibial tuberosity; and all of the associated supporting soft tissue such as retinaculum, peripatellar synovium, and the structure known as the synovial plica. Any pathological process involving these structures can ultimately be traced to an anatomical predisposition. Without anatomic predisposition, disorders of the extensor mechanism almost never occur, especially in the usual athletic setting. Predisposition alone, however, is often not enough to create problems unless accompanied by some acute injury process or, more commonly, repetitive overuse.

Historically speaking, thoughts have changed drastically during the 20th century about the role of kneecap problems in athletic injuries. Goldthwait,[5] during the first decade of the century, articulated beliefs that persisted as late as the 1960s. Those concepts included the idea that patellar problems afflicted only chubby, knock-kneed, teen-aged females—certainly not the vigorous male athlete. Hughston, in 1968, published a landmark article that helped to change that thinking.[6] He pointed out the prevalence of extensor mechanism disorders in male and female athletes alike. Since then, much of our thinking in orthopedics has solidified with regard to extensor mechanism disorders. On the other hand, substantial questions remain unanswered, especially with respect to sources of pain and the role of changes in joint pressure in the causation of this pathology.

The purpose of this chapter is to present a logical approach to disorders of the extensor mechanism of the knee so that the primary care physician can deal with them most effectively in an office. As in the preceding chapter, emphasis is on detailed history taking, careful physical examination, and nonsurgical treatment.

TAKING A HISTORY

Extensor mechanism disorders may present as a single traumatic occurrence or as a chronic overuse problem. In traumatic injuries, some patients will admit on careful questioning to having had previous mild symptoms. Others report no previous difficulties at all. The most likely acute injuries to the patella are instability episodes and osteochondral fractures. Instability may be in the form of an acute subluxation or of an acute dislocation. Obviously, these differ only in the degree of instability. Sometimes it is impossible to tell whether the patella has completely left its normal relationship to the femur and spontaneously reduced, or has continued to maintain partial contact with the articular surface of the trochlea.

Twisting is the typical mechanism of injury for any patellar instability. There may be a force delivered to the knee, usually along the lateral aspect, tending to force the knee into valgus. A patella, however, may subluxate or dislocate as a result of noncontact mechanisms as well. In either case, the athlete usually contracts the quadriceps violently. As in any musculotendinous unit, when the quadriceps is contracted it tries to make a straight line from the point of origin on the femur to the point of insertion into the tibial tuberosity. With the knee in valgus and the tibia in external rotation, the quadriceps tends to "bowstring," drawing the patella over the lateral side of the femoral condyle.

As discussed in the preceding chapter, the physician should press the patient for as many details as possible about the sensation experienced at the moment of injury. Most patients report immediate pain along the medial aspect of the knee. Many are able to state clearly that the patella "slipped." The instability usually causes enough "giving way" to force the athlete to fall. A knee held in flexion greater than 90°, which is accompanied by pain that is relieved when the knee is finally straightened out, suggests patellar dislocation. The athlete who happens to lie on the ground in such a way as to see the knee may report that the patella was over the lateral side of the joint. Others do not notice the laterally displaced patella but see instead the uncovered medial femoral condyle and swear that something popped out on the medial side of the knee. When someone finally extends the knee, whether the patient or someone else, there is usually a "clunk" and a sensation of something going back into place as well as relief from pain. Of course, in subluxation, reduction on knee extension should be absent.

The history of swelling may vary tremendously, depending to a great extent on the degree of congenital laxity of the patella. A patella may dislocate completely with surprisingly little damage to the supporting structures. In such cases, swelling may not be marked. Large swelling within the joint that occurs within 2 hours indicates a hemarthrosis and should alert a clinician to the possibility of the presence of one of the common osteochondral fractures occurring in episodes of patellar instability.

Acute patellar subluxation or dislocation may present a dramatic appearance and be easier to describe. The patient with a chronic or overuse problem of the extensor mechanism, however, is the one most often seen by the primary care physician. These difficulties can be equally disabling and equally challenging to the physician—sometimes more so.

Many of the guidelines provided in the preceding chapter are also relevant to taking a history in a patient with a chronic extensor mechanism disorder. The most common complaint will be pain, usually located around the anterior aspect of one or both knees. Swelling may also be noted, but it usually is relatively mild in comparison to that seen in acute episodes. Many patients notice cracking, popping, or other noises coming from the region of the kneecap. Transient catching episodes with the knee in full extension are typical of extensor mechanism problems. Instability or giving way of the knee when the athlete twists, pivots, or cuts is likewise common but often difficult to separate from ligamentous instability. Most symptoms reported by patients with tracking problems of the patella are nonspecific. Aside from the occasional patient who clearly states, "My kneecap slips out of place," most patients' complaints could be consistent with a half-dozen different knee disorders.

Two symptoms deserve special mention when dealing with problems of the kneecap: the pain that occurs after sitting for a long period of time with the knee flexed, and pain that increases when descending stairs or slopes. The greater the degree of knee flexion, the more force that is generated within the patellofemoral joint, even with sitting in a non-weight-bearing position. Though the exact mechanism of pain production is unclear, patients with any disorder of the extensor mechanism seem to experience more painful symptoms when forced to sit in a cramped position for a long time. Back seats of small cars, theater seats, and airline seats all cause havoc with symptomatic patellae, forcing the patient to stand and walk around or seek the aisle seat, where the knee can be extended for comfort. Biomechanically, descending stairs or slopes produces some of the highest forces within the extensor mechanism. The joint experiences force that is not simply equal to body weight but is actually several times greater, as the extensor mechanism works in an eccentric fashion to decelerate the body's momentum and control its decent. This problem with stairs can become sufficiently marked to force the patient with chronic extensor mechanism problems to choose to live in a ranch-style house rather than a multi-level one.

Most symptoms related to the extensor mechanism of the knee are nonspecific. The spontaneous onset of bilateral anterior knee pain, perhaps accompanied by mild swelling, is highly suggestive of patellar problems, especially if the pain is accentuated by sitting with the knee flexed or by descending stairs. The key to diagnosing extensor mechanism problems, however, is artful physical examination.

PHYSICAL FINDINGS

The general comments given in the preceding chapter regarding physical examination of the knee apply here as well: the importance of examining the patient in positions other than with the patient's lying flat on a table; watching the patient walk or run; comparing findings with those of the normal (or *more* normal) knee; and the gentleness with which the examination is done. Naturally, you will not examine a knee for *either* extensor mechanism problems or ligament and meniscal problems. Therefore, the examination process as outlined in this chapter and the preceding one must be integrated in your mind.

Observation on Standing

When examining a patient with a suspected tracking problem of the patella, carefully observe him or her in the standing posture. Look for exaggerated angular deformities from the front and the side views. Extreme valgus of the lower extremities has always been associated with extensor mechanism problems. Marked varus deformities, however, especially those in which the varus is sharply localized to the proximal tibia, can also be associated with kneecap problems. When looking at the knees from the side, the physician is interested mainly in the presence of congenital recurvatum of the knee. This indication of generalized joint laxity would perhaps make you expect to see some relative patellar hypermobility. Look carefully at the feet. Marked pronation may accentuate extensor mechanism difficulties; and treatment of hyperpronated feet may be beneficial to the patellar symptoms.

Most important of all the observations made of the patient in the standing position is detection of what has been called the "miserable malalignment syndrome." Stan James coined this term[9] to describe the patient who has rotational deformities of the legs and feet. Typically, this is a patient (Fig. 1) with marked femoral anteversion, so that, as the lower extremities come down from hip joints to knees, the femoral condyles are rotated internally, making the kneecaps face inward toward one another (so-called "squinting patellae"). This condition is most noticeable when the patient stands with feet parallel. The overall appearance of the legs will be that of a varus deformity, with most of the varus sharply localized to the proximal third of each tibia. There will also be concomitant external tibial torsion bilaterally, so that when the patient stands with kneecaps pointed straight ahead, the feet are externally rotated 45° or more. Finally, there is often pronation of both feet of a rather marked degree. This complicated deformity extending from the hip joints to the feet is indeed a malalignment of the extensor mechanism, and one that is not easily treated by any method, including surgery.

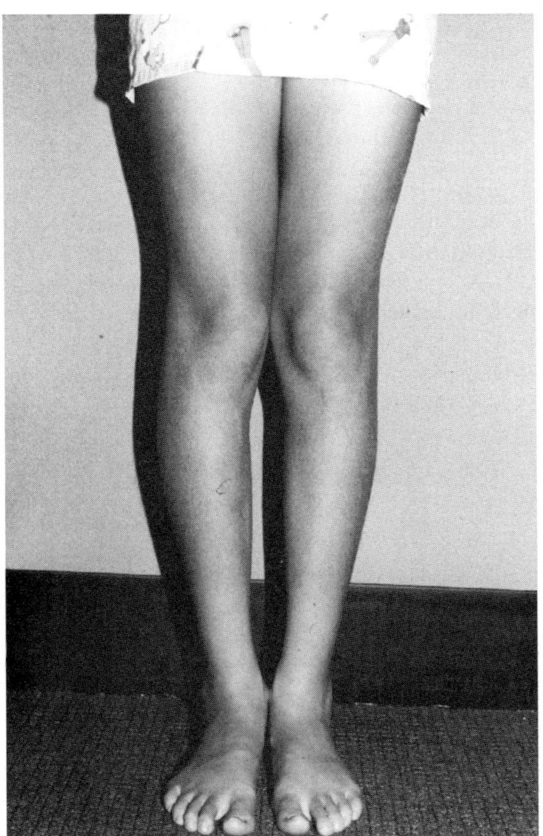

FIGURE 1. **Miserable malalignment syndrome:** The patient demonstrates femoral anteversion and external tibial torsion. When feet are parallel, kneecaps "squint" toward one another. When patellae point straight ahead, feet are markedly externally rotated.

Observation on Walking

While watching the patient walk in the hallway, you should pay particular attention to the patella and its movement. Look for any abnormal movements of the patella as it engages or disengages the trochlea. Also observe the position of the lower extremities. Does the patient throw his legs in some abnormal fashion to indicate one of the rotational deformities mentioned above? Also observe the foot mechanics and any part they may play in accentuating the problem.

Examination on Sitting

Next, have the patient sit on the side of the examination table with the knees flexed to 90°. Simply observe the patellae in their positions relative to the distal femora. When viewed from the side, the normal patella should sit very much on the distal end of the femur with the face of the patella pointing toward the wall in front of the patient. A wide range of proximal displacement (patella alta), or more rarely, distal displacement (patella baja) can be seen in this position. (Fig. 2) In patients with extreme patella alta, the face of the patella points almost straight up toward the ceiling. Any degree of patella alta is one of the congenital predispositions to extensor mechanism problems. As the patella is positioned more and more proximally, it loses much of the bony support of the femoral trochlea.

Looking at the knees from the front, the normal patella should be very much in the center of the knee as the patient sits with the two knees touching. Again, a spectrum of abnormal lateral postures of the patellae can be seen (Fig. 3). Lateral dis-

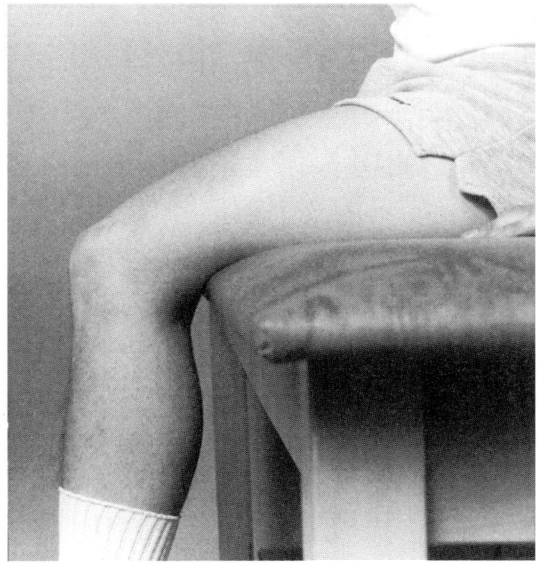

FIGURE 2. **Patella alta.** Knee viewed from the side demonstrates more proximal positioning of patella in relation to femur. The top of the patella interrupts the downslope of the thigh to give an appearance much like the lip of a ski jump.

placement is also considered to be one of the congenital predisposing findings. Most frequently, one will find a combination of both high and lateral posture of the patellae, the so-called "grasshopper eyes" appearance.

Tibial torsion may also be assessed with the patient in the sitting position. By standing above the patent's knees and sighting along the tibial tuberosity and anterior tibial crest, the physician can assess the relative position of an imaginary line connecting the medial and lateral malleoli of the ankle. Normal external tibial torsion has been reported[4] to range between zero and 40°.

The other observation that is easily made at this time is to look for Osgood-Schlatter changes of the tibial tuberosity. Enlargement of the tibial tuberosity is easily seen. Palpate the enlarged tibial tuberosity to ascertain whether it is also tender.

Now have the patient actively extend the knee from 90° flexion to full extension. Carefully watch the tracking of the patella as the knee comes into full extension. Usually, the patella shows a slight lateral deviation in the last few degrees of full knee extension. Abnormal patellae may show a marked lateral slide on terminal extension, however. Then palpate the patellofemoral joint as the patient goes through the same range of motion, feeling for crepitation that may be present. Finally, apply resistance to the knee extension with your opposite hand on the ankle while palpating the patellofemoral joint. Often in a patient with a diseased patella, forced knee extension against resistance creates pain.

Next, have the patient hold both knees actively in a position of 45° flexion. This is the best position in which to examine for presence of dysplasia of the vastus medialis obliquus muscle (VMO) (Fig. 4). Dysplasia of the VMO is probably the prime causative finding in all extensor mechanism disorders. We certainly consider it to be a major predisposition. If a patient shows a bulky, well-developed VMO in this position, your thinking may rightly be directed away from the extensor mechanism. Again, the presence of VMO dysplasia does not confirm a specific diagnosis, but merely shows a

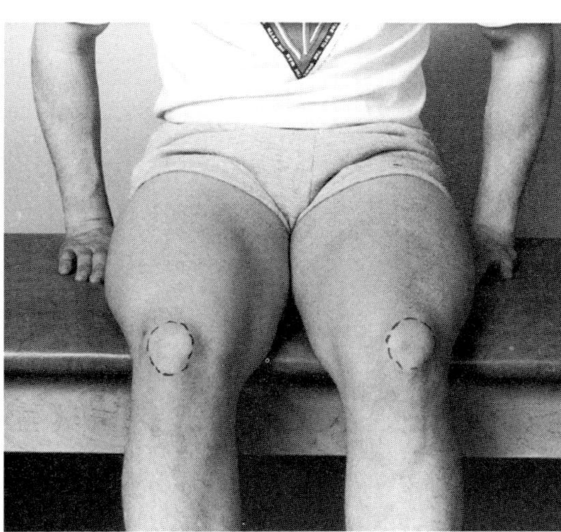

FIGURE 3. **Lateral positioning of patellae.** Knees viewed from front show lateral displacement of patellae. Kneecaps are tilted away from each other.

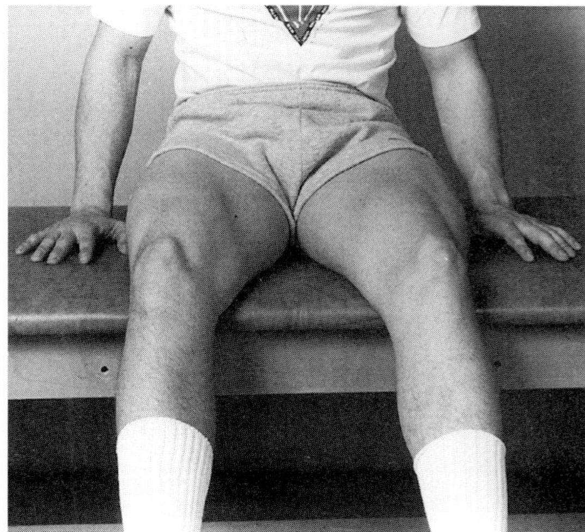

FIGURE 4. **Vastus medialis obliquus (VMO) dysplasia.** Patient sitting with knees held at 45° of flexion demonstrates lack of normal bulk of VMO along the proximal medial patella.

congenital predisposition to the various syndromes affecting the extensor mechanism.

Examination in Supine Position

Many of the findings noted in the previous chapter are also important in the patient with an extensor mechanism problem. For example, you should certainly palpate for effusion and check the range of motion of the knee. Some findings specifically relate to the extensor mechanism, however.

Next, compress the patella against the anterior aspect of the femur, causing the patella to glide both medially and laterally as well as proximally and distally. Not only will this give you some indication of the overall mobility of the patellofemoral joint, but it may also reveal a sensation of crepitation, which may be painful. Traditionally, it has been taught that painful crepitation from these maneuvers indicates chondromalacia of the patella. Flex the knee to 30° over a pillow or bolster, and then repeat this compression test. Often, both crepitation and pain will disappear in this position. If they were caused by true chondromalacia of the patella, they would not disappear. Many times crepitation and pain in the fully extended position come from compression of the patella against the supratrochlear soft tissues, because many patellae lie above the trochlea when the knee is fully extended.

You can next palpate around the entire extensor mechanism. Frequently, symptomatic patellae will be tender along their medial edges. Once again, this was thought to be caused by degenerative changes of the patellar articular surface. It is, however, more logical that such tenderness results from the soft tissues' being trapped between the examining finger and the patellar surface. By pressing down on the proximal pole of the patella, one can cause the patella to tilt its distal pole upward. Palpate along the entire inferior pole at the attachment of the patellar tendon. Patellar tendinitis is shown specifically by tenderness to palpation in this area (Fig. 5). Less commonly, tenderness occurs along the proximal edge of the patella at the attachment of the quadriceps tendon, thus indicating quadriceps tendinitis. In the patient with acute patellar dislocation, palpation could also be done along the entire course of the VMO to ascertain the point of injury. If the VMO has been ruptured from its insertion into the proximal medial portion of the patella, you may very easily discern a defect in that area that allows invagination of the skin and soft tissue almost into the interior of the joint.

Determine the alignment of the extensor mechanism by measuring the quadriceps angle, known as the "Q angle." The patient's knee must be fully extended with the quadriceps *contracted*. Center the pivot point of the goniometer over the patella. The proximal arm of the goniometer points to the anterior superior illiac spine and the goniometer's distal arm lies along the patellar tendon (Fig. 6). If the results of this measurement are greater than 10° in males, this is considered an abnormal Q angle. Because females normally have greater valgus of the knees, up to 15° is considered normal in women.[3]

Next, palpate for the presence of a pathological synovial plica by passively flexing and extending the knee from about 30 to 90° of flexion (Fig. 7). At the same time, the patella should be displaced

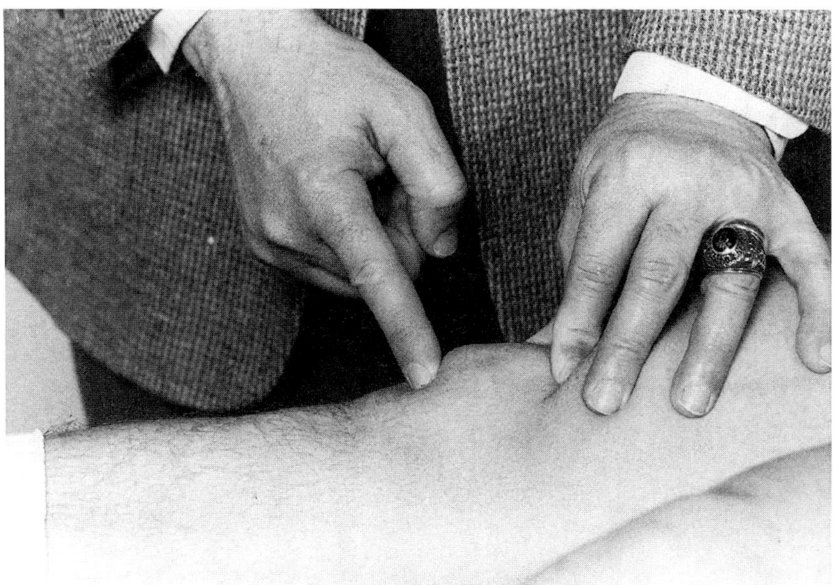

FIGURE 5. Patellar tendinitis. Pressure on proximal patellar pole will tilt distal pole upward. Patellar tendinitis is shown by tenderness along inferior edge at attachment of patellar tendon.

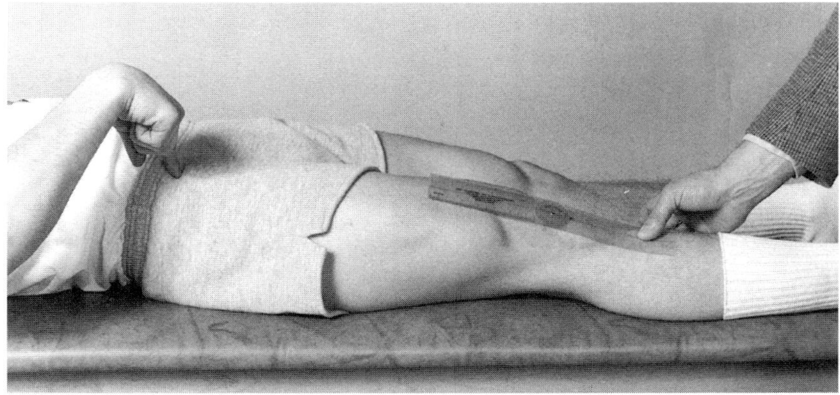

FIGURE 6. **Measuring for the quadriceps angle ("Q angle").** Angle is measured with knee extended and quadriceps contracted.

slightly medially and the fingers of the examining hand should be placed in the medial peripatellar region. With the quadriceps relaxed, a tender fold may often be palpated that recreates the familiar painful popping sensation that the patient feels.

The remaining part of the examination of the patella itself is in the lateral hypermobility test (as discussed in Chapter 21, Fig. 10). Remember that you are looking not only for hypermobility but also for apprehension, pain, and the patient's subjective

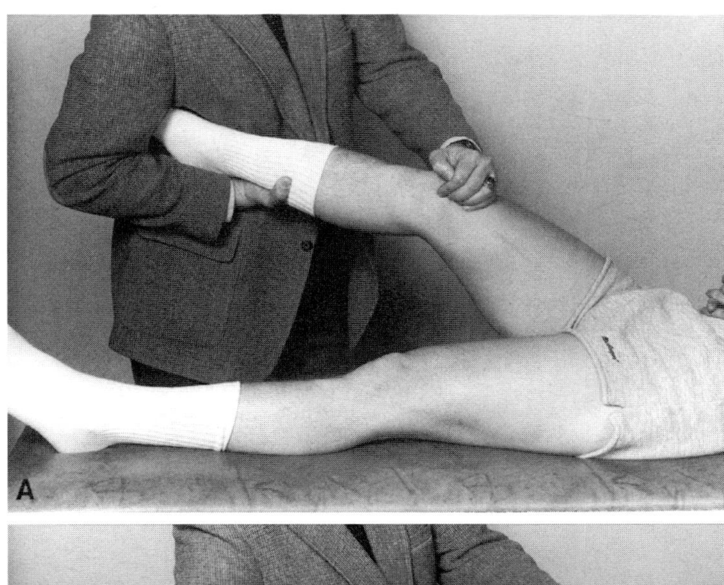

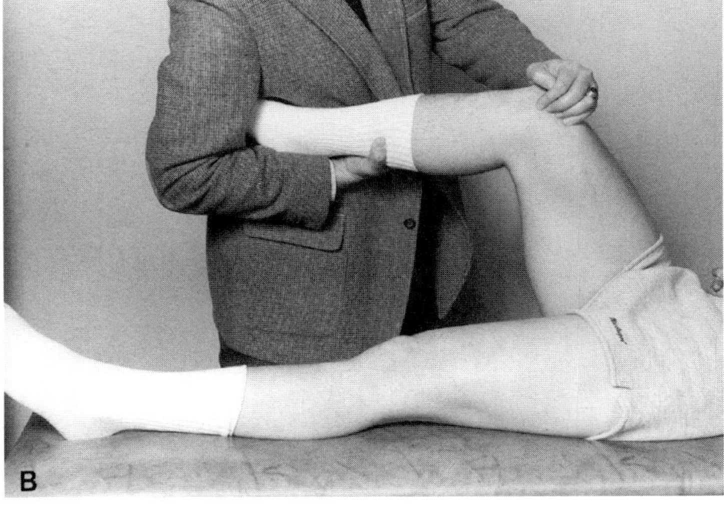

FIGURE 7. **Palpation for synovial plica.** Foot and tibia are internally rotated. Examiner's hand lies along lateral edge of patella, displacing patella medially. Fingers palpate medial patellofemoral joint while knee is passively moved from approximately 30° (A) to 90° (B) of flexion.

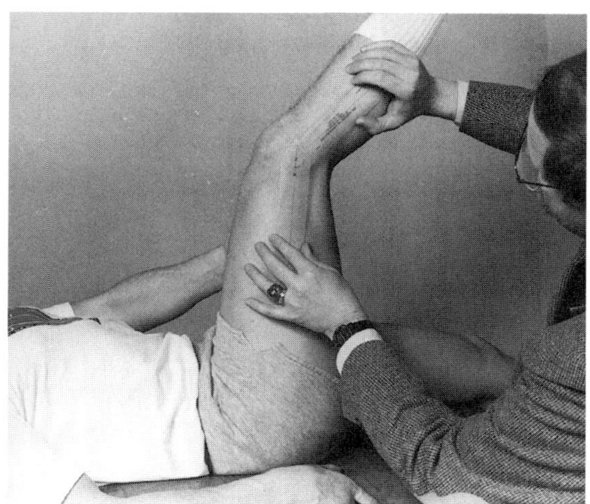

FIGURE 8. **Measuring hamstring tightness.** With patient supine and hip flexed 90°, knee should extend fully if hamstrings are flexible. If knee will not extend completely, residual knee flexion angle is measured and recorded as hamstring tightness.

report that this is a familiar feeling associated with the knee disability.

Other Examination

Quadriceps muscle tone and bulk may be checked, but measuring the thigh's circumference is not worth the effort. Muscle status can probably best be evaluated by simply observing the relative bulk of the musculature and palpating for any relative loss of tone.

Inflexibility in certain muscle groups is critically important in dealing with the extensor mechanism. Most common is tightness of the hamstrings. With the opposite leg fully extended, have the patient flex the hip to 90°. While maintaining the hip at 90°, see if he or she can fully extend the knee so that the entire leg is pointed straight up at the ceiling (Fig. 8). This indicates normal hamstring flexibility, at least in the general population. In certain athletes whose sport requires great flexibility, such as dancers and gymnasts, this is minimal flexibility. These athletes should be able to bring the entire leg into more flexion at the hip, with the leg coming toward the head. Lack of normal hamstring flexibility is shown in inability to extend the knee fully with the hip flexed to 90°.

The next most important muscle flexibility measurement to ascertain is that of the gastroc-soleus group along the posterior calf. With the knee fully extended and the foot slightly inverted, passively dorsiflex the ankle as far as possible (Fig. 9). In normally flexible calves, the foot should come to approximately 15° of dorsiflexion beyond neutral.

The third, and more often neglected, flexibility to assess is that of the quadriceps muscle group itself. Turn the patient to a prone position and acutely flex the knee, bringing the heel toward the buttock (Fig. 10). Lack of knee flexion in comparison to the uninjured side, obligatory flexion of the hip joints such that the anterior pelvis rises off the examination table, or simply the patient's report of increased "tightness" along the anterior thigh during this maneuver are all indications of quadriceps muscle tightness that should be stretched out.

Finally, evaluate the iliotibial band tightness using Ober's test (Fig. 11). Position the patient on his or her side with the leg to be tested up, and flex the untested hip and knee to 90°. Stand behind the patient and steady the pelvis with one hand. Flex the knee of the upper leg to 90° and bring the hip into full extension. With normal iliotibial band flexibility, the knee of the upper leg should be able to drop to near table level.

With the patient supine, hip range of motion should be evaluated. With the hip flexed to 90°, internal rotation that exceeds external rotation is an indication of some degree of femoral anteversion.

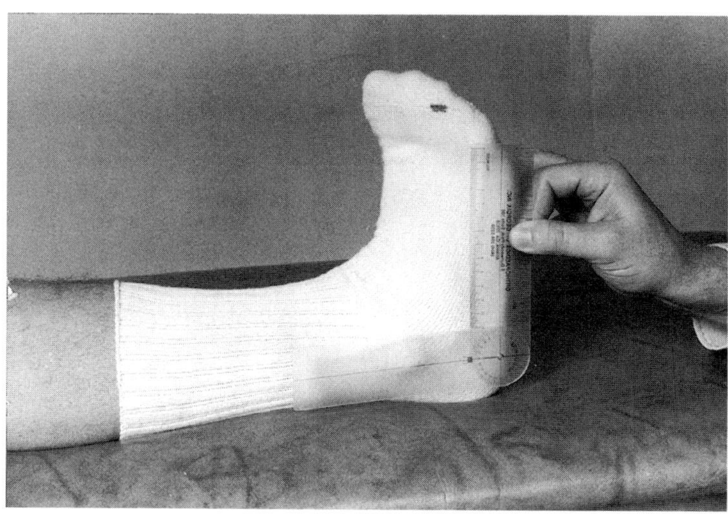

FIGURE 9. **Heel cord tightness measurement** with knee fully extended and foot slightly inverted. Ankle is dorsiflexed as far as possible. Normally flexible gastrocsoleus muscles should allow 15° of dorsiflexion past the neutral position.

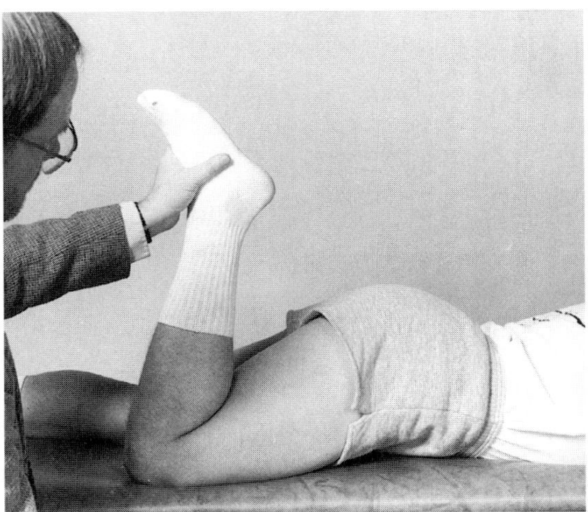

FIGURE 10. **Quadriceps flexibility measurement.** Patient is turned prone. Knee is flexed to bring heel as close to buttock as possible. Anterior pelvis rising off examination table, sensation of tightness along anterior thigh, or lack of knee flexion compared to opposite side may all indicate quadriceps tightness.

Radiographic Evaluation

Most radiographic evaluation is as discussed in the preceding chapter. More recently, however, we have started taking our lateral radiographs of the knee in 90° flexion (Fig. 12), which is the same position in which we assess patellar position clinically. A normally placed patella, that is, one with no patella alta, should be placed very nearly on the distal end of the femur, with its proximal pole approximately in line with the anterior femoral cortex.[14] Deviations from this norm are most easily seen in this 90° flexed lateral view. Various techniques have been described for measuring a radiographic film to determine patella alta and patella baja. The most commonly used is the method of Insall, Goldberg, and Salvati,[7] which expresses the greatest diagonal length of the patella as a ratio to the length of the patellar tendon (Fig. 13). This ratio should approximate 1.0. Deviations greater than 20% in either direction (less than 0.8 or greater than 1.2) indicate significant patella alta or patella baja. This ratio may be a little difficult to determine because of uncertainties in measuring the length of the patellar tendon on radiographic film, especially in determining the point of its attachment into the tibial tuberosity.

The most significant view in dealing with the patellofemoral joint is the infrapatellar, which must be done at 30° to 45° knee flexion. Although many different techniques exist,[14] any using flexion greater than 90° are not helpful.

Various abnormalities may be seen in the infrapatellar view, and are most easily seen when both knees have been x-rayed on the same cassette, allowing direct comparison. Relative deficiency of the lateral femoral condyle, allowing either lateral tilting or lateral subluxation of the patella, may be seen (Fig. 14). Like the clinical findings noted earlier, these radiographic findings may span a wide range, from mild to severe. Avulsion fractures along the medial edge of the patella are virtually pathognomonic for recurrent patellar dislocation (Fig. 15). Osteochondral fractures may likewise be seen.

Many different techniques for measurement of lateral tilting, lateral displacement, and lack of patellofemoral congruity have been described,[12] but

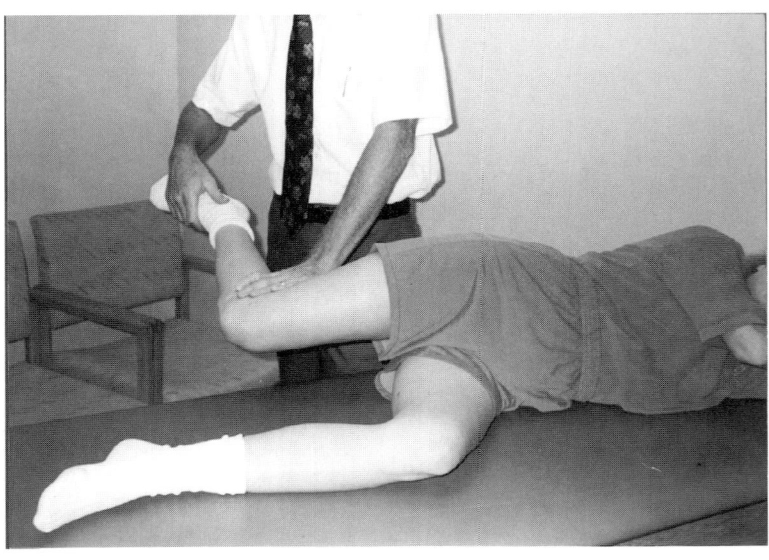

FIGURE 11. **Ober's test for iliotibial band tightness.** Normal flexibility should allow the patient's knee to drop to near table level. See text for details.

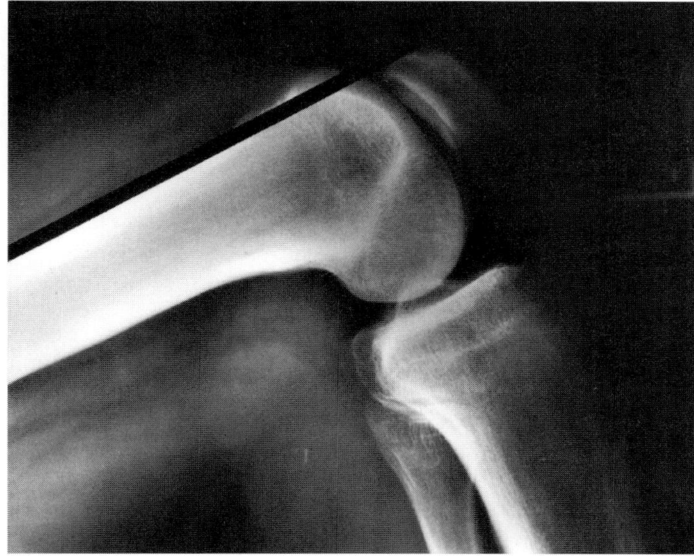

FIGURE 12. **Lateral knee radiograph at 90°.** Allows assessment of patella alta or patella baja. Proximal pole of patella should be in line with anterior femoral cortex.

are not helpful in office practice. Use the infrapatellar radiographic view for the information it readily provides. It may alert you to problems within the extensor mechanism that you had not suspected. You may be prompted to go back and examine the patellofemoral joint more carefully. It may show congenital predisposition that is present even on the asymptomatic side. However, to spend time drawing lines and measuring angles is generally not worth much. The final diagnosis lies in careful history taking and physical examination.

SPECIFIC PROBLEMS AND THEIR TREATMENT

Acute Patellar Instability

The athlete with an acute injury may have experienced an acute dislocation that persisted until reduced, an acute dislocation with spontaneous reduction, or an acute subluxation. Diagnosis of this situation is by taking a typical history and by confirmatory physical examination, which should show the usual predisposing physical findings (VMO dysplasia, high and lateral patella, increased Q angle) on the opposite uninjured knee, as well as swelling, tenderness over the medial supporting structures, and patellar hypermobility with associated apprehension and pain on the injured knee.

Treatment for the first-time patellar dislocation is controversial. Some authors point out that the injury to the medial supporting structure is like any other acute ligamentous knee injury and recommend immediate surgical repair.[2,13] We believe that surgery is necessary in only two settings: VMO rupture and large osteochondral fracture with loose body. If the VMO has been ruptured at its insertion, and a defect is palpable along the superomedial edge of the patella, then it is best handled by early surgical repair. This portion of the VMO does not heal well with simple closed treatment. In most patellar dislocations,

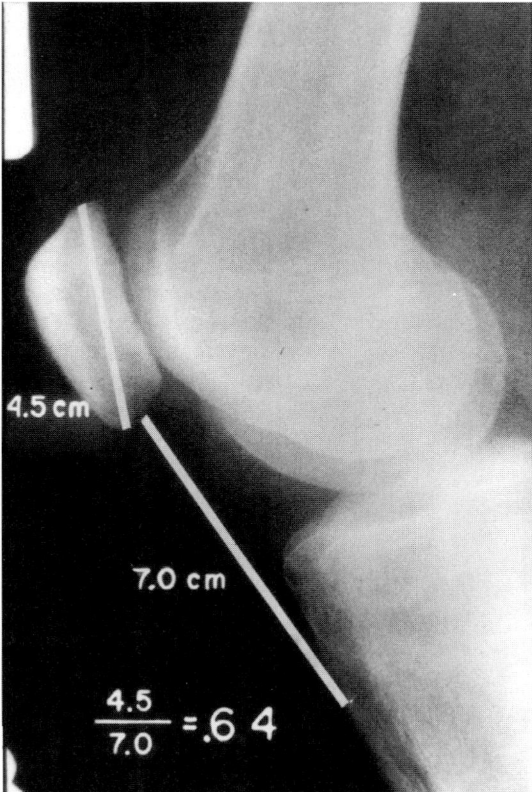

FIGURE 13. **Insall-Salvati method for measuring patella alta or patella baja.** Greatest diagonal length of patella as a ratio to length of patellar tendon should be 1.0 ± 0.2.

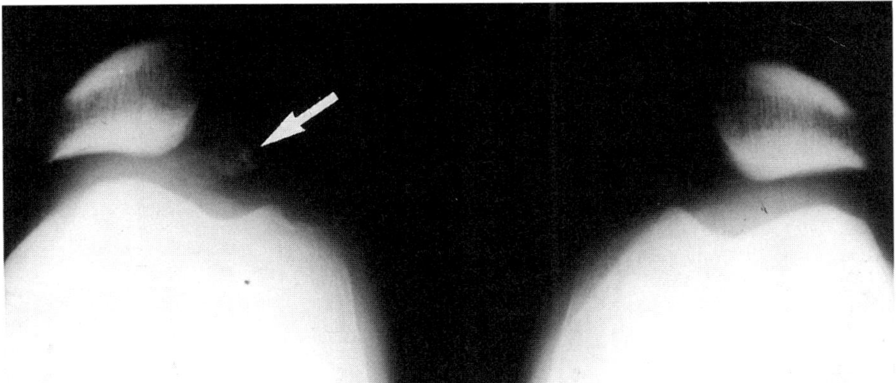

FIGURE 14. **Infrapatellar radiograph shows lateral tilting and lateral subluxation of both patellae.** Also seen is osteochondral fracture from acute injury (arrow).

however, the VMO has been injured either in its midsubstance or at its origin from the femur and medial intermuscular septum and is treated nonsurgically in the acute setting. If a large fracture is visible on radiograph, then surgery with removal or reattachment of the fracture fragment may be indicated as shown in the section on osteochondral fracture below.

Some patellae can dislocate with surprisingly little acute change in the soft tissues. Consequently, the majority of first dislocations of the patella can be handled with closed treatment. If a large, tense hemarthrosis develops, the knee can be aspirated for comfort, as described in the preceding chapter. For many decades, standard treatment for the first-time patellar dislocation included a cylinder cast extending from groin to malleoli with the knee in full extension. Immobilization was often continued for 6 weeks.

Current immobilization is much less stringent; casting is almost never used. A thick foam rubber or felt pad can be placed over the area of tenderness on the medial supporting structures to compress them snugly against their femoral attachment. A crescent-shaped foam rubber or felt pad can also be placed along the lateral edge of the patella to displace it more medially. A knee immobilizer is recommended on an individual basis to control pain and swelling. Crutches to allow partial weight bearing are encouraged in all our patients. Physical therapy and McConnell muscle re-education and taping techniques[10,14] are instituted early. Return to sporting activities is based on alleviation of symptoms and return to functional ability rather than a specific time frame. Diminished immobilization time and early introduction to physical therapy has dramatically reduced the degree of quadriceps atrophy and has allowed the patient more rapid return to daily functions and sporting activities.

Osteochondral Fractures

With any acute instability episode of the patella, an osteochondral fracture may occur, as Milgram[11] described the mechanism. As the patella either

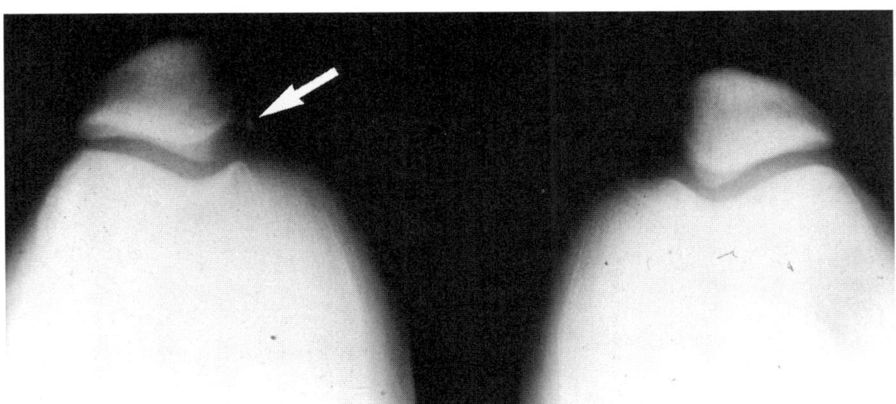

FIGURE 15. **Infrapatellar radiograph.** Avulsion fracture from medial edge of patella (arrow) is pathognomonic for recurrent patellar dislocation.

leaves or re-enters the femoral trochlea, a segment of bone and overlying articular cartilage may be sheared off, usually from either the lateral lip of the trochlea or the medial facet of the patella. Some of these fragments, if they contain sufficient bone, may be visible on initial radiograph. In other cases, evidence of such a fracture may only come through finding fat droplets in the bloody aspirate taken from the knee. Purely chondral fractures may not be apparent at all.

In sizable osteochondral fractures visible on radiograph or inferred by blood in the aspirate, orthopedic consultation is indicated. Arthroscopy of the knee may be necessary for large fractures. Occasionally a fragment must be reattached with internal fixation. Some smaller osteochondral fractures can simply be observed and treated later if symptomatic. This is, however, a decision that is probably best made by your orthopedic consultant.

Recurrent Patellar Subluxation

Many patients will present to your office with recurrent slipping of the kneecap and giving away of the knee, but they have never experienced an acute episode of major proportions, certainly not a complete patellar dislocation. Examination will show the typical predisposing physical findings as well as hypermobility and apprehension. The patient should be able to associate this feeling of apprehension with the feeling he or she gets when trying to pivot, twist, or cut during sports. The primary care physician may successfully help these patients by prescribing a detailed rehabilitative exercise program as well as the use of patellar taping or bracing. Remember that the rehabilitative program is not simple "quad sets and thigh squeezes." Rehabilitation does not focus merely on quadriceps strength, per se, but also on the quality of the quadriceps contraction beginning medially with the VMO and progressing laterally. Many times, biofeedback techniques are helpful in "re-educating" the quadriceps mechanism. Simple patellofemoral taping techniques (McConnell techniques)[10] also play an important role in conservative management of the patellofemoral joint and in many cases may eliminate the need for patellar bracing. Please see Chapter 5 for further details on these techniques. If this problem occurs in a younger individual, generalized growth and development with increased muscle bulk may also be a helpful factor. Certainly far greater than 50% of the patients with this problem should respond to nonsurgical treatment. If the patient still has significant functional disability after attempting rehabilitation and patellar taping or bracing, then orthopedic referral is indicated. Various surgical approaches to this problem are available. Arthroscopic lateral release has gained a reputation for providing relief in many patients. Open methods of extensor mechanism reconstruction have existed for many decades, however, and still tend to be helpful in the patient whose malalignment has not been helped by, or is not appropriate for, lateral release.

Chondromalacia Patella

Even though it has a precise pathological meaning, the term "chondromalacia patella" has come to be applied to any condition that creates painful symptoms around the kneecap, especially crepitation and tenderness. In truth, this is an extremely difficult diagnosis to make with certainty through purely clinical or radiographic means.[8,14] The term "chondromalacia patella" should be reserved for cases in which objective articular cartilage changes are seen on arthroscopy or magnetic resonance imaging (MRI).

Chondromalacia patella does *not* occur spontaneously, but is a patellar response to some abnormal mechanical situation, usually one of the syndromes of abnormal patellar tracking. If you believe strongly that your patient has chondromalacia, the appropriate treatment is, once again, thorough rehabilitative exercise, the use of patellar taping or bracing, and administration of NSAIDs. Rather than using the term "chondromalacia patella" willy-nilly, it is probably better to use the term "patellofemoral pain syndrome" or "extensor mechanism malalignment."

Patellofemoral Pain Syndromes

The opposite of patients with patellar instability problems are those with pain but without instability symptoms. Indeed, even though examination of these patients shows typical predisposing physical findings, one may not find any true hypermobility or apprehension on testing the patella. Actual mechanisms of pain production in these syndromes has not been completely elucidated. Logically, however, pain can be caused by inflammation of the peripatellar soft tissues such as the synovium. Undoubtedly, these patients are best treated with the three-part approach of rehabilitative exercises, patellar taping or bracing, and NSAID therapy. Patients who do not respond to this protocol may be candidates for surgery and should be referred. Arthroscopy may be helpful in determining the source of the symptoms and perhaps in treating these problems through such procedures as patellar chondroplasty, débridement of peripatellar synovium, or lateral retinacular release.

Synovial Plica

Somewhere in the spectrum of patellofemoral pain syndrome is the entity that has been variously known as the synovial plica, the suprapatellar plica, the medial shelf, and the plica synovialis mediopatellaris. The actual structure is a shelf of synovium extending into the joint and then doubled back upon itself, which is believed to be a remnant of the embryological division of the knee joint into three separate cavities: the medial, lateral, and suprapatellar pouches. As the embryo develops, these three fuse together, with resorption of the old wall separating them. This resorption may be more or less complete. The incompletely reabsorbed wall is believed to be found grossly as the synovial plica.

There may be a suprapatellar part to this structure. In fact, the suprapatellar pouch may still exist as a totally separate cavity, but more usually the more symptomatic part of the plica is the medial portion, which extends along the medial side of the patellofemoral joint. Frequency of such a medial shelf is unknown, but arthroscopy has demonstrated a large percentage of patients have some degree of plica. The question remains as to how large a shelf is significant. Some are seen to extend 1 cm or more beneath the medial facet of the patella and are undoubtedly symptomatic. Others are quite narrow, softer, and probably cause no trouble.

Diagnosing a synovial plica can be a clinical challenge. Typically, the patient with pathological plica has pain that greatly increases with sitting with the knee flexed for any long period. The patient usually learns to extend the knee to relieve the pain. Often, when the knee is extended after sitting, there is a definite "pop" that occurs over the medial aspect of the patellofemoral joint and is associated with relief of the painful symptom. The patient soon learns to extend the knee and pop it to gain relief. There may be mild recurrent knee swelling, and typically, intermittent catching episodes. Occasionally, the patient will find that placing the knee in a slight amount of flexion provides the most comfortable resting position.

Physical examination for a plica is as described above. Even though this synovial abnormality could be expected to occur in patients without the other typical predispositions to extensor mechanism problems, it seems that most symptomatic plicae occur in patients with some element of extensor mechanism malalignment. Often the plica is only part of the overall picture in any given patient.

Successful conservative treatment depends on how far the inflammatory process has progressed in the synovial structure itself. Early, mild inflammatory changes may be reversed by NSAIDs and use of extensor mechanism rehabilitative techniques. Ice massage and hydrocortisone phonophoresis may also be tried. Corticosteroid injection of the plica has also been described, but it is difficult to imagine how one could really be certain of injecting only this synovial fold.

If conservative treatment fails, surgical treatment may be undertaken with good prospect for success. In fact, a plica may be one of the few knee problems in which surgical treatment restores an essentially normal knee. This view is predicated on the thought that this entity is a functionless embryological remnant. On the other hand, if the plica is present with other extensor mechanism problems, arthroscopic excision may give only partial relief. Most often, even after plica excision, the patient finds it necessary to continue working on the extensor mechanism through rehabilitative exercise and perhaps with external support.

Fat Pad Impingement

Little information is available regarding infrapatellar fat pad impingement. Despite lack of recognition in the literature, this extensor mechanism problem is frequently seen in our office. The fat pad lies just posterior to the patellar tendon. When inflamed, it may extend proximally between the patella and femur and become impinged. This chronic impingement causes inflammation and hypertrophy of the fat pad. A vicious cycle evolves as hypertrophy leads to further impingement that again leads to further inflammation and hypertrophy.

In addition to the usual extensor mechanism complaints, these patients will also complain of a sharp pain in the anterior jointline just medial or lateral to the patellar tendon. Pain may come and go suddenly with intermittent impingement. In the very acute phase, the patient may actually appear to have a locked knee and lack terminal extension.

Fat pad impingement can be treated conservatively with physical therapy directed at the patellofemoral joint. Taping the patella so that the inferior pole is tilted anteriorly may also help. In our experience, corticosteroid injection into the fat pad has been of little benefit. Beyond conservative treatment, surgical options are limited. During arthroscopy, fat pad hypertrophy and impingement can be seen easily from the superolateral approach. The fat pad can be "debulked" during arthroscopy with the use of a power shaver.

Patellar Tendinitis ("Jumper's Knee")

Repetitive jumping in sports such as basketball and volleyball can create chronic inflammatory changes in the patellar tendon. The symptoms usually appear at the inferior pole of the patella where the patellar tendon attaches. Even though the entire patellar tendon may be ultimately involved by some degenerative process, only rarely are the symptoms or findings referred to the body of the tendon itself. Observation would indicate that this patellar tendinitis rarely, if ever, occurs in a knee without the congenital predisposing physical findings we have discussed. Usually patella alta and VMO dysplasia are prominent findings in the patient with jumper's knee. In addition, many of the factors known to aggravate other extensor mechanism disorders, such as inflexibility of the hamstrings, can greatly accentuate the symptoms of patellar tendinitis. Other than through a history of jumping sports, complaints of infrapatellar pain, and the presence of physical predisposition, the diagnosis of patellar tendinitis is made simply through palpation of the inferior pole of the patella (see Fig. 5). Point tenderness in this area confirms the suspected diagnosis.

Chronic patellar tendinitis can be terribly difficult to treat. Traditionally, VMO strengthening and stretching of the hamstrings, heel cords, and quadriceps have been used as rehabilitative techniques to deal with patellar tendinitis. Certainly they are important. More recently, work on the eccentric function of the quadriceps has been emphasized in dealing with this disorder.[3] It has also been pointed out that, through a biomechanical linkage with ankle mechanics, most patients with chronic patellar tendinitis also have demonstrable weakness of the ankle dorsiflexor muscles. Good success in treating patellar tendinitis has been reported with a program of eccentric strengthening of ankle dorsiflexors.[1] So far this appears to be our experience as well.

In addition to rehabilitative exercises, NSAIDs are certainly worth a try. External support of the extensor mechanism using patellar bracing may be beneficial although we have not found the straps manufactured specifically for patellar tendinitis of any help. Ice and deep friction massage to the inflamed area also seem to be helpful. Hydrocortisone phonophoresis or iontophoresis may likewise be tried. One should *never* be tempted to inject a corticosteroid into the patellar tendon, however, until all other techniques have been exhausted. To inject a major load bearing tendon such as the patellar tendon is to weaken it and to invite rupture. We use this technique only as a desperate last measure, and then only with the patient's understanding that he or she must refrain from activity for a protracted period. This option is best reserved for the orthopedic consultant.

Is there any surgical treatment to offer the patient with intractable patellar tendinitis? Magnetic resonance imaging (MRI) can document degenerative changes and chronic partial tears of the patellar tendon. A patient with this condition may be offered surgery, although none of the reported techniques seems very successful. Having been unsuccessful in all attempts to treat patellar tendinitis, you may wish to refer the patient for orthopedic consultation, realizing that débridement of chronic inflammatory tissue, excision of the inferior pole of the patella, releasing the peritendinous sheath, or some other surgical approach may be the only avenue remaining.

Osgood-Schlatter Disease

For many years, so-called Osgood-Schlatter disease was considered to be an osteochondrosis, that is, avascular necrosis of a growth center in the immature skeleton. More recent views identify Osgood-Schlatter disease as part of the spectrum of mechanical problems related to the extensor mechanism. Almost all young patients with this condition have evidence of some mechanical inefficiency of the extensor mechanism. Most often, this is a significant patella alta. Dysplasia of the VMO is difficult to judge in the typical age group with this condition because of general lack of musculoskeletal development at that age.

Diagnosis is not complicated; usually a history of insidious onset of pain in the region of one or both tibial tuberosities exists. Occasionally, there may be an acute episode superimposed on chronic symptoms, or less commonly, acute onset only, which may represent additional avulsion of the cartilage along the anterior aspect of the tibial tuberosity apophysis. In the chronic setting, this process occurs more gradually.

Radiographs may vary from normal, in the early stage, to later showing of separate bony ossicles loose within the patellar tendon substance. Almost all patients have marked inflexibility in hamstrings, heel cords, and quadriceps muscles.

The danger in treating Osgood-Schlatter disease lies in overtreatment. Although in the past, casts, cortisone injections, and complete cessation of normal childhood activities have been recommended, in general, none of this is necessary. Mechanical inefficiencies of the extensor mechanism should be treated by appropriate rehabilitative exercises. All inflexibility should be mitigated through stretching. As with patellar tendinitis, ankle dorsiflexion exercises are indicated if weakness can be demonstrated. Simple patellar support such as a neoprene rubber sleeve may be helpful. Local padding over the tender tuberosity can be used to prevent flareup of symptoms when the knee is struck against another object. NSAIDs may help relieve symptoms. Liberal use of icing techniques may also help. Throughout treatment, however, the patient may carry on with whatever physical activity is comfortable. In other words, although inactivity should not be *enforced,* it should be *advised* based on symptoms present. Full and normal activity may be returned to as symptoms recede. In the worst cases, the patient will have persistent enlargement of the tibial tuberosity. This may become intermittently painful in later life. If the patient does develop a loose ossicle within the substance of the patellar tendon, excision may be indicated. In such cases, simple excision of the ossicle without extensor mechanism reconstruction and correction of the patella alta may not suffice. More extensive reconstruction may be necessary, with a thorough postoperative rehabilitation program. None of these possibilities, however, is affected by letting the early adolescent go ahead with a normal lifestyle. No convincing evidence exists that the Osgood-Schlatter lesion leads to a disastrous consequence such as avulsion fracture of the tibial tuberosity.

SUMMARY

Disorders of the knee's extensor mechanism range broadly from primarily instability syndromes to those characterized solely by pain. All these syndromes originate in congenital predisposition. Some of these syndromes are simple and easy to manage. Most, however, are chronic or recurrent. Primary care physicians should become confident in their ability to assess such problems and have at their disposal a treatment plan that emphasizes rehabilitative exercise, simple physical modalities, anti-inflammatory medication, and bracing of the patella. When such treatment is made available to the patient, well over 50% of cases, and perhaps as many as 80 to 90% of cases, should be correctable.

REFERENCES

1. Black JE, Alten Sr: How I manage infrapatellar tendinitis. Phys Sportsmed 12:86–92, 1984.
2. Boring TH, O'Donoghue DH: Acute patellar dislocation: Results of immediate surgical repair. Clin Orthop 136: 182, 1978.
3. Curwin S, Stanish WD: Tendinitis; Its Etiology and Treatment. Lexington, MA, D.C. Heath, 1984.
4. Galland O, Walch G, Dejour H, Carret JP: An anatomical and radiological study of the femoropatellar articulation. Surg Radiol Anat 12:119–125, 1990.
5. Goldthwait JE: Permanent dislocation of the patella: WIth the report of eleven cases. Boston Med Surg J 150:169, 1904.
6. Hughston JC: Subluxation of the patella. J Bone Joint Surg 50A:1003, 1968.
7. Insall J, Goldberg V, Salvati E: Recurrent dislocation and the high-riding patella. Clin Orthop 88:67–69, 1972.
8. Insall J: "Chondromalacia patellae": Patellar malalignment syndrome. Orthop Clin North Am 10:117–127, 1979.
9. James SL: Chondromalacia of the patella in the adolescent. In Kennedy J.C. ed.: The Injured Adolescent Knee. Baltimore, Williams & Wilkins, 1979.
10. McConnell J: The management of chondromalacia patellae: A long term solution. Aust J Physiother 2:215–223, 1986.
11. Milgram JE: Tangential osteochondral fracture of the patella. J Bone Joint Surg 25:271, 1943.
12. Minkoff J, Fein L: The role of radiography in the evaluation and treatment of common anarthrotic disorders of the patellofemoral joint. Clin Sports Med 8:203–260, 1989.
13. Vainiopaa S, Laasonen E, Silvennoinen T, et al: Acute dislocation of patella. A prospective review of operative treatment. J Bone Joint Surg 72B:366–369, 1990.
14. Walsh WM: Patellofemoral Joint. In DeLee J, Drez D eds, Orthopaedic Sports Medicine: Principles and Practice. Philadelphia, W.B. Saunders Co, 1994, pp. 1163–1248.

23

Evaluation and Treatment of the Injured Ankle

Randall D. Neumann, M.D.

Ankle injuries, seen daily by family practitioners, physical therapists, and orthopedic surgeons are the most common conditions encountered in the treatment of the athlete.[7] Ankle sprains account for 25% of all athletic injuries[14] and 10–15% of all lost time in high school, college, and professional football.[7] As common as these injuries are, their evaluation and treatment are not uniform. Routine sprains have a high recovery rate, but some patients have chronic pain, swelling, and recurrent injury. Other conditions can mimic the classic ankle sprain, including peroneal tendinitis and subluxation, osteochondritis dessecans of the talus, and ankle impingement, thus making diagnosis difficult. Therefore, the management of ankle injury relies on a precise understanding of the mechanism of injury, a working knowledge of the anatomy, systematic evaluation, the clear ability to differentiate between the normal and pathologic, and principles of treatment including operative indications and rehabilitative techniques.

ANATOMY

The ankle mortise (Fig. 1) is formed by the distal articulation of the tibia, the fibula and the dome of the talus, and constitutes the hinge joint of the ankle. Range of motion is generally only in one plane, including plantar flexion and dorsiflexion. The subtalar joint, however, allows for the full range of inversion, eversion, supination, and pronation. The two joints often work together as a universal type joint with modifications in one affecting the biomechanics of normal activity of the other.

The medial malleolus is an extension of the distal tibia. The inner surface is covered with articular cartilage and articulates with the medial facet of the talus. There is a groove on the posterior surface where the posterior tibial tendon passes behind the malleolus and the tendon sheath is attached. The fibula provides the lateral support of the ankle. Just above the ankle joint the fibula sits in a groove formed by the broad anterior tubercle and a small posterior tubercle of the tibia. There is no articular surface between the distal tibia and fibula, even though there is considerable motion between these two bones. Articular cartilage covers the medial border of the fibula in the joint. The distal end tapers and has a posterior groove for the peroneal tendon. The talus is covered almost entirely by articular cartilage. The superior surface is convex from front to back and slightly concave from side to side. The dome of the talus is trapezoidal in shape and its anterior surface is an average of 3–4 mm wider than the posterior surface. The articular surfaces of the malleoli are also wider anteriorly and support the talus. The talus articulates with a navicular, calcaneus, tibia, and fibula.

The lateral ligamentous complex (Fig. 2) of the ankle consists of three ligaments: the anterior talofibular ligament blends with the lateral capsular structures of the ankle. It is approximately 5 mm wide and is 12–15 mm in length. It originates at the anterior border of the lateral malleolus and inserts into the body of the talus just anterior to the articular facet. The calcaneal fibular ligament is approximately 25 mm long and originates from the tip of the lateral malleolus and runs to the lateral side of the calcaneus. The posterior talofibular ligament is approximately 6 mm wide and approximately 9–12 mm in length. It originates posteriorly to the calcaneal fibular ligament. On the fibula it inserts into the lateral tubercle of the posterior process of the talus. The superficial aspect of the ligament provides a surface over which the peroneal tendons glide. It is confluent with the peroneal tendon sheath just as the anterior talofibular ligament blends with the anterior

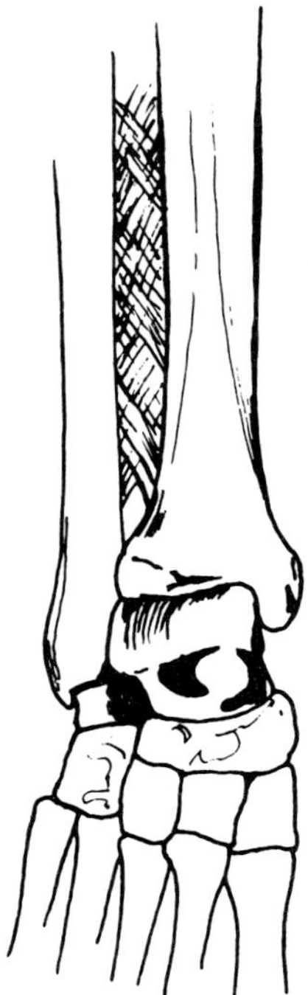

FIGURE 1. The ankle mortise is formed by the distal articulation of the tibia, the fibula, and the dome of the talus.

capsule of the ankle joint. Each of the ligaments plays a role in stabilizing the ankle joint, depending on the position of the foot and ankle. In a dorsiflexed position the anterior talofibular ligament is usually quite loose, whereas the posterior talofibular ligament is taut. In plantar flexion the converse occurs: the anterior talofibular ligament is taut and the posterior talofibular ligament becomes loose. The calcaneal fibular ligament generally restrains inversion of the calcaneus with respect to the fibula.

The deltoid ligament (Fig. 3) is the main stabilizing ligament on the medial side of the ankle. The deltoid ligament is divided into two portions: the superficial and the deep. The superficial deltoid takes origin off the anterior and posterior positions of the medial malleolus and inserts into the talus and calcaneus in a broad fan-shaped fashion. The deep deltoid (Fig. 4) takes origin from the same area, but is more horizontal in nature. This shorter and thicker ligament inserts into the medial wall of the nonarticular surface of the talus.

There are three distinct ligaments of the syndesmosis: (1) the anterior inferior tibiofibular ligament; (2) the posterior inferior tibiofibular ligament; and (3) the interosseous ligament. (Figs. 5A and B) The anterior inferior tibiofibular ligament runs obliquely from the anterior lateral tubercle of the tibia downward to the anterior distal fibular at approximately a 45° angle to the plafond. It is approximately 20 mm wide and 20–30 mm long. This ligament is the most commonly injured ligament in the syndesmotic sprains with diastasis. The posterior inferior tibiofibular ligament arises deep posteriorly on the posterior surface of the tibia at the posterior lateral tubercle and runs obliquely posteriorly and downwardly to the distal portion of the fibula. It is approximately 20 mm wide and 30 mm long. The interosseous ligament interconnects the tibia and fibula approximately 1–2 cm above the plafond. This is sometimes considered the primary bond between the tibia and fibula. As its course is superior, the interosseous ligament is continuous with the interosseous membrane and provides additional strength to the stabilizing effect of the syndesmosis ligaments.

The tendons around the ankle include that of the Achilles tendon, peroneal tendons, anterior and posterior tibial tendons, and the extensors and flexors of the foot. The peroneal tendons course from the lateral aspect of the leg to their insertion sites in the foot by passing around the lateral

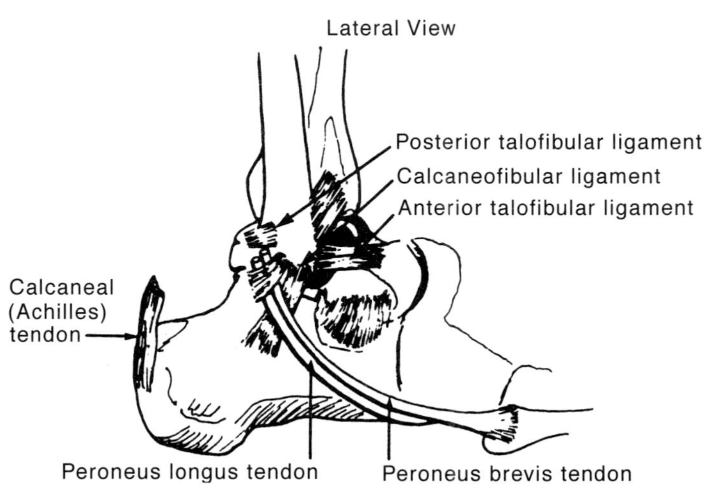

FIGURE 2. Lateral ankle ligaments.

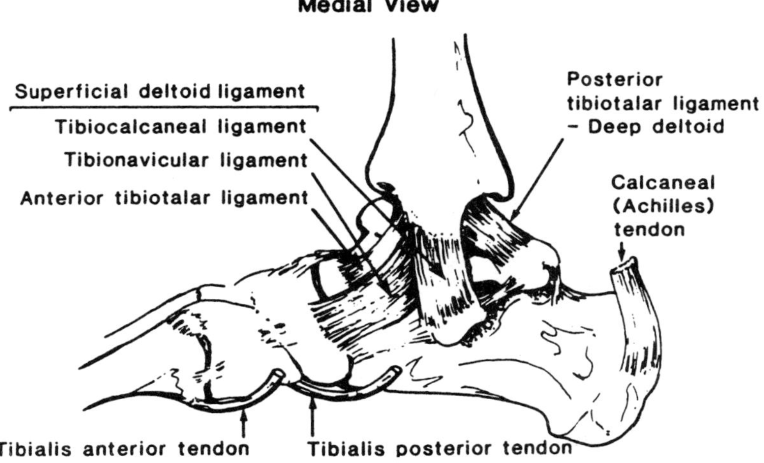

FIGURE 3. Medial ankle ligaments.

malleolus of the ankle with a fibro-osseous tunnel. This tunnel is bounded by the calcaneal fibular and posterior talofibular ligaments. The peroneal retinaculum on the superficial surface holds the peroneal tendons in its groove. The posterior tibialis tendon, flexor hallucis longus, and the flexor digitorum longus course along the posterior portion of the medial malleolus. The gastrocsoleus complex from the deep posterior compartment join to form the Achilles tendon. The Achilles tendon inserts superficially posteriorly on the calcaneus. The tendons that cross the ankle anteriorly include the anterior tibial tendon, extensor hallucis longus tendon, and the extensor digitorum longus with the peroneus tertius. The retinaculum superiorly includes the superior extensor retinaculum and the inferior extensor retinaculum. The tendons pass deep through these areas in their own separate compartments.

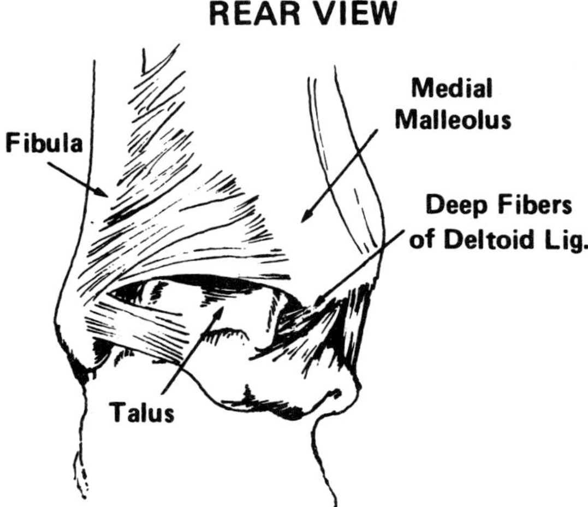

FIGURE 4. Posterior view of ankle demonstrates deep fibers of the deltoid ligament.

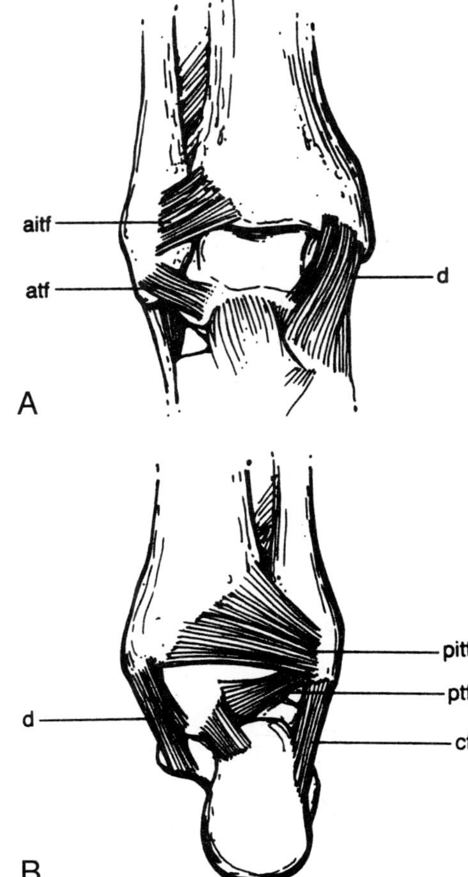

FIGURE 5. *A,* The tibiofibular syndesmosis from the front. Anterior inferior tibiofibular ligament, aitf; anterior talofibular ligament, atf; deltoid ligament, d. *B,* The tibiofibular syndesmosis from the back. Posteior inferior tibiofibular ligament, pitf; posterior talofibular ligament, ptf; calcaneofibular ligament, cf; deltoid ligament, d. (From DeLee JC, Drez D Jr (eds): Orthopaedic Sports Medicine: Principles and Practice, Vol. 2. Philadelphia, W.B. Saunders, 1994, with permission.)

The posterior tibial nerve, which is a branch of the sciatic nerve, enters the tarsal canal proximal to the ankle joint. The tarsal canal or tunnel is a fibro-osseous structure created by the tibia anterior and the posterior process of the talus and calcaneus laterally. The flexor retinaculum that creates the tarsal tunnel is intimately attached to the sheaths of the posterior tibialis, flexor hallucis, and flexor digitorum longus tendons. The posterior tibial nerve then splits into its three terminal branches: the medial plantar, the lateral plantar, and the medial calcaneal nerves. The posterior tibial artery courses along with the posterior tibial nerve and splits into the medial and lateral plantar arteries, forming the arch of blood supply for the foot. Anteriorly the dorsal pedis artery accompanies the deep peroneal nerve through the extensor retinaculum to end in the deep palmar arch.

CLINICAL EVALUATION

History

A complete history should be taken from a patient sustaining ankle injury or having symptoms about the ankle. The history should include all of the following points

1. Acute trauma. Was there a traumatic event, such as a motor vehicle accident or a pedestrian accident? These victims may have high-energy trauma with fracture of the tibia, fibula, talus, or calcaneus. If it was an athletic event, was it related to a twisting blow or to a rebounding or cutting injury? Some patients who have sustained a fall will have compression injuries to the joint with the possibility of osteochondral fractures. If the patient describes a tearing, popping or snapping, this certainly could be related to ligamentous injury. History should be obtained concerning the position of the foot at the time of injury, the direction of the force, any immediate swelling or ability to bear weight.

2. Has there been a previous injury? Those patients with chronic instability may complain of a chronic spraining of the ankle, locking of the joint, or instability. If there were many previous injuries, could this be related to degenerative joint disease, loose bodies, peroneal or posterior tibial tendinitis, or osteochondral fractures?

3. History of overuse symptoms? Patients with overuse problems, including stress fractures or tendinitis, may complain of pain, swelling, or instability after rigorous activity.

4. No traumatic event. These patients may have a history of redness and swelling that may tip the examiner off to a diagnosis such as degenerative arthritis, rheumatoid arthritis, or crystalline arthropathies.

5. Is pain present? The patient should be questioned for the onset of pain; whether it was immediate or delayed, whether intermittent or continuous, whether it diminishes or increases with activity, and its time of onset during the course of the day.

6. Swelling. Is the swelling in the medial to lateral planes, anterior or posterior planes, localized or diffused?

7. Effusion. Does the swelling occur in the joint, such that the patient notices fluid moving in the joint? This usually signifies intra-articular process including arthritis, loose bodies or osteochondral injury.

8. History of catching or locking. This generally signifies that the patient has loose bodies or osteochondritis dissecans. History should include where the locking occurs, what position the foot and ankle are in, and how often it does occur.

9. Functional activities. The patient should be questioned concerning the ability to walk, run, and climb stairs. Most patients with overuse symptoms will continue to be able to run, jump, and twist. Patients with instability may have instability with common daily activities.

10. Weakness. Does the patient feel as it the ankle is weak and will not support him or her, either from a muscular or a ligamentous standpoint? Often those patients with chronic ankle sprains will have radicular symptomatology and describe weakness of dorsiflexion or eversion.

11. Stiffness. Do patients have loss of range of motion or normal range of motion with a feeling of tightness or stiffness in the ankle?

12. Previous treatment. The patient should be questioned about treatment, including which modalities have been used, including heat and cold, compression or elevation, bandages, crutches, braces, or injections. The patients should also be questioned about other diagnostic tests performed.

13. General medical conditions. The patient should be queried about other medical conditions. Patients with radiculopathy can have weakness and complain of chronic instability of the ankle. Patients with generalized rheumatoid arthritis may have involvement in the ankle or subtalar joint. Patients with metastatic disease, although rare, may complain of distal tibial pain.

Physical Examination

The patient should be fully examined in standing, walking, and sitting positions. The ambulatory status of the patient should be evaluated. Does the patient walk with a limp? Does the patient use walking aids? Does the patient have braces? Are any deformities noticed during observation of walking? The ankle is observed in the sitting position for any lacerations, abrasions, or ecchymosis.

Swelling may be diffuse, but should be evaluated for its source. Range of motion is to be checked both passively and actively. Patients are examined for maximum passive and active dorsiflexion, and for plantar flexion. It is imperative that subtalar motion be evaluated for inversion and eversion. The bony anatomy should be palpated. Any tenderness is to be noted, along with its location. The anterior joint and medial and lateral malleoli are checked for any swelling and an effusion. With range of motion, crepitation may be felt as a snapping or popping sensation. Areas of tenderness should be checked with a Tinel sign. Neural entrapments may be seen in the tarsal tunnel, deep peroneal, and sural nerves. Stability tests including the talar tilt and anterior drawer are evaluated in those patients suspected of having instability. A complete neurologic examination of the lower extremity is required, including reflexes and sensory examination for deficits. The vascular status assessment should include capillary refill and the arterial pulses felt in the dorsal pedis and posterior tibial arteries. Strength testing should be done in the anterior tibial, posterior tibial, gastrocnemius soleus complex, and the peroneal tendons. The extensor hallucis longus, flexor hallucis longus, and toe flexors and extensors are all then checked for strength and function. The examination is completed by further examination of the cervical spine, lumbar spine, hip, or knee as indicated.

RADIOLOGY

A routine ankle series includes the anterior-posterior (AP) and, lateral views, and an internal oblique, more commonly known as the mortise, view. The AP view allows evaluation of the tibiotalar joint, the distal tibia, and fibula. The lateral view assesses the ankle for talocalcaneal relationships and joint congruity. Oblique views assess the ankle mortise, talar dome, and malleoli. This is the best view to assess the integrity of the ligamentous status.

Stress views of the ankle are commonly obtained to assess ligamentous stability in patients suspected of having soft tissue injury. Standard radiographs are generally normal except for the possibility of avulsion fractures. Anterior or lateral stress may be placed on the ankle and the appropriate radiographs taken. Discrepancies between the injured and normal side will commonly be seen.

Computed tomography (CT) is useful in evaluating the ankle in thin sections. Osteochondral lesions of the talus and loose bodies may be identified which may be more readily missed on standard radiographic films.

Nuclear bone scan is commonly used to evaluate tumor or tumor-like conditions, trauma, avascular necrosis, arthritis, infection, and pain of unknown cause. The most common agent is 99m technetium diphosphonate.[111] Indium-labeled white blood cell scanning is indicated for those patients thought to have infection.

CT has been used to assess a wide variety of clinical problems in the foot and ankle, including fractures, neoplasms, infections, foreign bodies, osteochondral injuries, tendon injuries, avascular necrosis, and congenital abnormalities. It is particularly useful in severe talar or ankle fractures; and is the primary means for diagnosing adult tarsal coalitions who are having symptoms of instability.

Magnetic resonance imaging (MRI) is superior in soft tissue detail to CT scan. It is considered to be the imaging modality of choice in the evaluation of soft tissue trauma for chronically diseased tendons such as that of the posterior tibialis and the Achilles tendon. It is superior to CT for the evaluation of osteomyelitis, avascular necrosis, and osteochondritis dissecans of the talus.

ACUTE LATERAL ANKLE SPRAINS

Lateral ligament sprains are by far the most common injury seen in sports.[7,8,14,18] The distribution is highest in basketball, volleyball, soccer, football, and other sports involving running and jumping activities.[14] Ankle sprains are generally lower in track, tennis, and swimming. Overall, ankle sprains constitute approximately 25% of all injuries in all sports.[7]

Mechanism. The most common cause of lateral ligamentous injury is the inversion sprain.[7,17] Typically, the foot and ankle are in a plantar-flexed position. The heel inverts and the forefoot adducts. In plantar flexion the anterior talofibular ligament is taut as the foot supinates, or "rolls," and the ligament is thereby torn.[20] With increased inversion, the calcaneal fibular ligament becomes taut and then tears. In the dorsiflexed position, the posterior talofibular ligament is taut and will tear with further inversion. Generally this is done in conjunction with the anterior talofibular and calcaneal fibular ligaments. In a study by Brostrom,[5] isolated tears in the anterior talofibular ligament were present in 65% of cases. A combination of the anterior talofibular ligament and calcaneal fibular ligament occurred in 20% of patients. The remainder included a combination of the inferior tibial fibular ligament, deltoid ligament, or posterior tibiofibular talofibular ligament.

Classification. Ankle sprains are classified according to their tearing, their injury to the ligament, or their instability. Traditionally, Grade I injuries involve ligament stretch. Generally, minimal swelling, tenderness, functional disability, or instability exist. Grade II injury is a partial tearing of the ligamentous complex. Pain is involved, along with tenderness over the involved ligament. Mild joint instability may be present. A Grade III ligament injury is a complete ligament rupture with marked swelling, hemorrhage, and tenderness. Disability is usually maximal. This classification system has been used for many years in the medical literature. Although it is imprecise, the prognosis is generally consistent for these injuries.

Clinical Evaluation. Patients generally give a history of "twisting," "rolling," or "spraining" of the ankle. Patients also describe an inversion injury occurring while jumping, cutting, or landing from a fall. Patients relate of rolling on the lateral border of the foot with a sensation that the fibula touches the ground. Most patients will be unable to bear weight initially, but may tolerate weight bearing as the pain subsides. Swelling may be present immediately, or may appear over the ensuing 3–4 hours. Swelling is generally localized over the anterior talofibular and calcaneal fibular ligaments. Some patients will gradually develop ecchymosis that can go to the lateral border of the foot and into the toes. Others may describe acute weakness or instability, such that they do not feel comfortable bearing weight on the extremity, mainly because of mechanical symptoms.

Examination will reveal varying degrees of difficulty in bearing weight. Swelling will be over the anterior talofibular ligament and over the lateral malleolus. A mild effusion may be present. Point tenderness is found just anterior to the fibular, over the anterior talofibular ligament, and distal to the tip over the calcaneal fibular ligament. Range of motion is diminished and is usually proportionate to the amount of swelling. Tenderness and swelling posterior to the malleolus should make the examiner suspicious of posterior fibular fractures and peroneal tendon subluxations or dislocations. Medial tenderness and swelling generally indicate a deltoid injury.

The patient should be tested provocatively with the anterior drawer test and talar tilt test. These may be quite difficult and painful if the problem is in the acute phase. The anterior drawer test (Fig. 6) is performed with the patient sitting. The heel is cupped with one hand while the tibia is stabilized with the opposite hand. The heel and foot are pulled forward while pushing posteriorly on the anterior portion of the distal tibia. Anterior laxity is identified and compared to the opposite extremity. This test confirms a tear in the anterior talofibular ligament. The talar tilt test (Fig. 7) is the inversion stress test. The calcaneus is again grasped with the examiner's hand. The tibia is stabilized. Inversion stress is then placed on the calcaneus. Generally, the test is positive if the examiner can feel any opening of the joint space. If positive, the talar tilt test generally signifies injury to the anterior talofibular ligament in combination with the calcaneal fibular ligament. Both of these tests may be graded as mild, moderate, or severe instability.

Radiographic Evaluation. Standard films should include the AP, lateral, and mortise views. In most ankle sprains, the radiographs will be normal. Some patients will have avulsion of the ligament off either the talus or the fibula. Small calcifications can be seen adjacent to the bony insertions. Special radiographs are also appropriate in those patients with suspected ligamentous injury. Radiographs are taken in the lateral plane doing the anterior-drawer test. In the anterior plane, a talar tilt test is then performed. Radiographs are then compared with their stress views on the normal extremity. With the anterior-drawer stress radiograph, anterior displacement is seen (Fig. 8). There is a widening of the posterior joint space and loss of congruity of the joint. The talar tilt or inversion stress radiograph is measured using the angle between two lines drawn

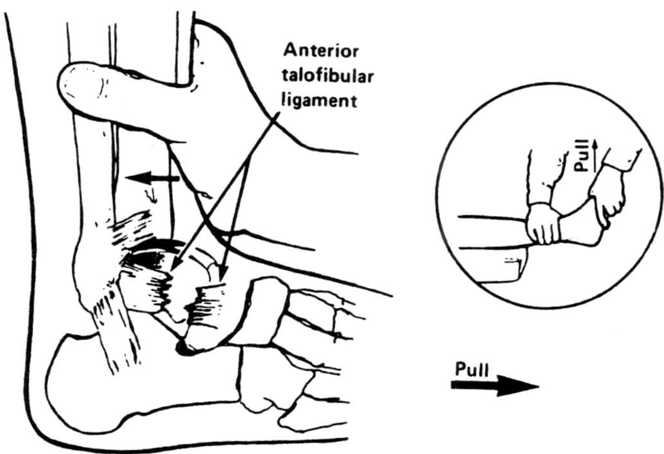

FIGURE 6. Anterior drawer test.

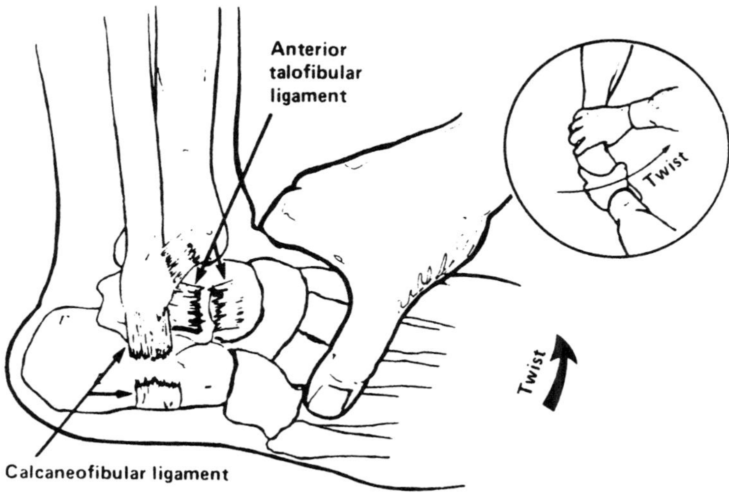

FIGURE 7. Talar tilt test.

to the tibial plafond and the talar dome (Fig. 9). During stress the talus may tilt as much as 30°. In general terms, if the measured side-to-side difference is greater than 10°, abnormal laxity is present.

Other diagnostic tests are sometimes used including ankle joint tomography, bone scans, CT scans, and MRI. If the diagnosis is in question and other forms of pathology are suspected, these tests may be performed. In those patients with straight forward ankle sprains Grades I through Grade III, however, further diagnostic tests are unwarranted.

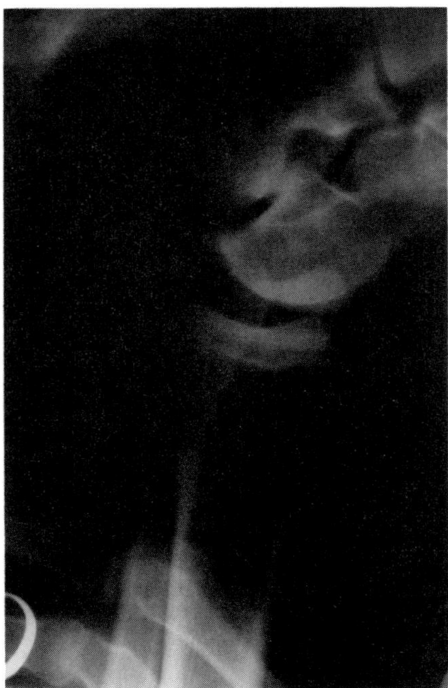

FIGURE 8. Lateral radiograph of the ankle demonstrating the anterior drawer stress radiograph.

Treatment. Treatment follows these principles. **PRICES** therapy is begun. This includes **Protection, Rest, Ice, Compression, Elevation, and Support.** Protection may be in the form of diminished weightbearing, crutches or other walking aids, braces, and casts. Rest therapy may be complete with elevation to relative rest for the milder cases. Patients should be asked to ice and compress the extremity. Elevation helps diminish the swelling. Range of mo-

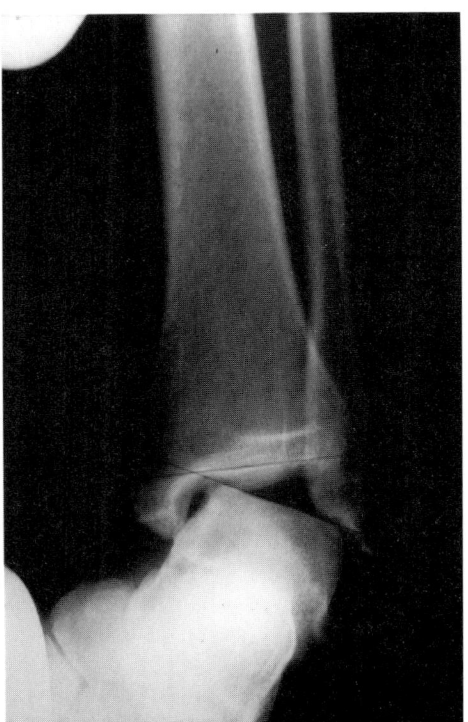

FIGURE 9. Anteroposterior radiograph of the ankle demonstrating the talar tilt stress radiograph.

tion exercises ought to begin as soon as the patient can tolerate them. Plantar flexion and dorsiflexion should be instituted when tolerated. Nonsteroidal anti-inflammatory drugs (NSAIDS) may help control pain and diminish the inflammatory response. As pain and swelling diminish and the range of motion increases, weightbearing may be advanced. External support using taping or bracing may be used while weightberaing. Patients are then started with stretching for flexibility in the Achilles, peroneal strengthening, heel and toe raises, and proprioceptive training using a slant- or a tilt- board. Functional training can progress when the patient has full range of motion, no pain, minimal swelling, and at least 85% strength. These include Thera-band exercises, single leg hopping, figure-of-eight drills, running backwards, carioca, zig-zag drills, and stair climbing. Sport-specific drills can be done when the functional activities are easily accomplished by the patient.

Other treatments exist including casting and surgical repair. Numerous studies have shown that functional treatment is comparable to operative treatment.[7,8,17] Surgical intervention for chronic ligamentous instability is also quite successful. It is my opinion that all ankle sprains should be treated functionally. Casting may be used for a short duration for patients with significant swelling and pain that inhibit range of motion and ambulation. Surgery should be reserved for patients with chronic ankle instability.

Prognostically, grade I and II injuries recover quickly, generally speaking within 7–14 days. Grade III sprains will vary in recovery time, depending on the amount of ligamentous damage, loss of range of motion, and swelling. Rehabilitation may slowly get the patients back to normal activities over a 6-week time frame.

SYNDESMOSIS INJURIES

The ankle syndesmosis includes the anterior tibiofibular ligament, posterior tibiofibular fibular ligament, and the interosseous ligament. Injuries occur with partial or complete rupture of these ligaments.[10] When complete rupture occurs, this is known as a tibia-fibula diastasis (Fig. 10 and also see Fig. 13). This can occur as an isolated injury but is most commonly seen with deltoid injuries and fractures. The mechanism of injury nearly always includes external rotation. The body, tibia, and fibula internally rotate on the planted foot. This causes external rotation forces on the ankle where the talus abuts the fibula. Tearing of the anterior talar tibiofibular ligament, interosseous, and posterior tibiofibular ligament will occur. (see Fig. 10) Straight abduction injuries where the force is applied laterally can also tear the syndesmosis. A deltoid injury or medial malleolus fracture generally occurs with this injury.[21] In sports, blows to the lateral portion of the ankle, such as a helmet injury, are often the inciting cause.

The clinical history is usually positive for external rotation or abduction injuries to the foot and ankle. Pain is located in or above the ankle and swelling is described in these areas. Examination reveals varying degrees of tenderness in the lateral ligamentous complex, anterior, and posterior syndesmosis. Forced external rotation or abduction commonly elicits pain. The squeeze test is performed. Proximal to the injury, the tibia and fibula are "squeezed," causing pain distally over the syndesmosis. A test must elicit the pain in the area of injury to be considered positive.

Radiographic films are generally normal or show subtle changes. Common views include the AP lateral and obliques. If calcification is present, this

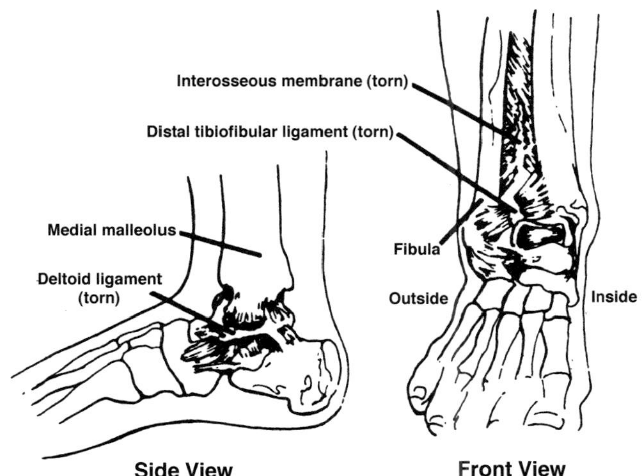

FIGURE 10. Injury to the syndesmosis from an external rotation injury.

signifies previous syndesmosis injury. In the AP view, the relationship of the fibula to the tibia must be scrutinized. In the normal anatomic relationship, 10 mm of overlap or less are found when measuring from the medial fibula to the lateral anterior process of the tibia. This overlap of these two bones should be 10 mm or less. Greater than 10 mm signifies shift of the fibula laterally, diagnosing a syndesmosis sprain. Also, the clear space between the fibula and tibia is normally less than 5 mm. If a greater distance is identified, diastasis again is present.

Treatment of Grade I and Grade II injuries, signifying partial tearing without displacement, should be treated with PRICES, NSAIDs, functional rehabilitation, and the occasional use of a splint. Taylor[23] found that these injuries take approximately 4 to 6 weeks for return to complete functional recovery. He also found that even though the patients had functional recovery, 36% had symptoms as long as 4 years after the injury. These symptoms included pain, swelling, and stiffness. Heterotopic ossification was present on 50% of follow-up radiographs. Grade III injuries are usually associated with other injuries around the ankle. They may, whoever, be isolated. Operative treatment is indicated for those patients who have greater than 5 mm of clear space between the fibula and tibia, with a diagnosis of syndesmosis rupture.[24] The fibula is approached laterally and overdrilled. A screw is then placed through the fibula into the tibia to recreate its anatomic position. This screw is left in place for 6–8 weeks while the patient is treated with casting and non-weightbearing. The screw is removed at 8 weeks and full rehabilitation is begun. Complications include screw fracture, fibular fracture, and heterotopic ossification with the above-mentioned symptoms.

CHRONIC ANKLE INSTABILITY

Chronic ankle instability is defined as a positive anterior drawer test or talar tilt test with at least 6 months after the index injury.[8] Up to 10% of patients with a lateral ligamentous injury will go on to have chronic symptoms. These include persistent synovitis or tendinitis, ankle stiffness, swelling, pain, muscle weakness, and giving way symptoms.[26] Patients' pain may be chronic or recurrent. Range of motion may be limited, but is usually normal.

Most patients complain of instability symptoms. These include instability while walking on uneven ground, instability with sports activity, and recurrent sprains with activities of daily living. These episodes of instability are generally followed by pain and swelling that is limited to less than 1 week. Patients are then able to regain all functional mobility and return to activities. Recurrent sprains may occur in 1 week to 1 year, depending on the activity of the patient.

Examination will generally show significant instability on stress testing. Anterior drawer tests may show an anterior sulcus present with significant anterior displacement of the talus in the ankle joint. Talar tilt will show demonstrable instability by clinical examination. Stress radiography generally shows a 6 mm side-to-side difference in the anterior drawer test, and a greater than 10° difference in the talar tilt test.

Functional instability is most likely a complex syndrome in which neural, muscular, and mechanical factors are involved. Treatment should therefore address these components. Ankle taping or bracing is used in the treatment of the mechanical and functional ankle instabilities. High-top shoes and laced ankle stabilizers in combination have been found to be the most effective prophylaxis against chronic ankle sprains.[8] Neuromuscular retraining should be done with a balance board and proprioceptive devices. Strengthening and flexibility exercises are used on a daily basis with resistive exercises from surgical tubing.

Operative indications for the treatment of chronic ankle instability include rehabilitation failure after one year, no improvement in muscle strength after rehabilitation, disability pain, chronic instability symptoms, 10° of increased talar tilt on inversion stress radiographs, or anterior drawer test results of 4 to 6 mm or more as compared with the opposite side.[8] Several types of reconstructive procedures are available. An anatomic reconstruction (Fig. 11) may be done of the anterior talofibular and calcaneal fibular ligaments. The elongated ligaments are divided approximately 5 mm from their fibular insertions. Multiple drill holes are then made in the bone and the ligament is reinserted into the bleeding bony bed. The fibular portion of the ligament is then imbricated over the distal portion. Treatment then consists of casting for 3 weeks followed by functional rehabilitation. The alternative approach is a tenodesis. The peroneus brevis is transected. This tendon is then used, with various techniques, to reconstruct the anterior talofibular ligament. This reconstruction is more time consuming and generally has some loss of motion postoperative, but has an excellent track record for stability. These reconstructions include the Evans procedure, the Watson-Jones procedure, and the Elmslie procedure and its modification by Chrisman and Snook. The Chrisman-Snook procedure (Fig. 12) is indicated for those patients who have concomitant subtalar instability. These procedures have a 90% success rate for chronic lateral ankle instability.

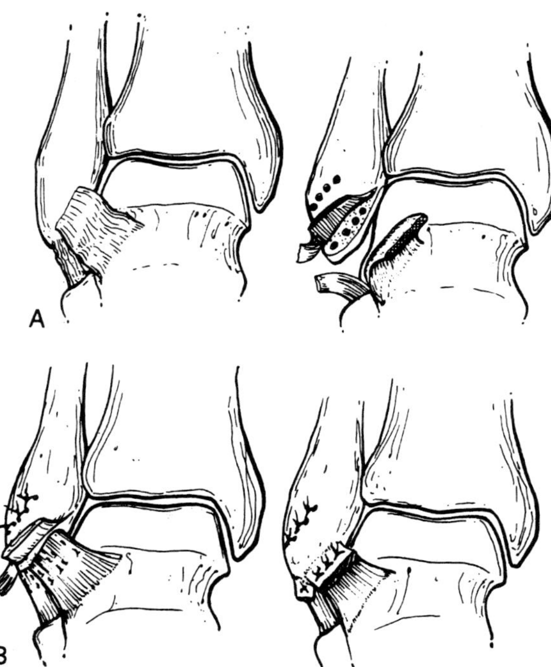

FIGURE 11. *A,* Anatomic reconstruction (delayed repair) of the anterior talofibular and calcaneofibular ligaments of the ankle. First, the elongated ligaments are divided at a point 3 to 5 millimeters from its fibular insertion. Then the bone surface on the distal end of the fibula is roughened to promote ligament healing, and drill holes are made through the distal fibula. *B,* Mattress sutures are used to fix the distal stump of the ligaments to the fibula. The sutures are tightened, holding the foot in dorsiflexion and eversion. Last, the proximal end of the ligament is imbricated over the distal portion. (From DeLee JC, Drez D Jr (eds): Orthopaedic Sports Medicine: Principles and Practice, Vol. 2. Philadelphia, W.B. Saunders, 1994, with permission.)

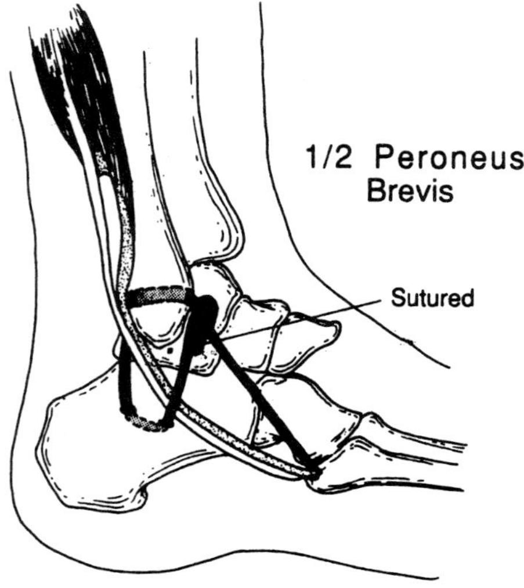

FIGURE 12. Chrisman-Snook procedure. (From Mann RA, Coughlin MJ (eds): Surgery of the Foot and Ankle, 6th ed., Vol. 2. St. Louis, Mosby, with permission.)

OSTEOCHONDRAL FRACTURE OF THE TALAR DOME

Osteochondral fracture of the talar dome is uncommon. Several terms describe it, including osteochondritis dissecans, transchondral fractures, osteochondral fractures, and talar dome fractures.[6] This lesion was originally felt to be secondary to avascular necrosis or similar to the osteochondritis dissecans of the knee. Most recently, experts believe that the lesion is not related to avascular necrosis and therefore not truly an osteochondritis dissecans, but is largely caused by a traumatic event.

These lesions occur in two locations, the more common of which is laterally on the talar dome. The second type is found medially along the posteromedial aspect of the talus. Medially the lesions are generally more cup-shaped, whereas the lateral lesions are wafer-shaped. Berndt and Harty classified four stages of the disease process.[4] Stage 1 is a small area of compressed subchondral bone. Stage 2 has partially detached fragments still located in its crater. Stage 3 manifests a completely detached fragment remaining in the talar crater. Stage 4 has a fragment loose and free-floating in the joint. Most authors believe that the osteochondral fractures of the talus are due to inversion injuries.[6,11] If the foot is plantarly flexed during inversion, a medial lesion results from compression of the medial talar dome by the tibia. On the other hand, if the foot is dorsiflexed, a lateral talar lesion results from shearing forces produced from striking the fibula.

Patients, who are predominantly athletic males in the second and third decades of life, generally present with a history of trauma to the ankle. Symptoms include persistent pain, swelling, and instability. When this lesion is detached, symptoms of catching and locking are quite common. Physical examination generally reveals a lack of findings, although small effusion may be found and tenderness may be present over the area of the lesion. Range of motion and stability are normal. Tenderness that is present may be palpable anterolaterally or posteromedially overlying the injuries.

Standard AP, lateral, and mortise views are essential for the diagnosis of osteochondral fracture of the talus. Although grades I and II injuries may not be noted radiographically, grades III and IV lesions are most certainly seen, but can easily be missed if little attention is placed on the talar domes (Fig. 13A). ^{99m}Technetium bone scans can be used to screen for those patients with undiagnosed posttraumatic disability and a suspicion of osteochondral lesions. MRI is, however, now the diagnostic method of choice. Changes from osteochondral fractures are easily detected on MRI, which is ap-

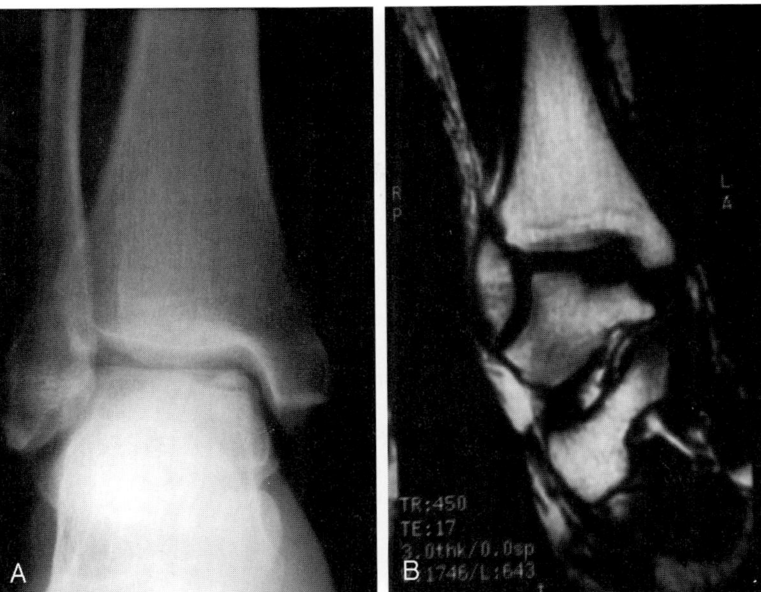

FIGURE 13. *A,* Radiograph showing a medial osteochondral fracture of the talus. *B,* Corresponding MRI.

propriate for staging the lesion by grade and size (Fig. 13B).

Treatment of stage 1 and 2 lesions that are acute without signs of nonunion, such as sclerosis, uneven joint surface, or arthritic changes, are treated with a short leg non-weightbearing cast until union is demonstrated. Patients may, at 6 weeks if partial union is found, be placed in a functional walker and given range of motion exercises to do. Those patients with grade IV lesions, meaning a loose fragment, should be treated operatively with arthroscopic removal. Lesions that are long standing show signs of sclerosis, fragmentation, and cystic degeneration and so should be treated operatively for attempts at repair. Arthroscopically the lesion is débrided to a bleeding bony surface.[1,11] The fracture is then reduced and held in place with bioabsorbable pins or bony pegs.[16] Patients are treated with passive and active range of motion exercises. Weightbearing is not allowed for 8–12 weeks. If the loose piece is fragmented, all loose bodies should be debrided and the bony base cleared of burring. Some evidence indicates fibrocartilage will form over the lesion. Such patients have a higher incidence of degenerative changes in the joint and may require subsequent ankle arthrodesis if symptoms continue.

ANKLE FRACTURES

Fractures that may be treated nonoperatively with closed techniques and casting must be differentiated from those requiring operative treatment. Ankle fractures are those involving the medial and lateral malleoli or tibial plafond of the ankle.[24] Various mechanisms, including external and internal rotation, vertical loading, abduction, and adduction are involved to give various characteristic fractures. Ultimately involvement may include the deltoid ligament, the lateral ligamentous complex, the syndesmosis, and the medial or lateral malleolus, along with a higher fibular fracture. These can occur in various combinations, depending on the mechanism of injury. Conservative treatment may be used for the following indications: single malleolar fracture without displacement, no widening apparent on the medial or lateral clear space between the talus and malleoli, intact syndesmosis, and small avulsion fractures. Operative indications include displaced malleolar fracture, bimalleolar fractures with 1–2 mm of displacement, fractures that involve talar tilt or widening of the clear space between the malleoli and talus, syndesmosis disruption, and fracture dislocation. Any athlete who is contemplating return to his or her sport and a vigorous lifestyle must have an anatomic reduction and internal fixation. Yablon[25] has shown that displacement of 1 mm of lateral shift of the talus in the mortise reduces the contract area of the ankle joint by 42%. Using this as a criterion, open reduction internal fixation should be contemplated if there is a shift of the talus enough to widen the clear space. Some authors[24] report as high as 85% of those having inadequately reduced fractures will later develop degenerative arthritis. Because of this high incidence, anatomic treatment of ankle fractures is essential.

PERONEAL TENDON SUBLUXATION

Subluxation or dislocation of the peroneal tendons is an uncommon injury, and is frequently misdiagnosed as a lateral ankle sprain.[9] Because this is often missed acutely, chronic symptoms of dislocation occur. Associated dislocation mainly results from sports and athletic activity. The most common sport is snow skiing,[13] followed by football, basketball, soccer and ice skating.

Anatomically, the peroneal tendons course behind the lateral malleolus to their insertions into the foot. A cartilaginous ridge is found lateral to the peroneal groove on the fibula. This forms a tunnel, with the roof being the superior peroneal retinaculum (Fig. 14). The floor of the tunnel includes the calcaneal fibular and posterior talofibular ligaments. The most common injury mechanism is a sudden dorsiflexion stress with a reflex contraction of the peroneal musculature. Several anatomic lesions are identified. Peroneal retinaculum may be stripped off the fibula with subsequent dislocation. The fibrous rim may be avulsed from the posterolateral aspect of the fibula without a fracture. Commonly, a bony avulsion with the entire retinacular sheath is displaced anteriorly (Fig. 15).

Patients usually present with a history of acute injury that generally involves forced dorsiflexion. Some patients will describe this as an ankle sprain, even though there is no history of eversion. Patients will complain of pain along the peroneal tendon sheath, with swelling along the course of the peroneal tendons. Examination shows minimal anterior pain or swelling. Symptoms originate from an area located posteriorly along the course of the peroneal tendon sheath. Ecchymosis and swelling is found posterior to the fibula, with maximal tenderness generally just posterior to the tip of the lateral malleolus. In the chronic state, patients may be able to visibly dislocate the tendon.

Routine radiographs are essential. Up to 40% of these patients will show the characteristic rim fracture that is seen adjacent to the lateral malleolus. CT and MRI scans have been recommended for evaluation to show the soft tissue structures, but these have been found to be unnecessary in most circumstances.

Controversy exists over the treatment of acute injuries. Two courses of treatment may be followed. The first is conservative. A well-molded short leg cast is applied and worn for 6 weeks. Success rate for treatment is greater than 60%. Because of the high failure rate, some authors recommend operative intervention with the direct surgical repair of the acute injury. Postoperatively the patients are treated with 6 weeks in a short leg walking cast, followed by 3–4 months of functional rehabilitation.

In those patients with chronic dislocation peroneal tendons, treatment is generally surgical. Multiple operations have been developed, including anatomical soft tissue reconstruction, bone block procedures that buttress the peroneal tendons, and tissue transfer procedures utilizing Achilles tendon to reconstruct the superior retinaculum. Recurrence following surgical treatment is rare.

PERONEAL TENDINITIS

Tendinitis of the peroneal tendons is commonly seen in patients who have had chronic ankle instability and recurrent sprains. Peroneal tendons pass through a fibro-osseus tunnel posterior to the lateral malleolus. Some authors believe that the stenosing tenosynovitis of these tendons occurs because of recurrent injury in these canals. Patients present with a history of pain posterior to the lateral malleolus. Swelling and aching are persistent and on a daily basis. With increased activities, pain may limit the patient's performance. Treatment consists of con-

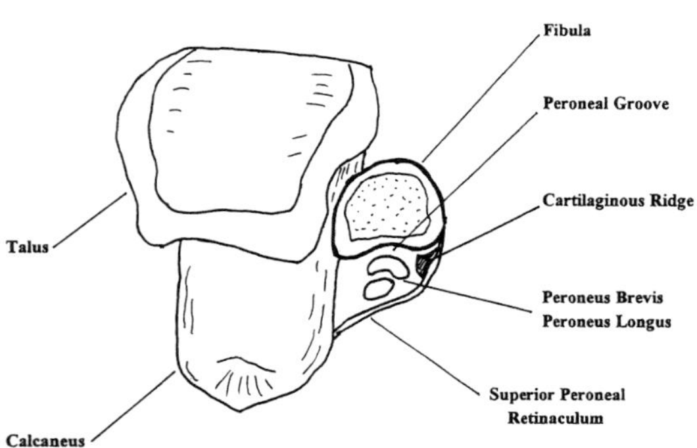

FIGURE 14. Normal peroneal tendon sheath with its anatomic relationships.

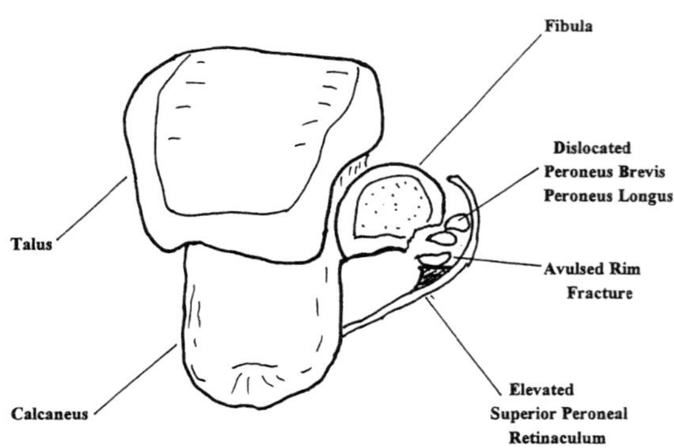

FIGURE 15. Dislocation of the peroneal tendons with an avulsed rim fracture and elevated peroneal retinaculum.

servative treatment with casting in the acute phase followed by functional rehabilitation and bracing. Those patients with persistent pain may require surgical debridement of the tendons. Occasionally, complete tears of the peroneus longus are identified. These tears are debrided and side-to-side anastomosis to the peroneus brevis is the treatment of choice. The tenosynovectomy will diminish the likelihood of recurrence.

POSTERIOR TIBIAL TENDINITIS

Tendinitis is quite common in the posterior tibial tendon. Most patients with this problem typically are women in their fourth through sixth decades. Symptoms include gradual onset of pain and burning posterior to the medial malleolus. Physical examination reveals swelling and tenderness over the posterior tibial tendon. If there appears to be loss of the longitudinal arch of the foot along with heel valgus or eversion, complete disruption of the posterior tibialis tendon is possible.[15] Most patients, however, with only tendinitis will have normal-appearing anatomy. Treatment consists of NSAIDs, bracing, or casting for several weeks to several months to alleviate swelling, flexibility and strengthening exercises, and orthotics for support of the longitudinal arch. Steroid injections should be avoided, because they are known to be associated with complete rupture of the tendon. Operative treatment may include tenosynovectomy, repair of longitudinal tears, or repair of reconstruction for chronic rupture of the tendon.[15]

MENISCOID LESIONS

Patients with persistent pain, swelling, and stiffness for months after ankle sprains may have developed a meniscoid lesion.[22] This is a soft tissue lesion laterally between the talus and the lateral malleolus. On arthroscopic examination it somewhat resembles a meniscus—thus its name.

Patients generally present with a history of inversion or other recurrent sprains. Most patients complain of anterior or anterolateral joint pain. They often feel the joint is unstable and has recurrent sprains. Occasionally, patients will complain of swelling in the ankle joint; and on examination, lateral swelling may be present. Patients generally have a normal range of motion with minimal effusion. They will have lateral tenderness anterior to the fibula or in the anterolateral joint. This lateral area is called the "lateral gutter."

Radiographic results generally are normal. An MRI may show this soft tissue lesion anterolaterally or in the lateral gutter.[22] The differential diagnosis includes chronic lateral ankle instability, loose bodies, synovitis, peroneal tendon subluxation, subtalar injury, osteochondritis dissecans, or syndesmosis sprain.

Treatment should be conservative for a minimum of 6 months. Most patients who diligently continue with functional rehabilitation during this time will have good symptomatic relief. If patients are adequately rehabilitated yet have no relief, arthroscopic debridement of the hypertrophic synovium or extensive fibrosis is done.[1] This should eliminate 90% of the patients' symptoms.

ANTERIOR IMPINGEMENT OF THE ANKLE

Anterior impingement of the ankle is characterized by bony[12] or ligamentous[2] impingement of the anterior tibia and the talus in dorsiflexion. The common characteristic is a bony exostosis that is seen best on lateral radiographs, with talar or anterior tibial spurring. This spurring is thought to develop because of years of impingement. Microfractures occur from the impingement with subsequent calcification and exostosis formation. This condition is seen after repetitive injury, and is common in runners and ballet dancers.

Patients generally present with a history of chronic ankle pain, commonly seen after exercise, running, or dancing. Most patients will be able to continue their activities, but will have pain afterwards. Examination usually shows minimal swelling with tenderness over the anterior ankle. The hallmark is loss of dorsiflexion and pain on forced dorsiflexion. Radiographs reveal an anterior osteophyte off the tibia at the ankle joint with a corresponding dorsal talar osteophyte (Fig. 16). Radiographs in full dorsiflexion may show abutment of these two exostoses.

Conservative treatment consists of NSAIDs, restricted extension with orthotics, or a heel lift. If patients have persistent pain, arthroscopic debridement of the exostosis usually alleviates symptoms.[19]

NERVE COMPRESSIONS

Tarsal tunnel syndrome,[3] a common cause of chronic ankle pain, has been extensively written about as a cause of pain in the ankle. The tarsal tunnel is a fibro-osseous tunnel formed by the flexor retinaculum posterior to the medial malleolus. The tunnel includes the tendons of the posterior tibialis, flexor digitor longus, flexor hallucis, and the posterior tibial artery and vein. The posterior tibial nerve is compressed and patients describe pain after injury with pain that is located posteriorly to the medial malleolus. Tinel's sign may be positive. Patients may complain of sensory deficits along the medial and lateral plantar nerves. Treatment is generally conservative, but occasionally surgical decompression is necessary.

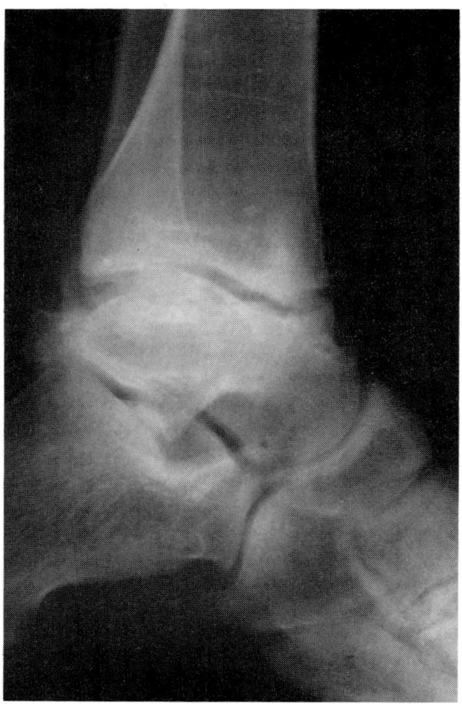

FIGURE16. Radiograph of anterior impingement of the ankle. Note both superior talar and anterior tibial osteophytes.

The deep peroneal nerve lies between the extensor digitorum longus and tibialis anterior muscles in the proximal one-third of the leg. It enters into the extensor retinaculum with the dorsal pedis artery. The deep peroneal nerve can be trapped under the inferior extensor retinaculum.[3] Such patients will complain of anterior ankle pain along with occasional radiation into the first webbed space. The pain usually occurs during athletic activities, but subsides with removal of the shoe and rest. Treatment consists of NSAIDs, heat, cold, and compression modalities, and flexibility exercises. Occasionally the retinacular ligament must partially be released at the anterior ankle joint to decompress the deep peroneal nerve.

The sural nerve runs between the heads of the gastrocnemius muscle and penetrates the deep aponeurosis approximately halfway down the leg. It travels along the border of the Achilles tendon laterally next to the short saphenous vein. The sural nerve runs inferior to the peroneal sheath in a subcutaneous position at the ankle. Sural nerve entrapment can occur anywhere along its course. Recurrent ankle sprains can lead to fibrosis and subsequent nerve entrapment.[3] Patients usually give a history of an acute twisting injury or recurrent ankle sprain. Symptoms include shooting pain and paresthesias. Pain will be described along the fibula or distal to the tip of the fibula. Treatment again is symptomatic with NSAIDs and the occasional use of a steroid injection. Rarely will surgical exploration be necessary unless it is felt that entrapment by surgical scar or fibrosis exists.

CONCLUSION

The majority of ankle injuries will present to the primary care physician. With a solid understanding of the anatomy, mechanism of injury, and the intervention techniques, most of these injuries will resolve and the patients' return to play will be successful. Consultation is advised if the diagnosis is unclear, or if symptomatology or clinical findings persist, or the rehabilitation is nonprogressive. A solid differential diagnosis will avoid misclassifying osteochondral fractures as chronic sprains, or mistaking a strain or tendinitis for a fracture. Finally, the continuous care provided by a family physician will identify a problem before an irreversible or poor result is established.

REFERENCES

1. Baker CL, Graham JM: Current concepts in ankle arthroscopy. Orthopedics 16:1027–1035, 1993.
2. Bassett FH, Gates HS, Billys JB, et al: Talar impingement by the anterior inferior tibiofibular ligament. J Bone Joint Surg 72A(1):55–59, 1990.
3. Baxter DE: Functional nerve disorders in the athlete's foot, ankle, and leg. The Instructional Course Lectures. Am Acad Orthop Surg 42:185–193, 1993.
4. Berndt AL, Harty M: Transchondral fractures (osteochondritis dissecans) of the talus. Am J Bone Joint Surg 41:988–1020, 1959.
5. Brostom L: Sprained ankles I: Anatomic lesions and recent sprains. Acta Orthop Scand Suppl 128:483–495, 1964.
6. Bryant DD, Siegel MG: Osteochondritis dissecans of the talus: a new technique for arthroscopic drilling. J Arthroscop Rel Surg 9:238–241, 1993.
7. DeMaio M, Paine R, Drex, D Jr: Chronic lateral ankle instability inversion sprains, part I. Orthopedics 15:87–96, 1992.
8. DeMaio M, Paine R, Drex, D Jr: Chronic lateral ankle instability inversion sprains, part II. Orthopedics 15(2): 241–248, 1992.
9. Eckert WR, Davis EA: Acute rupture peroneal retinaculum. Am J Bone Joint Surg 58A:670–673, 1976.
10. Edwards GS, DeLee JC: Ankle diastasis without fracture. Foot Ankle 4:305–312, 1984.
11. Ewing JW: Arthroscopic management of transchondral talar dome fractures (osteochondritis dissecans) and anterior impingement lesions of the ankle. Clin Sports Med 10:677–687, 1991.
12. Ferkel RD, Karzel RP, DelPizzo W, et al: Arthroscopic treatment of anterolateral impingement of the ankle. Am J Sports Med 19:440–446, 1991.
13. Fritschy D: Unusual ankle injury in top skiers. Am J Sports Med 17:282–286, 1989.
14. Garrick JM: The frequency of injury, mechanism of injury, and epidemiology of ankle sprains. AM J Sports Med 5:241–242, 1977.
15. Johnson KA: Tibialis posterior tendon rupture. Clin Orthop 177:140–147, 1983.

16. Kristensen G, Lind T, Lavard P, Olsen PA: Fracture stage IV of the lateral talar dome treated arthroscopically using Biofix for fixation. J Arthroscop Rel Surg 6:242–244, 1990.
17. Lassiter, Jr TE, Malone TR, Garrett WE: Injury to the lateral ligaments of the ankle. Orthop Clin North Am 20: 629–640, 1989.
18. Mack RP: Ankle injuries in athletics. Clin Sports Med 1:71–84, 1982.
19. Ogilvie-Harris DJ: Anterior impingement of the ankle treated by arthorscopic removal of bony spurs. Br J Bone Joint Surg 75B:437–440, 1993.
20. Rasmussen O: Stability of the ankle joint: Analysis of the function and traumatology of the ankle ligaments. Acta Orthop Scand Suppl 211:1–75, 1985.
21. Stiehl JB: Complex ankle fracture dislocations with syndesmodic diastasis. Orthop Rev 14:499–507, 1990.
22. Stone JW, Guhl JF: Meniscoid lesions of the ankle. Clin Sports Med 10:661–676, 1991.
23. Taylor DC, Englehardt DL, Bassett FH III: Syndesmosis sprains of the ankle: The influence of heterotopic ossification. Am J Sports Med 20:146–150, 1992.
24. VanderGriend RA, Savoie FH, Hughes JL: Fractures of the ankle. In Rockwood CA Jr, Green DP, Wilkins KE, et al (eds): Rockwood & Green's Fractures in Adults, 3rd ed, Philadelphia, J.B. Lippincott, 1991, pp 1993–2039.
25. Yablon IG, Heller FG, Shous L: The key role of the lateral malleolus in displaced fractures of the ankle. Am J Bone Joint Surg 59:169, 1977.
26. Zimmer TJ: Chronic and recurrent ankle sprains. Clin Sports Med 10:653–659, 1991.

24

Overuse Syndromes in Runners

Walter B. Franz, III, M.D.

GENERAL PRINCIPLES

Physical exertion in America has moved from the workplace to the swimming pools, tennis courts, and tracks of our communities. During the Industrial Revolution, human labor accounted for 30% of the energy used in factories and farms. It now accounts for less than 1%.[59] As work-centered human activity decreased, leisure and fitness intensive activity increased markedly. An estimated 30 million Americans run recreationally or competitively and approximately 36% of these runners will sustain an injury of some type in their running career.[19] (See Second Opinion I.)

As an entry point into the health care system, the primary care physician is often faced with diagnosis and treatment of runners' injuries, regardless of the physician's specialty or background. In approximately 65% of injuries when the primary care physician is knowledgeable about this subject, no addition consultation may be needed.[62]

Overuse Syndromes: A Functional Definition

Overuse syndromes are chronic musculoskeletal syndromes that occur when an excess of injury over repair exists in exercised tissue. If stresses continue unabated, inflammation in tissue can accumulate and an athlete can overload the capacity of tissue to compensate and repair, thus resulting in injury.[42]

Overuse syndromes involve chronic tissue stress occurring during repetitive activities, and the tissues affected are usually biomechanically critical anatomic structures. Lower extremities in runners are the structures most stressed, because they are responsible for locomotion, shock absorption, and surface adaptation. The capacity of the lower extremities to repair after-running-induced stress is limited by the necessity in using the lower extremities extensively in activities of daily life.

Runners endure injuries and the rigors of training for a variety of reasons, the most notable being improved physical fitness and decreased cardiovascular risk factors,[33] reduced stress,[45,48] prolonged life[51] lost weight.[21] In contrast, runners stop running more often due to switching to another form of exercise to save time rather than injury, because most runners feel that it is better to run while hurting than not to run at all.[32] With the vast popularity of running as well as its strong association with modification and amelioration of cardiovascular risk factors, it is not surprising that runners will avoid any encounter that may decrease their chosen activity. The injured runner will appreciate a health professional who has an approach of returning a runner to exercise as soon as clinically appropriate.

Pathophysiology of Overuse

Pathologically, overuse syndromes in runners start as microtrauma to localized tissue areas that are under biomechanical stress. As inflammation develops faster than the tissue's capacity for self-repair, macroscopic irritation and damage culminate in tissue disruption.[26,42] Ideally at the onset of symptoms in very early overuse (Grades I and II), the runner should evaluate his or her training program for possible errors or deficiencies (Table 1). The same "drive" that motivates athletes to run likely will encourage an attempt to "run through" the pain, however. Most patients will not seek medical advice until more advanced injuries are present, as in Grade III or IV overuse. At this time pain limits competitive effectiveness, and some interruption of the patient's training activities is inevitable in order to allow tissue repair.[42] During this period of enforced rest, the patient should be taught the warning symptoms of early overuse and be encouraged not to follow the inappropriate, and overused, dictum, "no pain, no gain."

TABLE 1. Staging of Overuse Syndromes

Grade	Symptoms
Grade I	Post activity soreness Duration of symptoms less than two weeks Generalized tenderness
Grade II	Pain during end of running and immediately after Duration of symptoms greater than two weeks Localized pain, minimal inflammation
Grade III	Pain during early training Duration of symptoms greater than three weeks Point tenderness, definite objective tissue inflammatory signs (erythema, edema, crepitus)
Grade IV	Pain with activities other than training, severity of which prohibits training or competition Grade III symptoms plus—Disfunction of injured structure, muscle atrophy, tissue breakdown

Adapted from McKeag DB, Primary Care 11:43, 1984.

Epidemiology of Overuse Syndromes in Runners (OSR) (See Second Opinion II)

Epidemiologically, the most significant factor in OSR is excessive mileage during training.[6,32,53] A linear relationship exists between injury rates in runners and mileage run[53] (Fig. 1). From a practical standpoint, once the 30-mile-per-week training threshold is reached, the yearly injury rate exceeds 20%/yr for females and 15% for males.[53] Numerous other factors have been epidemiologically examined with respect to runners' injuries such as age and sex of the runner, the effect of terrain upon running injuries, and the benefit of stretching and warm-up activities upon injury incidence. Although all of these factors may have direct importance in individual cases, the mileage run becomes most important. "Over-mileage," however, may be a relative, rather than an absolute, concept. For instance, total mileage run per week does not take into account how rapidly this level of mileage was achieved; and although relatively few total miles per week have been run, the pace of advancement may have been excessively ambitious.[6] Specific guidelines on how often and to what degree weekly mileage should be advanced may be difficult to find. In general, a greater than 10% increase of weekly mileage should be avoided.[1] From a pathophysiologic approach, an increase in training mileage should not be accompanied by more than the lowest grade of overuse symptoms.

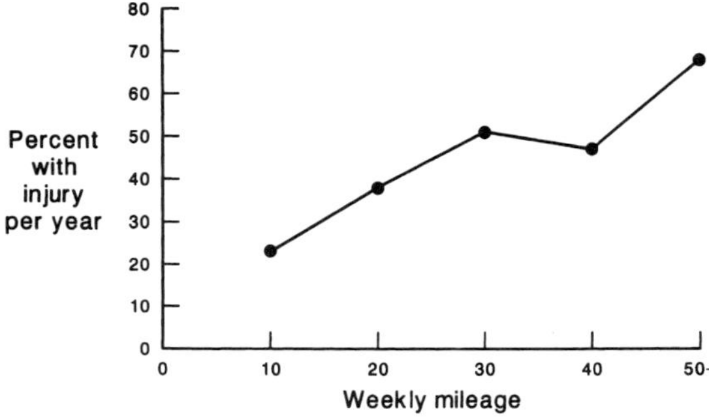

FIGURE 1. Percentage of runners, male and female, injured during one year per weekly mileage run. (Adapted from Koplan JP, et al: JAMA 248:3118, 1982.)

Basic Biomechanics of Running[2,29,30,39] (See Second Opinion III)

Forces generated by an average runner during even a leisurely jog are astounding. For each mile run, each foot contacts the runner surface approximately 1000 times. At initial foot contact the lower extremity is required to absorb and dissipate forces 2 to 3 times body weight. In a one-mile jog, several tons of force per foot are accumulated and then multiplied by the several miles per day many runners run.[16] Exact biomechanical analysis of walking, running, and sprinting is beyond the scope of this chapter, but understanding the basic components of running biomechanics is helpful to the primary care physician in comprehending OSR.

Two basic phases of gait exist in running, the support phase during which the reference foot contacts the surface, and the recovery phase during which the reference foot is airborne and following through in preparation for recontact. The percentage of the gait cycle delegated to the support phase or the recovery phase varies greatly from walking to running and sprinting. The walking gait generally does not have a prolonged recovery phase because there is no time when a limb is airborne; therefore, the amount of time in the support phase is longer and allows for excellent shock absorption and dissipation (Fig. 2). Time available for shock absorption in the runner's support phase decreases to approximately 50% of that of walking, and the recovery phase is lengthened. As speed increases and a sprinting stance is assumed, the support phase is further shortened to approximately a third of the time compared to walking.[39] Careful gait analysis of the runner has shown that when speed increases to the point of sprinting, the athlete runs continually on his or her toes. Because of high speed, insufficient time exists for the lower extremities to absorb shock other than to absorb some ground contact forces by ankle dorsiflexion. An analogy has been suggested—that the sprinter is using his or her legs

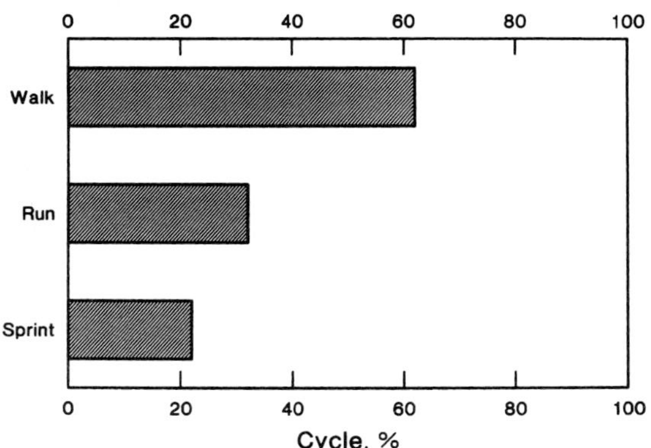

FIGURE 2. Comparison of time available for support phase in walking, running, and sprinting. (Adapted from Mann RA, Hagy J: Am J Sports Med 8:345, 1980).

as if they were spokes on a wheel rather than as a flexible, adaptive structure.[29]

It is helpful to review a normal running gait cycle, and for reference purposes the right foot will be described (Fig. 3). With foot contact, (Fig. 3.1) the support phase begins. The hip is initially in extension and slight internal rotation. The knee is slightly flexed and in most runners the foot initially makes contact in a supinated position. The supinated foot is a relatively firm, rigid base to support surface contact and eventual propulsion. The contact stage takes approximately 25% of the time of the total support phase. Then the foot rapidly pronates (Fig. 3.2) into an unstable but highly shock-absorbing and flexible structure to allow for surface adaptation. The subtalar joint is anatomically responsible for pronation, whereas shock is absorbed by the foot in general.[68]

If the foot cannot pronate adequately, an increase in foot-strike force will be transmitted proximally, leading to possible overuse symptoms. If the foot pronates excessively, the resulting hypermobility can likewise lead to injury. This occurs primarily because motion is also occurring in the transverse plane during midstance with internal tibial torsion occurring concomitant with subtalar-joint pronation. If excessive torque is transmitted proximally in the kinetic chain, referred OSR can result at some distance from the anatomic site of dysfunction.

The midstance phase encompasses the middle 50% of the support phase. During this segment, the center of gravity of the body moves over the foot because of hip extension and forward momentum. Ideally, the foot should be in a neutral position, neutral to the calcaneus and perpendicular to the metatarsals. At the end of the midstance phase, a 10° forward swing occurs on the foot in order to start heel lift for the eventual takeoff stage (Fig. 3.3). The foot also dorsiflexes slightly to enhance heel lift.

During the end of the midstance phase, the tibia rotates externally and the subtalar joint supinates, changing the foot to a rigid structure in preparation for takeoff. During the take-off or toe-off phases, the last 25% of contact phase, the heel rises, the knee extends, and plantar flexion occurs at the ankle. The very forceful extension of the knee and plantar flexion of the foot propels the body with the center of gravity moving up and forward (Fig. 3.4).

The rigid lever generated by supination of the subtalar joint accommodates the intense muscular activity of takeoff. Ideally the propulsive forces extend vectorally toward the ball of the foot and first ray. (Fig. 3.5)

In this simplistic overview of running biomechanics, it must be appreciated that upper body structures are also playing a role in the running gait cycle. Generally the arms are synchronous with the contralateral lower limb and the trunk rotates away from the supporting limb. The trunk should be nearly erect; and if it is not, as occurs with fatigue, there is less time to accelerate the foot backwards during the descent phase, with resulting increased force on foot strike.[39]

Further attention may now be directed to the biomechanics of the subtalar joint (STJ) (Fig. 4). Ideally the STJ, when in neutral position, should allow the tibia, talus, and calcaneus to be in direct alignment, and a line drawn through these structures should be perpendicular to the metatarsals as they contact the supporting surface (Fig. 4).[68] Mild deviation from ideal STJ alignment is probably well tolerated by most runners, as is abnormal frontal plane movement at the STJ. With the enormous forces generated by running, however, even a small

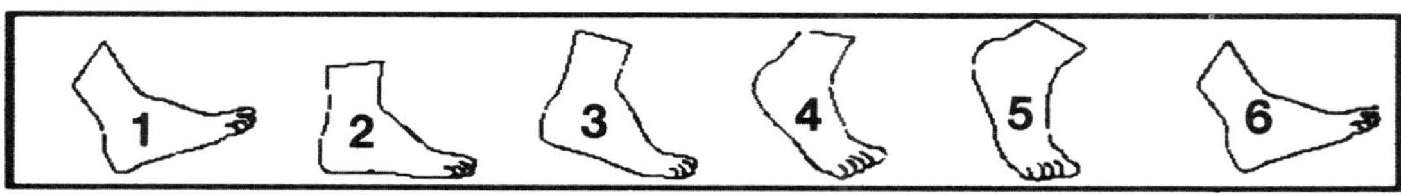

FIGURE 3. Stylized biomechanics of the running foot. 1.*Heel strike.* Foot in supinated position, initial surface contact, beginning of support phase. 2. *Midstance.* Foot pronated to adapt to surface and to dissipate shock. Center of gravity over STJ. Tibia internally rotates. 3. *Late midstance.* Center of gravity anterior to STJ. Heel lift with dorsiflexion of foot. 4. *Early toe-off.* Foot re-supinates to allow rigid lever for propulsion. External rotation of tibia. 5. *Toe off.* Propulsion of limb. 6. *Recovery phase.* Foot airborne, begins to swing posteriorly in preparation for new gait cycle.

variation from ideal STJ motion or alignment may generate chronic stress.

APPROACH TO THE INJURED PATIENT

History of Present Injury

The history of a patient with a presumed overuse syndrome should include several units. The first unit is concerned with the traditional aspects of any patient encounter, i.e., when the symptoms were first noted, what structures are injured, characterization of the pain, what treatment has already been provided, and so forth. The second unit is the pertinent past medical and orthopedic history. This should be obtained in detail, including all injuries self-treated by the patient.

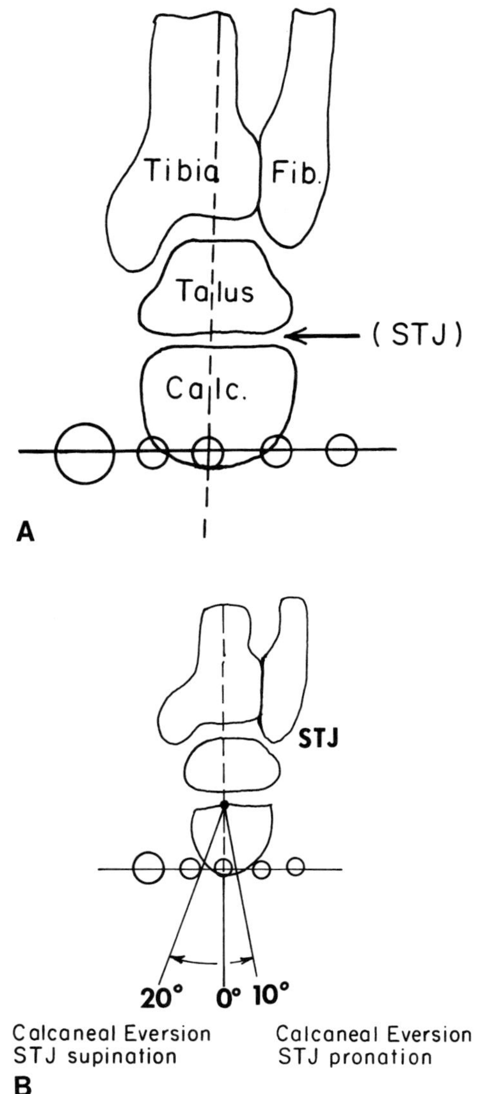

FIGURE 4. *A. The theoretical ideal: the neutral subtalar joint (STJ).* In this position tibia, talus, and calcaneus are in alignment. The metatarsals are perpendicular. *B,* Motions about the subtalar joint (STJ) Total range of motion = 30°.

The third unit should include questions about specific training practices. In the competitive runner, practices such as interval training may be undertaken to build speed and strength in addition to the long, slow distance training most joggers prefer. Interval training commonly introduces fast or sprint running at a pace greater than normally seen in racing. Because the biomechanical strain of sprinting is greater, injury may occur.[5] Careful inquiry should be made about the total weekly mileage as well as recent changes in miles run or intensity of running because this is such an important epidemiological factor in OSR. Such inquiry should include a compendium of the patient's history in competition. The patient should be encouraged to describe a typical training session in detail.

Because of differences in shock absorption, the type of surface upon which the runner trained should be asked. The surface grade should be noted, because if the patient has recently switched to hill training, additional stress may have been placed upon previously unstressed structures. For instance, uphill running may overstress the gastroc-Achilles tendon system and downhill running may stress tibial stabilizers such as the plantaris muscle, or overstress the anterior tibialis muscle group.

A frequently omitted but important item in the history is learning which side of the roadway the runner trains on. Consistently running on a banked roadway or track will cause excessive pronation of the upper foot and excessive supination of the lower (Fig. 5).[64]

Careful scrutiny should be made of "leisure" sports in which the patient participates. Much time can be spent dissecting the training practices of a runner without finding specific factors that indicate the diagnosis of an overuse syndrome only to learn that the patient has taken up other sports that the patient does not view as competitive or fitness-oriented, but which may be contributing to an injury. A typical example is the runner who also participates in racquet sports where excessive strain may be caused by the necessary quick lateral motions. Therefore, a combination of sports may place more strain on a lower extremity structure than any of the individual activities taken alone. Many athletes now include resistance training in their personal fitness programs. Such training, especially that involving full quadriceps extensions, squats, or hamstring strengthening exercises, should be noted because ligamental strain, muscle injury,and tendinitis may result from overzealous resistance work.

The history should also focus on footwear. This includes both the patient's training footwear, speci-

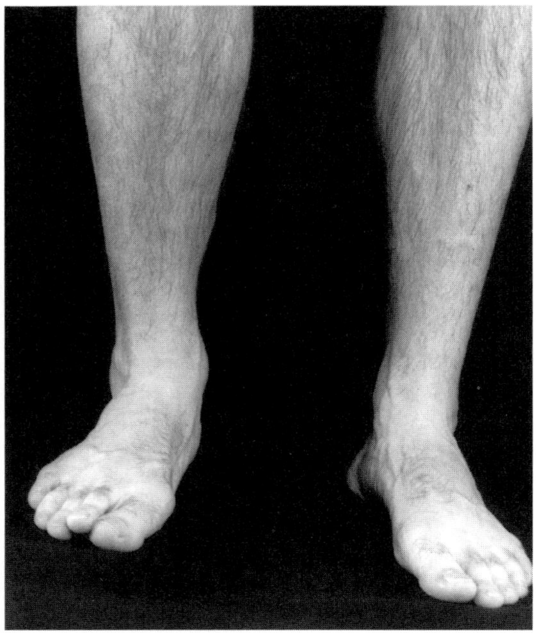

FIGURE 5. Effect of banked surface on biomechanics. Subject is exhibiting internal rotation and pronation of uphill (right) tibia and foot and external rotation and supination of downhill (left) foot.

fically how often a patient changes footwear, to what degree wear is apparent before a change, and whether or not the patient trains extensively in repaired rather than replaced shoes. Extensively repaired shoes may lose their shock-absorbing function due to midsole fatigue. The use of racing footwear should be noted because racing flats may have little heel lift or shock-absorbing capacity and should only be used primarily for highly competitive situations and not for general training. It is also prudent to question the patient about footwear worn recreationally or during work. Many patients run only a few minutes a day, whereas they may walk, work, climb stairs, dance, and stand for several hours a day in ill-fitting, poorly shock-absorbing footwear.

Physical and Biomechanical Examination[2,28,29,52,68]

The physical examination of the runner with an overuse syndrome centers on three major areas: (1) the specific physical examination of the injured anatomical area; (2) examination of the patient for any biomechanical abnormalities that could have caused the injury or might lead to injuries in the future; and (3) the dynamic or functional examination.

First examine the joints above and below an injured area or joint. Document the neurovascular status of tissue distal to the injury. Compare the injured area to the contralateral uninjured area or joint. If possible, have the patient localize the precise area of greatest symptomology. (I prefer to have the patient mark this area for me with an ink pen.)

A systematic approach is used for the biomechanical examination. With the patient standing, first examine general muscular development, noting the quadriceps, particularly the vastus medialis group. Deficiency in the vastus medialis muscle may lead to abnormal patellar tracking. Observing the rear of the patient, attention should be paid to any evidence of pelvic tilt, which may suggest a leg-length discrepancy. If there is a question of leg-length discrepancy, the patient may be placed supine and leg length measured from the anterior-superior iliac spine to the medial malleolus. A true anatomically short lower extremity will usually have compensatory supination of the foot on the short extremity and pronation of the foot on the normal or longer extremity. A greater than 1/4" difference in leg lengths may be sufficient to warrant an appropriate correction.

Again examine the standing patient in the frontal plane to note varum or valgum deformities of the femur and tibia. Generally a valgum deformity of the femur is accompanied by genu varum and varum deformity of the femur by genu valgum. These frontal plane deformities tend to cause considerable alteration of foot planting and side-to-side sway during running. The coxa vara-genu valgum combination is especially problematic with respect to overpronation as well as medial joint strain in the knee. Tibial varum is a relatively common condition found on the biomechanical examination. This will be noted by the patient's knees' being far apart when the feet are in juxtaposition. The patient can then be asked to assume his or her most comfortable normal stance. Careful attention should be directed to whether or not the patellas are centered toward the examiner, turned in toward each other, or deviated laterally. Deviation from reasonable patellar alignment may indicate a risk for a tracking abnormality. If not already determined, the range of motion of the kinetic chain joints (ankle, knee, hip) should be determined bilaterally.

To examine the STJ, place the patient prone and palpate medially and laterally over the talus, moving the foot until there is an equal protrusion of the talus on each side. The subtalar joint should be in the neutral or biomechanically ideal position. At this point note the relationship of a line bisecting the calcaneus and tibia (Fig. 6). In most cases the calcaneus will be in a slight varus position, i.e. no greater than 4° in relationship to the lower leg (Fig. 7A). The angular positioning of the forefoot from the rearfoot is then determined by providing plantar force to the fourth and fifth metatarsals until re-

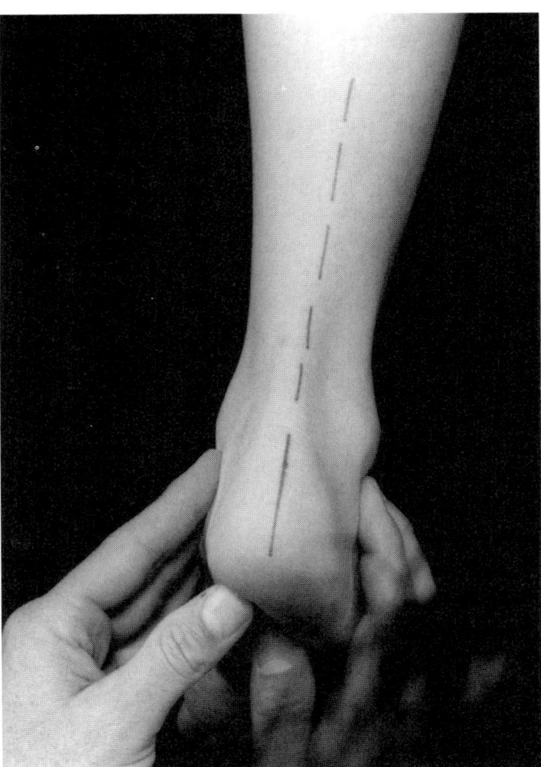

FIGURE 6. Determining the "neutral" subtalar joint. The patient is prone and the talar neutral position is being determined.

sistance is felt (Fig. 7B). When resistance occurs, draw an imaginary line from the head of the fifth metatarsal to the head of the first and then determine if this line deviates from a perpendicular relationship with a line bisecting the calcaneus. If the relationship is a perpendicular one, then no different exists between alignment of the forefoot to hindfoot. If there is a forefoot varus or valgus difference, this should be noted. Forefoot valgus is commonly found in the cavus foot. Forefoot varus may require increased pronation to adequately contact the surface while running.[29,68]

Physical examination of any runner presenting with an overuse syndrome is not complete without an examination of the patient's footwear.[9,16] The patient should always be encouraged to bring along running footwear, which may demonstrate the patient's biomechanics by its specific wear pattern. The normal wear pattern for most biomechanically sound runners includes wear on the outside or lateral aspect of the heel, which represents initial foot strike, and wear over the first metatarsal and ball of the foot, representing normal toeoff. In many runners the wear pattern may be normal, but it may be obvious that the running shoes are badly overworn. Once the lateral heel sole is thin to the point of showing midsole, the shock-absorbing capacity of many shoes will be exhausted. In addition, overwear of the lateral aspect of the heel will allow ex-

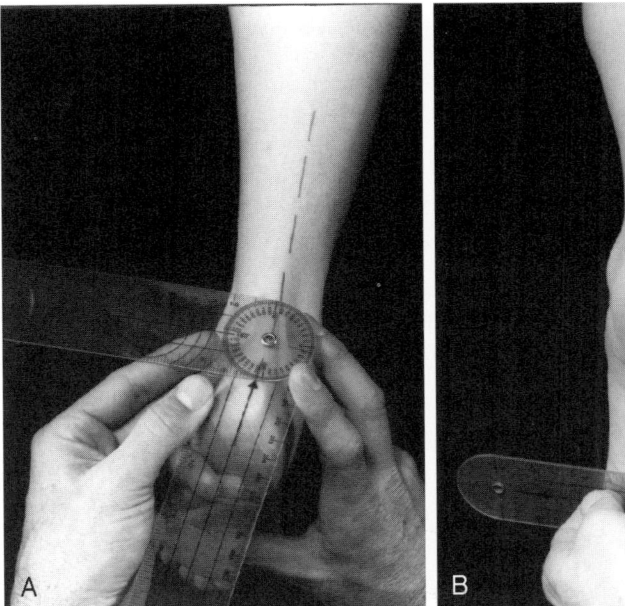

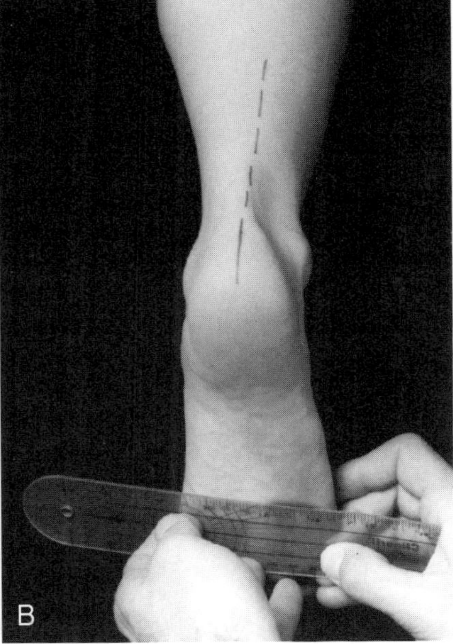

FIGURE 7A. The subtalar joint neutral position has been determined and its angular deviation from the perpendicular is measured. This subject shows minimal varus displacement.

FIGURE 7B. Determining forefoot angular deviation from the ideal. This subject has a slight varus of the forefoot.

cessive supination of the foot at the time of heel contact. It is also important to examine the everyday footwear of the patient, because in many cases the patient will have appropriate athletic footwear but overworn everyday shoes.

The dynamic or functional part of the physical exam consists of having the patient demonstrate normal gait, any movements which reliably reproduce symptoms, and if necessary an examination of the patient's running gait by direct observation or with the aid of a video recording while on a treadmill. Most OSR will not require this sophistication however, and the office exam should suffice.

The importance of biomechanical abnormalities found on exam should always be balanced by the relevance and magnitude of the abnormality. As in any patient examination, an abnormality may be of prime causation of may be simply an incidental finding.

GENERAL TREATMENT PRINCIPLES

The initial step in the treatment of OSR is classification of the degree of overuse. Classification of the extent of overuse will help both physician and patient evaluate treatment effectiveness and training modification.[42] The McKeag scale (see Table 1) is a classification of overuse in terms of severity and symptoms and goes beyond the simple utility of an accurate record in the patient's history.[42] This involves the patient in noting overuse symptoms, when they occur and to what degree, and engages the patient in the diagnosis and treatment of the problem, thereby making the patient an active participant in therapy and prophylaxis. Such cooperation is essential, because the goal of the treatment of OSR is to make the patient the prime factor in rehabilitation and modification of training or competitive practices that may have caused the injury.

Rest[26,30,42,61]

Paramount in the treatment of OSR is rest, because the basic etiology of overuse injuries is the inability of the normal repair mechanisms to compensate for inflammation generated during activity. Rest, however, is a generic term and must be properly prescribed. The more severe the overuse the more likely that more stringent rest is needed. Likewise in the sedentary individual, cessation rather than modification of activity may be necessary; whereas in the elite athlete, "rest" may mean a decrease in training mileage, with modification rather than cessation of training.

Both recreational and competitive runners may benefit from adopting a training activity with less biomechanical strain but that maintains aerobic fitness and strength. For many runners, this will be a non-weight-bearing activity such as swimming. Bicycling may also be utilized in specific instances if it is pain-free. For athletes who must maintain a high level of competitive performance, training may need to be divided into several smaller training sessions per day, with rest and rehabilitation in between.

Whenever rest is prescribed, it must be done with the goals and preferences of the patient in mind. If not, the athlete will view rest as a mandated cessation of a desired activity and perhaps an unwelcome side effect of consulting a physician and therefore a treatment to be avoided. If, however, rest is presented to the patient as a way of decreasing inflammation of an injured structure, and if an ancillary activity is provided that allows the patient to remain active and fit, he or she will likely accept rest as a useful adjunct of therapy.

Cryotherapy[31,43,61] (See Second Opinion IV)

Application of ice or other forms of cryotherapy to injured structures in overuse syndromes is generally used in any situation involving acute inflammation. Cryotherapy inhibits inflammation directly and increases the tensile strength of injured tissue. The athlete may apply the ice for 20 minutes or to his tolerance for discomfort and then allow tissue rewarming and reapplication. Ice is most useful in the acute and early treatment phase of overuse syndromes to decrease swelling and as an adjunct therapy to decrease pain and inhibit inflammation during rehabilitation. Contraindications to cryotherapy include any medical condition in the patient that inhibits the sensory nerve supply such as diabetes, vascular disease, use of local anesthetics, or with any medical condition that would place the patient at risk of cold injury. Heat is best used in rehabilitation to increase tissue flexibility and elasticity and to encourage stretching. It should not be applied acutely or in suspected compartment syndromes, because heat may increase compartment volume and further compromise circulation.

Compression and elevation of the injured structure are combined with cryotherapy. Compression decreases edema and prevent accumulation of inflammatory products in the tissue. Elevation likewise decreases edema, promotes venous and lymphatic flow, and localizes concentrations of inflammatory debris in tissue.

Pharmacologic Treatment

Nonsteroidal anti-inflammatory drugs (NSAIDs) are useful both acutely and chronically in OSR. These drugs basically act by inhibiting prostaglandin synthesis, which interrupts the cascade of inflammatory response in injured tissue. Pain relief during the longer term use of these agents generally signifies decreased inflammation as well as the initial "pain killing" mechanism of action. Use of a specific NSAID depends on cost, convenience of dosing, and side effects. Agents generally need 2 weeks for full effect.

Injectable corticosteroids, often mixed with a local anesthetic, are indicated when more conservative methods of treating soft tissue injuries have been exhausted. Steroids should not be injected into tendons, because direct injection into these structures may induce structural weakening and ultimately cause rupture.[54] Because some systemic absorption will occur with injectable corticosteroids, they should be used cautiously. The possibility of introducing infection should always be considered, especially if joint injection is planned, and the risks and benefits of joint injection should be carefully weighed in this situation.

Orthotics[11,16,18,30] (See Second Opinion V)

Orthotics are insets of rubber, plastic, or other molded materials inserted into the shoe to alter or counteract biomechanical abnormalities in overuse syndromes. Orthotics balance the foot and direct its biomechanics toward the ideal neutral position to inhibit excessive pronation or supination.

An orthotic will best suit, the patient when a definitive biomechanical abnormality is found that is directly implicated in the overuse syndrome being experienced by the patient. Considerable knowledge of orthotics and their biomechanical use is needed in the proper construction and application of devices to limit STJ abnormalities. It is important to realize that many runners will have abnormalities on biomechanical examination but will be symptom-free. In these patients the use of orthotics may themselves cause symptoms, and therefore such treatment is inappropriate.

Shoes[2,9,16,20] (See Second Opinion VI)

A component of any treatment program for OSR is the prescription of proper footwear. The major footwear problem of most runners is overworn shoes, followed by footwear inappropriate for a specific biomechanical abnormality. Runners accumulating more than 25 miles/week should change shoes every 3 months; those accumulating fewer than 25 miles/week should change shoes every 4 to 6 months.[20] The basic functions of any quality "running" shoe are shock absorption, foot control, and provision of good traction and protection (Fig. 8).

The soles of good running shoes should be carbonized to provide longer wear. Waffle/style construction of the sole will allow greater shock absorption. A widened heel with a heel lift provides for enhanced shock absorption and less stress upon the Achilles tendon.

The last or curve of the sole of the shoe should generally conform to the patient's own foot shape. In general, most patients will do well with a relatively straight last. The runner with a high arch or cavus foot may benefit from a more C-shaped or curved last. The shoes should be comfortably snug but allow for a mild increase in volume of the foot during running.

Heel control to limit excessive heel motion can be accomplished by purchasing a shoe with a firm heel counter or cup. A good controlling shoe will not wobble when standing on one foot.[20] Padding around the Achilles tendon in good quality shoes provides less direct trauma to the Achilles tendon. A meshed upper portion decreases heat and moisture buildup in the shoe. Many manufacturers now provide information on shoes that have been selectively designed to control common foot abnormalities such as overpronation at the STJ. If these biomechanical abnormalities are thought to play a role in a particular patient's overuse syndrome, it would be reasonable to prescribe a particular shoe type.

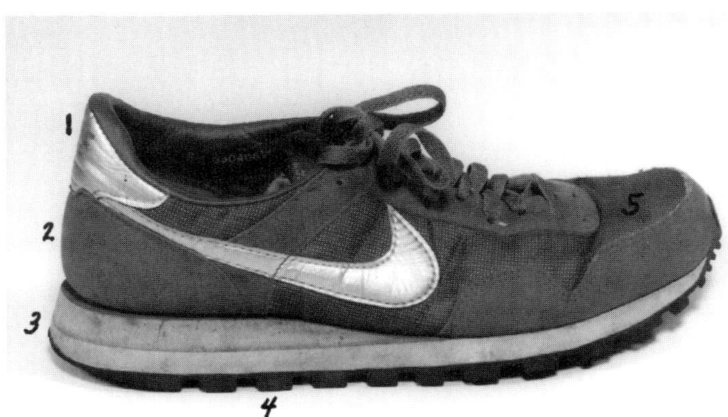

FIGURE 8. Running shoe anatomy: **1,** Achilles tendon pad; **2,** heel counter for form heel control; **3,** heel lift to decrease Achilles tendon tension and add shock absorption; **4,** carbonated waffle sole to provide increased shock absorption, traction and excellent wear characteristics; **5,** nylon mesh upper to promote ventilation, decrease shoe weight and provide flexibility.

Training Practice (see Second Opinion VII)

The training protocols of runners will likely be as varied as the individuals themselves; therefore, the health professional should be familiar with the basic principles of training that serve runners of all levels and allow a proper training foundation.

A warm-up period is essential for proper training and prevention of injury and overuse. Physiologically an appropriate warm-up session allows increased muscle temperature, enhances oxygen release from hemoglobin, increases blood flow by a vasodilatory effect in muscle, and decreases blood viscosity.[35] A proper warm-up also enhances muscular contraction and speed of neuromuscular transmission, which improves the reaction time to stimuli. The final benefit of the warm-up period is that tissue elasticity increases along with decreased viscosity of synovial fluid, thereby allowing greater flexibility and gains to be made from stretching. Almost any activity which promotes a smooth warm-up without excessive stretching of muscle or joints is permitted. Many runners warm up by using a walk-jog pattern. An appropriate warmup in this instance would be alternating a jog for 220 yards with walking 20 yards for approximately a half mile.[35]

Immediately after the warm-up, gentle nonballistic stretching should be done. Many specific muscle stretching techniques and regimens have been devised, but a general guideline for any stretching program for runners is to pay careful attention to the hamstring and gastrocnemius muscle group and to the iliotibial band, because excessive tightness in any of these muscles and connective tissues may lead to specific overuse syndromes. Proprioceptive exercises that involve stretching also seem important to facilitate enhanced neuromuscular efficiency.[59] Stretching must be done greatly and never past the point of minimal discomfort, because excessive pain may represent tissue injury and not enhanced flexibility.[62]

Following the training period an active rather than passive cool-down period is recommended to facilitate removal of lactate from tissue; this is to allow heart rate and respiration to decrease to pre-exercise levels and to allow further stretching of warm flexible muscles. The simplest cool-down procedure is walking, perhaps interrupted by short periods of stretching. Other athletes may prefer to ride an exercise bike at low RPMs or do jog/walk intervals. It is probably not critical how an athlete cools down but that a cool-down period is undertaken.

In-depth review of other training practices such as resistance training and cross-training is beyond the purpose of this chapter. The professional dealing with athletes who run, however, must be familiar with these general principles.

Basically, resistance training has two purposes; one strengthens the muscle groups used in running and the other is an adjunct to general fitness. Two examples are the strengthening of the vastus medialis group with short-arc quadriceps extension exercises and then, abdominal crunches to improve abdominal wall strength and to serve as a prophylaxis against low back pain.

Cross-training generally involves the participation in other high aerobic demand activities which usually do not have a high potential for lower extremity overuse, two examples of which are swimming and biking.

Inclusion of resistance training and cross-training into a running program is highly individualized. Some athletes regularly include these activities; others use them only during periods of rehabilitation or as a rest from running. Most authorities encourage runners to include these practices in their training routines.

Training Goals (See Second Opinion VIII)

As noted, the most common etiologic factor in overuse syndrome is overtraining.[32,53] When a patient is seen for an overuse syndrome, one of the most important factors related to treatment and rehabilitation is reevaluation of training practices and goals, which may change greatly the rate of injury recurrence with little or no change in fitness.

Case Report

A 30-year-old man suffered from chronic bilateral Achilles tendinitis of two years' duration. At the time of presentation to his physician, the patient had been running approximately 20-22 miles/week at a 7 1/2 min/mile pace. To increase fitness, the patient was alternating running with competitive soccer. When asked what the basic goals of his personal fitness program were, he listed them as: (1) to maintain fitness and modify cardiovascular risk; (2) to maintain a high enough fitness level to be competitive in soccer; and (3) to continue a fitness program but to decrease the chronicity of the Achilles tendinitis. The history disclosed running on hard, unyielding concrete roadway and asphalt.

This athlete's running shoes were of good quality but badly overworn, and his everyday footwear had a badly worn sole and heel. Physical and biomechanical examination disclosed a relatively high-arched foot with severe tenderness of both Achilles tendons and a tendency for the calcaneus to be in varum with the talus in the neutral position. It was suggested to the patient that he decrease his mileage significantly and purchase new street and running shoes; but the patient was reluctant to decrease his training or to limit his competitive soccer.

The main reason that the patient refused to decrease his training mileage was that he felt he would suffer in terms of cardiovascular fitness. The patient was then asked to undergo a cardiovascular fitness evaluation, which disclosed a functional aerobic capacity of 140% for his age group. With this information, the patient acknowledged that his current program was producing excellent fitness but also overuse. The patient agreed to decrease total mileage run and to minimize his soccer. A frequent recheck of the patient's fitness level disclosed that his fitness was maintained but the Grade III overuse syndrome of Achilles tendinitis decreased to a minimal Grade I.

In this case no change in fitness was noted with decreasing mileage run per week, whereas the overuse problems were rapidly ameliorated. Alternative goals for a similar patient might be to participate in another sport activity such as swimming or bicycling to maintain fitness while allowing the running-induced injury to heal.

SPECIFIC OVERUSE INJURIES OF RUNNERS

For the practicing physician, overuse injuries will not present as a training problem or as a biomechanical abnormality, but rather as pain or dysfunction of a specific body party which is interfering with running. Any lower extremity structure can be affected in a runner. Therefore, the list of possible injuries is almost inexhaustible. In this section common major overuse syndromes associated with running are presented.

Knee: Patellar Pain Syndrome

Pain in and around the knee is the most common overuse complaint and site of injury of runners.[6,29,32,44,49] Patellar pain syndrome or "runner's knee" is the most common knee OSR.[6] Many authorities would term this syndrome chondromalacia patella, but true chondromalacia or frank degeneration of the articular surface of the patella with fibrillation of the surface occurs only in the most severe forms of this syndrome.[10,44] Patellar pain syndrome is discussed in Chapter 22.

Iliotibial Band Syndrome (ITB)[2,26,29,37]

Iliotibial band friction syndrome is the most common cause of lateral knee pain in runners. Anatomically, the iliotibial band is a fascial band that extends from the iliac crest and inserts on the lateral tibial tubercle, also known and Gerdy's tubercle. The iliotibial band also receives contributions from the tensor fascia lata and the gluteus maximus muscles. With hip flexion and extension, the band is pulled anteriorly and posteriorly, and with repeated movement the band may impinge and develop friction with the lateral femoral condyle.[37]

Etiology. Biomechanical abnormalities associated with ITB suggest that any abnormality increasing the varus stress about the knee possibly will cause increased iliotibial band friction. Common findings include genu varum, cavus feet, footwear excessively worn on the lateral heel, and runners with overpronation leading to increased internal rotation of the knee and increased knee retinaculum tension laterally.[29,37]

ITB may result from a single severe running session or a sudden increase in running distance. Downhill running is often implicated because of the increased stride length of downhill running, which increases lateral tissue tension about the knee.

History. The patient first notes pain laterally around the knee after exercise. This pain is usually not initially limiting and running may be continued. Pain then develops during running, eventually leading to severe cases in which pain occurs during daily activities, especially going up and down stairs and during other sports. The patient often finds that walking with a stiff knee in full extension is pain-free.

Physical Examination. Physical examination demonstrates tenderness laterally 2 cm above the joint space over the lateral femoral condyle (Fig. 9). Crepitus may be noted over the area of pain. Palpa-

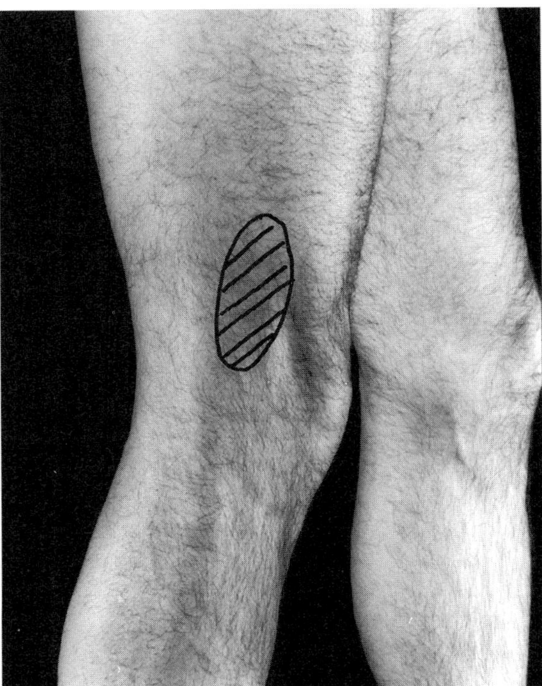

FIGURE 9. Location of pain laterally in iliotibial band syndrome.

tion of the iliotibial band with flexion and extension of the hip will reproduce the pain. Ober's test may also be utilized to detect increased iliotibial band tension, which may be causing excessive pressure on the lateral femoral condyle.[28,52]

Therapy and Rehabilitation. Immediate therapy consists of ice, NSAIDs, and elimination of harmful training practices such as running on hills, banked tracks, and slanted roads. Using running shoes with enhanced shock-absorption characteristics and free from lateral heel wear is also appropriate. Correction of leg-length imbalance with heel lifts and inhibition of overpronation of the foot to decrease internal tibial torsion may be warranted. Iliotibial band stretching (Fig. 10) should be emphasized, as well as encouraging the patient to exercise only to the beginning of pain to prevent further inflammation. The use of corticosteroids applied by phonophoresis or iontophoresis often markedly reduces inflammation. Some clinicians emphasize the use of injectable steroids for painful friction areas, but it has been found that more conservative therapy helps in more than 80% of cases of ITB, with 50% of patients being improved in 3 weeks or less of conservative therapy.[37] After 12 or more months of conservative therapy without improvement, a surgical approach consisting of releasing posterior iliotibial band fibers concomitant with, or releasing iliotible band fibers from, the lateral retinaculum of the knee and patella is recommended if the runner must continue in rigorous competition.[37]

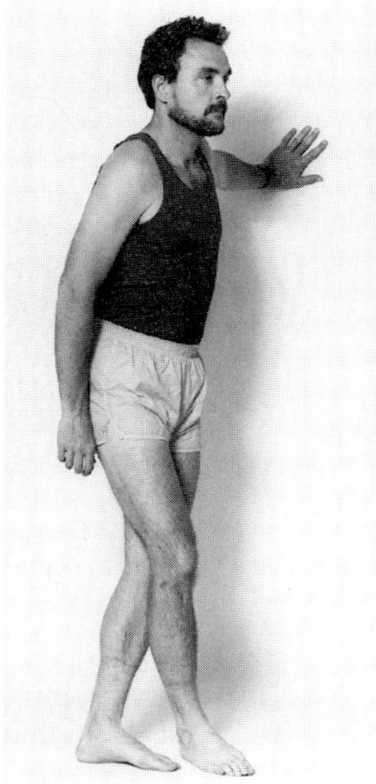

FIGURE 10. Iliotibial band stretching. The subject is applying a varus stretch to the left iliotibial band by leaning gently into a wall.

Lower Leg Pain Syndromes (LLPS)[2,26,29,69]

Generically, LLPS describes a group of overuse syndromes consisting of pain distal to the knee and proximal to the ankle. Because of the great number of muscular, osseous, ligamental, and tendinous structures involved in the lower leg, it would be impossible to describe all the potential overuse problems that arise. The majority of patients, however, will have one of a few distinct syndromes attributable to overuse in the lower leg. The main difficulty for the diagnostician is distinguishing benign condition such as "shin splints" from the orthopedic emergency of acute compartment syndrome. The term shin splints[2,5,17,29] refers to a syndrome consisting of pain along the inner distal two-thirds of the tibial shaft. LLPS also includes the most common source of osseous injury in the runner, that is, tibial stress fracture. Each of the main components of LLPS is described below.

Etiology. The pathophysiology and biomechanical etiology of this syndrome cause some disagreement among authorities, with some believing that this syndrome is caused by excessive stress placed on the interosseous membrane between the tibia and the fibula as a result of excessive activity of the posterior tibialis muscle, causing periostitis and periosteal stress reaction.[11] Others feel that the periostitis originates from the area of the soleus muscle after excessive activity.[17]

History. Regardless of the muscle group involved, this syndrome usually presents with gradual increase in soreness and pain after running, then progresses to pain during activities such as walking. The pain has a dull, aching quality and typically is located over the posterior medial border of the tibia in the distal portion of the middle third.[3] Athletes involved in court or field sports often develop shin splints, probably caused by athletic footwear with poor shock absorption.

Physical Examination. Physical examination discloses pain over the area described above. The pain is usually bilateral and relatively diffuse. Point tenderness should evoke suspicion of a stress fracture. The most common biomechanical abnormalities found on examination of the patient include excessive heel valgus and excessive forefoot pronation. Excessive pronation will increase internal tibial torsion that stresses the interosseous membrane and provokes increased activity of the tibialis posterior muscle.

Therapy and Rehabilitation (See Second Opinion IX). Therapy and rehabilitation consist of relative or total rest, ice, anti-inflammatory medication, heel-cord and hamstring stretching, and strengthening the dorsiflexion of the foot. As improvement of initial symptoms becomes evident, the patient may return to training with an emphasis on running on a soft flat surface with shoes of proper flexibility and shock absorption. If a biomechanical anomaly such as overpronation is noted, an orthotic, or in milder cases a simple arch support, should be used. Prophylaxis of shin splints consists mainly of the factors noted above plus careful attention of the detection of the recurrence of symptoms and immediate modification of training practices. A useful addition to training programs for runners bothered by chronic exacerbations of shin splints is to shift some of their training program to swimming and bicycling, which maintain aerobic conditioning without biomechanical overload.

Stress Fractures[41]

Stress fracture as a clinical entity may have been described as early as 1855, some 40 years before the first clinical use of radiographs, but perhaps more succinctly in 1939 when Roberts and Vogt defined pseudofracture of the tibia.[56] The tibia is the most common site of stress fractures in runners; but because a stress fracture may occur in any lower extremity osseous structure, the diagnosis must be entertained if the history or examination suggests pain from bone (Fig. 11).

Etiology. Stress fractures are caused by repeated compression or similar stress on bone or with excessive periosteal traction. As repetitive stress is applied to bone, remodeling and repair may be sufficient, and transition from microscopic to macroscopic fracture may occur. Careful serial analyses of bone stress reactions indicate that the bone initially at risk for stress fracture is on one cortical side of the diaphysis. With increasingly severe osseous inflammation, the stress becomes circumferential, but no frank displacement of bony cortex occurs. If bony stress continues, displaced fracture may occur through the diaphysis.[25] Three-fourths of lower extremity stress fractures probably result from training errors, most notably poor shock-absorbing shoes, excessive mileage, training with another type

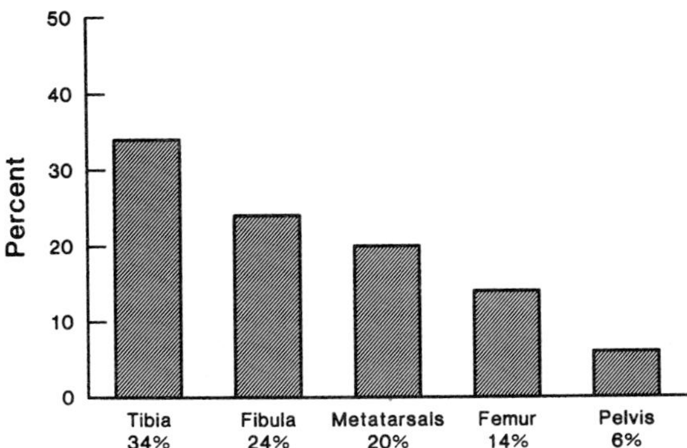

FIGURE 11. Most common bones involved with stress fractures in 1000 runners. (From McBryde AM: Clin Sports Med 4:737 Oct 1985.)

of lower extremity injury that changes normal biomechanics, or training normally despite a known biomechanically abnormal gait.[12,41]

Besides the obvious compressive forces that may cause microtrauma, another suggested etiology for stress fracture of the tibia is that which occurs when a bowing effect develops with forceful muscle contractions, i.e., in the gastrocnemius group.[14]

History. The patient complains of pain initially after running, which progresses to pain while running progressively short distances.[8] As sufficient microtrauma accumulates, pain occurs during nontraining activities and finally at rest. The pain is usually unilateral and may become disabling. If the patient is female, further important historical factors must be sought. (See Second Opinion X.)

Physical Examination. Physical examination generally discloses localized tenderness over an osseous area. If the tibia is involved, pain commonly is noted over the medial tibial diaphysis. In more dramatic cases, evidence of periosteal reaction, such as swelling or increased warmth, may be felt by palpation.[25] A tuning fork applied over the region of a suspected fracture may evoke pain, but should not cause pain with shin splints. Pelvic stress fractures may be noted by ipsilateral pain when the patient is standing on one leg.[60]

The most common biomechanical abnormality found in hyperpronation with excessive varus alignment of the lower leg and foot.[69] Ancillary testing such as plain radiographs and bone scans plays a prominent role in early detection and diagnosis of stress fractures. Two to six weeks are generally required from the onset of pain to visible plain radiographic changes.[23] The earliest changes are periosteal reactions or small linear unilateral cortical defects perpendicular to the diaphysis. Many mild stress fractures occur without causing any apparent changes on standard radiographs. Technetium polyphosphate scanning of the tibia with multiple views is especially useful, because the agent will concentrate in an area of high blood flow and metabolic activity, such as that seen with bony remodeling in a stress fracture.[22] One of the main advantages of radionuclide bone scanning for stress fractures is its great sensitivity and specificity.[22,25]

Although modalities such as ultrasound and thermography may play a role in delineation of stress fractures, radionuclide scanning provides the highest percentage of detection.[25] Within one week after development of symptoms, radionuclide scanning is usually positive for a stress fracture.[41] This capacity for early detection has clinical utility in that stress fractures detected early, before circumferential diaphyseal injury has taken place, heal in about one half the time required for a circumferential lesion.[8]

Therapy and Rehabilitation. Therapy for stress fractures depends largely on the site of the fracture and the "criticalness" of the bone involved. For the uncomplicated tibial stress fracture with noncircumferential involvement of the diaphysis, healing may be expected in 4–6 weeks.[8,69] In a circumferential lesion, healing may be delayed for 8–14 weeks.[8] In general it is prudent to advise the patient to take a relatively long period of rest from exercise because stress fractures tend to become recalcitrant or recurrent. Additionally, when stress fractures become complete fractures, there are high rates of delayed union and nonunion. Treatment of tibial stress fractures other than those of the tibial plateau involves decreasing training mileage to a pain-free level if the patient must continue to run. If the patient is willing, it might be best to switch to nonimpact aerobic sports such as swimming or bicycling. The patient should be placed in enhanced shock-absorbing footwear for both training and daily activities, and soft surfaces should be used for running with no sprinting or exercise on banked surfaces.[41,69] Recalcitrant cases of stress fracture of the tibia should be carefully examined for pathologic fractures, tumor, or infection.[41] If no other complicating factors are noted, casting and non-weight-bearing management may be used for resolution of the fracture.

Compartment Syndrome

Compartment syndrome (CS) is one of the true orthopedic emergencies that may confront the primary care physician when dealing with overuse syndromes.[2] The most important type is the acute anterior compartment syndrome, although any fascial compartment in the lower extremity may be involved in a potentially catastrophic event.[2] CS occurs when excessive muscle activity leads to an increased interstitial and muscle volume of as much as 20%.[13] The fascial compartments of the lower extremity are rigid containers; therefore, as muscle volume increases, compartment pressure rises, promoting first venous stasis and then frank ischemia. The ischemic muscle tissue releases inflammatory mediators that increase compartmental edema and tissue pressure. There is a vicious cycle of further tissue hypoxia, and increased edema. When ischemia and hypoxia become insurmountable, tissue necrosis occurs.

Etiology. Direct trauma such as a contusion, a sprain, strain, or unusually excessive prolonged exercise can all lead to acute CS.[67] Chronic CS can also occur in endurance athletes, but the cascade of overuse to tissue swelling to ischemia may not occur to an extreme degree. In these individuals, symptoms may be noted during or immediately after exercise.

History. The usual history suggests a patient who undergoes extreme exercise with progressive leg pain. In anterior CS, the pain is usually in the anterior tibial region as a result of overuse of the anterior tibialis group,but it also can occur laterally, representing overuse of the perinei muscles or, more rarely, as posterior calf pain implicating overuse of the posterior tibialis. Because the anterior compartment syndrome is the most common, the physician should be especially alert for acute anterior lower extremity pain. The patient may have noted paresthesias distally and usually will have noted progressive inability to walk properly.[67] Chronic CS patients note a pattern of pain corresponding to the particular muscular compartment involved. The symptoms are usually relieved with cessation of exercise.

Physical Examination. Physical examination of the patient will reveal weakness in the involved musculature. The muscles are tender, swollen, and tense; passive movement or stretching evokes pain. For anterior CS, loss of foot dorsiflexion and decreased sensory appreciation in the toe web between the first and second toes is noted.[26,55] The dorsalis pedis pulse is usually normal, unless previous vascular disease has been present.[55] Increased compartment pressures can be recorded by catheterized measurements with a manometer.[46] Wick pressures greater than 30 mm Hg along with appropriate clinical findings suggest a diagnosis of CS.[67] In chronic anterior CS, recurrent pain reproducible with activity will be noted in the anterior lower extremity. Diagnosis of this condition may be difficult unless anterior compartment pressures are measured during or after exercise.

Therapy and Rehabilitation. Treatment for acute anterior CS warrants immediate orthopedic consultation. Pending consultation, the patient should be put at rest. The use of ice to the lower extremity is controversial because the patient's sensation may be impaired and because tissue already under ischemic threat may be further injured. Prompt correction of any circulatory abnormality such as dehydration should be implemented. In acute cases where clinical examination or intracompartmental pressure analyses suggest impending tissue necrosis, fasciotomy should be done immediately.[55] In chronic CS after other diagnoses have been ruled out, surgical release of the anterior compartment accomplished by a 1 to 1 1/2" incision over the midportion of the tibia medially may be required.[1]

Prophylaxis of future compartmental problems should be aimed at correcting any problems of biomechanics or training. Because CS often arises after an episode of acute severe training or competition, training and competitive goals may need to be redefined. CS of the anterior muscle group can also be provoked by toe or hill running. Such training practices may need to be modified.

Ankle and Foot Syndromes

The most common overuse syndromes of the ankle and foot are Achilles tendinitis and plantar fasciitis. Although neither syndrome is as dramatic as syndromes that occur more proximally, both are notable for their frustrating chronicity.

Achilles Tendinitis[2,6,7]

Etiology. Increased stress of the Achilles tendon results from a variety of factors, including excessive pronation, a cavus foot, or a short rigid Achilles tendon. Moderate to severe forefoot varus may be found in most runners with severe symptoms.[6] Up to 75% of runners with significant Achilles tendinitis will have training errors, usually involving hill running, excessive mileage, or interval training featuring sprinting bursts.[6,26] Runners who participate in jumping sports also are at risk.[34]

History. Achilles tendinitis presents as pain over the Achilles tendon and posterior heel (Fig. 12). The pain is usually most prominent 2 to 3 cm proximal to the insertion of the Achilles tendon on the calcaneus.[7] In early Achilles tendinitis, pain occurs at the onset of running or sprinting. As inflammation becomes more chronic, the patient typically may note severe stiffness and pain of the Achilles tendon upon arising from bed. The pain may be particularly severe at the onset of a training period but will abate somewhat as the training session progresses. A training history usually discloses high mileage, but tendinitis does also occur in sprinters.[34]

Physical Examination. Physical examination discloses mild to excruciating pain over the Achilles tendon, usually at the base of the tendon and extending up to the level of the malleoli. Tendon and peritenon are often thickened. Severe cases may include visible swelling and inflammation as well as palpable crepitus. Loss of dorsiflexion caused by tendon stiffness is a common finding (normal >25°).[34] Some difficulty in differentiating Achilles tendinitis from retrocalcaneal bursitis may be noted. If tenderness is found more proximally on the tendon, the diagnosis is most likely tendonitis. Further diagnostic accuracy may also be achieved when the foot is plantar flexed forcibly against resistance or when having the patient perform toe walking. Ancillary testing such as radiography is usually not needed, but in chronic cases may show calcification in the body of the tendon or a spur at the insertion of the tendon into the calcaneus. These spurs are usually of no significance.

Further testing is useful if partial or complete rupture of the Achilles tendon is suspected. Such testing, including xeroradiography or nuclear magnetic resonance scanning of the tendon, may determine tendon integrity or rupture in difficult cases. Such rupture may be suspected in severe chronic overuse and a history of paroxysmal pain when exercising. Immediate physical examination in these cases, utilizing Thompson's test (forceful squeezing of the gastrocnemius muscle with the patient lying prone) may show no plantar flexion of the foot, thereby indicating complete tendon rupture.[26] (See Second Opinion XI.)

Therapy and Rehabilitation. Therapy and rehabilitation of Achilles tendinitis consists of the measures usually employed for overuse syndromes. More specifically, ice before and after training may be especially useful. A heel lift of at least 1/2″ should be present in the running shoe. Increased padding in the heel counter may decrease friction and provide better cushioning for the Achilles tendon. If excessive pronation is present, orthotics may provide better control of the STJ and reduce recurrent stress. Because the Achilles tendon is not enclosed in a definitive tendon sheath, attempts to inject steroids into

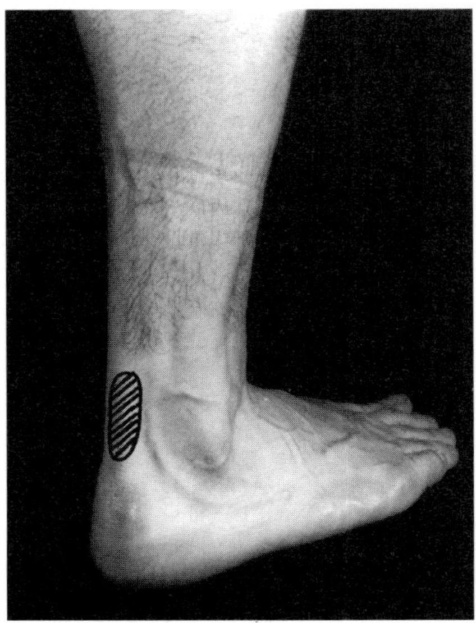

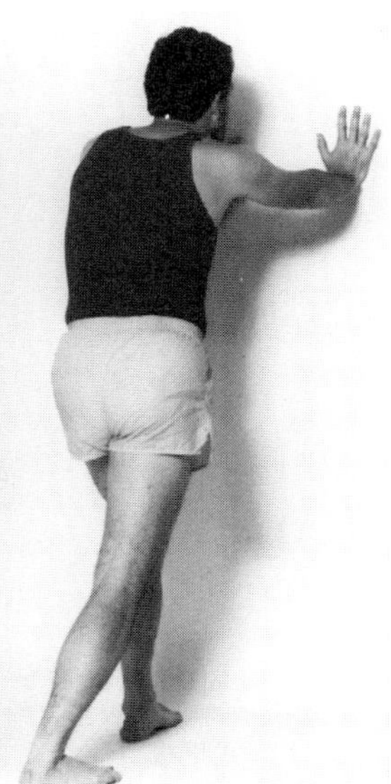

FIGURE 12. **Left,** Location of pain is directly over tendon, most notably at the level of the malleoli. **Right,** Achilles-gastrocnemius stretch. The subject is stretching the right gastroc-Achilles unit by leaning into a wall.

the peritenon region may be dangerous, because the injection may be directly into the tendon itself.[54] Injections into the tendon may weaken the tendon structure enough that rupture may occur during further training. Prophylaxis of Achilles tendinitis is carried out by careful analysis of any biomechanical abnormalities thus increasing soleus and gastrocnemius strength and flexibility and revising the training schedule until symptoms are minimal.[66]

Plantar Fasciitis[2,26,29,69]

Etiology. Plantar fasciitis presents as sharp, shooting pain in the arch and medial aspect of the foot (Fig. 13). Biomechanically, this syndrome results from repetitive microtrauma to the plantar fascia secondary to increased traction at the insertion of the fascia on the calcaneus. Such increased tension occurs most commonly in the high arch or cavus foot, creating a bowstring effect upon the fascia. Plantar fasciitis is also seen in excessive pronators and in runners who participate in ancillary activities (e.g., dance or sports requiring jumping) that encourage extreme foot plantar flexion with concomitant metatarsal-phalangeal dorsiflexion.[40]

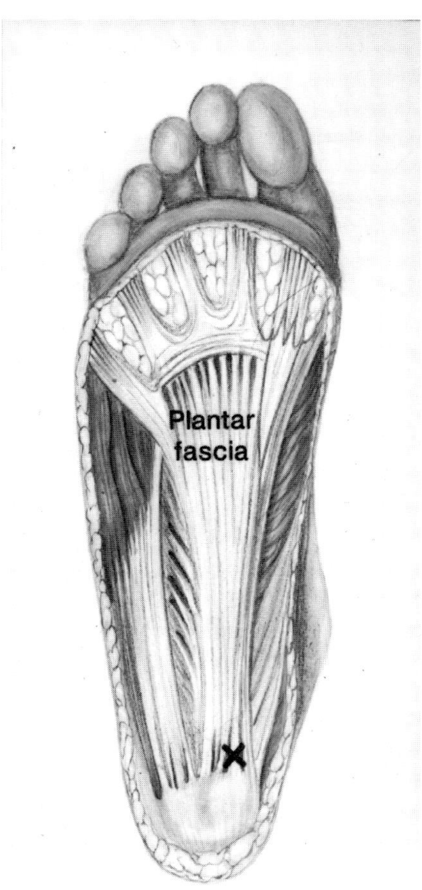

FIGURE 13. Plantar fascia, plantar fasciitis. The plantar's fascia serves as a stabilizer of the arch. The pain of plantar fasciitis may occur along the fascia but especially over its insertion into the calcaneus (x). (Reprinted from Mayo Clinic Health Letter with permission of Mayo Clinic, Rochester, Minnesota 55905.)

History. The patient usually first notices pain with activity or especially upon arising. This syndrome may progress to pain during walking or any maneuver that involves stretching of the plantar fascia.

Physical Examination. Physical examination discloses point tenderness of the fascia at its origin at the middle of the distal edge of the plantar surface of the calcaneus. The pain can usually be easily reproduced in the office if the examiner stretches the plantar fascia or has the patient walk on his/her toes.[26]

Ancillary testing is usually not necessary, but radiographs of the foot may disclose a calcaneal spur.[18] It is controversial whether calcaneal spurs actually contribute to plantar fasciitis. Most authorities suggest that calcaneal spurs are not implicated in plantar fasciitis.

Therapy and Rehabilitation. Treatment involves practices standard for OSR. Therapy should include massage of the plantar fasciitis and application of ice to trigger areas. Rehabilitation includes strengthening intrinsic foot musculature to aid the plantar fasciitis during foot stabilization;[40] for example by picking up marbles off carpet with the toes. Prophylaxis involves decreasing arch stretch with an orthotic or arch support, especially in patients with cavus feet. Patients with overpronation may be treated with a orthotic to limit abnormal motion. Excessive metatarsophalangeal dorsiflexion can be diminished by a stiffer sole in the forefoot.[40] Almost all runners benefit from added cushioning over the calcaneus. Steroid injection at the origin of the plantar fascia may be effective although it is painful. One theory is that it works mainly by weakening the plantar fascia, thus leading to its disruption.

In the young runner, calcaneal pain similar to that noted in plantar fasciitis may occur with Sever's disease in which inflammation of the calcaneal epiphysis occurs. Heel cord stretching generally is therapeutic. Persistent calcaneal pain that does not respond to treatment directed at plantar fasciitis may be indicative of stress fracture of the calcaneus, and investigation should be directed toward this possibility.

Less common overuse syndromes of the foot should also be considered in the differential diagnosis of plantar fasciitis. Most important among these are stress fracture of the calcaneus or the metatarsal. Pain over the lateral midfoot just anterior to the calcaneus could represent cuboid syndrome, peroneus longus tendinitis, or plantar nerve entrapment. Pain between the proximal phalanges of the toes suggests interdigital, or Morton's neuromas.[18,39]

SECOND OPINION I HOW MUCH IS ENOUGH AND HOW MUCH IS TOO MUCH?

The central question for many health professionals dealing with runners with overuse injuries is the root cause of the injury. To answer this, Dr. Morris Mellion in a recent editorial in *Heart Disease and Stroke* suggests that the health professional closely examine the motivation, the amount of exercise being done, and the goals of the exercising patient. Dr. Mellion raises the following points:

(1) About one-half of our patients exercise, but the most common reason is for weight control and weight loss, not necessarily for fitness.

(2) As professionals, we all are aware of the need to motivate the sedentary patients to exercise. But what about the "overmotivated" patient who feels "if a little exercise is good, a lot must be better."

(3) Recently research has been devoted to what "a little" exercise means. For most patients, both the American Heart Association and the American College of Sports Medicine suggest that a training level at 50% of a person's maximum exercise capacity for 20 to 30 minutes three times per week is likely beneficial. Exercise at lower intensity may also be acceptable but must be done for a longer training session. "More" may simply be "too much."

As professionals we must understand the difference between "exercising for health" and "exercising for fitness" or performance. "Exercising for health" may require as little as 700 calories per week additional activity.

(4) The CDC now (1993) recommends that we look at physical activity and not just pure exercise as providing a health benefit. This concept includes walking to and from work, manual and not machine-assisted labor at home or work place, and leisure activities that promote recreation and exercise. The CDC suggests to us and our patients that these activities total about 30 minutes per day.

(5) Finally Dr. Mellion emphasizes the importance of "gradual accommodation to exercise" and the avoidance of "exercise addiction." He suggests that 2 days per week be scheduled for regular *rest* and not exercise.

This editorial is an excellent source for advice to our patients who exercise and for educating ourselves.

Reference: Mellion MB: Editorial. Heart Dis Stroke 3:2–4, 1994.

SECOND OPINION II EPIDEMIOLOGY OF OVERUSE SYNDROME IN RUNNERS (OSR)

Walter and Hart in their prospective 1-year study of 1000 runners agree with the amount of mileage run as the prime etiological factor in OSR. In their study, injury was not associated with pace, running surface, hill running, or the experience of the runner. The lowest risk groups for OSR averaged 10 to 19 miles per week, and the highest risk group averaged 30 to 40 miles per week. At this level there was a 50% higher risk for injury.

Reference: Walter SD, Hart LE, et al: Ontario Cohort Study of Running-Related Injuries. Arch Intern Med 149:11, 1989.

SECOND OPINION III BIOMECHANICS

Nuber emphasizes the enormous forces encountered at foot strike by the runner. At heel strike, forces greater than 200% body weight occur. For a 150-lb runner running 1 mile, 110 tons per each foot accumulate. Walking generates approximately 60 to 65 tons per foot. The main difference between the two means of locomotion is the double limb support phase of walking.

Although great emphasis is placed on movement of the subtalar joint (STJ) in the frontal plane, the STJ is a mortise joint with horizontal and transverse vectors of motion. For instance, foot dorsiflexion stabilizes the arch and helps invert the hind foot in the late stance phase. This allows the foot to be a rigid lever as a whole and aids in toe off. The forefoot usually escapes discussion in analyses of biomechanics of the foot. It is important to note that tarsal-metatarsal (T-MT) joints 1 and 5 flex, extend, and supinate and pronate. The remaining T-MT joints flex and extend only. Extension of the T-MTJs promotes plantar fascia tension and arch stabilization.

Reference: Nuber GW: Biomechanics. Clin Sports Med 7:1, 1988.

SECOND OPINION IV CRYOTHERAPY

Although crytotherapy is almost universally safe if a few precautions are observed, Covington and Basset warn clinicians that serious complications can occur. They report six cases of peripheral nerve damage after cryotherapy, all of which occurred in healthy athletes who would be assumed to be at low risk for complications from cryotherapy. The authors suggest that to avoid nerve damage with cryotherapy the following precautions be observed:

(1) Restrict the use of ice to 20 minutes or less.

(2) Always use an insulator between ice and skin.

(3) Use caution when applying ice to patients who are very lean with little subcutaneous adipose tissue.

(4) Avoid ice application over areas of major nerves.

(5) Do not use compression simultaneously with ice.

(6) If you are providing field treatment of injuries, consider commercially-available chemical cold packs. The temperatures yielded by these items are above the 50°F threshold of temperature-related damage to nerves.

Reference: Covington DB, Bassett EH: When cryotherapy injures. Physician Sportsmed 21 (3):1993.

SECOND OPINION V ORTHOTICS

Redford and colleagues agree that primary care clinicians should use caution in prescribing rigid orthotics. They stress, however, that the clinician should be familiar with soft orthotics because these devices will often help their patients' problems. Examples of soft orthotics include soft pads placed over corns, callouses, and bunions, and metatarsal pads. A little additional expertise is needed to treat medial arch pain with a properly fitted insert, but this is well into the "learning curve" of the interested clinician.

These authors stress that even if a clinician is not going to prescribe orthotics, the clinician should know the basics of a good foot exam, be able to measure leg length, and be able to examine a shoe for appropriate and abnormal wear patterns. This is a good introductory article.

Reference: Redbord JB, Reinberg RP, Wu KK: Foot orthoses: For your patients? Patient Care 27:87–106, 1993.

SECOND OPINION VI SHOES

Prescribing proper footwear is critical for athletic performance, injury prevention, and treatment. Wichmann and Martin interviewed several expert professionals about athletic footwear and found these suggestions for primary care practitioners:

(1) Patients who participate in sport more than 3 times per week should use sport-specific footwear.

(2) Patients should be fitted for shoes at the end of the a training session when feet are most swollen.

(3) Shoe length should provide a thumb's breadth between the great toe tip and the end of the shoe.

(4) Women's shoes are typically 1/4″ to 1/2″ narrower than their male counterpart's. Women should use extra care in selecting the width of their shoes.

(5) As an adjunct to width selection, cut out an index card profile of the widest part of the foot. Use this as a sizing insert. If the insert buckles in a trial shoe, it is too tight.

(6) Runners should change shoes every 3 to 6 months or after every 300 to 500 miles of running.

(7) Comfort, not theory, should guide shoe selection. When in doubt, "if the shoe fits, wear it!"

Reference: Wichman S, Martin DR: Athletic shoes: Finding the right fit. Physician Sportsmed 21(3):1993.

SECOND OPINION VII TRAINING PRACTICES

Wes Emmert deals with athletes of all ages and capabilities. He cites the following points as the most important factors for health professionals to be aware of when discussing training with runners.

(1) No one seems to stretch enough. The basic stretching program for a runner should be static stretching of the hamstrings, quadriceps, gastrocnemius, and lumbar spine muscles. Athletes should view stretching as an integral part of injury prevention, not as a preparticipation ritual.

(2) Approach resistance training as a whole body work out. Use resistance which can be tolerated for a 10 to 12 repetition set. Stress movement of the resistance through a full range of motion. Aim for at least two resistance sessions per week. Increase resistance as accommodation occurs. Mild overload, not overuse, is essential.

(3) For the beginning runner, work up to a 2-mile jog at a "conversational" pace and advance training mileage or increase the intensity or pace slowly. Running 4 or 5 days per seek for 2 miles may be enough for most fitness-seeking runners. Early in a program, include cross-training to keep variety in your training and to avoid lower extremity injury. Biking and the use of a flotation vest for "pool running" are suggested activities. If a runner becomes interested in long distance running or going beyond running for fitness alone, consult with a trainer or at least contact a local running club for advice. This will help avoid errors in training and prevent injury.

Wes Emmert was Head Strength and Conditioning Coach at Boston College. He received his undergraduate education at Michigan State University and did graduate work in exercise science at the University of Nebraska. Wes is a certified member of the National Athletic Trainers Association and National Strength and Conditioning Association. He has published several articles on strength and conditioning and frequently lectures on a number of health and fitness topics. He is currently the

Athletic Director at the Rochester Athletic Club, Rochester, Minnesota.

SECOND OPINION VIII MARTY LUHMAN, MARATHONER, ROCHESTER, MN

"I was doing a lot of couch potatoing," says Marty Luhman of his exercise level after retiring from the Air Force ten years ago. He had not run more than a mile or two at a time, but he decided to use running as a means of remaining fit. He literally started with running a few blocks before being able to run 1 mile after 2 months of training. After building up to 15 miles/week, he decided to try to run a marathon. After 4 years of training, he was able to reach the 50 mi/week level at age 45 and began to run marathons. At age 51 he reached another milestone by having run 50 marathons in 50 states.

I recently asked Mr. Luhman for his opinions on injury prevention, training, and injury treatment. His response was "The best program for prevention is stretch, rest, and ice. I work on quadriceps strengthening because I have had a knee operated on (meniscectomy, 1968). For every hour I run, I devote an hour to stretching and rehab activities. I also stop to stretch during a run.

I run from 35 to 40 mi/week in the winter and up to 60 mi/week for marathon training. When I run over 60 mi/week, I notice overuse. I'll use my bike and cross-train to avoid overuse stress. To run a marathon, you should build up to making a 2 to 2 1/2 hour run every week! Do not hesitate to rest if tired.

Yes, I have had injuries. I have sprained my ankles running in the winter and slipping. I have had iliotibial band syndrome, and I missed 9 months of running when I had a stress fracture. When I hurt I do not run, but I do not stop training. I became a biker during my stress fracture rehab; now I can use it as a cross-training tool."

Mr. Luhman enjoys his running. He has not been injury-free; but because he has an outstanding appreciation of how to take care of himself, he heals and perseveres. He runs for enjoyment and fitness, never for "time."

SECOND OPINION IX SHIN SPLINTS

Stretching of both anterior and posterior lower leg muscle groups is important for rehabilitation of "shin splints." Specifically the gastrocsoleus, anterior and posterior tibial muscles, and the peroneus group should be focused upon. Encourage the patient to stretch the selected muscle to its limit of pain-free tension and then hold for up to 60 seconds. Do 10 REPS several times a day. Add resistance with rubber tubing after pain-free full range of motion is achieved. Alternatively, isometrically exercise the muscles with a partner's resistance.

Reference: Fick DS, Albright JP, Murray BP: Relieving painful "shin splints." Physician Sportsmed 20(12):1992.

SECOND OPINION X WOMEN AND STRESS FRACTURES

It is well established that female athletes have more stress fractures than their male cohorts. Hackeling and Richmond review the current etiologies and suggest that the common thread is a decrease in bone-mineral density in these women. The primary causes appear to be the following:

- estrogen deficiency secondary to menstrual dysfunction
- late menarche and heavy exercise
- cigarette smoking, which lowers estrogen levels
- eating disorders and poor nutritional practices

These factors need attention for the appropriate diagnosis, treatment, and prophylaxis of stress fractures in women. The authors suggest the following:

- gradual increases in training loads and careful balance of body weight and weekly mileage
- strict observation of no smoking
- daily calcium intake greater than 800 mg
- use of oral contraceptives in amenorrheic athletes
- couseling athletes and coaches about eating disorders, nutrition, and body image

Reference: Hackeling TA, Richmond JC: Women and stress fractures. Female Patient 18:63–66, 1993.

SECOND OPINION XI ACHILLES TENDINITIS (AT)

Leach, Schepsis, and Takai recommend 3–6 weeks of running and jumping cessation for their patients with AT. Substituting water running, swimming, and biking can help their patients stay fit. To increase foot dorsiflexion, they suggest slow, painless stretching with five to six repetitions. Strengthening of the gastroc soleus muscles is accomplished by dorsiflexing against an elastic cord and when the patient is pain-free, then advancing to toe stands.

Recalcitrant cases of tendinitis may need surgery, including partial resection of the posterior superior aspect of the calcaneus.

Reference: Leach RE, Schepsis AA, Takai HE: Achilles tendinitis. Physician Sportsmed 19(8):1991.

REFERENCES

1. Apple DF: End stage running problems. Clin Sports Med 4:657, 1985.
2. Brody DM: Running injuries. Clin Symp 32:2, 1980.
3. Calabrese LH, Rooney TW: The use of nonsteroidal anti-inflammatory drugs in sports. Physician Sportsmed 14: 89, 1986.
4. Chrisman OD, Snook-Gregory J, Anderson MD, Wilson TC: Aspirin against degeneration of human cartilage. Clin Orthop 84:193, 1972.
5. Clancy WG: Runners' injuries, Part 1. Am J Sports Med 8:138, 1980.
6. Clement DB, Taunton JE, et al: A survey of overuse running injuries. Physician Sportsmed 9:47, 1981.
7. Clement DB, Taunton JE, Smart GW: Achilles tendinitis and peritendinotis: etiology and treatment. Am J Sports Med 12:179, 1984.
8. Collier BD, Johnson RP, et al: Scintigraphic diagnosis of stress-induced in complete fractures of the proximal tibia. J Trauma 24:156, 1984.
9. Cook SD, Kester MA, et al: Biomechanics of running shoe performance. Clin Sports Med 4:619, 1985.
10. Cox JS: Patellofemoral problems in runners. Clin Sports Med 4:669, 1985.
11. D'Ambrosia R: Orthotic devices in running injuries. Clin Sports Med 4:611, 1985.
12. Daffner RH, Martinez S, et al: Stress fractures of the proximal tibia in runners. Diagn Radiol 142:63, 1982.
13. Detmer DE: Chronic leg pain. Am J Sports Med 8:141, 1980.
14. Devas MV: Stress fractures of the tibia in athletes or "shin soreness." J Bone Joint Surg 40B:227, 1958.
15. Devereaux M, Parr G, et al: The diagnosis of stress fractures in athletes. JAMA 252:531, 1984.
16. Drez D: Running footwear. Am J Sports Med 8:140, 1980.
17. Dumont M, Lamourex F, et al: Diagnosis and followup of shin splint syndrome with TC 99m MDP bone scintigraphy. J Trauma 24:156, 1984.
18. Eggold JF: Orthotics in the prevention of runner's overuse injuries. Physician Sportsmed 9:125, 1981.
19. Falkel J: Methods of training. Clin Phys Ther 10:1986.
20. Festa S, Schuster R: Ask the experts what the doctor says. Runner 9:61, 1986.
21. Franklin BA, Rubenfire M: Losing weight through exercise. JAMA 244:377, 1980.
22. Geslien, CE, Thrall JH, et al: Early detection of stress fractures using 99M TC polyphosphate. Radiology 121:683, 1976.
23. Giladi M, Ziv Y, et al: Comparison between radiography, bone scan, and ultrasound in the diagnosis of stress fractures. Milit Med 149:459, 1984.
24. Grana W, Kriegshauser LA: Scientific basis of extensor mechanism disorder. Clin Sports Med 4:247, 1985.
25. Hallel T, Amit S, Seycl D: Fatigue fractures of tibial and femoral shaft in solders. Clin Orthop 118:35, 1976.
26. Harvey JS: Overuse syndromes in young athletes. Pediatr Clin North Am 29:1369, 1982.
27. Hasting AW: The fitness boom. Medical World News, 1984, p 44.
28. Hoppenfeld S: Physical Examination of the Spine and Extremities. Norwalk, CT, Appleton-Century-Crofts, 1976.
29. James SL, Bates BT, Osternig LR: Injuries to runners. Am Sports Med 6:40, 1978.
30. James SL, Brubaker CE: Biomechanics of running. Orthop Clin North Am 4:605, 1973.
31. Knight KL: I.C.E. Phys Sports Med 10:137, 1982.
32. Koplan JP, Powell KE, Sikes RK, et al: An epidemiologic study of the benefits and risks of running. JAMA 248:3118, 1982.
33. LaPorte RE, Dearwater MS, et al: Cardiovascular fitness: Is it really necessary? Physician Sportsmed 13:145, 1985.
34. Leach RE, Schepsis AA, Takai HE: Achilles tendinitis. Physician Sportsmed 19:8, 1991.
35. Leard JS, Guifogle JE: Physiologic basis of warm up and cool down. Clin Phys Ther 10:81, 1986.
36. Levine J: Chondromalacia patella. Phys Sportsmed 7:41, 1979.
37. Lindenberg G, Rinshaw R, Noakes T: Iliotibial band function syndrome in runners. Physician Sportsmed 12:118, 1984.
38. Lutter LD: The knee and running. Clin Sports Med 4:685, 1985.
39. Mann RA, Hagy J: Biomechanics of walking, running, and sprinting. Am J Sports Med 8:345, 1980.
40. Marshall P: The rehabilitation of overuse foot injuries in athletes and dancers. Clin Sports Med 7:1, 1988.
41. McBryde AM: Stress fractures in runners. Clin Sports Med 4:737, 1985.
42. McKeag DB: The concept of overuse. Prim Care 11:43, 1984.
43. McMaster W. Cryotherapy. Physician Sportsmed 10:112, 1982.
44. Mindess RC, Kramer D: Chondromalacia patella: Diagnosis and treatment. Fam Pract Res J 8:26, 1986.
45. Monahan T: Exercise and depression: Swapping sweat for serenity. Physician Sportsmed 14:192, 1986.
46. Mubarah SJ, Haryens AR, Owne CA, et al: The wick catheter technique for measurement of intramuscular pressure. J Bone Joint Surg 58A:1016, 1976.
47. Murphy P: Warming up before stretching advised. Physician Sportsmed 14:45, 1986.
48. Nash H: Can exercise make us immune to disease? Physician Sportsmed 14:250, 1986.
49. Newell SG, Brainvell ST: Overuse injuries to the knee in runners. Physician Sportsmed (12):1984.
50. Newell AG, Woodle A: Cuboid syndrome. Physician Sportsmed 9:71, 1981.
51. Paffenbarger RS, Hyde RT, et al: Physical activity all-cause mortality and mortality and longevity of college alumni. N Engl J Med 314:605, 1986.
52. Polley HF, Hinder GG: Rheumatologic Interviewing and Physical Examination of the Joints, 2nd ed. Philadelphia, W.B. Saunders, 1978.
53. Powell KE, Kohl HW, et al: An epidemiological perspective on the causes of running injuries. Physician Sportsmed 14:100, 1986.
54. Reilly DT, Martens M: Experimental analysis of the quadriceps muscle force and patello-femoral joint reaction force for various activities. Acta Orthop Scand 43:126, 1972.
55. Reneman RS: The anterior and lateral compartment syndrome of the leg due to intensive use of muscles. Clin Orthop 113:69, 1975.
56. Roberts SM, Vogt EC: Pseudofracture of the tibia. J Bone Joint Surg 21:891, 1939.
57. Roy S, Irvin R: Injuries to the running athlete. Sports Med 412, 1983.
58. Rubin BD, Collins HR: Runner's knee. Physician Sportsmed 8:49, 1980.
59. Sady SP, Wortman M, Blanke D: Proprioceptive neuromuscular facilitation. Arch Phys Med Rehab 63:261, 1982.
60. Sallis RE, Jones K: Stress fractures in athletes. Postgrad Med 89:6, 199.
61. Scott S: Current concepts in the rehabilitation of the injured athlete. Mayo Clinic Proc 59:77, 1984.
62. Shyne K: To stretch or not to stretch. Physician Sportsmed 10:1982.
63. Simon HB: Current topics in medicine I. Scientific American Medicine, 1984.

64. Smith WB: Environmental factors in running. Am J Sports Med 8:138, 1980.
65. Stamford B: Training distance and injury in runners. Physician Sportsmed 12:160, 1984.
66. Stanish WD, Curwin S, Rubinovich M: Tendinitis: The analysis and treatment for running. Clin Sports Med 4:593, 1985.
67. Stuart MJ, Karaju TK: Acute compartment syndrome. Physician Sportsmed 22:3, 1994.
68. Subotnich SI, Newell SG: Podiatric Sports Medicine. Mount Kisco, NY, Futura, 1975.
69. Taunton JE, Clement DB, Webber D: Lower extremity stress fractures in athletes. Physician Sportsmed 9:77, 1981.

25

Foot Problems in Athletes

Timothy C. Fitzgibbons, M.D.
Bernard G. Keown, M.D.
Colleen Sampson, L.P.N.
David Burton, Cert. Pedorthist

Although the ankle has clearly been shown to be the joint most often injured in sports activities, there is no question that associated foot problems, especially hindfoot problems, are closely related. There is almost no sports activity in which the foot is not in jeopardy. Whether it be the obvious strenuous sports of basketball or tennis or a less demanding sport such as ping-pong, extensive use of the feet is required. Complaints of discomfort and disability of the foot are commonly heard in the office.

We believe strongly that the primary treatment of most foot problems (including sports related foot problems) is nonsurgical. This places the primary treatment commonly in the hands of the patient's family physician or the team physician covering the individual sport. A basic knowledge of the anatomy, clinical evaluation techniques, and basic treatment principles is required.

This chapter will begin with a review of the anatomy of the foot. It will then progress through evaluation of the patient including careful history-taking, physical examination, and finally recommendations for diagnostic studies. General principles as well as specific treatments for individual problems will be discussed. The chapter will end with suggestions and "pointers" from Colleen Sampson, a nurse specializing in office foot and ankle care techniques. Dave Burton, a Certified Pedorthist, will also discuss shoe modification and shoe fitting techniques that will help in the office management of sports-related foot problems.

ANATOMY

For purposes of discussion in this chapter, the foot is divided into the forefoot, the midfoot, and the hindfoot (Fig. 1). The forefoot includes all structures extending from the base of the metatarsals to the toes. The midfoot includes all structures from the talonavicular and calcaneal cuboid joints to the tarsal metatarsal joints. The hindfoot includes all structures and problems from the ankle joint to the talonavicular and calcaneal cuboid joints. Because the ankle joint itself was addressed in a previous chapter, it will not be included in this section.

The Forefoot

The forefoot includes all five metatarsals with their corresponding metatarsophalangeal (MTP) joints and associated ligamentous and tendinous structures. There are three phalanges in all lesser toes but only two phalanges in the great toe. Sesamoid bones are ossifications in the flexor tendons with articular surfaces. These bones have developed to give a mechanical advantage to toe flexion. Two are normally present in the great toe MTP joint, but other sesamoids can be seen in various parts of the foot.

The toenail is, of course, part of the forefoot. Because injuries to the toenail and specifically ingrown toenails can be a problem in sports, a discussion of treatment of toenail problems is included later in the chapter. The anatomy of the toenail is shown in Figure 2.

The Midfoot

The midfoot includes the talonavicular and calcaneal cuboid joints as well as the three cuneiforms and the articulations at the tarsometatarsal joints. Although the important anatomic landmarks in the midfoot are mainly bone and joint structures, one must remember that there are multiple small sensory nerve branches in the subcutaneous tissues that are frequently injured in sporting activities.

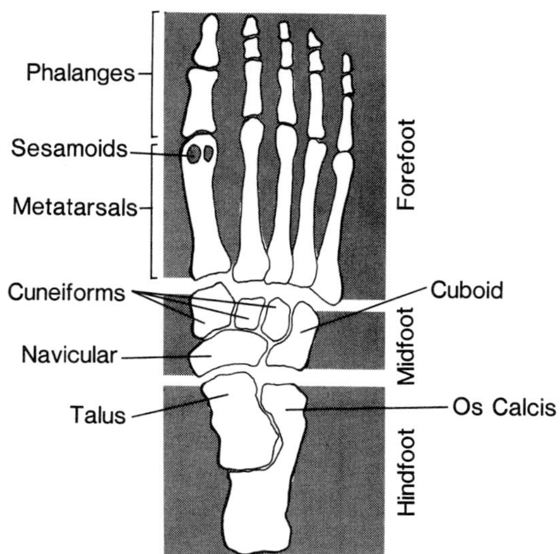

FIGURE 1. Dorsal view showing hindfoot, midfoot, and forefoot.

The Hindfoot

The hindfoot is composed of the talus and calcaneus and three important joints: subtalar joint (talocalcaneal), talonavicular, and calcaneal cuboid. Also of importance is the plantar fascia, which attaches to the calcaneus and extends along the entire plantar aspect of the foot to the toes. The posterior tibial tendon, flexor hallucis longus tendon, flexor digitorum longus tendon, and posterior tibial nerve and vessels traverse the medial aspect of the hindfoot (Fig. 3). On the lateral aspect of the hindfoot the peroneal tendons traverse behind the fibula with the peroneus brevis tendon attaching to the base of the fifth metatarsal and the peroneus longus tendon diving into the plantar aspect of the foot (Fig. 4).

CLINICAL EVALUATION

The clinical evaluation of any sport-related foot problem should follow the basic guidelines set out for the general evaluation of any foot or ankle problem. A satisfactory history must be obtained: factors such as the time of onset, main complaint, location and severity of symptoms, and factors increasing and relieving the symptoms should be ascertained. Any prior treatment and its effectiveness should be determined. The localization and description of the pain must be clarified. Any associated numbness, paresthesias, or weakness should be documented. Deformity and changes in skin color or temperature must be noted. It is important to know whether the patient has developed a limp or gait abnormality. Other important points in the history include preexisting musculoskeletal disorders such as the associated problems of the knee or hip. It is important to know if there has been a discrepancy of leg length in the past. Any problems with the spine or pelvis should be noted. Also any congenital abnormalities or preexisting inflammatory or infectious disorders must be listed.

The physical examination of any sports-related foot problem should include six basic steps. Physical examination should also systematically examine the foot by region (Fig. 5). These regions include the forefoot, midfoot, and hindfoot. It is also important to evaluate the patient in both weight-bearing and non–weight-bearing positions if at all possible.

The inspection part of the evaluation includes a visual observation of swelling, masses, joint effusion, and any changes in the skin or nails. Deformities of the foot and toes should be looked for carefully. Deformities such as hallux valgus, splay foot, hammertoe, or clawtoe should be evaluated. Bony prominences must also be observed. Any evidence of prominences of the calcaneus, such as a pump bump, should be noted.

Hands on palpation includes evaluation for tendon subluxation, atrophy, hyperkeratotic lesions, and any localized areas of tenderness. Effusion of joints should also be evaluated. Muscle contraction against resistance should be evaluated.

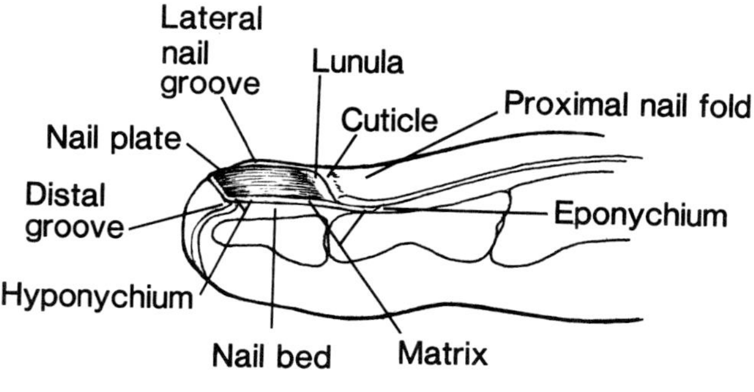

FIGURE 2. Toenail anatomy.

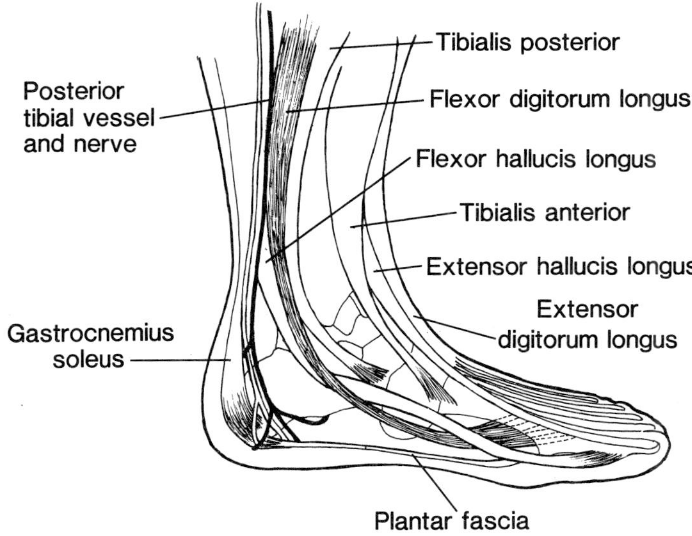

FIGURE 3. Medial aspect of foot and ankle.

Functional evaluation includes active and passive range of motion of all of the joints of the foot. Observation for any pain or crepitus during this evaluation should be documented. Neurovascular evaluation in the sports-related foot problem mainly would be done to evaluate any injury to the peripheral sensory nerves. This is especially common in midfoot and anterior hindfoot injuries.

As noted, it is important to observe patients in a weight-bearing functional mode. Observation of gait is important when possible.

Finally, special clinical tests are sometimes helpful, such as the single and double heel rise test indicative of posterior tibial tendon rupture. Patients with posterior tibial tendon rupture are unable to stabilize their hindfoot in the normal varus position when stepping on the toes. This can be demonstrated stepping on one foot alone or on both feet. Another common clinical test is the Thompson test, which is a squeezing of the calf to look for plantar flexion of the foot (see Figs. 16*A* and *B*). A positive test with no plantar flexion indicates an Achilles tendon rupture. In summary, there is no substitute for a good history and physical examination in the evaluation of sports injuries of the foot. Listening to the patient and careful observation are the hallmarks of diagnosis.

GENERAL DIAGNOSTIC STUDIES

In the acutely injured patient there is almost no time when at least a plain non–weight-bearing x-ray of the foot is not indicated. At the least, AP, lateral, and oblique views of the affected foot should be obtained. In the chronic or subacute pa-

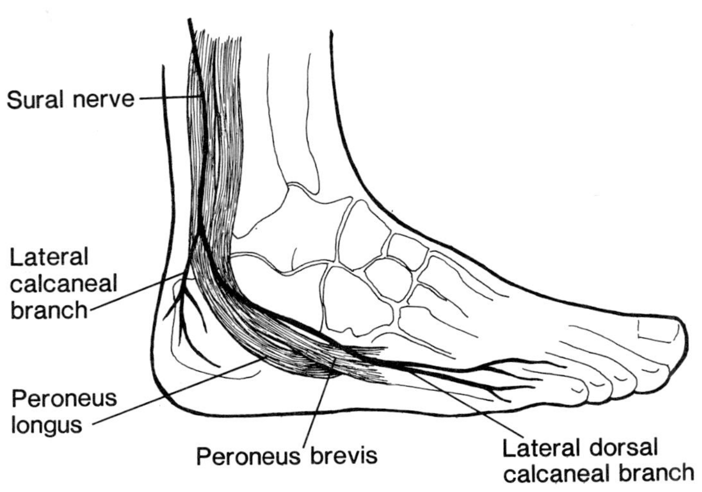

FIGURE 4. Lateral aspect of foot and ankle.

Physical Examination - Six Steps	Physical Examination By Region
•Inspection	•Ankle
•Palpation	•Hindfoot
•Functional evaluation	•Midfoot
•Neurovascular evaluation	•Forefoot
•Gait	
•Special clinical tests	

FIGURE 5. Physical examination.

tient, a standing AP and lateral of both feet with or without an oblique is preferred (Figs. 6 and 7). Not only does this x-ray give information in a weight-bearing or functional position, it also allows comparison with the opposite nonaffected extremity.

Newer diagnostic imaging techniques such as CT and MRI are justified in some circumstances but usually are not considered appropriate as a routine first-line diagnostic studies.

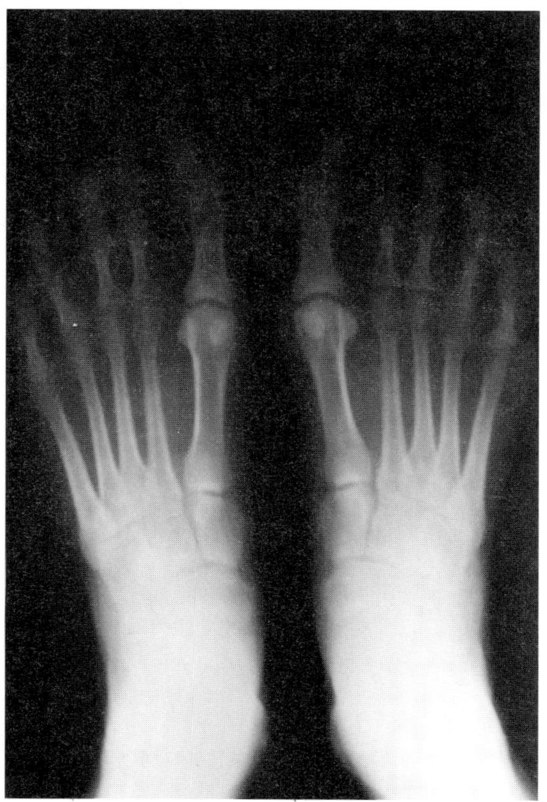

FIGURE 6. Standing AP x-ray of both feet.

SPECIFIC CLINICAL PROBLEMS AND INJURIES

Injuries to the Toenails

Toenail Avulsions. Injuries to the toenails are common, especially in sports in which shoes are not worn. However, any sport requiring running and cutting can cause trauma to the toenails. The toe most often affected is the great toe.

Acute injuries to the toenails usually involve complete or partial avulsion of the nail. When feasible, the nail should be preserved. Trimming the nail back to a stable margin with appropriate wound care will usually suffice. Taping the nail for protection can also be helpful.

Ingrown Toenail. Ingrown toenails are common in adolescence and therefore are commonly encountered in the adolescent athlete. When possible, conservative nonsurgical treatment should be used. Most ingrown toenails actually can be looked at as "overgrowth of the soft tissue over the nail" rather than a true ingrowing of the nail. On the tibial side this usually occurs because of hyperpronation of the great toe. On the fibular side it tends to occur because of pressure of the great toe against the second toe. Techniques to try to relieve these forces that promote ingrown toenail inflammation, such as spacers between the toes and the use of wide toe box shoes, should always be recommended. Once the inflammation occurs, twice-a-day soaking with a "soft tissue teasing technique" can be dramatic (Figs. 8 and 9). When these conservative measures fail, marginal nail excision is the usual surgical treatment of choice.

Subungual Hematoma. A common sports-related office complaint is the development of a dark or blackened area underneath a toenail. Far and away, the most common cause is a subungual hematoma. This can occur with just the excessive forces of pronation and pressure against the shoe encountered in sports such as tennis or racquetball. One must always

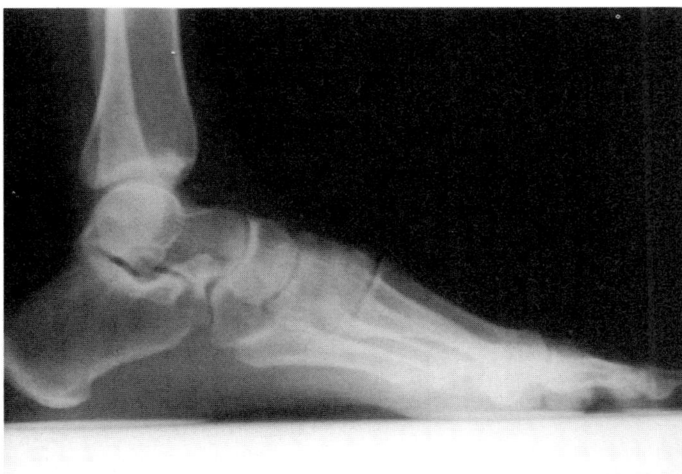

FIGURE 7. Standing lateral x-ray of foot.

be concerned about the possibility of underlying neoplasm, such as subungual melanoma or glomus tumor. However, the much more common explanation is subungual hematoma. If the patient clearly has had preexisting trauma, then these lesions can be observed. Patients should be informed that it can take months for these to slowly resolve. If they do not resolve, exploration and biopsy may be necessary.

Problems of the Great Toe

Turf Toe. Perhaps no sports-related foot injury has received more attention than "turf toe."[4,5,6,40,43] Although some controversy exists over the exact definition, in this discussion turf toe refers to symptoms that occur at the MTP joint as a result of hyperdorsiflexion (extension), hyperplantarflexion, or valgus injuries. The most common injury is hyperextension with plantar capsular involvement. Treatment of the acute injury is nonoperative. For the minor injuries, simple rest, ice therapy, and elevation may be all that is necessary. Stiffening of the sole of the shoe is used to prevent future injury. Various methods are available to stiffen the sole of the athlete's shoe. Figure 35 demonstrates the use of an extended steel shank built into the sole of the shoe. Another method is to use turf toe plates or stiff inlays that can be placed directly in the shoe. These inlays, although easier to use, are not always tolerated by the athlete and, therefore, a formal modification of the sole of the shoe is sometimes necessary. For the

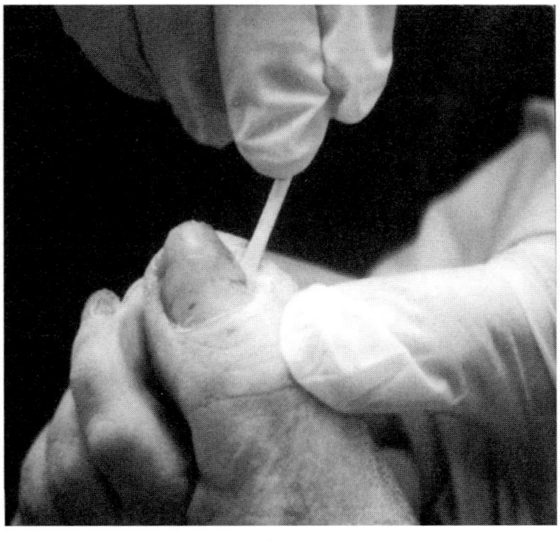

FIGURE 8. Soak the foot for 20 minutes in plain warm water. The tissues will be soft and pliable to work with. Then "tease" the tissue back away from the nail with a manicure stick.

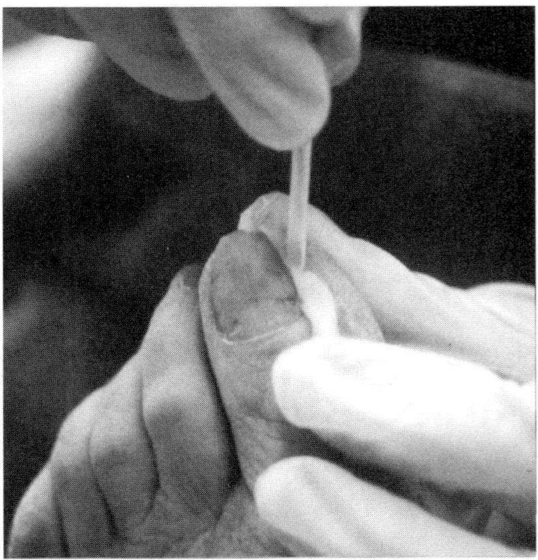

FIGURE 9. Take a strand of a cottonball and wet it with plain warm water. Roll it slightly until cylindrical. Tuck cotton strand along the border of the nail. Blot out excess moisture and trim the ends if necessary. Do this twice daily until the inflammation settles down.

more severe cases, formal physical therapy, non–weight-bearing with crutches, and even plaster immobilization may be necessary.

Depending on the type of injury, taping may be used to counter the forces that caused the initial injury. If the injury was hyperdorsiflexion, taping is used to keep the toe from dorsiflexing. If the injury was hyperplantarflexion, then the reverse taping technique is used. Coker et al. studied a group of athletes and concluded that turf toe involved an injury to the great toe MTP joint complex which was probably related to shoe construction and types of playing surfaces.[8] They felt that the incidence was increasing and that surgery was indicated only when specific disruptions occurred such as fractures of the sesamoids or specific tendon or capsular tears.

Hallux Rigidus. Hallux rigidus is a premature degenerative arthritis that occurs at the great toe MTP joint.[17] The classic patient is the man aged 30–50 who presents to the physician's office complaining of a "bump" on the top of his great toe MTP joint. He also complains of a lack of dorsiflexion of the toe and thus an inability to walk with a normal gait. A common complaint is that the patient can no longer "walk 18 holes of golf."

X-rays show a spur on the dorsum of the distal first metatarsal (Fig. 10). The amount of true degenerative arthritis in the joint is variable. Initial treatment is to minimize the forces of dorsiflexion across the great toe MTP joint. This is accomplished with stiffening of the sole of the shoe or the use of the new lightweight stiff Vibram type soles. Surgery may be helpful in advanced cases. Initial surgical treatment is aimed at removing enough distal metatarsal to allow more dorsiflexion of the joint. If this fails, the definitive treatment recommended is arthrodesis of the joint. Use of Silastic implants or total toe replacements are not recommended because of the common complications encountered. These complications can be devastating and make any possible advantages of replacement surgery not worth the risk.

Miscellaneous Forefoot Problems

Painful Bunions, Bunionettes, and Corns. The great toe bunion is a painful bursa on the medial aspect of the MTP joint occurring because of shoe pressure. The bunionette is the same type of bursal formation on the lateral aspect of the fifth metatarsophalangeal joint. Corns are skin changes on the tops of the toes or between the toes secondary to pressure of the toes against the top of the shoe or toes against each other. The common denominator in all these problems is pressure against a bony prominence. For that reason, any measure that alleviates pressure of the shoe against bony prominences usually cures these problems. Patients with preexisting above-described deformities who are involved in sports will have pressure-related problems. The primary treatment should be shoe modification and different techniques will be discussed later in this chapter. Surgical intervention is justified in cases failing conservative treatment. However, athletes, especially elite athletes, should be warned that some motion, and thus performance, may be lost with surgery.

Metatarsalgia. Metatarsalgia is pain in the ball of the foot secondary to excess pressure against all or some of the metatarsal heads. This can be especially problematic in runners who are "toe runners." Treatment is directed at alleviating the force concentrations to this area of the foot and usually can be accomplished with soft inlays in the shoes or changes in the type of sole of the shoe.

Metatarsal and Phalangeal (Toe) Fractures. Metatarsal and phalangeal (toe) fractures that occur in sports are treated in the same manner as any other similar fractures would be treated. In the lesser toes, except for an occasional dislocation or interarticular fracture, nonsurgical treatment is almost always indicated. This usually involves an initial period of rest followed by stiffening of the soles of the shoes and taping of the toes. Fractures involving the great

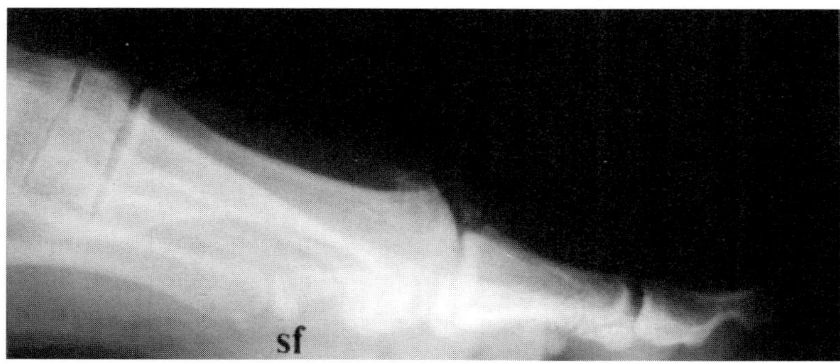

FIGURE 10. Lateral x-ray of patient with hallux rigidus and dorsal bunion. See the large spur formation formed on the dorsum of the distal metatarsal and also, in this severe case, a secondary spur which has formed on the proximal dorsal portion of the proximal phalanx.

toe are more aggressively treated with occasional open reduction and internal fixation. Most metatarsal fractures can be treated with a temporary wooden shoe followed by a stiff walking or tennis shoe. Casting is only occasionally necessary. A major exception to this is the fracture of the base of the fifth metatarsal, which will be discussed under a separate section.

Interdigital Neuroma. Interdigital neuroma is a thickening of the distal branches of the plantar nerve usually at the bifurcation into digital nerves to the inner aspects of two adjoining toes (Fig. 11). This entity, commonly called Morton's neuroma, is usually caused by either compressive trauma of two metatarsal heads against this nerve or a tethering that occurs just distal to the transverse metatarsal ligament. Classic symptoms are burning of two adjoining toes, a feeling of a mass in the plantar aspect of the foot at the intermetatarsal level, and relief of symptoms with removal of the shoes. This problem usually occurs in women who chronically wear high-heeled narrow toebox shoes. Interdigital neuroma, however, can occur in athletes, especially runners. Treatment usually consists of wide toebox shoes, anti-inflammatories, physical therapy, injections, various shoe modifications, and surgical excision as a last resort.

Stress Fractures. Stress fractures do not occur with sudden acute trauma but rather with repetitive trauma such as in running sports.[18,33,34] Patients usually complain of an initial vague ache followed by progressive swelling and discomfort. Initial x-rays may be negative. Bone scanning may be of benefit. For metatarsal stress fractures, treatment primarily consists of rest, use of stiff-soled shoes, and time. Only occasionally is immobilization with a cast necessary. For other bones, casting and occasional surgery may be necessary. Common bones of the foot affected: metatarsal, sesamoids, navicular, and occasionally the cuboid.

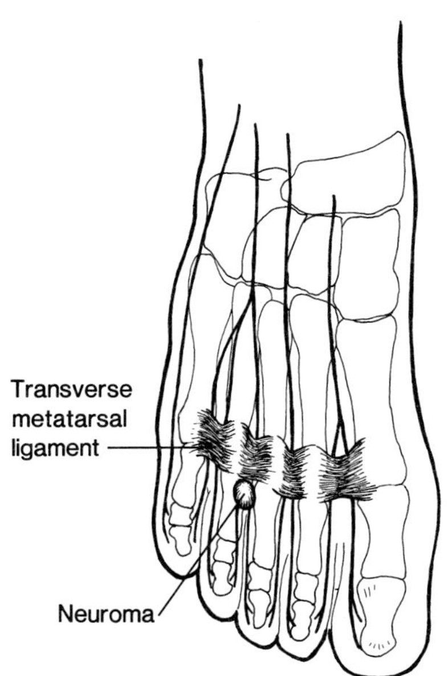

FIGURE 11. Interdigital neuroma.

Sesamoiditis and Sesamoid Fractures. The sesamoid bones of the metatarsophalangeal joint are subject to heavy repetitive loads. They are therefore vulnerable to both acute and chronic injury.[9,32,35] Acute injuries of the sesamoids usually involve soft-tissue inflammation or sesamoid fracture. These fractures are usually of the avulsion type. Chronic injuries include sesamoiditis, stress fracture, avascular necrosis, and even degenerative arthritis. Sesamoiditis refers to inflammation associated with chondromalacia of the articular surface as well as synovitis. Any patient with pain in the plantar aspect of the great toe MTP joint should be suspect for sesamoid injury or inflammation. Differential diagnosis can be accomplished with plain x-rays, tomograms, and CT, MRI, and bone scans. Treatment of sesamoid problems, however, is initially the same regardless of the diagnosis. Ice therapy, elevation, anti-inflammatory medications, and rest, usually through a period of partial weight-bearing, are indicated. As symptoms improve, measures to decrease the pressure with sports activities should be used. Surgery for chronic sesamoid problems is occasionally justified but usually only if nonsurgical treatment has failed. Conservative measures should be tried for a long period of time, usually for at least a year before considering surgery.

Midfoot

Tarsometatarsal and other Midfoot Sprains. Pain in the midfoot after athletic injury is not uncommon.[39] Symptoms can localize at various regions of the tarsometatarsal joint as well as the intercuneiform and navicular cuneiform joints. Most of these injuries are soft tissue inflammation and ligamentous sprains, and most are self-limited and can be treated with rest, antiinflammatory medication, and local physical treatment. Activities can be gradually resumed; use of a stiff-soled shoe may be helpful.

Of importance with tarsometatarsal injuries is the recognition of a Lisfranc's fracture dislocation.[11] Standing x-rays of both feet allow comparison of the tarsometatarsal articulations. Any evidence of a difference from one side to the other should alert the physician of the possibility of a more significant Lisfranc's injury. In chronic injuries, localized injections may be of benefit. With severe tarsometatarsal and midfoot sprains, short-term casting and non–weight-bearing status can also be justified.

Superficial Contusion of the Midfoot and the Anterior Hindfoot. Any injury involving a direct blow to the skin and and subcutaneous tissue of the midfoot or more proximally in the anterior hindfoot can cause either temporary or permanent neural injury.[14,38] This involves the superficial cutaneous nerve branches. Symptoms usually are consistent with the injury, with paresthesias into the dorsum of the forefoot, especially into the toes (Fig. 12). Neuroma formation occasionally can be present. The most significant physical finding is a positive percussion test at the level of the injury causing paresthesias distally. Although most of these cases can be treated nonsurgically with shoe decompression, surgical decompression occasionally is warranted for refractory cases.

Stress Fracture of the Navicular. Stress fractures of the navicular are a well-described injury especially in the adolescent athlete.[20] Any young athlete with persistent pain in or around the navicular should be suspected for a stress fracture. Diagnosis can be extremely difficult, as plain AP x-rays often are not diagnostic. Localized views of the navicular or more sophisticated testing such as bone scanning or CT may be necessary. Treatment initially consists of cast immobilization followed by gradual resumption of activities. Patients who are refractory to treatment may require cancellous screw fixation and bone grafting.

Avulsion Fracture of the Base of the Fifth Metatarsal (Jones' Fracture). Because of the blood supply to the base of the fifth metatarsal, any fracture in this area can be fraught with delayed union or nonunion.[24,28,46,47] The peroneus brevis tendon attaches to the base of the fifth metatarsal. Inversion injuries of the ankle and hindfoot may easily cause an avulsion fracture of the base of the fifth metatarsal. When this fracture involves only the most proximal portion and represents a small fragment, it is a benign injury. Most of these can be treated with a stiff-soled shoe. Casting is not usually necessary. However, those fractures of the base of the fifth metatarsal that extend to the proximal diaphysis are a different injury (Fig. 13). Because of the blood supply difficulties described above, these fractures are prone to delayed union and even nonunion. Many such fractures present as incomplete stress fractures and appear benign. However, the patients continue to have symptoms throughout the season, and delay in diagnosis is common. These fractures usually heal with early immobilization and casting, but it can take a long time. In elite athletes, recent evidence has shown that early cannulated screw fixation can speed recovery and is sometimes justified. One must weigh the risks of surgery with the benefits of early healing.

Hindfoot

Peroneal Tendinitis and Subluxation. Since acute inversion injuries of the hindfoot and chronic varus stresses on the hindfoot are common in athletics, peroneal tendon injuries and subluxation must be discussed.[1,12,15,23,26,36,41,44] Subluxation of

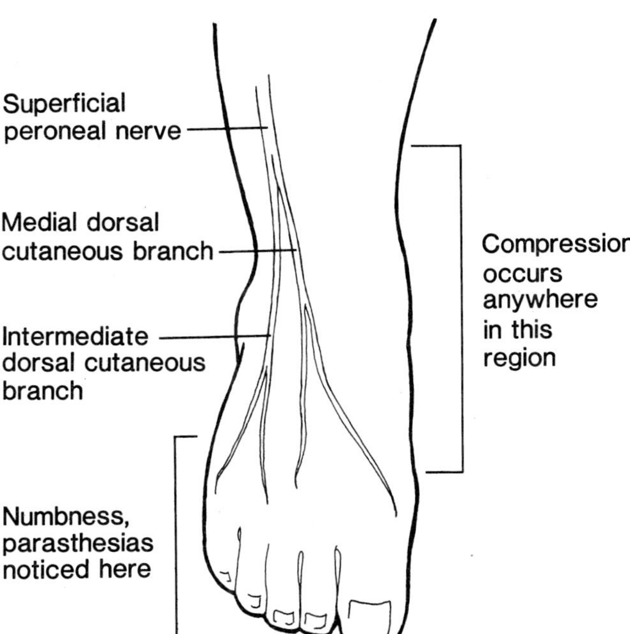

FIGURE 12. Nerve contusions.

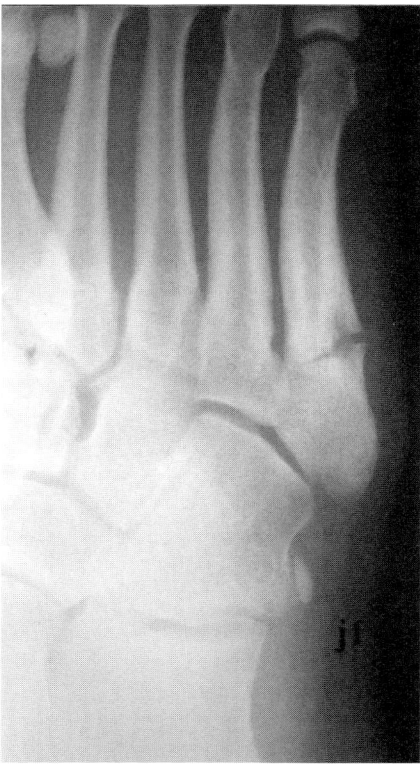

FIGURE 13. X-ray of Jones' fracture.

the peroneal tendons may occur in the acute patient after an injury damaging the retinaculum. Some patients, however, because of the shallowness of the peroneal groove behind the fibula, develop symptoms spontaneously. These patients commonly have bilateral symptoms. Treatment of peroneal subluxation is initially nonsurgical with the usual acute anti-inflammatory treatment followed by different types of padding and taping techniques to prevent the recurrent subluxation. If, however, the subluxation continues and is painful, then surgical intervention is warranted. Surgery involves reconstruction of the retinaculum or various procedures to deepen the peroneal groove.

Peroneal tendinitis and partial and complete peroneal tendon ruptures are probably more commonly seen. There have been many recent descriptions in the literature of patients with lateral ankle injuries and symptoms that do not respond to treatment. Many of these patients have been found to have partial tears or avulsions of the peroneal tendons. MRI is the test of choice for signal changes in the peroneal tendon. Initial treatment is nonsurgical with physical therapy, anti-inflammatory medications, and occasionally injections into the peroneal tendon sheath (not into the tendon itself). However, when conservative treatment fails, exploration of the peroneal tendons with repair or tenodesis may be justified.

Medial Hindfoot Tendinitis. Any patient with persistent medial ankle and medial hindfoot pain and tenderness should be suspected for medial hindfoot tendinitis. The tendons involved are the posterior tibial tendon, which attaches to the medial navicular; the flexor digitorum tendon, which is just posterior to the posterior tibial tendon; and the flexor hallucis longus tendon. Treatment of these is similar to that for the peroneal tendonitises, with physical therapy, anti-inflammatory medications, and occasionally injection into the tendon sheath. Medial wedges in the athlete's shoe and occasionally soft inlays in the shoe may also be of benefit. Patients with posterior tibial tendinitis tend to have an associated flexible flatfoot. Also, an accessory naviular bone commonly is seen. These patients may have a prominent bony deformity on the medial aspect of their foot at which a bursa can form and show signs of occasional acute fluid accumulation and discoloration. Beware of the use of a hard arch support in these patients, as the pressure of this bony prominence against the hard arch support can make the problem worse. If these patients fail nonsurgical treatment, then an MRI may be obtained to look at the status of the tendon; occasional tendon sheath release with cast immobilization is warranted.

Injections in either the medial or lateral hindfoot tendon should be done with great caution. Injection into the tendon itself can precipitate tendon rupture in time and therefore should be avoided. Any injection should be done only once or twice and should be into the tendon sheath and not actually into the tendon.

Tarsal Tunnel Syndrome. On the medial aspect of the hindfoot the posterior tibial nerve traverses posterior to the medial tendons, underneath the flexor retinaculum, and enters the plantar aspect of the foot. At the level of the flexor retinaculum it branches into the medial plantar and lateral plantar nerves. Multiple branches of the lateral plantar nerve innervate areas of the heel (Fig. 14). Compression of the posterior tibial nerve has classically given symptoms of numbness in the plantar aspect of the foot but has very commonly mimicked the symptoms of classic plantar fascitis and plantar heel pain. Much has been written recently about the first branch of the lateral plantar nerve and its branch to the abductor digiti minimi as a cause of heel pain.[38] In patients for whom plantar fascitis treatment has failed, tarsal tunnel syndrome or compressive injuries to branches of the posterior tibial nerve should be considered. Treatment, however, should be nonsurgical for an extended period of time because recent reports have shown that the surgical treatment of tarsal tunnel release is not particularly successful, and to some extent "the cure may be worse than the disease."[46]

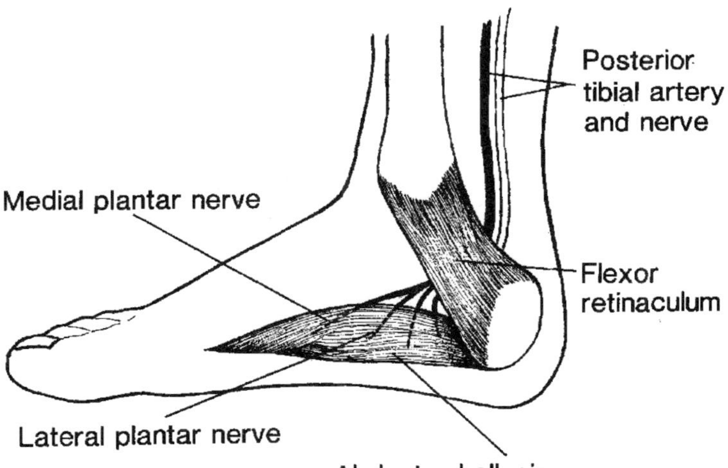

FIGURE 14. Branches of the posterior tibial nerve—medial foot and ankle.

Plantar Fasciitis. One of the most common athletic problems encountered is pain on the plantar aspect of the foot in the region of the plantar fascial attachment to the calcaneus.[3] The classic symptoms are pain on first arising in the morning, some relief of symptoms with walking and stretching of the foot, recurrence of symptoms after rising from a sitting position during the day, and localization to the plantar aspect of the heel usually more medial than lateral. It is extremely common and is quite analogous to the lateral epicondylitis (tennis elbow) seen in the upper extremity. Although many of these patients on x-ray are found to have calcification at or near the plantar fascial attachment to the calcaneus (heel spur), most authorities do not feel this calcification is significant. Rather, the pain occurs because of the stretching of the plantar fascia at an inflamed area. These problems almost invariably fade away with time but unfortunately it can take months or even years for the symptoms to disappear completely. The role of the physician is to control the symptoms and make the athlete comfortable enough to perform while nature takes its course. Surgical intervention, which should be considered only after prolonged nonsurgical treatment, includes release of the plantar fascia with or without decompression of the branches of the posterior tibial nerve.

Nonsurgical treatment includes antiinflammatory medication, various types of heel cups, physical therapy, and injections of cortisone. Our recent experience with formal physical therapy as a treatment of plantar fasciitis has shown that modality treatments, such as ultrasound and steroid phonophoresis, are helpful on a short-term basis.[25] Long-term relief seemed to be best accomplished with plantar fascial and Achilles' tendon stretching and a good home program.

Pump Bump Syndrome. A common complaint among young athletes is the development of a painful bursa on the posterior aspect of the heel usually just superior and lateral to the attachment of the Achilles' tendon (Fig. 15). This adventitial bursa or thickening of the skin and subcutaneous tissue develops from pressure of the shoe against a prominent posterior superior calcaneal tuberosity. Treatment includes physical therapy, antiinflammatory medication, shoe modification aimed at taking the

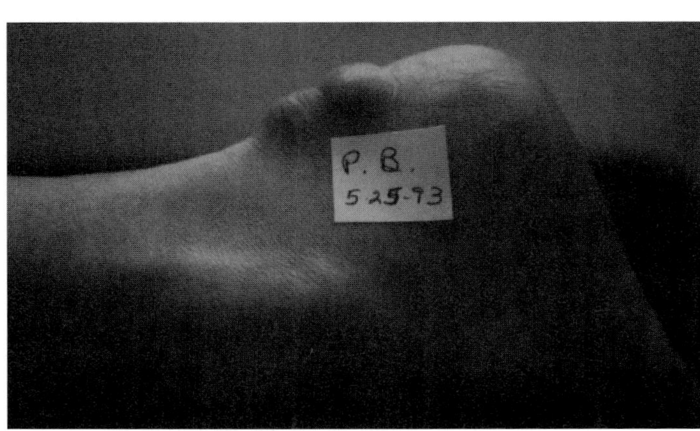

FIGURE 15. Pump bump.

pressure of the counter of the shoe away from this bony prominence. This can be accomplished with heel lifts to elevate the foot away from the counter or by splitting and padding this posterior counter. If nonsurgical treatment fails, surgical removal of a generous portion of the posterior superior calcaneal tuberosity is indicated. Risks of surgery, of course, involve wound healing problems and rupture of the Achilles' tendon; therefore, surgery should not be entered into lightly.

Retrocalcaneal Bursitis. Retrocalcaneal bursitis can present with symptoms very similar to the previously described pump bump syndrome. These patients, however, usually localize symptoms to an area slightly more superior and in more proximity to the Achilles' tendon. They also tend to have symptoms more related to Achilles' tendon function. Treatment is usually nonsurgical with antiinflammatory medications and physical treatment. Occasional injection into the retrocalcaneal bursa (not in the Achilles' tendon) may be justified. If nonsurgical treatment fails, surgical excision can be considered.

Achilles' Tendinitis and Rupture. One of the more common and frustrating problems of the hindfoot is the development of Achilles' tendinitis, Achilles' prerupture symptoms, and of course ultimately Achilles' tendon rupture.[7,16,19,21,27] Beware of the middle-aged athlete who begins to complain of discomfort either in the mid-calf or Achilles' tendon area as this may be nature's warning of impending rupture. Symptoms may be localized in the calf, along the Achilles' tendon itself, or even at the attachment to the calcaneus. Treatment includes rest, physical therapy, Achilles' tendon stretching exercise, heel lifts, and sometimes even cast immobilization. If symptoms persist, an MRI may be justified to ascertain signal changes consistent with partial rupture or intrasubstance tearing. In certain patients exploration of the tendons through a posterior incision may be justified.

Rupture of the Achilles' tendon may present the physician with a diagnostic challenge and a treatment recommendation challenge. In patients with incomplete rupture some plantar flexion may still be possible even with a significant injury. The Thompson test or squeezing the calf and watching for plantar flexion of the foot is very helpful (Fig. 16A and B). This is done with the patient prone with both feet hanging over the end of the table. Both calves are squeezed equally, and the amount of plantar flexion that occurs is compared. If it is absent or diminished on the affected side, this is a positive Thompson test. MRI may also be helpful in determining rupture of the Achilles' tendon. In terms of treatment, there are two schools of thought, both with good statistical evidence of good results. Nonsurgical treatment includes cast immobilization with the foot in plantar flexion for an extended period of time. Part of this cast immobilization period is with a long-leg cast and part with a short-leg cast. Usually, a total of 3 months of immobilization is required. The patient is then protected for six months to a year with heel lifts in the shoe. Physical therapy is usually helpful. The statistical results in comparison with surgery are very similar. There is a slightly higher rerupture rate and some question of a decrease in the eventual strength of the tendon. For the middle-aged amateur athlete this is certainly a viable option and should be presented to all patients.

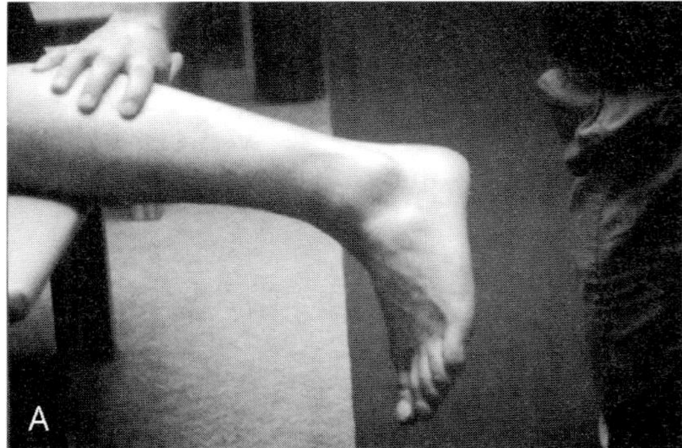

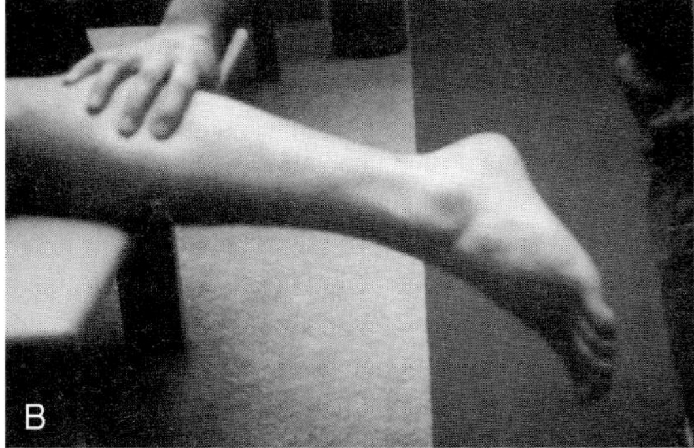

FIGURE 16. *A,* With the patient prone and the foot hanging over the table and the calf not being squeezed the foot is in neutral position. *B,*Upon squeezing the calf muscles, the foot plantar flexes. In a patient with an Achilles' tendon rupture, squeezing of the calf would not produce plantar flexion of the foot and thus would be a positive test.

Surgical treatment involves exploration of the tendon and repair as necessary. The immobilization time after surgery varies but in general is slightly shorter than the nonsurgical treated patients. Complications include wound healing and infection. Careful presentation of the pros and cons of both forms of treatment must be given to all patients with an Achilles' tendon rupture. Most orthopedists involved with sports medicine recommend a repair for those very active athletes with Achilles' tendon ruptures.

PRACTICAL OFFICE AND SHOE MODIFICATION FOR ATHLETIC INJURIES OF THE FOOT

Along with the physician, trainer, and physical therapist, other allied medical personnel can be helpful. In foot and ankle problems, these people are the certified pedorthist and the foot and ankle nurse. A certified pedorthist has special training and certification in making shoe modifications as prescribed by a physician. In our practice, Colleen Sampson, LPN, has special training in foot and ankle problems and has been extremely helpful in teaching patients practical treatment measures for athletic foot and ankle problems. Dave Burton is a Certified Pedorthist who has been extremely helpful in fabrication of shoes and shoe modification to help injured athletes in our practice. The following section includes some of these practical office and shoe modification measures.

OFFICE DEVICES FOR COMMON FOOT PROBLEMS

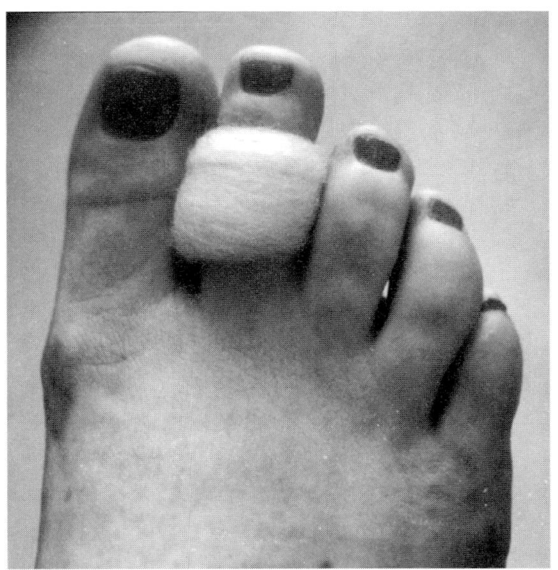

FIGURE 17. Lambs' wool helps to relieve hammertoes, corns, etc. Also absorbs perspiration. May be used when "buddy taping" fractured toes to prevent maceration.

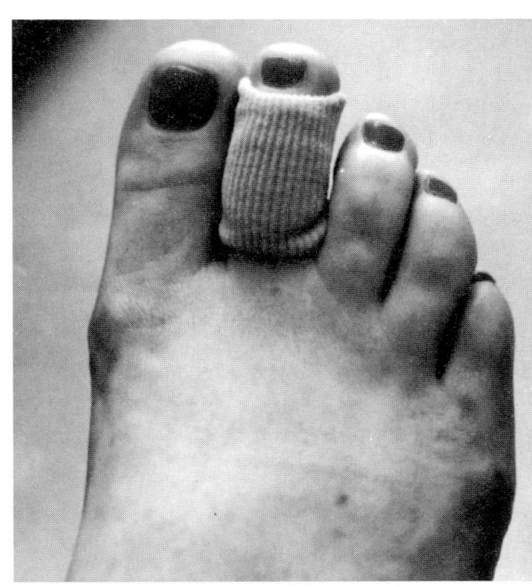

FIGURE 18. Silopad toe pads relieve the pressure of hammertoes, corns, soft corns, etc.

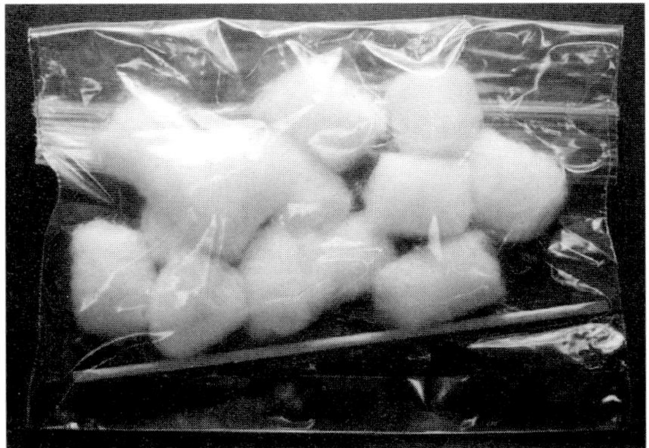

FIGURE 19. Toenial kit consists of cotton balls and a manicure (orange) stick.

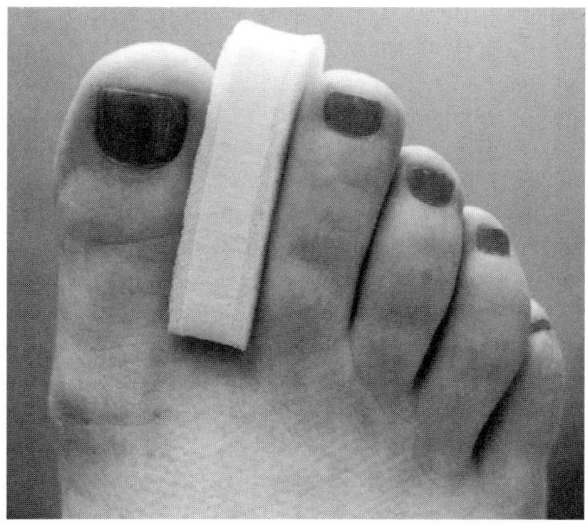

FIGURE 20. Toe separators, for relief of soft corns and to maintain alignment for bunions.

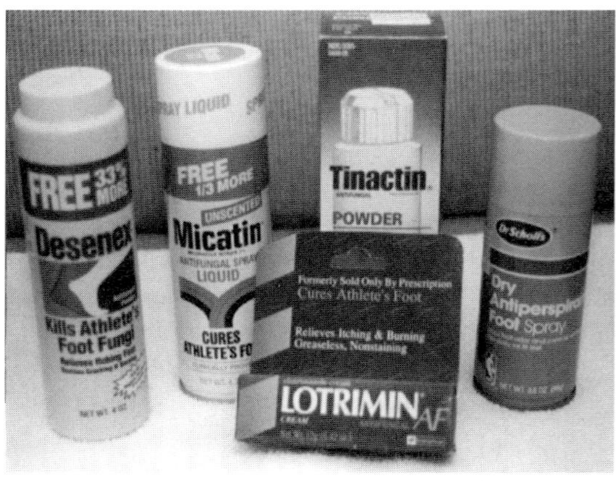

FIGURE 21. Over-the-counter products available for common fungal infections of the foot.

TREATMENT OF PLANTAR FASCITIS

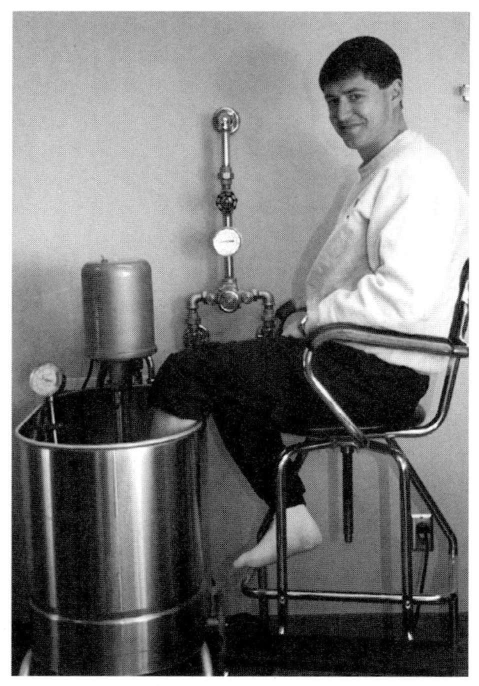

FIGURE 22. Whirlpool. One of the many modalities helpful in sports injuries, including plantar fascitis.

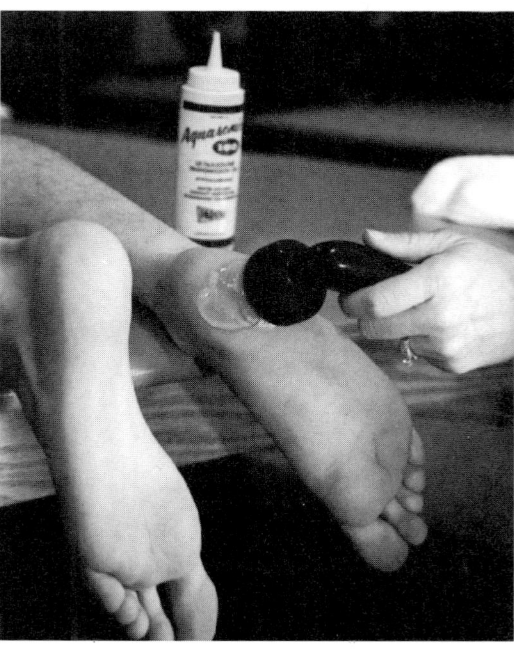

FIGURE 23. Ultrasound may be used for an inflammatory problems in the foot, including plantar fascitis.

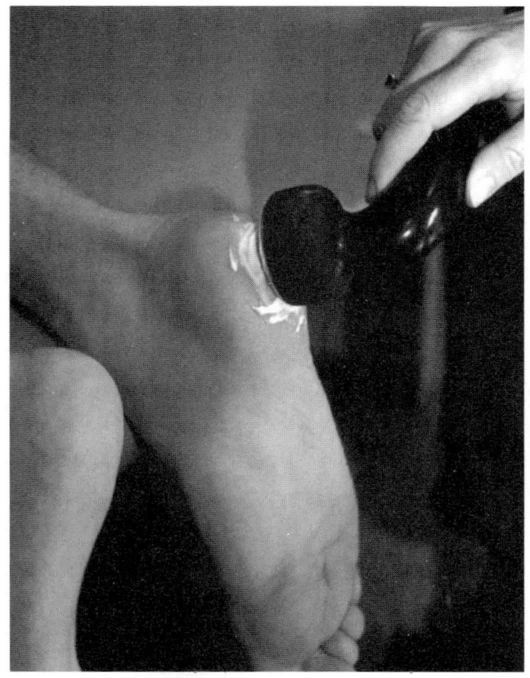

FIGURE 24. Steroid phonophoresis—10% hydrocortisone cream mixed with ultrasound gel. Small amount of gylcerin added for consistency. This is prepared by a pharmacist.

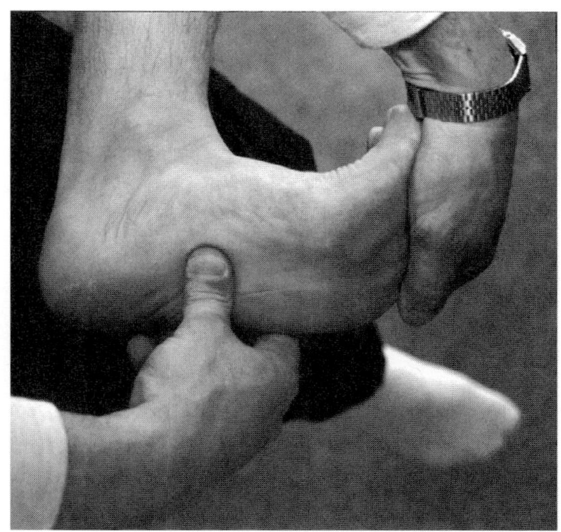

FIGURE 25. Plantar fascial stretching.

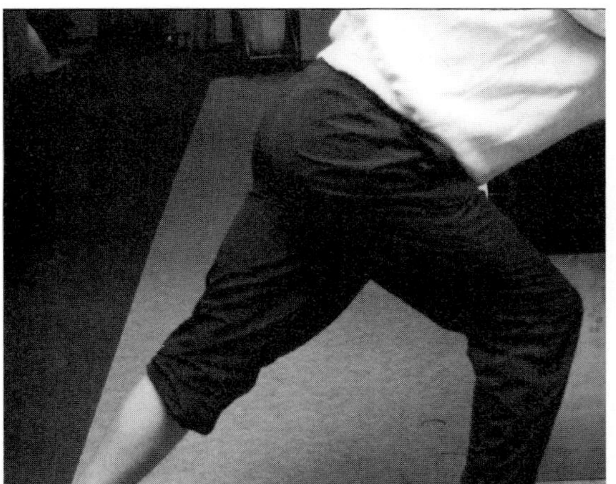

FIGURE 26. Achilles' tendon and gastrocnemius stretching (to isolate the Achilles' tendon for stretching, the knee should be flexed).

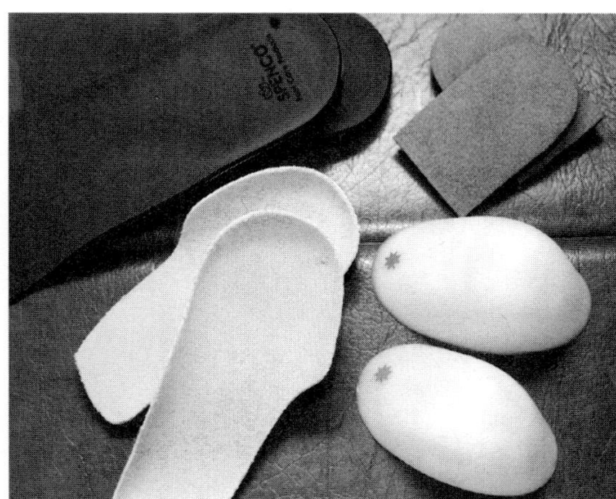

FIGURE 27. Heel cups/pads are useful for mild plantar fascitis, "heel spur," and general cushioning effect.

SHOE MODIFICATIONS AND SHOE TYPES

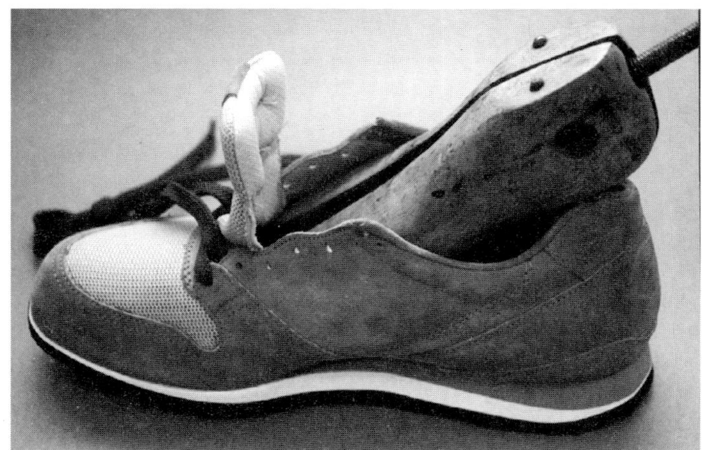

FIGURE 28. Shoe stretcher, used to widen the toe box area or to raise the instep of the shoe when one foot is larger or swelling is present in one foot.

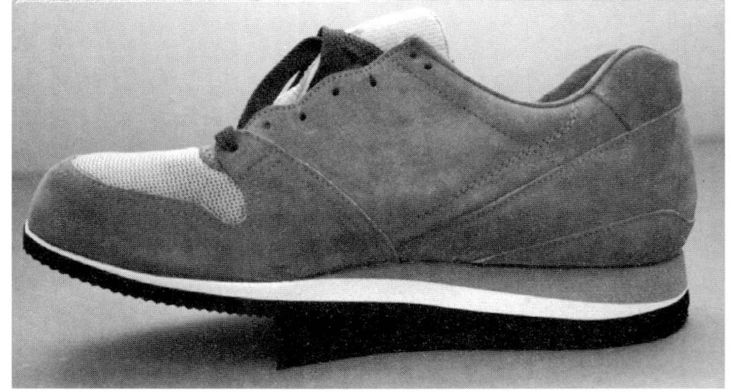

FIGURE 29. Metatarsal bar, used for sesamoiditis and metatarsalgia. The shoes can be modified in several ways to relieve forefoot pain.

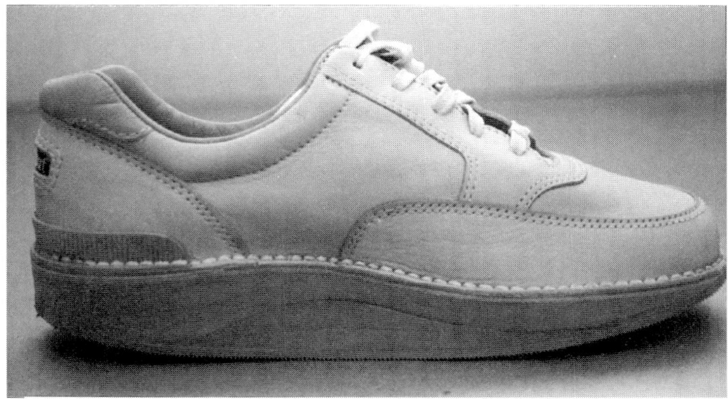

FIGURE 30. Mid-foot roller sole, used to limit ankle motion for arthritis of the subtalar joint or mid-foot. It is more effective with custom-molded inlays.

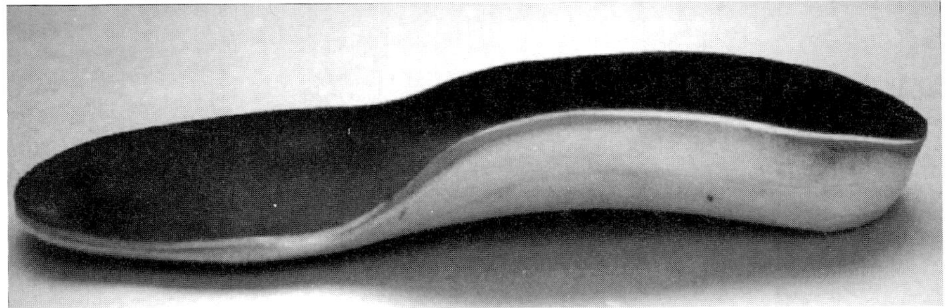

FIGURE 31. Custom-molded inlay with medial reinforcement, used for posterior tibial tendon dysfunction, arthritis, diabetes, prominent metatarsal heads or dropped metatarsal heads. It should be used with a shoe that has an extended medial counter and a broad, flat heel base. It may also be used with the mid-foot roller for ankle/mid-foot arthritis.

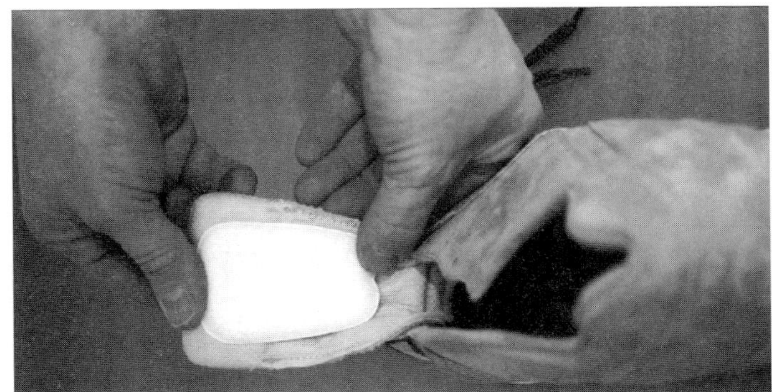

FIGURE 32. Self-adhesive tongue pad, used to tighten the overall fit of a shoe by forcing the heel further back into the counter of the shoe. It may be cut out to relieve prominent bony areas of the dorsum of the mid-foot or cut and placed anywhere that localized padding is required.

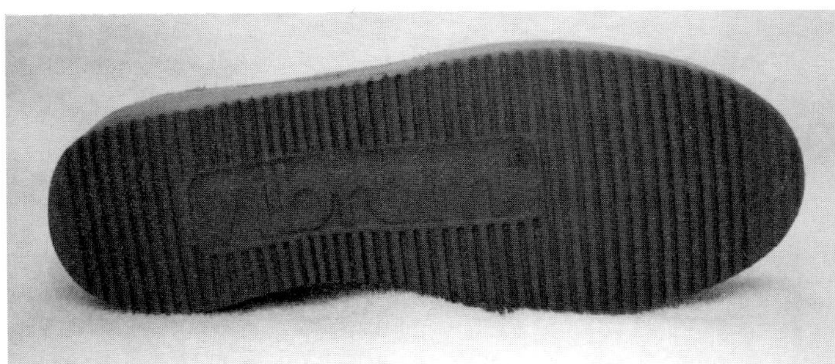

FIGURE 33. Vibram sole provides cushion and good traction, and is useful in shoe modifications.

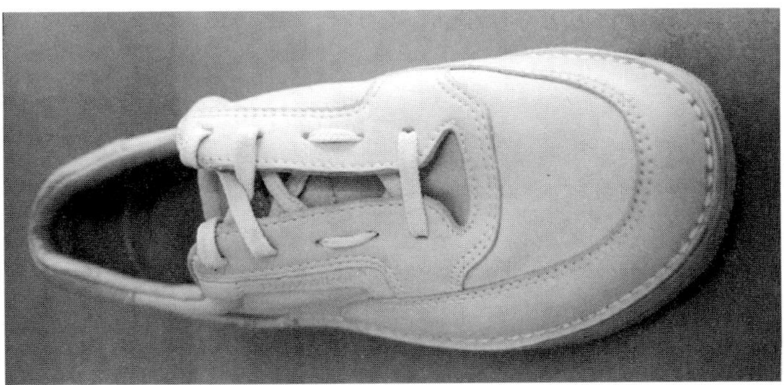

FIGURE 34. Skip an eyelet. This is used with a cut-out tongue pad to lessen pressure due to laces overriding prominent bony areas on the dorsum of the mid-foot.

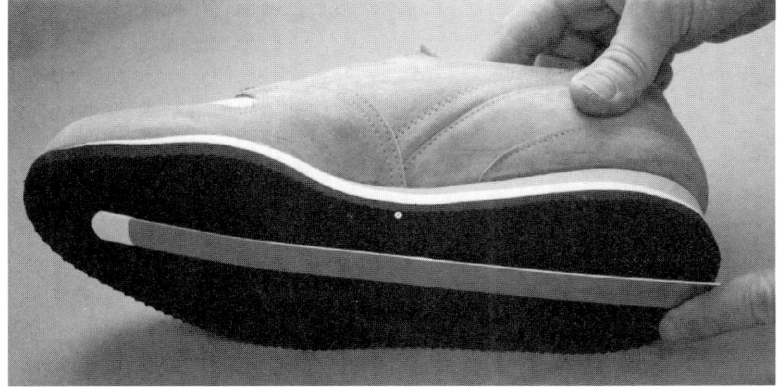

FIGURE 35. Addition of an extended steel shank to the shoe, used to limit motion in the joints of the entire foot. This especially limits flexion of the great toe at push off. It is useful for hallux rigidus or fractures of the metatarsals. It may be used as either flat sole to promote a flat-footed gait or with the mid-foot roller if some heel rise can be tolerated.

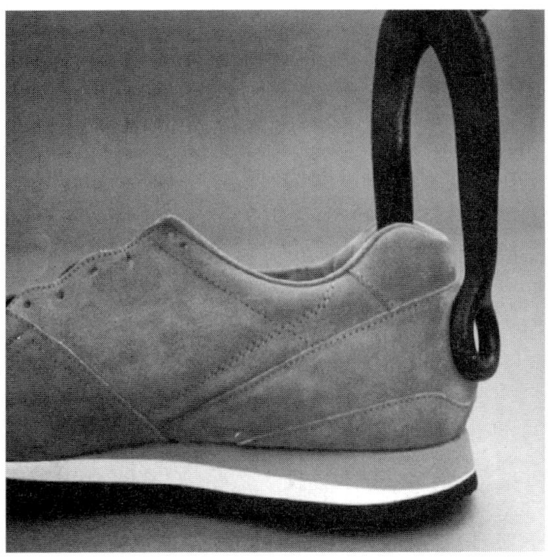

FIGURE 36. Ball and ring stretcher—"cobblers goose," used to make permanent round depressions in bunion areas, counters of shoes for pump bumps, toe boxes for hammertoes, and anywhere corns develop. It is the tool used most often to "custom fit" a shoe.

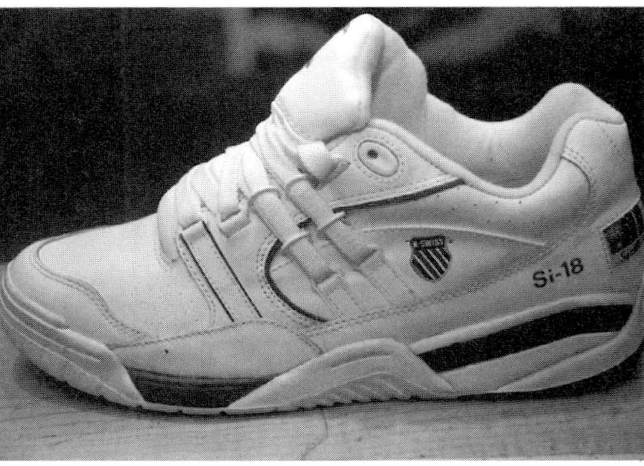

FIGURE 37. Tennis shoe. This shoe needs to have good medial and lateral support for side-to-side movements in tennis. The sole must be flexible in the forefoot for quick forward movements.

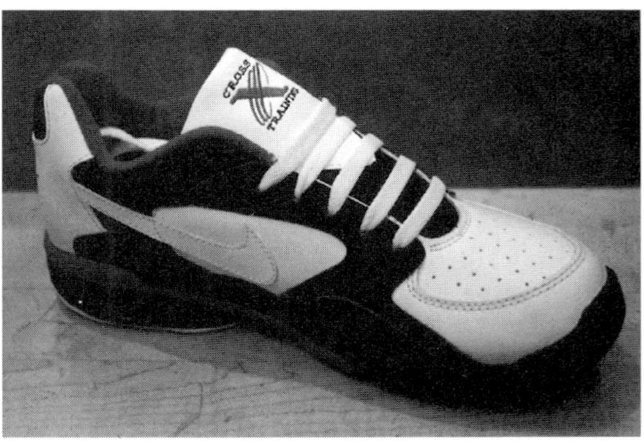

FIGURE 38. Cross-trainer shoe. This shoe can be used for more than one sport. It has a flexible forefoot for running and also the lateral stability needed for tennis or aerobics.

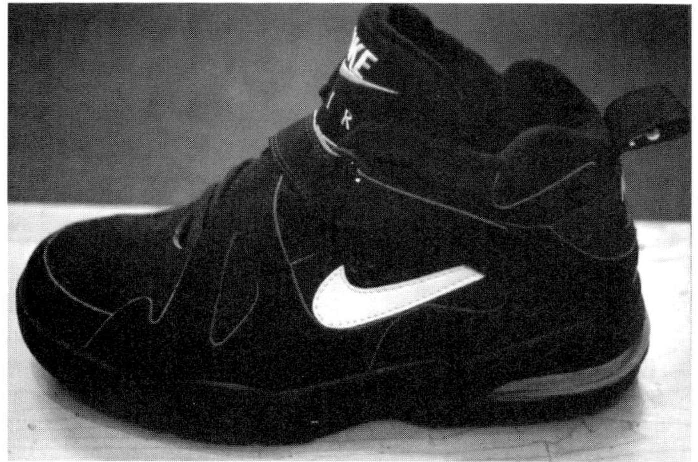

FIGURE 39. Basketball shoe. It has a thick, stiff sole for stability when running. To help prevent ankle sprains and give extra support, a high top is recommended.

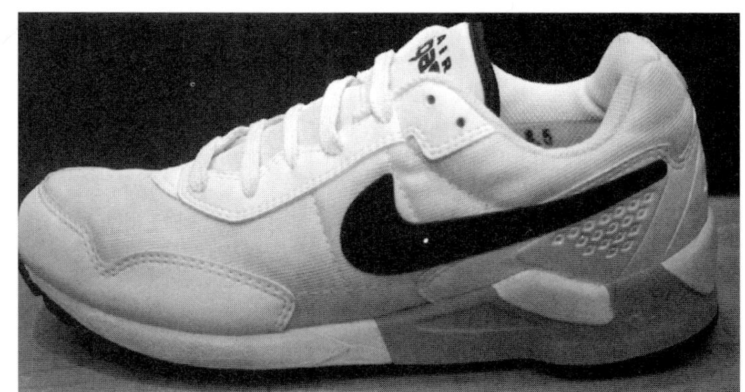

FIGURE 40. Running shoe. This shoe has additional cushion for shock absorption to help prevent shin splints, heel pain, etc. Also, needs good heel control.

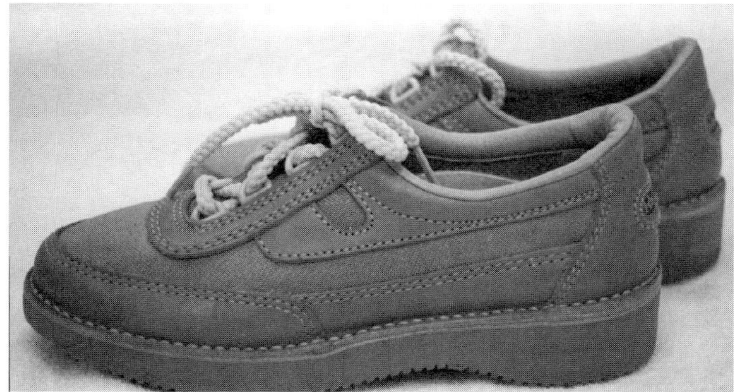

FIGURE 41. Walking shoe. It must be lightweight with extra cushioning in the heel area and under the ball of the foot. Walking shoes have more rigidity in the forefoot so that you roll off your toes. A rounded sole is recommended.

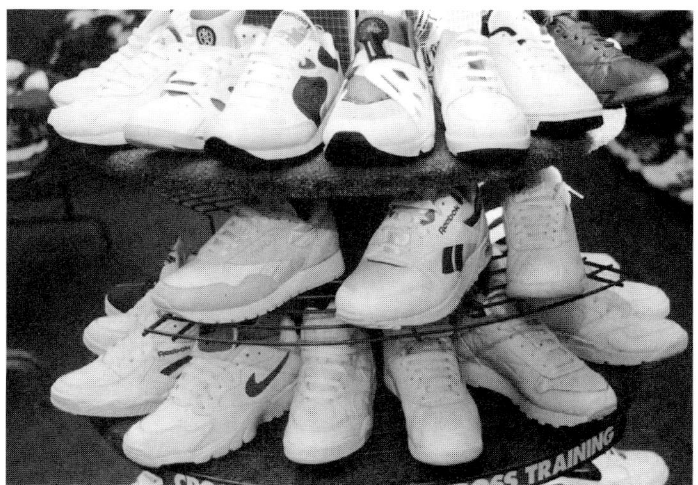

FIGURE 42. Assorted athletic shoes.

REFERENCES

1. Andersen E: Stenosing peroneal tenosynovitis symptomatically simulating ankle instability. Am J Sports Med 15: 258–259, 1987.
2. Caine D, Cochrane B, Caine C, et al: An epidemiologic investigation of injuries affecting young competitive female gymnasts. Am J Sports Med 17:811–820, 1989.
3. Clancy WG Jr: Tendinitis and plantar fasciitis in runners. In D'Ambrosia RD, Drez D Jr (eds): Prevention and Treatment of Running Injuries, 2nd ed., Thorofare, NJ, Charles B Slack, 1989, pp 121–131.
4. Clanton TO, Butler JE, Eggert A: Injuries to the metatarsophalangeal joints in athletes. Foot Ankle 7:162–176, 1986.
5. Clanton TO, Butler JE, Eggert A: Injuries to the metatarsophalangeal joints in athletes. Foot Ankle 7:162–176, 1986.
6. Clanton TO, Eggert KE, Pivarnik JM, et al: First metatarsophalangeal joint range of motion as a factor in turf toe injuries. Graduate thesis.
7. Clement DB, Taunton JE, Smart GW: Achilles' tendinitis and peritendinitis: etiology and treatment. Am J Sports Med 12:179–184, 1984.
8. Coker TP, Arnold JA, Weber DL: Traumatic lesions of the metatarsophalangeal joint of the great toe in athletes. Am J Sports Med 6:326–334, 1978.
9. Couglin MJ: Sesamoid pain: causes and surgical treatment. Instr Course Lect 39:23–35, 1990.
10. Drez D Jr: Therapeutic Modalities for Sports Injuries. St. Louis, Mosby-Year Book, 1989.
11. Faciszewski T, Burks RT, Manaster BJ: Subtle injuries of the Lisfranc joint. J Bone Joint Surg 72A:1419–1522, 1990.
12. Frey CC, Shereff MJ: Tendon injuries about the ankle in athletes. Clin Sport Med 7:103–118, 1988.
13. Gould J: Operative Foot Surgery. Philadelphia, W. B. Saunders, 1994, p 899–986.
14. Gould J: Treatment of the painful injured nerve in continuity. In Gilberman RH (ed): Operative Nerve Repair and Reconstruction. Philadelphia, J.B. Lippincott, 1991.
15. Gould N: Technique tips: Footings: Repair of dislocating peroneal tendons. Foot Ankle 6:208–213, 1986.
16. Hattrup SJ, Johnson KA: A review of ruptures of the Achilles' tendon. Foot Ankle 6:34–38, 1985.
17. Hawkins BJ, Haddad RJ: Hallux rigidus. Clin Sports Med 7:37–49, 1988.
18. Hershman EB, Mailly T: Stress fractures. Clin Sports Med 9:183–214, 1990
19. Holmes GB Jr, Mann RA, Wells L: Epidemiologic factors associated with rupture of the Achilles' tendon. Contemp Orthop 23:327–331, 1991.
20. Hunter L: Stress fractures of the tarsal navicular. Am J Sports Med 9:217–219, 1981.
21. Jacobs D, Martens M, Van Audekercke R, et al: Comparison of conservative and operative treatment of Achilles' tendon rupture. Am J Sports Med 6:107–111, 1978.
22. Jahss M: Disorders of the Foot and Ankle: Medical and Surgical Management. Philadelphia, WB Saunders, 1991, pp 2415–2465.
23. Jones DC: Bucket handle tears of the peroneus brevis. American Orthopaedic Foot and Ankle Society Meeting, Santa Fe, NM, July 17, 1987.
24. Kavanaugh JH, Bower TD, Mann RV: The Jones' fractures revisited. J Bone Surg 60A:776–782, 1978.
25. Kile T, Fitzgibbons TC: Physical therapy treatment for plantar fascitis: is it cost effective? Presented AOFAS Summer Meeting, 1994.
26. Kojima Y, Kataoka Y, Suzuki S, et al: Dislocation of the peroneal tendons in neonates and infants. Clin Orthop 266:180–184, 1991.
27. Leach RE, James S, Wasilewski S: Achilles' Tendinitis, Am J Sports Med 9:93–98, 1981.
28. Lehman RC, Torg JS, Pavlov H, DeLee JC: Fractures of the base of the fifth metatarsal distal to the tuberosity: a review. Foot Ankle 7:245–252, 1987.
29. Lillich JS, Baxter DE: Common forefoot problems in runners. Foot Ankle 7:149–150, 1986.
30. Lysholm J, Wiklander J: Injuries in runners, Am J Sports Med 15:168–171, 1987.
31. Mann R, Coughlin M: Surgery of the Foot and Ankle, 6th ed., Mosby, 1993, vol. 2, pp 1095–1276.
32. McBride AM, Anderson, RV: Sesamoid foot problems in the athlete. Clin Sports Med 7:51–60, 1988.
33. McBryde AM: Stress fracture in athletes. J Sports Med 5:212–217, 1976.
34. McBryde AM: Stress fractures in runners. Clin Sports Med 4:737–752, 1985.
35. McBryde AM, Anderson RB: Sesamoid foot problems in the athlete. Clin Sports Med 7:51–60, 1988.
36. McLennan JG: Treatment of acute and chronic luxations of the peroneal tendons. Am J Sports Med 8:432–436, 1980.
37. Mellion MB: Common cycling injuries: management and prevention, Sports Med 11(1):52–70, 1991.
38. Murphy PC, Baxter DE: Nerve entrapment of the foot and ankle in runners. Clin Sports Med 4:753, 1985.
39. Resch S, Stenström A: The treatment of tarsometatarsal injuries. Foot Ankle 11(3):117–123, 1990.
40. Rodeo SA, O'Brien S, Warren RF, et al: Turf-toe: an analysis of metatarsophalangeal joint sprains in professional football players. Am J Sports Med 18:280–285, 1990.
41. Sammarco GJ, DiRaimondo CV: Chronic peroneus brevis tendon lesions. Foot Ankle 9:163–170, 1989.
42. Sammarco GJ, Drez D Jr, Elkus RA, et al: Symposium: overuse syndromes of the leg, foot, and ankle in athletes. Contemp Orthop 12:67–93, 1986.
43. Sammarco GJ: How I manage turf toe. Phys Sportsmed 16:113–118, 1988.
44. Sobel M, Bohne WHO, Levy ME: Longitudinal attrition of the peroneus brevis tendon in the fibular groove: An anatomic study. Foot Ankle 11(3):124–128, 1990.
45. Trevino S, Gould N, Korson R: Surgical treatment of stenosing tenosynovitis at the ankle. Foot Ankle 2:37–45, 1981.
46. Torg JS, Baldini FC, Zelko RR, et al: Fractures of the base of the fifth metatarsal distal to the tuberosity. J Bone Joint Surg 66A:209–214, 1984.
47. Zogby RG, Baker BE: A review of nonoperative treatment of Jones' fracture. Am J Sports Med 15:304–307, 1987.

26

Taping and Bracing

Ronnie D. Hald, P.T., A.T.C.
Denise M. Fandel, M.S., A.T.C.

A frequent question asked by the injured athlete to the sportsmedicine practitioner is "How should I protect this injury once I return to play'?" The answer should result from a decision-making process, dependent on several factors. One of these factors is the knowledge and awareness of what is available. In this chapter, the sportsmedicine practitioner is exposed to numerous taping techniques and braces that may be beneficial in meeting the needs of athletic patients. It is not the authors' intent to teach competence in the techniques of taping or the designing of a brace; however, some detailed examples are presented to aid the discussion. The ability of the physician to identify and evaluate the options will facilitate prescription of the optimal method of support and protection. This understanding will also assist in communication to coaches, athletic trainers, and therapists working with the athlete, thus encouraging the team approach, a necessary component of optimal patient care.

SELECTION CONSIDERATIONS

Before considering common methods of athletic injury support, it is helpful to discuss factors involved in making an appropriate selection, including: (1) diagnosis of injury, (2) goals to be accomplished by taping or bracing, (3) resources available, (4) sport and position of the athlete, (5) the athlete's acceptance of the technique, (6) research findings, and (7) personal preferences. The investigation of these factors and their interaction will assist in determining the best choice.

Diagnosis of Injury. The location, nature, and severity of injury often dictate the suitability of providing external support. For instance, most shoulder problems are not helped by taping or bracing because restriction of range of motion leads to decreased function and possibly to secondary problems. The ankle, however, with its inherent skeletal stability, may be more readily supported externally. The acuteness and severity of injury may dictate more aggressive treatment than taping or bracing. Some chronic injuries may be helped by decreasing the effect of biomechanical forces present in repetitive activities e.g., long distance running or racquet sports. A referral to, and input from, an orthopedist may be beneficial.

Goals of Taping and Bracing. Taping and bracing can be divided into three main categories: (1) prophylactic; (2) rehabilitative; and (3) functional. Prophylactic supports reduce the incidence or severity of injury to uninjured normal anatomy or to fully rehabilitated injuries. Rehabilitative taping or bracing protects injuries during healing. Functional braces and taping are used to protect against reinjury following rehabilitation and surgical reconstruction. A taping procedure or brace effective for prevention may not be suitable as an adjunct to rehabilitation. Taping or bracing does not substitute for the need for complete rehabilitation. A helpful concept to understand this is that of "earning the brace" by completing rehabilitation. Taping may help support injured tissues during rehabilitation; and as such is a means to an end, not the end in itself. If taping or bracing cannot provide any additional benefit, it is probably best to do without it.

Resources Available. Even though a certain taping technique may be ideal for a particular problem, it will not help if no trainer or other individual skilled in its application is available to the athlete. This is why many braces are often used. Once the athlete is properly instructed in the brace's application, no additional expertise is needed. There are also financial considerations such as the cost of taping in labor and supplies, and the oftentimes considerable expense of a brace. With custom made braces, there may be a delay until the brace is available for the athlete's use. Coaches and trainers should be approached to determine which options are feasible. In the case of younger athletes, parents should be made involved when financial or insurance issues need clarification.

Sport and Position. A taping or bracing effective for an athlete in one sport may not be suitable for another in that sport, not even the same athlete in another sport. Each sport has its own physical requirements, equipment, environment, and rules that will affect, and many times govern, the selection of protective support for injuries. In some sports, an athlete's particular position or event may need to be considered. Taping may have to be tailored to allow the athlete to perform his or her function, but still to provide adequate protection. Braces must be made of materials that will not endanger the other participants.

Athlete's Acceptance. If the athlete feels that taping or a brace is uncomfortable or decreases performance, the attempt to support the site of an injury will fail. Involving the athlete in the decision-making process and providing choices, where possible, can reduce the risk of nonacceptance. If an appropriate choice is made, a very real effect of taping or bracing following injury is the psychological assistance to the athlete's confidence upon returning to competition.

Research Findings. Research about what does and does not work is still in the developmental stage. Many methods and devices that have been used for years are only now being tested rigorously. With respect to new techniques or products, it is probably better to keep an open mind but to be skeptical. As research is completed, clinical experience continues to have significant bearing in the decision-making process.

Personal Preference. After gaining clinical experience with various taping techniques and braces, one usually begins to have certain favorites. There is nothing wrong with relying on personal experience when the athlete is looking for expert answers, as long as each case is viewed on an individual basis.

IMPLEMENTATION

Once a method of support is selected, the choice needs to be made known to all parties involved. Information must also be shared. To evaluate the effectiveness of the support as part of the treatment plan, a follow-up visit should be scheduled.

Communication. During selection, lines of communication have been formed among the physician, the athlete, the athlete's coach, athletic trainer, and parents of the athlete. This encourages compliance, promotes safe return of the athlete to the sport, and encourages good working relationships among the professionals involved. This sort of communication is also very helpful to the team physician.

Education. It should be made clear that taping or bracing is only one part of a total care plan. All concerned should learn what is intended to be accomplished by taping or bracing. In some cases the taping procedure will need to be taught to a coach or athletic trainer by an individual familiar with it. Preventive measures to protect skin from being injured by frequent taping should be encouraged. With bracing, the athlete will need to be shown how to put on the brace properly. This may include an anatomy lesson to locate the joint lines and show how the straps must be placed to make the brace most effective. The athlete must be able to put on and take off the brace independently before leaving the clinic. Instructions about care and preventive maintenance should also be reviewed to maximize the life of the brace. Written instructions on application and care, if not available, should be developed.

Follow-up. The appropriate time to schedule a follow-up visit when an athlete has been cleared to resume the sport is at the conclusion of the sport's season. This allows the physician and rehabilitation team to reassess the effectiveness of the support, determine its continued need, and encourage "prehabilitation" of deficits before the next season. In multisport athletes, change in the type of taping or bracing may be necessary. For those involved in research, this also provides an opportunity to acquire data.

PRINCIPLES OF TAPING

To be proficient in taping, one must practice, practice, practice. Anyone who has attempted to learn how to tape knows how true this statement is. Exposure to some common techniques, however, can assist the primary care practitioner to provide a complete treatment plan and to communicate with professionals personally more skilled in these procedures.

Application. One of the most common mistakes made by the novice is using too much tape. Every piece of tape should have a distinct purpose—more is not better. Other common problems include continuous application of tape and the forcing of tape in a desired direction; both these errors may restrict circulation. A better approach consists of tearing smaller strips more often and in considering the contours of body parts. Learning how to tear tape and adapting use of a two-dimensional tool to a three-dimensional body part are basic skills. A good taper keeps in mind the need to restrict undesired motion yet to allow wanted motion. A tape support is made effective by bridging across the injury and duplicating the anatomy needing support; strength is developed by weaving the strips, overlapping them by at least half the width of the tape.

Tape Selection. Correct selection of the best tape for the job is important. The size of the body part determines the appropriate tape width. The tape must adhere well to the athlete's skin and have adequate tensile strength to provide the necessary support. Some tapes are elastic to increase ease of application or desired movement, yet also to provide adequate injury protection; of course this increases the cost of the tape. Of importance to the taper is how the tape unwinds from the roll and how easily it tears. Learning how to tear tape is the most basic skill to be acquired by the novice taper. Some tapes do not tear at all and will require cutting between application of strips.

Skin Care. Frequent taping of skin can lead to problems that are, however, preventable. Shaving hair not only increases the effectiveness of taping but also reduces the irritation and buildup of residue that can lead to infection. Skin to be taped should be protected by application of a taping base (usually containing tincture of benzoin) that also increases the adherent qualities of the tape. A tape underwrap of thin polyester urethane foam decreases skin problems and increases the athlete's comfort. This adds another interface, however, between the tape and the needing support. A lubricant placed in areas that may be pinched with movement within the taping, such as the lace and heel areas of the ankle, can prevent or at least decrease irritation. Using appropriate scissors or cutters to remove the tape should be taught to the athlete. Scissors with pointed tips should be avoided. Following practice, the skin must be thoroughly cleansed and treated if necessary. Failure to do so can lead to skin breakdown and wounds that may prevent further taping. Some individuals may develop allergic reactions to certain products or materials used in taping, and solutions to this problem must be found. If not, taping may need to be abandoned in favor of some other form of support and protection.

Procedures

This section describes and presents some common uses of tape to support athletic injuries. It is not intended to be complete or exhaustive but rather to indicate current practice.

Buddy Taping. This method splints an injured finger to an adjacent one to restrict varus and valgus forces (Fig. 1A). For additional support, felt or foam may be placed between the fingers being taped (Fig. 1B). Because it is important to allow interphalangeal motion, it is best to avoid using the index and little fingers as a splint, unless, of course, either finger is involved.

Thumb Figure-of-Eight. Hyperflexion injuries are supported by circling around the wrist and the thumb in a figure-of-eight pattern (Fib. 1C).

Thumb Checkrein. Hyperextension injuries to the thumb may be remedied by the use of a Checkrein between the thumb and index finger (Fig. 1D). Please note that use of this taping can injure the metacarpophalangeal joint of the index finger.[7]

Wrist Taping. Circumferential strips about the wrist may limit excursion of the carpals (Fig. 1E). In cases of dorsal impingement such as seen in the gymnast or tennis player, the incorporation of a foam "block" into this taping is often helpful.

Elbow Hyperextension Taping. With the athlete's elbow placed in slight flexion, fanning strips are placed anterior to the elbow joint between anchors about the upper arm and forearm (Fig. 2A). This taping can also be modified to provide medial (Fig. 2B) or lateral support.

Shoulder Taping. Although taping has been used for some shoulder injuries, we feel that the restriction of motion required to provide adequate support decreases function to a point where rehabilitation may be necessary.

Hip and Groin Taping. These areas are better supported by the use of elastic wraps using a figure-of-eight pattern about the waist and upper thigh. Because these areas are rarely taped, no further discussion is necessary. Again, it is important to question the problem of decreased function to achieve the desired support.

Medial (or Lateral) Knee Taping. Fanning strips across the medial (or lateral) aspect of the knee joint across anchors about the thigh and calf may reduce the effect of valgus (or varus) stress. Figure 3 demonstrates a taping to support the medial ligaments of the knee.

McConnell Patellofemoral Taping. Jenny McConnell, an Australian physiotherapist, has documented a program for decreasing the pain and dysfunction associated with malalignment of the patella. The program deals most specifically with retraining the poor ratio of vastus medial oblique (VMO) to vastus lateralis (VL) muscle contraction and coordination found in persons with patellofemoral pain. The taping technique is used in the early stages of the patellofemoral rehabilitation process. Although successful in reducing pain, this taping technique is probably the most frequently abused part of the program. When used properly, it is applied only after a very thorough evaluation by someone trained in the technique. It is accompanied by a comprehensive retraining of the extensor mechanism, concentrating on muscle re-education through the use of biofeedback training.

If improperly applied, however, the tape can increase pain and apply harmfully compressive forces on the patella. The technique described here provides the practitioner with information on how the taping and rehabilitation be helpful for patients, but is not intended to "train" anyone in the use of the tape. In-

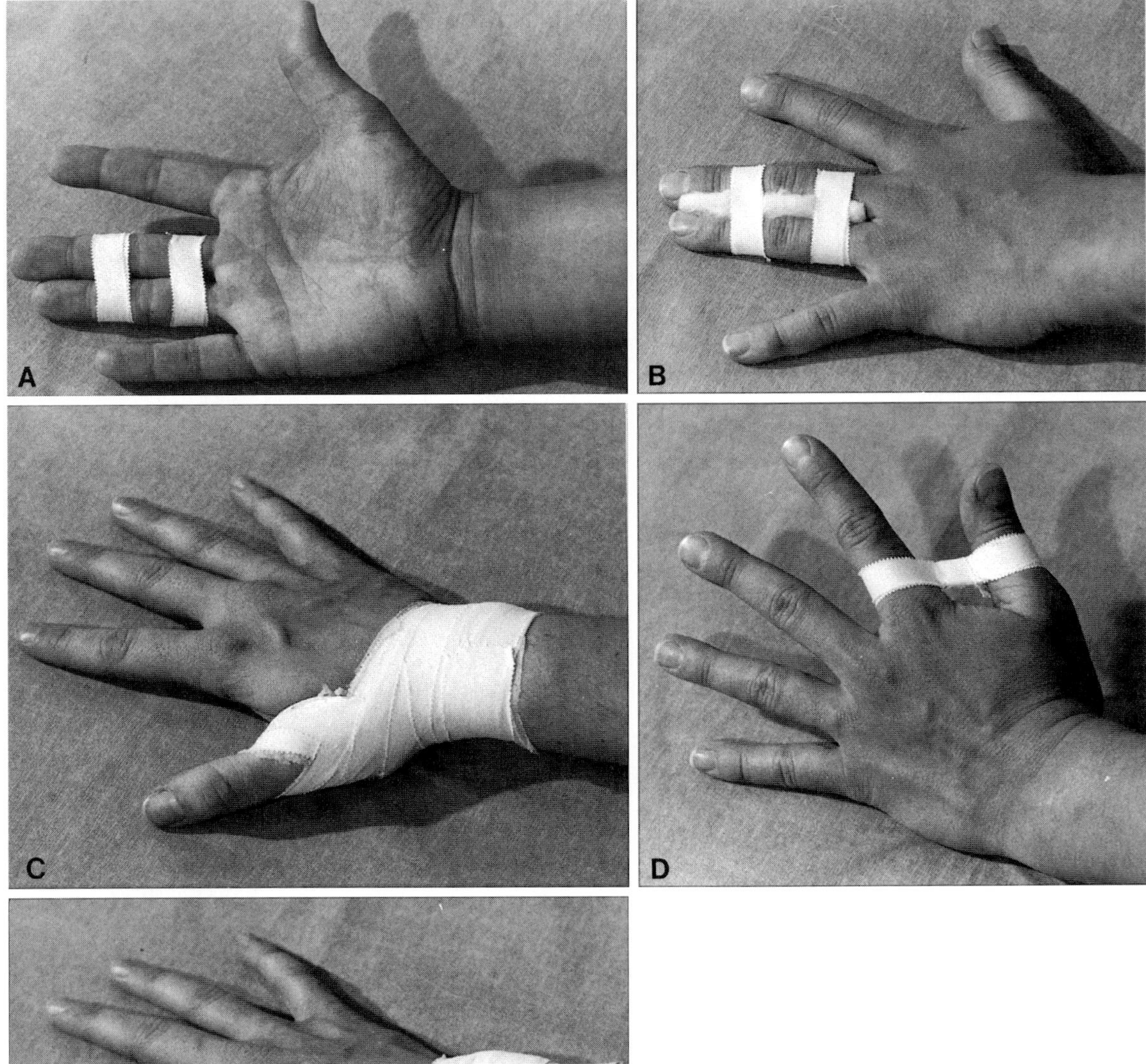

FIGURE 1. *A,* Buddy taping. *B,* Buddy taping with felt/foam insert. *C,* Thumb figure-of-eight. *D,* Thumb checkrein. *E,* Wrist taping.

struction in the evaluation and rehabilitation theory and technique is essential for the best use of the tape.

Technique. There are three basic taping strips in the technique: tilt, glide, and rotation. The use of each is dependent upon the evaluation of the patellar alignment. The taping strips are applied in the order of most serious malalignment to least. Again, the knowledge of the evaluation technique is essential in understanding the taping technique. In this technique, more is not necessarily better. After applying each strip of tape, the quality of pain improvement is assessed. Once the quality of pain has diminished as completely as possible, the application of additional strips is not necessary.

The taping technique uses two unique products, CoverRoll (Biersdorf, Inc, Norwalk, CT) and Leukotape P, a brown sports tape (Biersdorf, Inc, Norwalk, CT). CoverRoll is a special tape that pro-

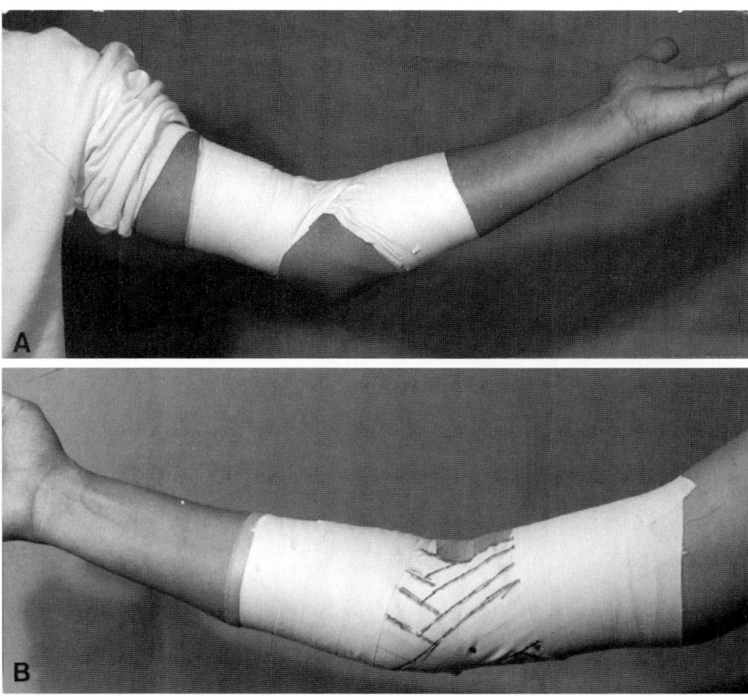

FIGURE 2. *A,* Elbow hyperextension taping. *B,* Medial elbow taping.

tects the skin from the brown sports tape while providing an anchor. It is important that the brown tape not be applied directly to the skin. In people whose skin is sensitive to the Leukotape P, CoverRoll can be used to correct malalignments. The Leukotape P has a higher fiber density than traditional white athletic adhesive tape. Some people have tried substituting other tapes with less success. Although both CoverRoll and Leukotape P are expensive, they are necessary to achieve the full benefit of the McConnell taping techniques.

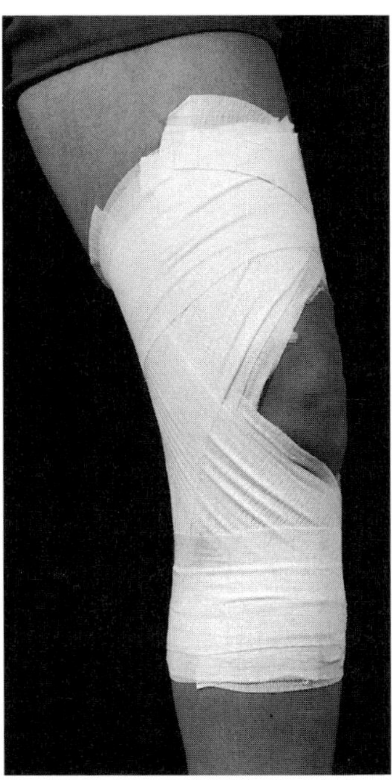

FIGURE 3. Medial knee taping.

Before any of the malalignment strips are applied, the area must be prepared. After the area is shaved and any lotion removed, CoverRoll is applied (Fig. 4a) to serve as an anchor for the Leukotape P. Hypa-Fix is affixed from the lateral patellar facet medially to a point between the tendons marking the popliteal fossa. As the tape is applied, the athlete lifts the soft tissues of the hamstrings and creates a "pucker" in the skin. This technique is also used on subsequent strips of brown tape (Leukotape P).

The tilt strip provides stretching of the lateral retinacular fibers of the quadriceps and the iliotibial band. It also will lift the inferior patellar facet to a more neutral position (Fig. 4b). The tape is applied at a point marking the midline of the patella and on the upper half of the patella. This strip can be applied with the knee in a position allowing a significant amount of flexion. Properly applied this strip will also decrease the stress on the medial patellar facet, the VMO and vastus medialis (VM) and the infrapatellar fat pad. Often a significant portion of (PFJ) symptoms stems from the VMO's being weakened because of constant stretching. The VMO is thereby inhibited from proper function, resulting in the VL's overpowering the proper joint mechanics and creating a lateral glide of the patella.

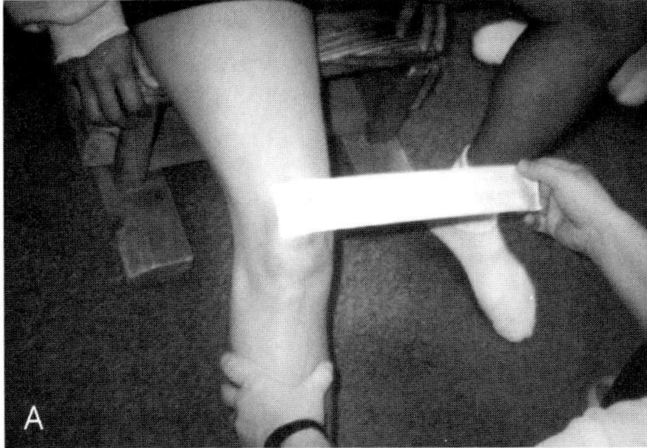

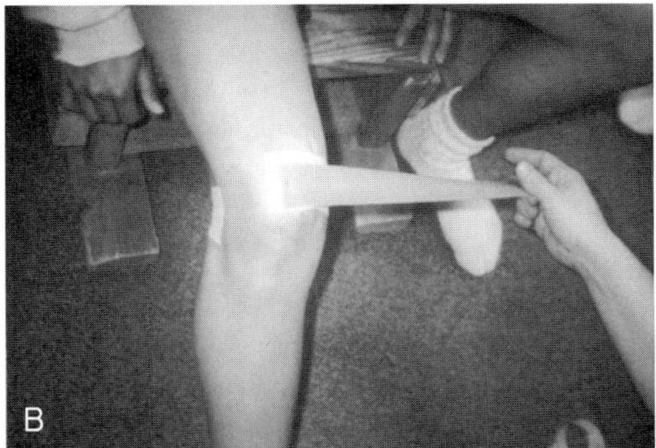

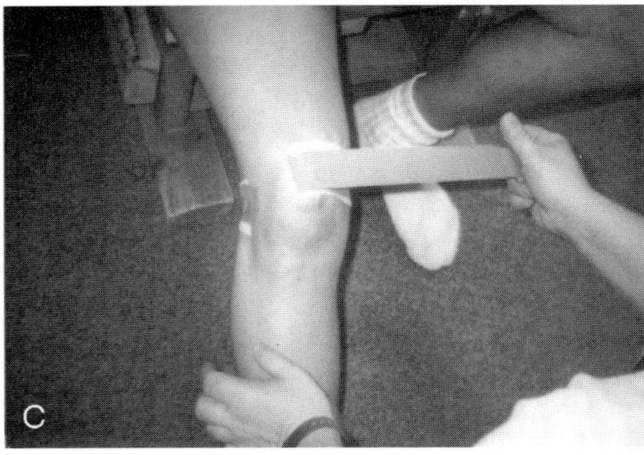

FIGURE 4. *A,* CoverRoll application. *B,* Tilt strip application. *C,* Glide strip application.

The glide strip (Fig. 4c) will provide secondary support for the proper placement of the patella in the groove. The strip provides additional stimulus to the VMO through proper placement additional stimulus to the VMO through proper placement of the patella. This strip is only applied if the tilt strip has not significantly decreased patellofemoral pain. It must be applied with the knee in extension so the posterior aspect of the patella is not placed in contact with the lateral femoral condyle. The technique described in the previous paragraph is also used on this strip. It is critical that the "pucker" at the medial patellar margin be emphasized.

A rotation strip, if necessary, will align the superior and inferior patellar poles with the long axis of the femur. The tape is applied at the inferior patellar facet, where the patella is grasped and rotated to align the long axis of the patella with the long axis of the femur.

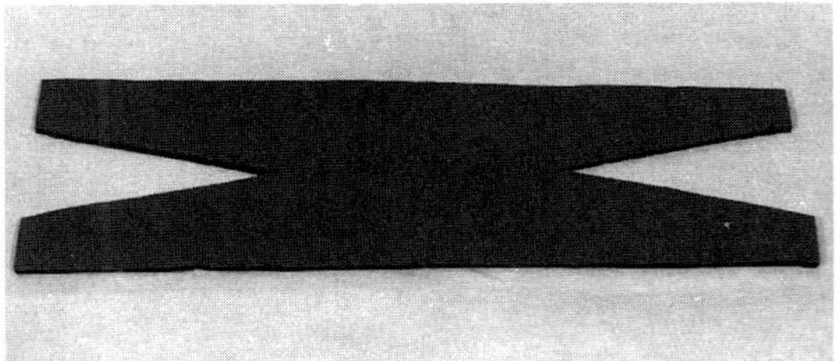

FIGURE 5. Neoprene support for the ACL taping.

Once again, proper materials, technique, and rehabilitative exercises can significantly reduce the amount of patellofemoral pain. The practitioner using the McConnell technique is strongly encouraged to learn the theory underlying it through outside coursework.

The next three taping procedures are presented in a step-by-step manner, because they are not easily demonstrated by a single photograph. They address areas were external support is most often considered.

Knee Anterior Cruciate Ligament (ACL) Taping. The Duke Simpson knee strapping has often been touted: "If this strapping fails to hold a knee from further sprain, no brace or other contrivance will."[32] In a modification of this strapping, Ross[28] developed an effective method to limit hyperextension of the knee, a major consideration in anterior cruciate ligament injury. The modification shown here[32] uses a four-tailed piece of neoprene rubber, 15″ × 6″ with 5″ × 3″ triangular cutouts (Fig. 5). Tape adherent and underwrap are applied (Fig. 6A), the neoprene support is placed in the popliteal space (Fig. 6B) and then covered by underwrap (Fig. 6C). This enables the athlete to reuse the neoprene. Using 3″ elastic tape, a laterally revulsive circumferential anchor is placed about the calf. The tape is drawn laterally and upwardly across the lateral joint line (Fig. 6D). A circumferential anchor about the thigh is then placed. Continuing on the medial side, the tape is drawn downwardly across the medial joint line (Fig. 6E), around the calf, then upwardly across the medial joint line again. This creates a medial "X" configuration, which covers the neoprene support (Fig. 6F). After passing the tape around the thigh, then down across the lateral joint line, the lateral "X" is completed (Fig. 6G). After again passing behind the calf, the tape is pulled laterally, then upwardly and posteriorly (Fig. 6H). This action should enclose the popliteal space, a practice usually avoided because of complications to the circulatory system. The use of the neoprene support, however, seems to mitigate this problem. After completing a finishing

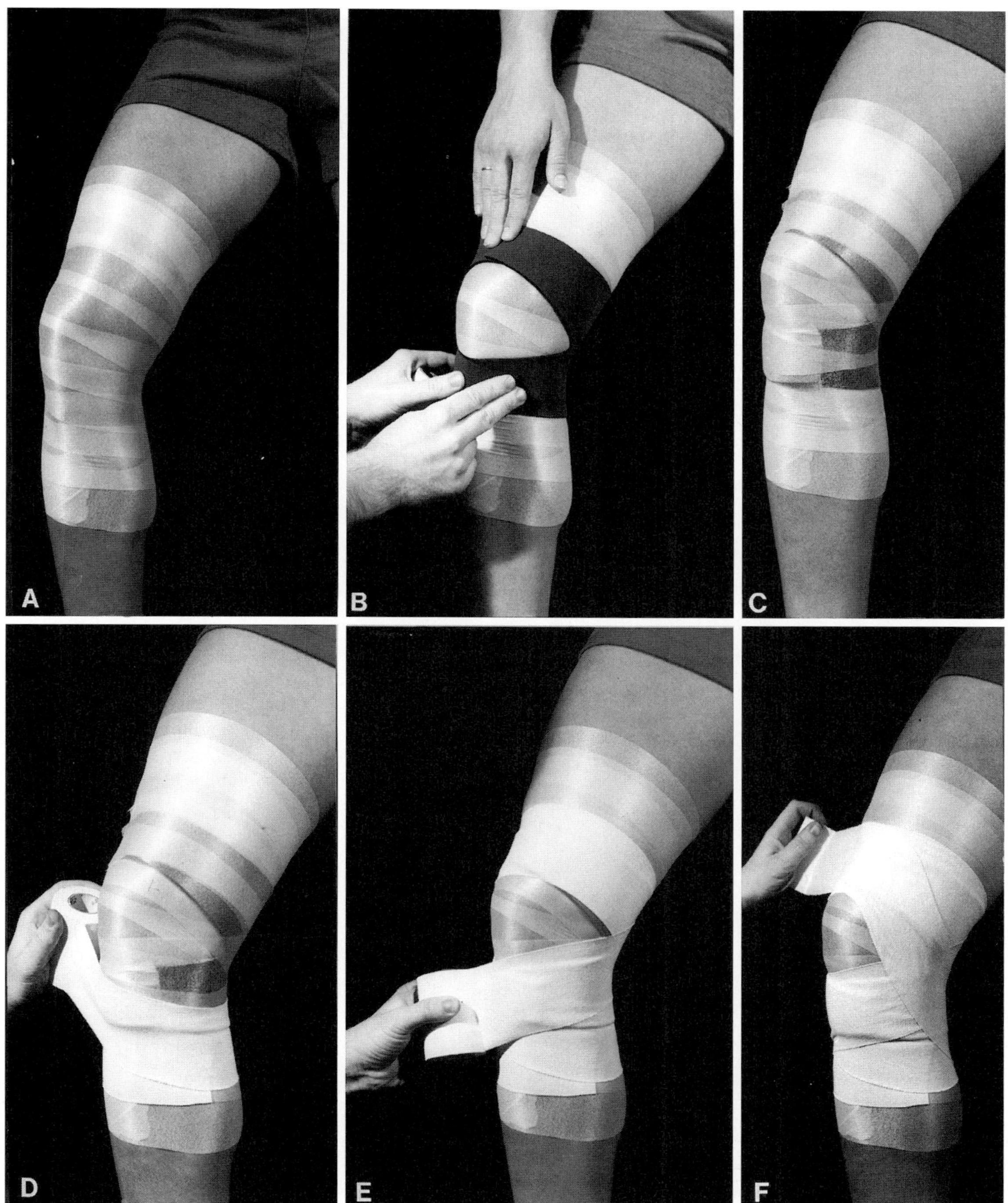

FIGURE 6. ACL taping.

anchor about the thigh, the tape is cut (Fig. 6I), and cloth adhesive tape placed about the thigh and calf to anchor the elastic tape (Fig. 6J). These anchors and the edges of the elastic tape should be applied directly to the skin. Cutting the calf portion of the taping posteriorly allows for expansion of the gastrocnemius musculature (Fig. 6K). This gap is closed with cloth adhesive tape to finish the taping. In order to reuse the neoprene support, this taping is removed strip by strip upon conclusion of activity.

Ankle Taping. Although there are probably about as many taping techniques for the ankle as there are athletic trainers, a basic method that incorporates some of the most common methods will be

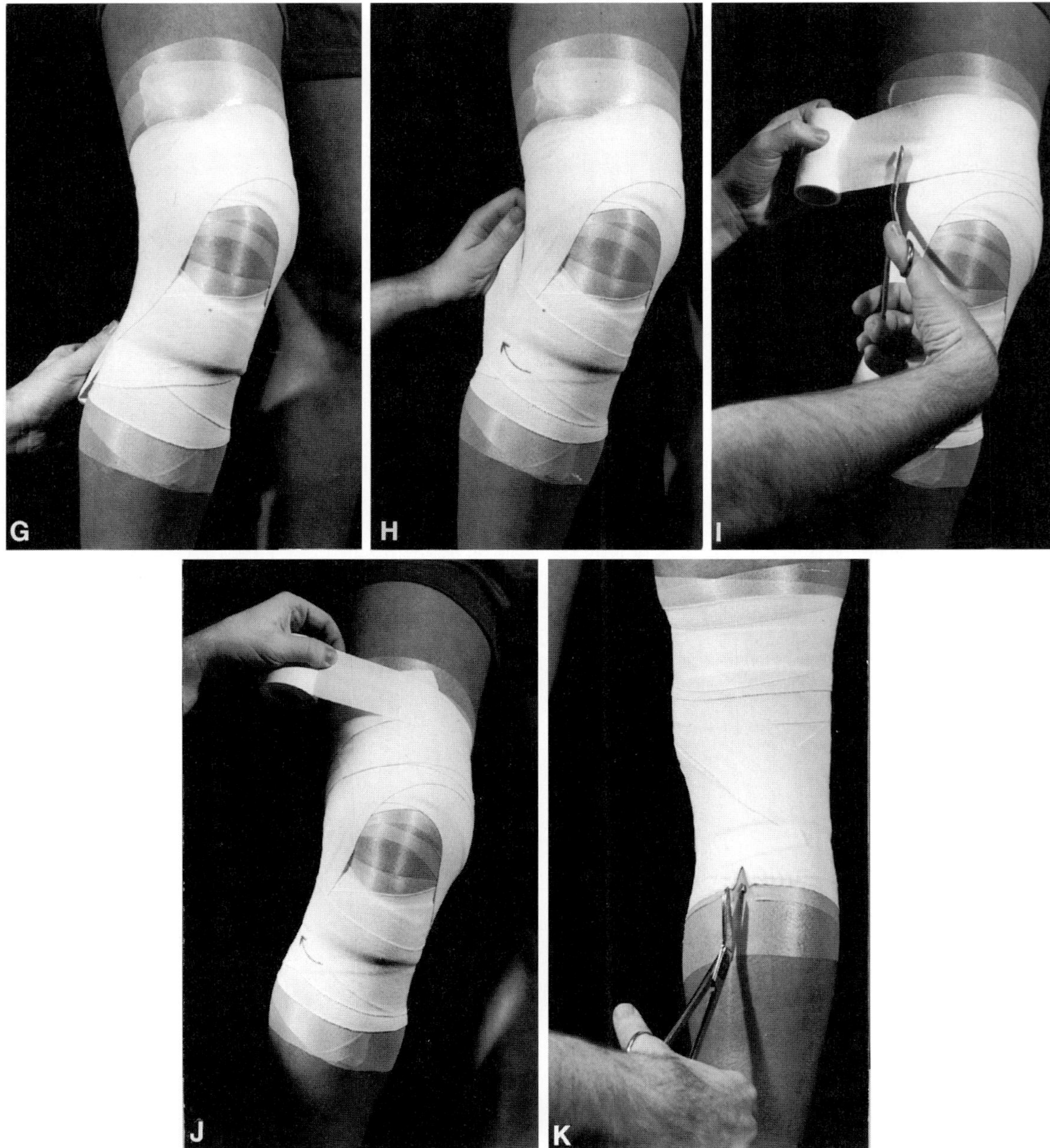

FIGURE 6. *(Continued).* ACL taping.

described here. To meet the goal of the taping—preventive, rehabilitative, or supportive for a functional return of a rehabilitated ankle injury—the basic steps are adapted by the experienced taper. The athlete's ankles should be positioned at a right angle of plantar/dorsiflexion with neutral inversion/eversion. Hair should be shaved to allow maximal support. Heel-and-lace pads made of gauze or similar protective material with lubrication are applied to the heel-and-lace areas to guard against blisters and tape cuts (Fig. 7A). Tape adherent and underwrap are then applied (Fig. 7B). Underwrap may be omitted to provide additional support, especially for more serious injuries, but special care of the skin will then be required. Anchor strips around the calf at the level of the musculotendinous junction of the gastrocnemius and around the arch are applied (Fig. 7C). The arch anchor must be placed proximally to the base of the fifth metatarsal to avoid discomfort as the foot spreads during weightbearing. A "stirrup" strip is placed on the calf anchor medially, passing beneath the heel posterior to the malleoli and pulling laterally to the other side of the calf anchor (Fig. 7D). In an ever-

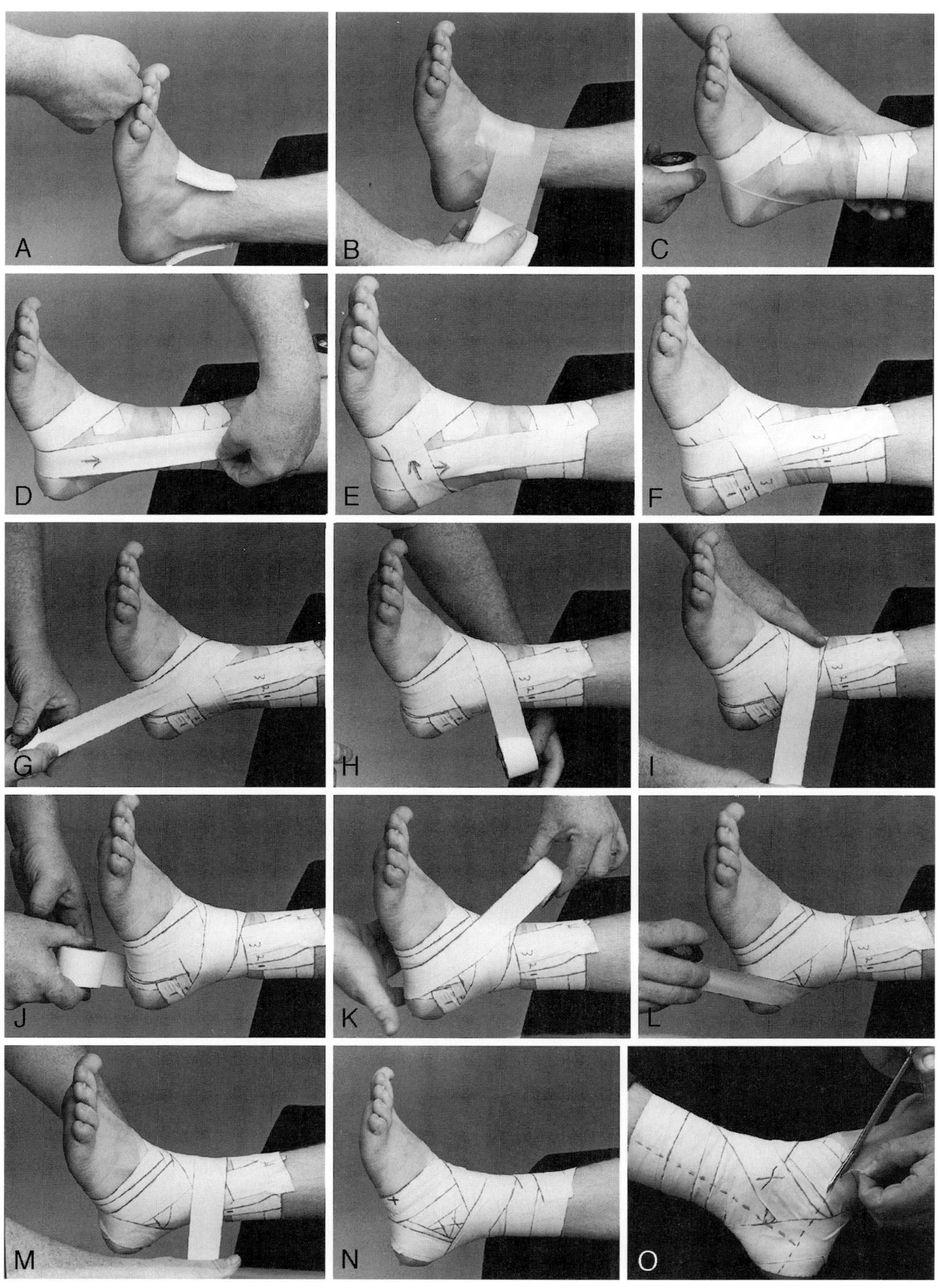

FIGURE 7A-O. Ankle taping.

sion sprain, the stirrup is placed with equal tension medially and laterally. Perpendicular to the stirrup, a "horseshoe" starting and finishing on the arch anchor (Fig. 7E) is applied distal to the malleoli. Stirrups and horseshoes are repeated twice more, overlapping the previous strip by half the tape's width. This completes the "basketweave" (Fig. 7F).

A "figure-of-eight" may be applied to restrict plantar flexion. In the present example, it begins on the outside of the foot, angling under it (Fig. 7H)."Heel locks" are used to restrict inversion/eversion. A medial heel lock, which restricts inversion, begins in the lace area (Fig. 7I) and angles behind and across the medial aspect of the heel (Fig. 7J), then under the heel to return to the lace area (Fig. 7K). A lateral heel lock is performed in the opposite direction, angling across the lateral aspect of the heel (Fig. 7L). These maneuvers may be repeated as necessary to obtain the desired support. Circular strips are placed about the lower leg, overlapping distally to proximally to eliminate open spaces that may cause skin irritation or blisters (Fig. 7M). Anchors may be repeated to close, thus decreasing the number of free tape ends exposed that may roll up when the athlete puts on socks. The completed bandage must be inspected for wrinkles and gaps, and then the athlete should be questioned to determine the adequacy of the support and comfort of the wrapping. (Fig. 7N). Ankle strapping is removed using blunt-nosed bandage scissors or a tape cutter to cut along the medial aspect, posterior to the medial malleolus (Fig. 7O). Various extra padding may be incorporated into the taping, such as an "L" pad along the lateral malleolus for subluxation of the peroneal tendons, or a dorsal "block" in the lace area to restrict dorsiflexion in cases of anterior impingement.

Questions are frequently asked about the value of preventive ankle taping. A review of the literature by Metcalf and Denegar[23] highlights several points. With exercise, the initial restriction of range of motion is considerably reduced, but restricting the extreme ranges of motion responsible for ankle injury does appear to be adequate. Some believe that the restriction of ankle movement may increase the incidence of knee injuries, but this has been refuted by research. Ankle taping does not affect athletic performance. There is some evidence, however, to show that the protective effect of taping is caused by increased proprioceptive input. It also appears that the use of ankle taping to prevent reinjury to ankles previously injured is more easily defended. There is less benefit from the use of reusable cloth ankle wrapping or the wearing of a hightop shoe. The greatest issue is in the cost savings. Until it is conclusively proven that the cost of labor and supplies needed to provide protective taping outweighs the cost of preventable injury, the decision of whether or not to tape rely on professional opinion and budget considerations.

Arch Figure-of-Eight. This taping method may be effective to control excessive pronation, to decrease stress on the plantar fascia, and to give an adjunctive treatment for shin splint. Due to the increase perspiration of the soles of the feet, it is almost mandatory to apply this taping without the use of underwrap. An anchor strip is placed loosely around the metatarsal heads (Fig. 8A). Half of the figure-of-eight is performed by starting at the base of the great toe, angling across the longitudinal arch, around the heel, and returning the base of the great toe (Fig. 8B). The other half is similar, using the base of the little toe as the starting and finishing point (Fig. 8C). These steps are repeated once or twice (Fig. 8D). Next horizontal strips are placed, pulling medially, from the heel to the ball of the foot (Fig. 8E). A "low dye" strip-4 is begun at the base of the little toe, passed behind the heel, and then ended at the base of the great toe (Fig. 8F). A closing anchor is placed on the dorsum of the foot over the original anchor (Fig. 8G). Care must be taken to allow for the expansion of the foot upon weightbearing.

Achilles' Tendon Taping. This technique uses anchors created with elastic tape around the arch of the foot and the calf to give support to the musculotendinous structure (Fig. 9). The athlete's ankle is taped in a position of slight plantar flexion, thus restricting excessive dorsiflexion.

Turf-Toe Taping. Strips are taped between anchors around the great toe and the arch to prevent flexion and extension of the great toe (Fig. 10).

BRACING

The primary care practitioner can be overwhelmed with choices when attempting to choose a brace. The marketing of braces is full of unsubstantiated claims, no guarantees, but many disclaimers of liability. Often the athlete may already have a brace or know where to borrow one. The physician's role then is to evaluate critically the brace's effectiveness. With more products available every day, it is probably more important to recognize certain features of the widely-used braces.

Bracing—Pros and Cons

Bracing has several advantages over taping. First and foremost is the ability to provide protection or support to athletes who do not have access to a person skilled in athletic taping techniques. After the initial investment, braces may be more cost effective. In certain conditions, a brace or orthotic device can provide a means of support not available from taping. Although most braces are more convenient,

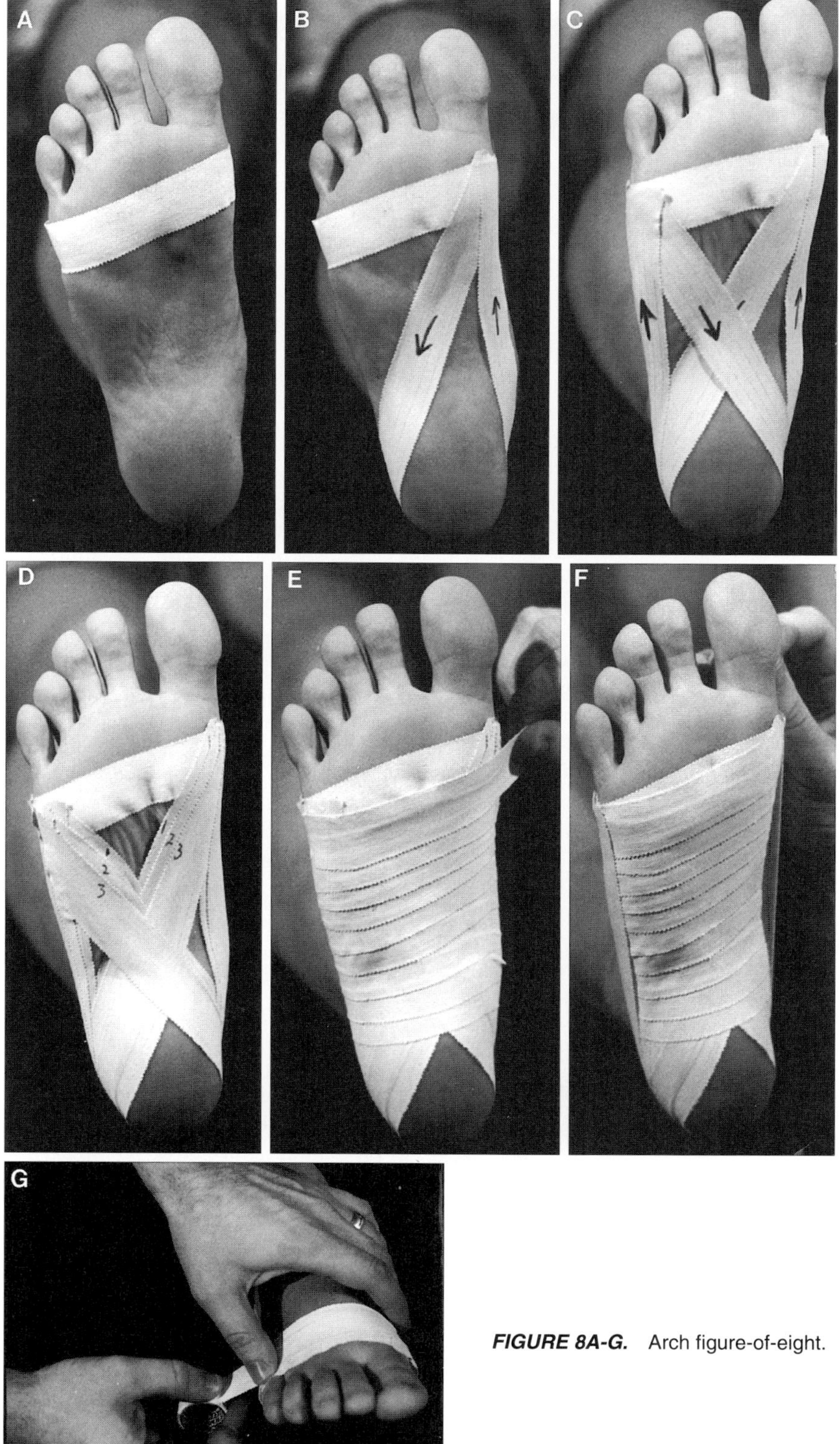

FIGURE 8A-G. Arch figure-of-eight.

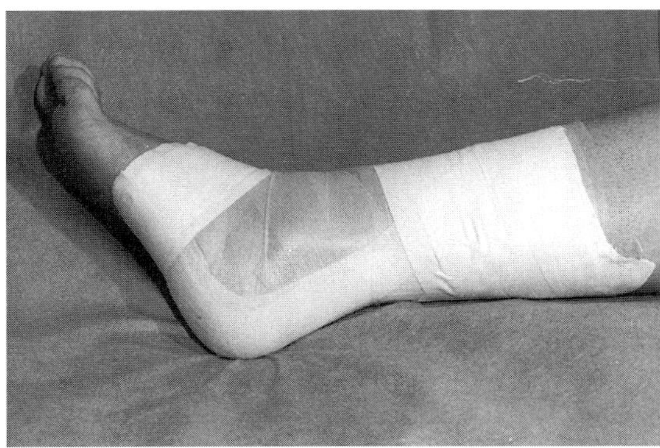

FIGURE 9. Achilles tendon taping.

drawbacks do exist. Because of the additional contact and lack of adhesion to the skin, migration of the appliance can occur during vigorous activity. This movement may cause the brace to fail to provide support and also to cause decreased athletic performance or other problems. Tape-adhesion, anti-migration straps, or specially designed undergarments may help. The most common complaint made by the athlete is the weight necessary in some braces to provide adequate protection. During wear-and-tear, Velcro fasteners tend to fail and release, straps or buckles break, and elastic stretches out. The athlete who is waiting for replacement parts cannot participate safely. Another problem is sizing—what do you do with athletes who are between sizes or who have body proportions that differ from that of the brace's design. Custom-made braces are available but are generally more expensive. The best advice is to select devices carefully and to prepare to deal with the problems that may arise from the braces prescribed to treat the patient. This is an area where the physician may need to seek the advice of the trainer, sports therapist, or orthotist.

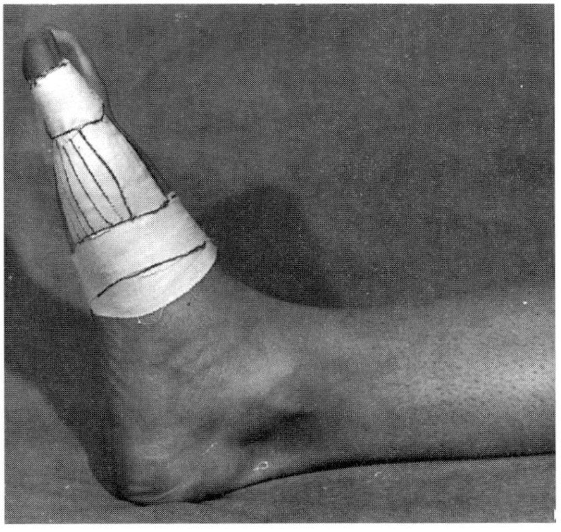

FIGURE 10. Turf-toe taping.

SUGGESTIONS FROM OUR PRACTICE

Tennis Elbow Strap

Epicondylitis is most commonly seen in athletes who participate in racquet sports, baseball, and softball who perform repeated forearm pronation and supination movements. The sports medicine practitioner can supplement and augment the rehabilitation program with a Velcro or elastic strap combination brace often called a "tennis elbow strap" or "counter-force brace" (Fig. 11). There are many available braces of this type, designed to reduce the contractile force of the extensor musculature, which causes irritation inflammation at or near the radiohumeral joint.

Silicone Rubber Wrist/Hand Cast

Some hand and wrist injuries requiring immobilization may be sufficiently supported so that participation in sports is permitted, even in collision sports such as football. By fabricating a playing cast out of various silicone rubber compounds, the injury can be adequately protected without subjecting other participants to risk from a brace made of an unyielding material. Details of their construction are found in the references.[4] A product called Soft-Cast has been introduced by 3M. This material provides the practitioner with a much quicker method of applying a rubber cast. Rules have been changed in high school competition to allow for plaster or fiberglass casts to be used in competition provided they are covered with padding. One must check the applicable rules to determine which option is possible for the specific injury.

Lateral Prophylactic Knee Braces

Prophylactic lateral knee braces (Fig. 12), designed to lessen the severity of lateral-impact valgus force injuries, are still in relative infancy both in design and implementation. Recent research has raised questions about the possibility of such braces "preloading" knee structures and predisposing the

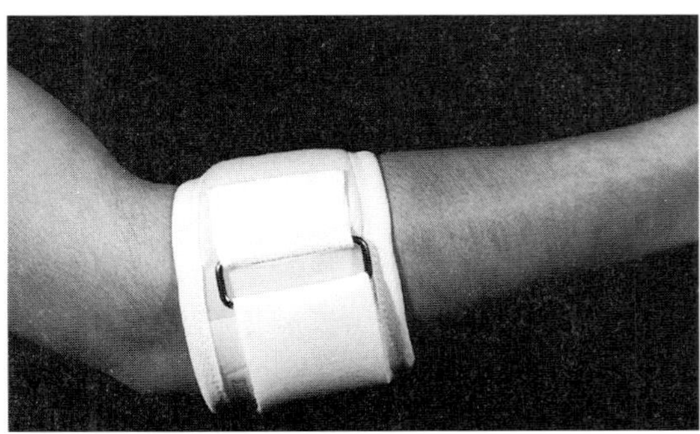

FIGURE 11. Tennis elbow counter-force brace.

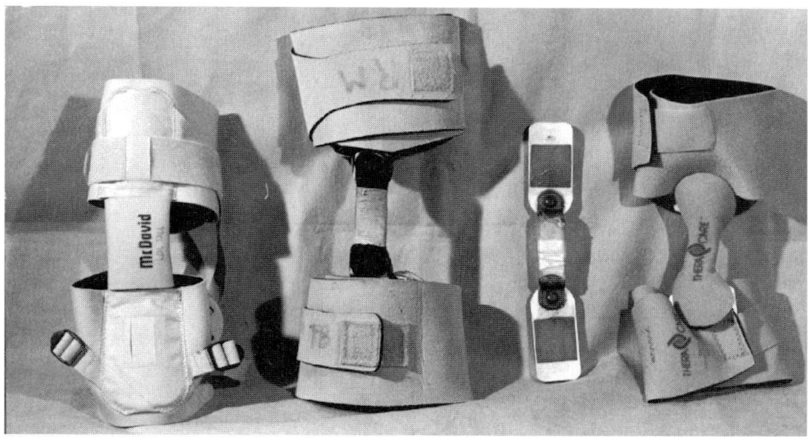

FIGURE 12. Examples of lateral prophylactic knee braces.

wearer to an increased risk of ligament injuries. Brace migration is a major problem as is compliance of the athlete in proper positioning and care of the brace, both essential to the success and effectiveness by: (1) shaving the skin as described for taping; (2) using a taping adherent; (3) using the audiovisual aids, (i.e., videotapes and posters, supplied by the manufacturers to teach proper application and as daily reminders; (4) daily checking of positioning by coaches and trainers; and (5) weekly checking on upkeep by coaches, parents, equipment managers, trainers, and players. With lateral prophylactic knee braces, as with all braces, there is no guarantee that an injury will not occur, but rather an assumption that, by design, lateral impact injuries may be less severe. A practical problem faced by the sports medicine practitioner is caused by the popularity of the braces, often based on anecdotal reports of bent braces that "saved" a player from injury. Research has not, however, substantiated this claim. Hewson et al.[16] found that in collegiate football players there appeared to be no reduction in the number of knee injuries after the adoption of lateral prophylactic knee braces and subsequent rule changes. With respect to their effect on performance, Prentice and Toriscelli found a significant decrease in 40 yard-dash times while wearing the braces but no decrease in agility or backward running.[27] We now feel that time and money might be better spent on preventive conditioning than for braces. Lateral knee braces may have a function at the end of a total rehabilitation program, but the popular notion that lateral knee braces are "better than nothing," in view of recent research to the contrary for athletes without injury, may require rethinking.

Functional Knee Braces

Another recent development is that of functional knee braces. These are designed to provide support to knees made unstable by injury or to provide additional protection following surgery to correct such instabilities. Some of these braces are ready-made in sizes to provide for immediate fit. Others require custom construction based on some form of cast molding or measurement of the athlete's leg. Considering the conditions being addressed and the cost of these devices, professional evaluation by an orthopedist essential. Attempts to support anterior cruciate injuries usually involve some form of hyperextension stop through the use of controlled hinges. The rotational component is controlled through the use of straps or fitted shells (Fig. 13). These braces also provide support to other knee structures. Some studies have investigated the relative effectiveness of these braces,[1,5,14] but no brace has been found to completely control the knee in all situations.

Knee Braces for Patellofemoral Pain Syndromes

Peripatellar pain and dysfunction resulting from anatomical causes, otherwise known as extensor mechanism malalignment (EMM), is being more accurately diagnosed and treated as knowledge of patellofemoral mechanics is widened by research. We have found success with two types of braces in assisting the athlete to return to full function: the Palumbo lateral patella stabilizing brace (DynOrthotics, Vienna, VA) and the neoprene rubber sleeve with patellar cutout. The Palumbo brace (Fig. 14) combines the support of an elastic sleeve with patellar cutout with a lateral buttress strap designed to dynamically decrease excessive lateral tracking of the patella, which is commonly responsible for the pain experienced by patients with EMM. Lysholm and associates[20] reported that during isokinetic testing of patients with EMM in braced and unbraced conditions, strength measurements increased whereas pain decreased during the test with the patellofemoral joint braced. Neoprene braces provide uniform compres-

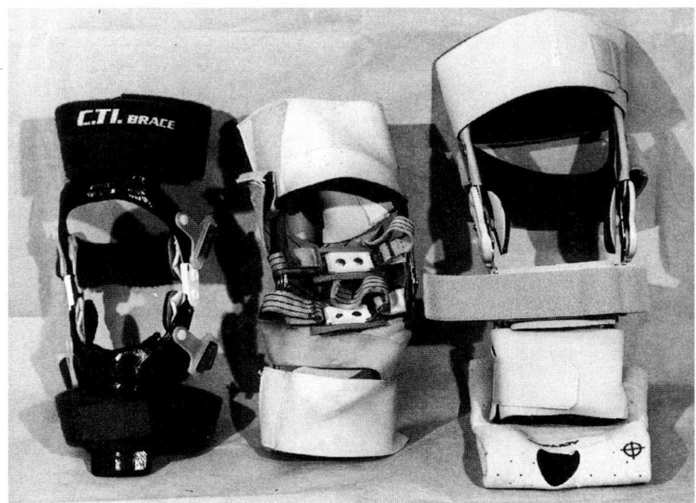

FIGURE 13. Examples of functional knee braces.

sion and allow for nearly normal range of motion of the knee (Figs. 14 and 15). It is essential that the athlete with EMM or patellar tendinitis ("jumper's knee") be fitted with a sleeve with a patellar cutout. This is necessary to allow full range of motion, support, proper tracking, and to decrease compression of the patellofemoral joint during activity. There are numerous brands available, some with a lateral buttress, for the physician and the athlete to choose from, but always keeping in mind the required patellar cutout.

Knee Sleeves

Sleeves can be used to provide compression of the knee (Fig. 15) as well as other soft tissue areas, such as calf musculature, the quadriceps, and the hamstrings. They are often made of elastic or Spandex, will provide even compression, and may promote local tissue healing. Neoprene is also used for these purposes. It differs from elastic and Spandex in its ability to retain body heat, thereby increasing the sense of warmth that sometimes makes the athlete who suffers from tendinitis more comfortable. The devices also provide some relief from pain caused by sensory stimulation. Patients wearing them report a feeling of security, probably due to increased proprioceptive input. As discussed previously, when a sleeve is used at the knee, it is important to use a brace with a patellar cutout to decrease irritation to those prone to EMM.

Ankle Braces

Ankle braces are available commercially which provide the sports medicine practitioner with variety and flexibility to the individual athlete and to support the site of injury. Slip-on elastic braces are best even when compression is desired, i.e., to de-

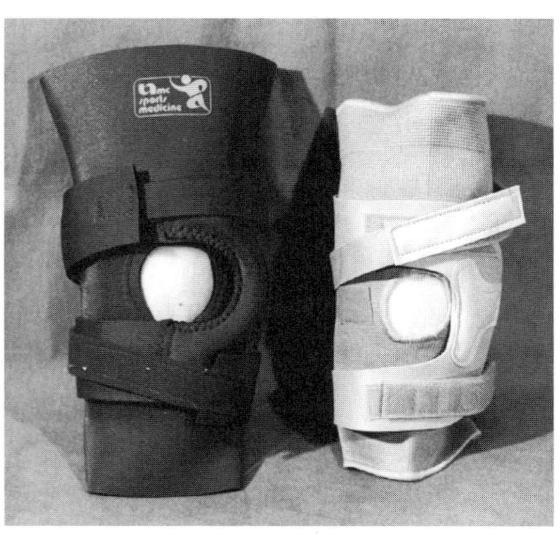

FIGURE 14. Palumbo braces, neoprene (left) and elastic (right).

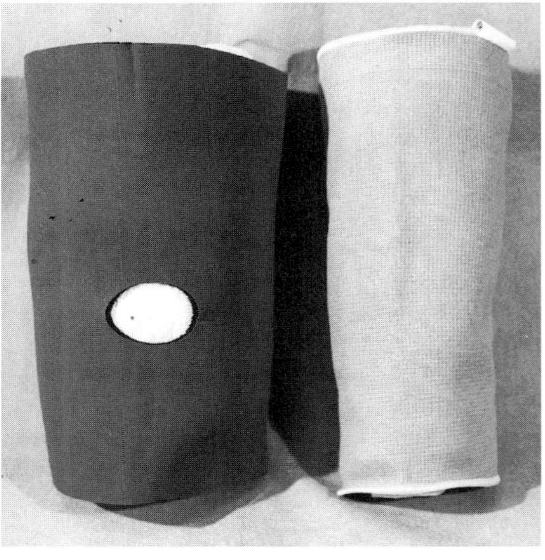

FIGURE 15. Knee sleeves, neoprene (left) and elastic (right).

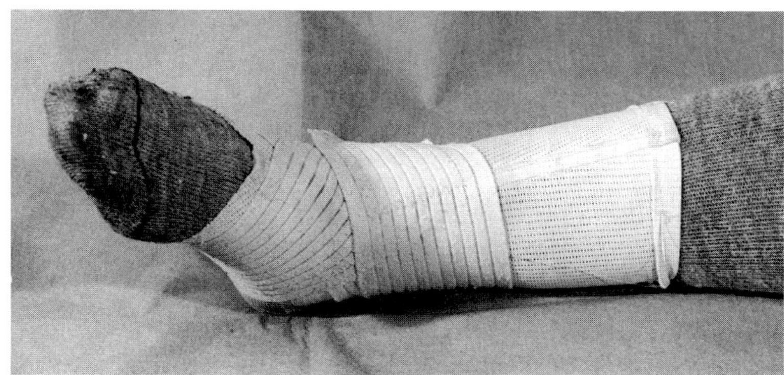

FIGURE 16. Elastic ankle support.

crease edema. They do not, however, restrict inversion or eversion enough to be considered as giving prophylactic support. Certain manufacturers, e.g., Stromgren, combine the comfort of even compression by using Spandex, elastic, and Velcro strap combinations to restrict inversion or eversion (Fig. 16). We have found them easier to manage during break-in; they are also a better alternative than the slip-on ankle brace. A third type of prophylactic support for the ankle is made in a lace-up style (Fig. 17). These braces often have both medial and lateral stays, thus providing increased restriction of movement related to inversion or eversion. In considering the use of these braces, one might also think of them as an alternative or adjunct to ankle taping, especially if a competent taper is not readily available. Bunch and colleagues[8] compared the comfort and effectiveness of ankle taping to five different commercially available ankle braces. Initial comfort and support were highest in the freshly taped ankle. After 20 minutes of inversion exercises, however, "two of the lace-on braces offered the same level of support as the tape."[8] The report concluded that, at the end of their conservative 20-minute test, there was no difference in the level of support for the top two lace-on style braces (Swede-O, Mikros 9-in.) and taping.

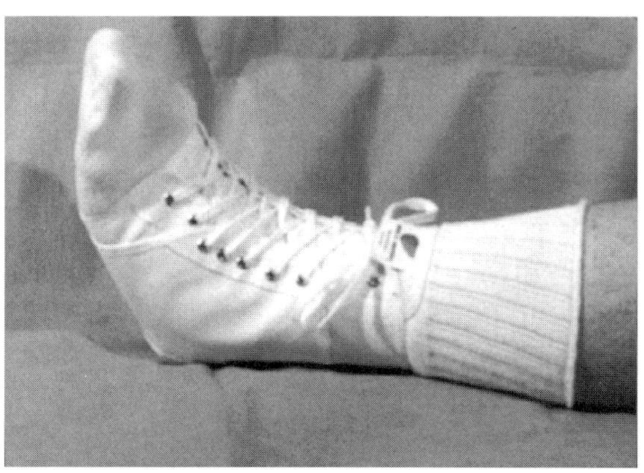

FIGURE 17. Lace-up ankle support.

Air Cast

The air cast can be of great use to the physician, therapist, and trainer from early in the rehabilitation program to the late stages preceding return to functional activity for the athlete with a moderate to severe ankle injury. Stover[29] described the use of a semirigid support in case studies of seven athletic patients. The air cast is similar in its design and principles for use to the semi-rigid material previously described (Fig. 18). It provides a milking effect upon weightbearing, which appears to decrease post-traumatic edema. With the addition of an air bag lining, it allows for an earlier return to functional activities, decreases unwanted excessive inversion and eversion, and protects the already injured ligament and soft tissues from reinjury or further injury, thereby decreasing rehabilitation time." We have found that air casts are easy to use and fit into most athletic footwear. Their application is easily taught and followed and the athlete's confidence in the race is increased with their use. Even when combined with ankle taping, the appliance does not significantly decrease speed or lessen jumping ability.

SHOE INSERTS

Although not truly braces, orthotics are commonly used to aid in the treatment of athletic injury. Orthotics are defined here as devices placed in the athlete's shoe to balance the foot during activity. External support in the area of orthotics requires careful selection by both practitioner and athlete, always being conscious of the demands of the activity, ease of application, and adaptability to the athlete's condition.

Soft Orthotics

Sometimes used before the permanent orthotic returns from the laboratory, soft orthotics can also be purchased over the counter (Fig. 19). They are relatively easy to adapt to and have a high compli-

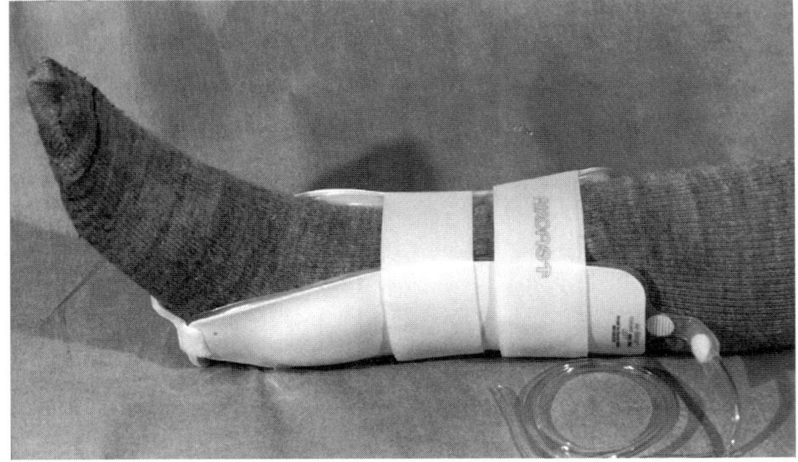

FIGURE 18. Air cast with pressure adjustment tube attached.

ance among athletes. Care must be taken in not using a "cure for all" orthotic that may treat more than one condition, thus predisposing the normal foot structures to injury.

Hard Orthotics

Sometimes more difficult to get accustomed to initially, these devices are usually custom fitted for the specific condition, but some over-the-counter varieties exist (Fig. 19). They hold up well and are often the key to solving the mystery of pain within the kinetic chain of the body. They should be used only in patients involved in straight ahead running.

Semirigid Orthotics

These devices attempt to provide the support of hard orthotics but are designed to balance the feet of athletes involved in sports requiring agility (see Fig. 19). Because each sport has its own skill requirements, the orthotic selected must reflect such differences.

Sorbothane Insoles

Sorbothane is often used to decrease impact forces (Fig. 20). Insoles made of it are easy to use, but do not attempt to correct or alter foot mechanics.

Heel Cups

Soft heel cups, e.g., Tulis, are highly recommended for the athlete with a "heel bruise" or "heel pain" after other possibilities have been ruled out. The appliances help to decrease impact and to improve the shock absorption of the fat pad of the calcaneus.

Metatarsal and Longitudinal Arch Pads

Metatarsal (Fig. 21) and longitudinal (Fig. 22) arch pads, when applied to the footwear and not the

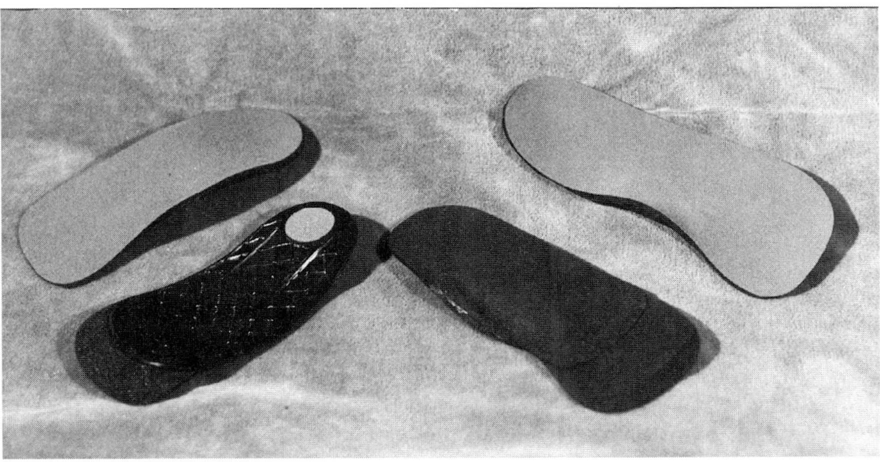

FIGURE 19. Spenco arch supports, rigid (left) and semi-rigid (right).

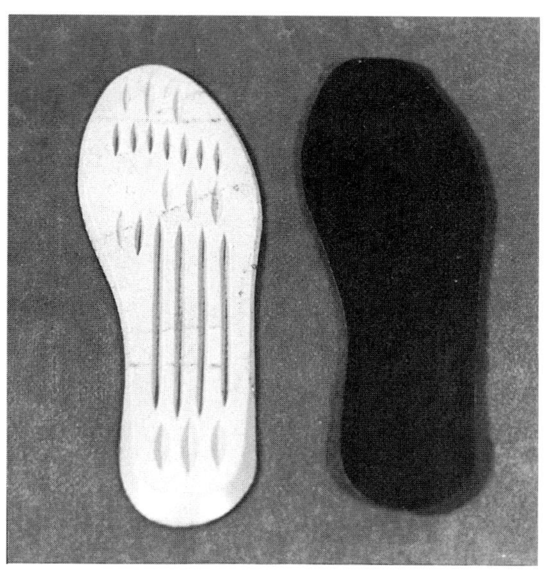

FIGURE 20. Sorbathane insoles.

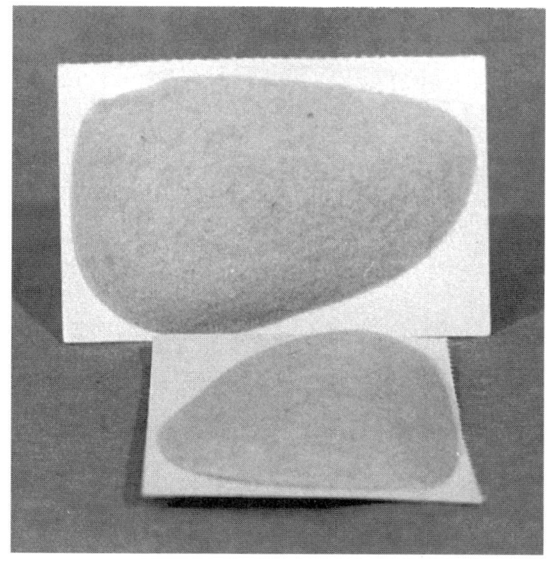

FIGURE 21. Metatarsal arch pads.

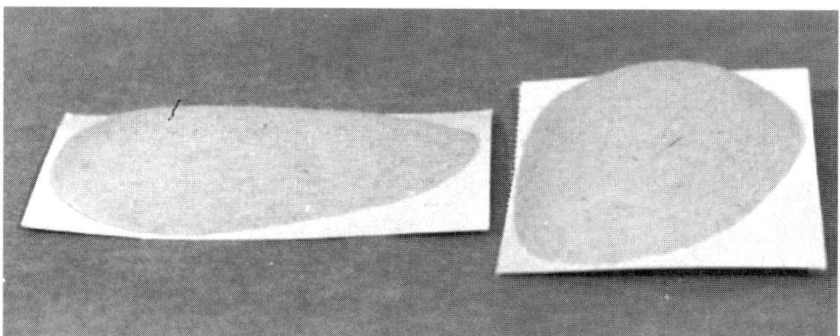

FIGURE 22. Longitudinal arch pads.

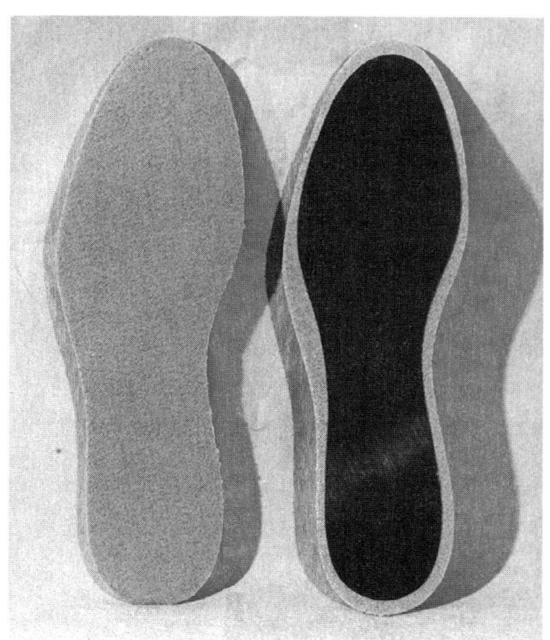

FIGURE 23. Steel shoe inserts.

foot, provide very good support to the ligamentous, bony, and muscular structures that help to form the arches of the feet. They also provide some symptomatic relief for painful foot conditions. They can also be applied directly to the skin, following the previously given principles of taping.

Steel Shoe Inserts

These help manage metatarsal fractures and turf toe. In certain brands of football turf shoes, they are standard and are incorporated directly into the insole liner (Fig. 23).

SUMMARY

Further research and development on external support of athletic injuries is much needed. Until the results of such rigorous studies are conclusive, decisions about taping and bracing will continue to depend on anecdotal information. Being aware of what is available, keeping abreast of new developments and analyzing them carefully, and talking to others who have experience in their use can assist the sports medicine practitioner in selecting a method of support. Taping and bracing can decrease the risk of reinjury, especially when performed under the supervision of people who are skilled and knowledgeable in these methods. Because of the inherent nature of sport, it is paramount that the practitioner give no guarantees. Placing an emphasis on complete rehabilitation and individualizing the choice of taping or bracing will allow the athletic patient to safely resume activity.

REFERENCES

1. Albright JP, Powell JW, Smith W, et al: Medial collateral ligament knee sprains in college football. Brace wear preferences and injury risk. Am J Sports Med 22:2, 1994.
2. Albright JP, Powell JW, Smith W, et al: Medial collateral ligament knee sprains in college football. Effectiveness of preventative braces. Am J Sports Med 22:12, 1994.
3. Barrett JR, Tanji JL, Drake C, et al: High versus low-top shoes for the prevention of ankle sprains in basketball players. Am J Sports Med 21:582, 1993.
4. Bassett FH, Malone T, Gilcrist RA: A protective splint of rubber. Am J Sports Med 7:358, 1979.
5. Beck C, Drez D. Young J, et al: Instrumented testing of functional knee braces. Am J Sports Med 14:253, 1986.
6. Borsa PA, Lephart SM, Fu FH: Muscular and functional performance characteristics of individuals wearing prophylactic knee braces. JOSPT 28:336, 1993.
7. Bradley JA: The modified rubber playing cast. Phys Sports Med 10:1h8, 1982.
8. Bunch RP, Bednarski K, Holland D, Macinanti R: Ankle joint support: A comparison of reuseable lace-on braces with taping and bracing. Physician SportMed 13:59, 1985.
9. Burks RT, Bean BG, Marcus R, Barker HB: Analysis of athletic performance with prophylactic ankle devices. Am J Sports Med 19:104, 1991.
10. Distefano V, Nixon JE: An improved method of taping. J Sports Med 2:209, 1974.
11. Doughtie M.: The use of RTV-11 silicone rubber for a carpal navicular fracture. Athletic Training 14:146, 1979.
12. Feuerbach JW, Grabiner MD: Effect of the Aircast on unilateral postural control: Amplitude and frequency variables. JOSPT 7:149, 1993.
13. Feuerbach JW, Grabiner MD, Koh TJ, Weiker GG: Effect of an ankle orthosis and ankle ligament anaesthesia on ankle joint proprioception. Am J Sports Med 22:223, 1993.
14. Functional knee braces help stabilize medial collateral ligament. Orthop Today 6:1, 1986.
15. Garrick JG, Requa RK: Role of external support in the prevention of ankle sprains. Med Sci Sports 5:200, 1973.
16. Hewson GF, Mendini RA, Wang JB: Prophylactic knee bracing in college football. Am J Sports Med 14:262, 1986.
17. Knee braces to prevent injuries in football: A round table. Physician Sportsmed 14:108, 1986.
18. Laughman RK, Carr TA, Chao EY, et al: Three dimensional kinematics of the taped ankle before and after exercise. Am J Sports Med 8:425, 1980.
19. Libera D: Ankle taping, wrapping, and injury prevention. Athletic Training 7:73, 1972.
20. Lysholm J, Nordin M, Ekstrand J, Gilquist J: The effects of a patella brace on performance in knee extension strength test in patients with patellar pain. Am J Sports Med 12:110, 1984.
21. McConnell JS: The management of chondromalacia patellae: A long term solution. Aust J Physiother 32:(4), 1986.
22. McConnell JS: Training the vastus medialis obliques in the management of patellofemoral pain. Proceedings of the Tenth International Congress of the WCPT, Sydney, Australia, 5:1987.
23. Metcalf GR, Denegar CR: A critical review of ankle taping. Athletic Training 18:121, 1983.
24. Nirschl RP: The etiology and treatment of tennis elbow. J Sports Med 2:308, 1974.
25. Palumbo PM: Dynamic patellar brace: A new orthosis in the management of patello-femoral disorders. A preliminary report. Am J Sports Med 9:45, 1981.
26. Peppard A: Thumb taping. Physician Sportsmed 10:139, 1982.
27. Prentice WE, Toriscelli T: The effects of lateral knee stabilizing braces on running speed and agility. Athletic Training 21:113, 1986.
28. Ross SE: The supportive effect of modified Duke Simpson strapping. Athletic Training 13:206, 1978.
29. Stover C: A functional semirigid support system for ankle injuries. Physician Sportsmed 7(5):71, 1979.
30. Stover CN: Air stirrup management of ankle injuries in the athlete. Am J Sports Med 8:360, 1980.
31. Thorndike A: Athletic Injuries: Prevention, Diagnosis and Treatment. Philadelphia, Lea & Febiger, 1948.
32. Weber JE: Personal communication. 1987.
33. Whitesel J, Newell SG: Modified low-dye strapping. Physician Sportsmed 8(9):129. 1980.

RECOMMENDED READING

Arnheim DD, Prentice WE: Modern Principles of Athletic Training, 8th ed. St. Louis, C. V. Mosby, 1993.

Athletic Uses of Adhesive Tape. New Brunswick, NJ, Johnson & Johnson Products, 1981.

Cerney JV: Complete Book of Athletic Taping Techniques. West Nyack, NY, Parker Publishing, 1972.

Austin K, Gwynne-Brett K, Marshall S: Illustrated Guide to Taping Techniques. London, Mosby-Year Book Europe Limited, 1994.

27

Bicycling Injuries: Prevention, Diagnosis, and Treatment

Morris B. Mellion M.D.

The popularity of the bicycle both as a recreational vehicle and as a mode of transportation is skyrocketing. The total number of U.S. bicyclists has risen from 72 million in 1983 to 99 million in 1992. The number of adults riding regularly has risen from 10 million to 31 million in the same period, and the number of bicycle commuters has gone from 1.5 million to 4.3 million. Similarly, the number of bicycle racers has expanded from 40,000 to 250,000.[3]

Since Americans won four bicycle gold medals in the 1984 Los Angeles Olympics and American Greg Lemond won the Tour de France three times, bicycle fever has risen even higher in the United States. Lance Armstrong's world championship victory in his first full year of professional bicycle racing and Julie Furtado's undefeated season in mountain bike competition have fueled American interest in bicycling.

During the 1980s the bicycle itself changed. Traditional 1, 3, and 10 speed bicycles have been replaced by 18, 21, and even 24 speed bikes. The dropped-handlebar road bike has been surpassed in popularity by a variety of mountain, or all-terrain, bikes and hybrids. Bicycling has become a $3.5 billion per year industry[19] with 11.6 million bicycles sold annually.[3] Californian Michael Sinyard began the transformation of the American bicycle industry when he manufactured the Stumpjumper, the first mountain bike, in 1981. The number of mountain bike riders has risen from 200,000 in 1983 to 25 million in 1992.[3]

With this increase in riding enthusiasm, there is also an increase in trauma. U.S. Consumer Product Safety Commission data from 1991 reveals that 601,172 bicyclists were treated for injuries in U.S. hospitals. Of these, 96% were treated in emergency rooms and released, and 4% were hospitalized. There were 841 fatalities, which represents approximately 2% of all traffic deaths. Seventy percent of bicyclists injured and 80% of bicyclists killed were male. Two-thirds of the injured were under 14 years of age.[3] The most common traumatic injuries involve the face and head, wrist, knee, ankle, and foot; the majority are soft-tissue injuries.[23,61,72,128] Traumatic injuries to bicyclists will generally be treated using standard approaches, which are well described in the trauma literature.

Physicians will also be faced with the challenge of diagnosing and treating nontraumatic problems arising from bicycling. The main focus of this chapter is these nontraumatic or overuse syndromes associated with bicycle riding, with more limited emphasis on traumatic injury. In order to treat and rehabilitate the injured cyclist, the physician needs a working knowledge of bicycle anatomy, proper technique for fitting the bicycle to the rider, proper riding technique, and bicycle safety equipment. The first section of the chapter focuses on these issues; the second is devoted to the commonly encountered overuse problems and injuries. It focuses on diagnosis and treatment, mechanical, as well as medical.

THE MODERN BICYCLE

"In order to prevent and treat bicycle injuries effectively physicians should understand: (a) the basic design and function of common bicycles; (b) the relationship of improper bicycle "fit" to injuries; and (c) the potential of various forms of serious riding and racing for injury."[80]

The conceptual origins of the modern bicycle date back to ancient China, Egypt, and India; but the development of the chain-driven rear wheel in the late 1880s and of the gear changing system in 1932 contributed to the bicycle as we know it.[36] The

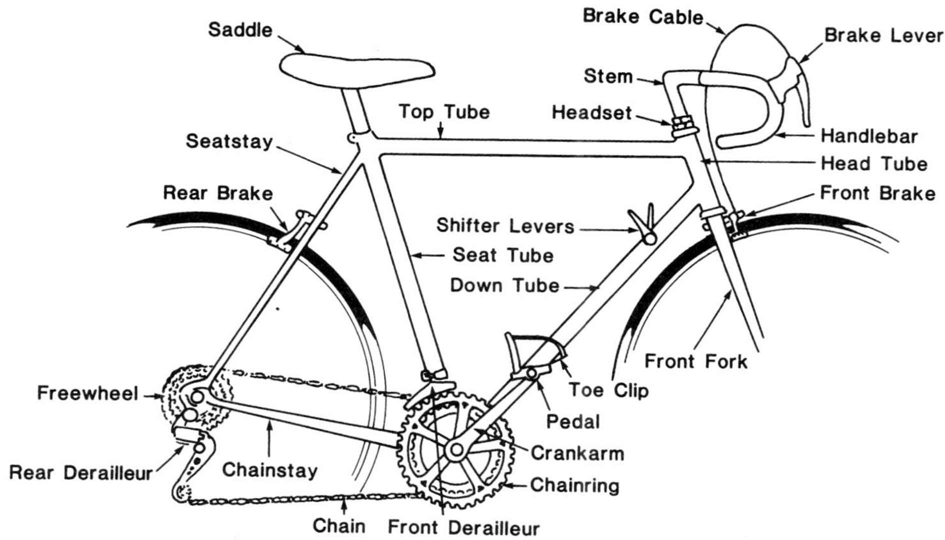

FIGURE 1. Anatomy and terminology of a modern bicycle.

dropped handlebars of the road bike became popular both because of their aerodynamic advantage[67] and because the dropped bar posture contributes to increased oxygen uptake, work output, and pulmonary ventilation.[37] The all-terrain bicycle was originally developed for off-road riding, but it has become increasingly popular because it allows experienced riders access to an almost unlimited variety of terrain and it provides a comfortable, forgiving vehicle for entry level cyclists.

Bicycle Anatomy

Physicians treating cyclists need a working knowledge of the "anatomy and terminology" of the bicycle. The modern bicycle consists of a frame ("frame set") and attached components including handlebars brakes and wheels pedals and gears. (Fig. 1) Most components of the bicycle can be changed, but a good frame is essential. Materials used in frame composition are changing drastically. The old steel frame has been replaced in the performance bicycle by a lighter, more resilient, and durable chrome-magnesium alloy, aluminum, and carbon fiber composites. The result is a stronger, lighter, better-handling bicycle.

The bicycle frame is shaped like a diamond lying on its side (Fig. 2). Racing bicycles have more upright geometry with steeper angles to the diamond. This configuration produces a stiffer frame, which

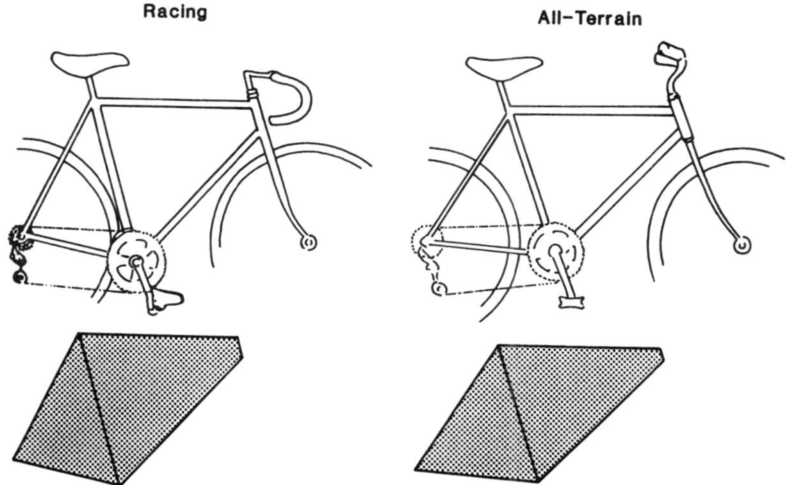

FIGURE 2. The bicycle frame is shaped like a diamond lying on its side. Racing bicycles have more upright geometry with steeper angles to the diamond. All terrain bicycles have somewhat flatter geometry with more shallow angles. Touring bicycles are generally in between.

is more responsive when turning and more efficient in converting the rider's energy into forward motion. Touring bicycles have a longer wheel base, which produces a somewhat flatter geometry. Their configuration produces more shock absorption with some sacrifice in cornering ability. All-terrain bicycles have an even flatter geometry, which results in better shock absorption on the rough surfaces of trails and unpaved roads. Recent developments in structural materials and engineering techniques allow even greater improvement in shock absorbency with less changes in geometry than were previously necessary.

All-terrain bicycles are heavier, lower-geared bicycles with wide balloon tires and upright handlebars. They are designed to be ridden in rough or hilly terrain. These bicycles typically weigh 28 to 35 lb, compared to 19 to 22 lb for road bikes. Mountain bikes come equipped with relatively wide 26″ diameter wheels, compared with the narrow 27″ wheels on road bikes. Because of the increased weight, the differences in wheel dimensions and gearing systems, and the less aerodynamic upright riding position, mountain bikes are considerably slower than road bikes when ridden on smooth terrain.

The newest group of bicycles to achieve popularity have been hybrids. They are bicycles with a combination of features from the road bike and all-terrain models. Hybrids are intermediate in weight and tire width, with either 26 or 27″ wheels. They generally have mountain-bike style handlebars, but their geometry is somewhat more upright like the road bike. They provide the comfort and upright riding position of the mountain bike in a faster, lighter model.

Fitting the Bicycle

If a bicycle is ridden for only short distances at low intensity, fit is not a very important consideration. The longer and more intense the riding, however, the more important fit becomes. For high-performance cycling and long-distance riding, proper fit is essential for the prevention of overuse injuries. The most efficient method to provide accurate fit for the serious cyclist is to use a commercial system such as a Fit Kit or ProBike Fit. These are systems of measuring the rider and predicting proper bicycle size and fit based on accumulated data. An optional component of the Fit Kit is the rotational adjustment device (RAD) which may be used to provide an accurate cleat adjustment for riders with cleated shoes or step-in pedals.

For most riders a commercial system is not necessary to make the proper frame selection and basic fit adjustments. The following guidelines provide sufficient information for the serious cyclist to set up a bicycle properly. Subsequent adjustments may be to fine tune the bicycle to the rider. There are six basic aspects of bicycle fit: frame size, seat height, seat position, handlebar reach, handlebar height, and handlebar width.

To determine the proper frame size of a bicycle, the rider should straddle the top of the bicycle with both feet flat on the ground wearing riding shoes. (Fig. 3) For racing, triathlon, criterium, and touring bicycles there should be a 1 to 2″ space between the rider's crotch and the top tube. For mountain bikes and hybrids, the clearance should be 3 to 6″ with the higher end of the scale being safer for use on extremely rough terrain. Another technique for determining frame size is to measure inseam height (Fig. 4) and multiply by .65 for road bikes and .52 for mountain bikes.[24]

There are many scientific and quasi-scientific methods for determining seat height;[16,74,80,127,130,145] three will be discussed. First, the inseam method multiplies the crotch-to-floor measurement of inseam by 1.06 to 1.09 to obtain the seat height measured from the top of the saddle to the top of the pedal, when the crank arm is at 6-o'clock, i.e., "dead-bottom center" position. The actual setting within this range should be fine tuned to the individual rider. Research has demonstrated that within this range, there is only a minimal effect from variations of seat height on force application.[10,16,74]

The second method sets the saddle height so that there is 25 to 30° of knee flexion when the saddle is in a neutral fore-aft position and the pedal is at dead bottom center (Figure 5).[54] The third method is

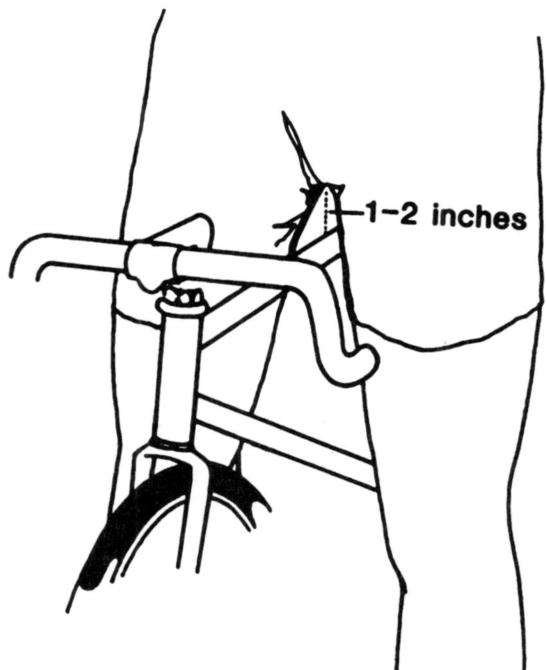

FIGURE 3. Proper frame size. Allow 1 to 2 inches between crotch and top frame tube for road bikes and 3 to 6 inches for hybrid and mountain bikes.

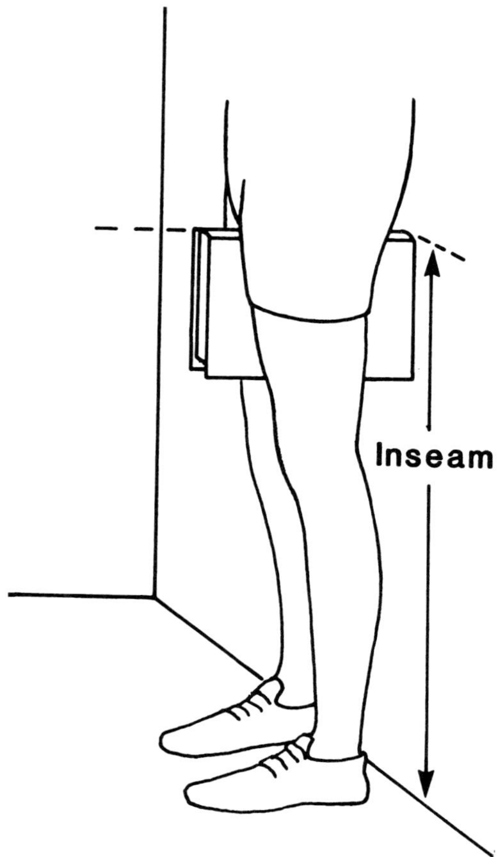

FIGURE 4. Seat height by inseam method. With rider wearing cycling shoes, measure inseam (floor to crotch) and multiply by 1.06 to 1.09 to obtain seat height range.

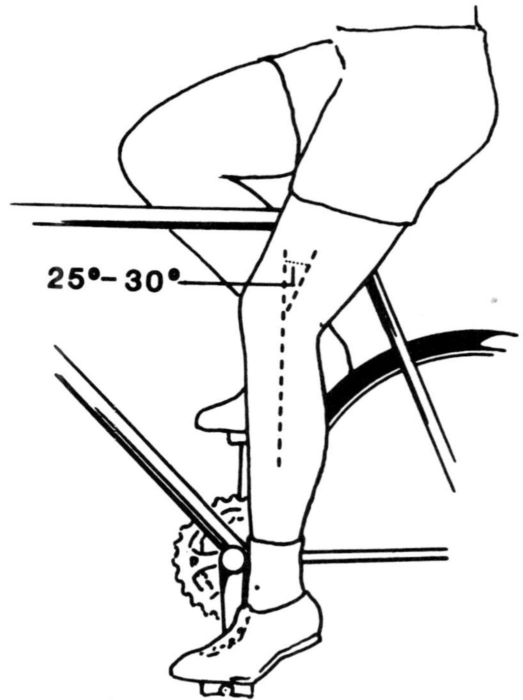

FIGURE 5. Proper seat height may be evaluated by measuring the amount of knee flexion with the foot at dead bottom center of the pedaling stroke (6 o'clock). There should be 25 to 30° flexion of the extended leg. The rider's ankle should be at the same angle that it usually is at dead bottom center in the rider's normal

known as "rocking in the saddle." Raise the seat to the point at which the rider must rock from side to side in order to pedal; then lower it in increments of ¼" until the rocking is unnecessary. All seat height formulas are estimates, and much fine tuning will be necessary.

The formulas have several pitfalls. They do not account for foot length or for riding style. An individual with a foot disproportionately large for leg length, who rides with a predominantly toe-down style might require a longer frame. Saddle compressibility and rider weight vary as well, so that a heavier rider on a more compressible saddle might have an effectively shorter seat height than that obtained by measurement. Another factor is the effect of a wide variety of clipless pedals on the distance between the sole of the riding shoe and the pedal spindle. The rider's solution is to fine tune seat height by making adjustments of ¼" at a time and maintaining the adjustment level for 2 to 3 rides at a time. Highly experienced riders may want to make adjustments as small as ⅛".

The fore and aft saddle position is adjusted by moving the bicycle saddle on the pair of rails that connect it to the seat post. These rails allow approximately 1½" adjustment range. With the rider in the saddle and the pedals at the 3- and 9-o'clock positions, the seat should be adjusted so that a plumb line dropped from the front edge of the patella should fall to the end of the crank arm (Fig. 6).[16,54] This is virtually the same position as in previous recommendations, so that a plumb line dropped from the tibial tubercle would intersect the axle of the pedal.[30,80,82]

Saddle angle should be set using a carpenter's level placed along the longitudinal axis of the saddle. One anatomical difference between male and female riders is the angle of the pubic arch in relation to the saddle angle. In the male the arch of the pubic symphysis is higher and allows enough clearance above the nose of the saddle for the rider to tolerate a saddle which is level or angled slightly upward in front. The shallower female pubic arch may cause the soft tissue of the perineum to press against the nose of the saddle. Consequently, most women may prefer to have the saddle level or tilted slightly downward. Others attempt to compensate by riding with a more upright posture to shift the weight from the anterior perineum.[16,22]

Handlebar height should be adjusted for recreational riders so that the handlebars are equal to or

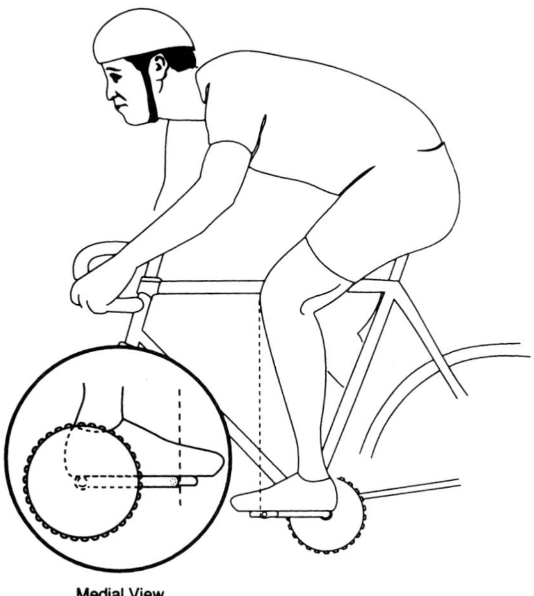

FIGURE 6. Seat position relative to the pedals is determined by putting the pedals at the 3 o'clock and 9 o'clock positions, with the ball of the foot firmly on the pedal. A plumb line drop from the middle of the anterior surface of the patella should fall at the front edge of the crank arm.

1″ below the level of the top of the seat. More experienced riders may want a lower position to improve aerodynamics. Time trialists and other short-distance racers may place the stem 3 to 4″ or more below the saddle height. Taller riders may want the difference between saddle height and the top of the handlebars to be greater to accommodate longer arms. The handlebars on mountain bikes should be 1 to 2″ below the top of the saddle to help put weight on the front wheel.[64]

Handlebar reach is the distance from the front of the saddle to the center of the transverse part of the handlebar. Proper handlebar reach can be estimated by placing the elbow at the front of the saddle with the olecranon touching the anterior aspect of the seat. The tips of the fingers should just touch the handlebar for proper distance (Fig. 7). Reach can be adjusted by exchanging the handlebar stem for one with longer or shorter extension (Fig. 8).[76,82,95,130]

One further consideration is the width of the handlebars. Handlebar width on the road bike should equal shoulder width measured between the lateral borders of the acromions. For mountain bikes, handlebar width should be determined empirically by what feels most comfortable to the rider. Narrower handlebars provide quicker steering, and wider bars give more control at slower speeds.[64]

A new form of handlebar called the aero bar has been used extensively in both triathlon and ultraendurance riding because it reduces aerodynamic drag.[66] More recently, it has found niches in time trialing and bicycle touring. It provides an aerodynamic body position resembling a downhill ski racing tuck which can be maintained for long periods. (Fig. 9). It also takes the rider's weight off the hands and reduces the incidence of nerve entrapment problems in the wrists. The aero bar height is set significantly lower than the seat height in an attempt to get the rider's back flattened to a position roughly parallel to the ground. There were questions about whether this tucked in position re-

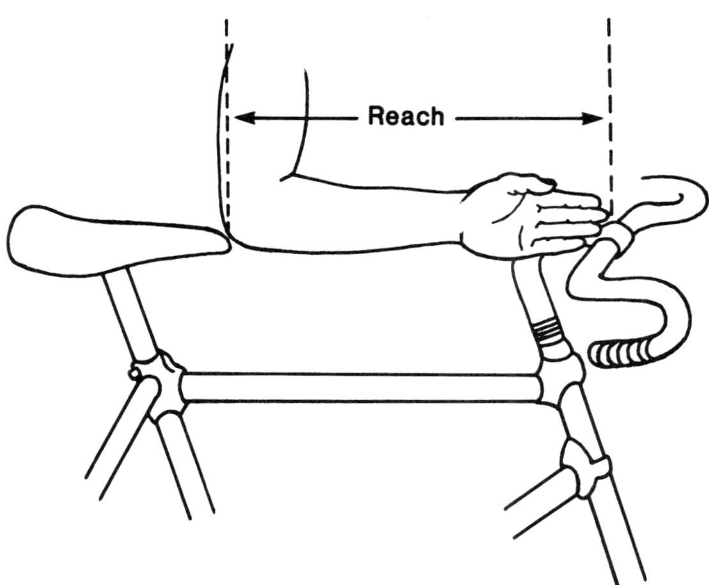

FIGURE 7. Handlebar height should be adjusted so that the handlebars are equal to or just below the level of the top of the seat. Proper reach is determined by placing the elbow at the front of the seat with the fingers extended; the finger tips should just touch the handlebars.

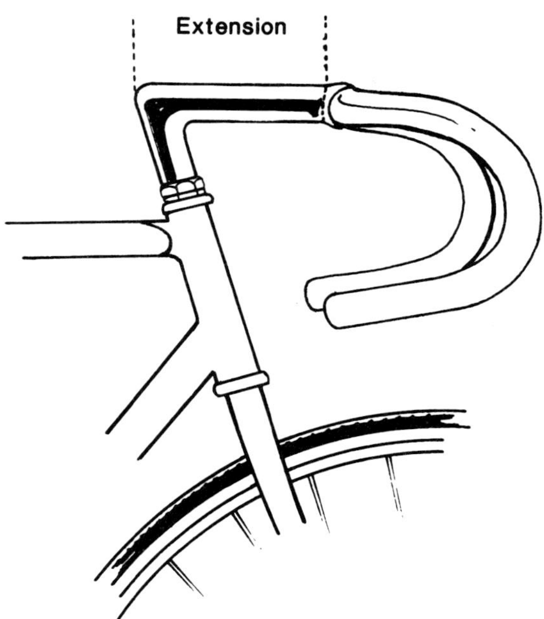

FIGURE 8. Extension is the horizontal length of the handlebar stem. It can be changed only by replacing the stem.

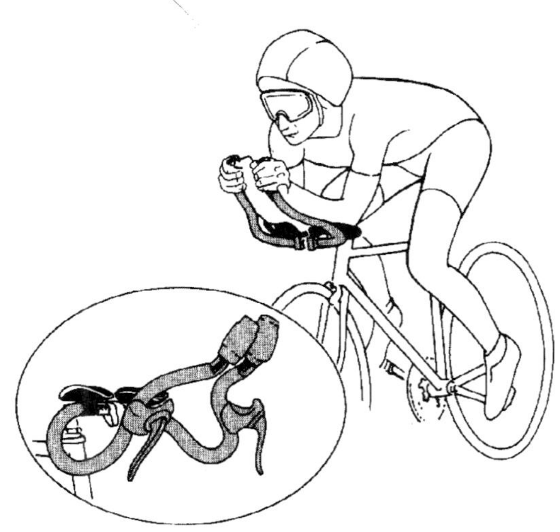

FIGURE 9. The aero bar is designed to permit the rider to maintain a highly aerodynamic position for a prolonged time. (From Mellion MB: Common cycling injuries: Management and prevention, Sports Med 11:52–70, 1991, with permission.)

stricted breathing capacity and oxygen consumption, but research has demonstrated no impaired response to high intensity exercise in the aero bar position.[2,27,59,91]

Riders with leg-length discrepancies need a special fit. In general the bicycle should be fit to the long leg with special corrections made for the short leg. Tibial leg-length discrepancies can be corrected with lifts or shims installed between the pedal and the shoe and cyclist orthotics. Femoral leg-length discrepancies, on the other hand, require a combination of lifts, shims, or orthotics with a modification of the foot position on the pedal. The long leg should be moved a few millimeters forward and the short leg a few millimeters back[54] (Table 2, p. 369).

Pedalling and Gearing

The cyclist functions best when riding with only a narrow range of pedal resistance to effort. The modern bicycle allows the cyclist to pedal comfortably with a relatively constant pedal resistance at a rather uniform cadence (cadence = pedal revolutions per minute [rpm]) by shifting through a range of 10 to 24 "speeds" or gears. Power is transmitted from the gears attached to the pedal crank by a chain composed of evenly spaced links to the gears connected to the rear wheel, which drives the bike. (Figure 10*A*) Because the gear teeth must be evenly spaced and of uniform size in order to mesh with the chain, the size of a gear may be expressed by its number of teeth. The front gears are attached to the "crank," or axle, around which the rider pedals. Virtually all road bicycles, all-terrain bicycles, and hybrids have a "large chain ring" and a "small chain ring" attached to the crank. Touring, all-terrain, and hybrid bicycles also have a very small chain ring, known as a "granny," attached to the crank as well. It is used for climbing steep hills. The rear wheel gears are smaller and are assembled in a cluster of 5 to 8 cogs (individual gears), known as a "free wheel" or "cassette." This gear set is mounted to the right of the rear wheel on the same axle.

To change the gears in use, the rider moves shift levers (see Fig. 1) The front shift lever controls the front derailleur, which moves the chain from one chain ring to another. The rear shift lever controls the rear derailleur, which moves the chain from one cog of the free wheel or cassette to another. The gear ratio (Fig. 10*B*) is the ratio of the size of the chain wheel in use to that of the free wheel or cassette cog in use:

$$\text{Gear ratio} = \frac{\text{number of teeth on chain wheel}}{\text{number of teeth on free wheel cog}}$$

A higher gear ratio, therefore, results in greater pedal resistance in a given riding condition than a lower gear ratio. Traditionally, racers and other serious bicyclists have multiplied the gear ratio by the diameter of the rear wheel to obtain a ratio called gear inches:

$$\text{Gear inches} = \text{Gear ratio} \times \text{rear wheel diameter.}$$

To complete the sequence and obtain the distance traveled per pedal revolution, simply multiply gear inches by π (.31416):

A

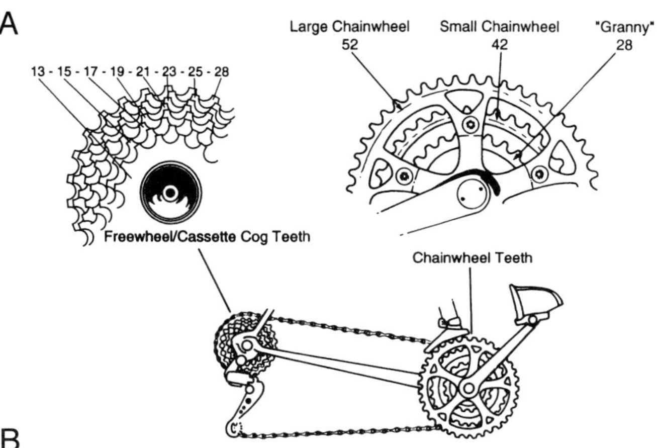

FIGURE 10. *A,* Modern bicycle gearing. This example is from a touring with 3 chainwheels on the crank and 8 cogs on the freewheel/cassette. *B,* Calculation of some typical gear ratios using the gearing illustrated in Figure 10A.

B

	GEAR RATIO	GEAR INCHES
EXAMPLES	$= \frac{\text{\# of teeth on chainwheel}}{\text{\# of teeth on freewheel cog}}$	= gear ratio x wheel dia.
VERY HIGH GEAR	$\frac{52}{13} = 4$	4X27 = 108
LOWER GEAR	$\frac{52}{26} = 2$	2X27 = 54
VERY LOW GEAR	$\frac{28}{28} = 1$	1X27 = 27

$$\text{Distance} = \text{Gear inches} \times \pi.$$

Table 1 provides general guidelines for selection of proper gears.

The human body can cope successfully with a narrow range of resistance to the effort of bicycling. Major sources of resistance include the inertia of the bicycle and rider, the rolling resistance of the bicycle tires on the road surface, the weight of the rider moving against an uphill grade, wind, and the friction of air.[67,69] Approximately 90% of the energy expended to ride at 20 mph on a calm day is used to overcome the friction of the bicycle and rider against still air.[67,70] Moreover, the reduction in strength, force, and efficiency of fatigued muscles after a long, hard ride is the equivalent of an additional source of resistance to movement. Riding in a high gear with too much pedal resistance at too low a cadence is second only to improper bicycle fit as a cause of overuse problems in cyclists. Inexperienced or overzealous riders tend to use gears that are too high for the rider's strength and ability; resulting forces on the legs and feet may cause a variety of overuse injuries.

Higher gear ratios result in greater pedal resistance in a given riding condition. They require greater muscle strength and conditioning and cause increased stress on the cyclist's hips, knees, and feet. The inexperienced or less fit cyclist will find it easier and safer to ride at a more moderate gear ratio with, perhaps, a slightly higher cadence.

Optimal bicycling cadence varies with: (1) the type of riding or racing; (2) the skill, strength and endurance of the athlete; and (3) the workload.

TABLE 1. **General Use of Gear Ratios**

Gear Inches	Use
27–35 (or lower)	Very low gears. Used for climbing steep hills. Also used for touring hilly terrain with heavily loaded bicycle.
36–44	Low gears. Used for climbing hills or riding into a severe headwind.
45–60	Slightly low gears. Used for riding on level ground. Effort may be maintained for a long time.
61–85	Standard gears. Used for riding on level ground. Effort may be maintained for a long time.
86–108	High gears. Used for high speed riding. Used when riding downhill or riding with a strong tailwind.
>108	Special gearing, not available on most bicycles.

When viewed in terms of gross efficiency, expressed as work performed/energy cost, optimal cadence is 60 to 80 rpm for moderate to high workloads and may increase to as much as 100 rpm for exceptionally high workloads.[21,38,47,111] Optimal cadence in terms of perceived exertion is 60 to 100 rpm, with 80 rpm the optimal peak.[21,47,73] To prevent a high lactate concentration, optimal cadence is also 60 to 100 rpm with an 80 rpm optimal peak.[8,21] Racers often ride at a higher cadence of 90 to 110 rpm, which may be mechanically more efficient.[38,49,57,93,96,142] There has been a growing trend for racers traveling at relatively steady speeds to ride at a somewhat lower cadence in order to preserve energy. Higher cadence riding is more appropriate for events like the criterium, where the speed is up and down; and the higher cadence allows more efficient acceleration.[29] In this setting the racer is willing to sacrifice efficiency for speed. Finally, the choice of optimal cadence may vary with the individual's percentage of fast-twitch versus slow-twitch muscle fibers. Riders with a higher percentage of slow-twitch fibers in the vastus lateralis are often more efficient at a relatively lower cadence.[101,117]

CLOTHING AND PROTECTIVE EQUIPMENT

The brightly colored clothing and specialized protective equipment that bicyclists use are much more than a display of fashion. These items are designed to help prevent injury. The uninitiated may think that the rider's garb is merely an in-group identification symbol; but, in fact, the helmet, riding pants, and gloves may be just the protection a beginner needs for his or her first long ride. The bright colors are more than fashion. They are designed to "advertise" the rider's presence in traffic or on the highway in order to avoid accidents. Reflective tape may be added to helmets and clothing for dawn, dusk, or night riding.

The Helmet

The most important protective device for a bicyclist is the helmet. Three-fourths of the bicycle-related deaths in the United States are due to head injuries, and in the vast majority of these cases, the riders were not wearing helmets. Bicycle helmets are generally very effective in absorbing and spreading shock and in preventing serious head injuries.[4,28,121,126,134]

Helmets are now required in all United States Cycling Federation, National Off-Road Bicycle Association, and Triathlon Federation USA competitions. Similarly, they should be required in any organized ride or race. The best advice about bicycle helmets is never to ride without one.

Modern bicycle helmets are made of high density expanded polystyrene or polyurethane foam which crushes on impact to absorb the shock of a severe blow. More rubbery or resilient materials may produce a recoil which may magnify the injury rather than protect against it.[4]

If a bicycle helmet has been crushed while protecting a rider, it should be replaced. Many helmet manufacturers have developed replacement programs through which they will replace a damaged helmet for a relatively small fee.

There are three national safety organizations that currently test helmets in the United States. The American National Standards Institute (ANSI) and The Snell Memorial Foundation have been testing helmets for many years. The ANSI Z90.1 and the Snell B-90 standards have served bicyclists well and have represented the minimum safety level for bicycle helmets. A new Snell B-95 standard will take effect with the 1995 model helmets and will require that helmets cover more of the head, absorb additional impact, and have a strap-retention system that holds the helmet firmly in place on the head.[144] The American Society for Testing and Materials will also promulgate standards for 1995.

Most current helmets are one of two types, "no-shell" or "mini-shell." The no-shell helmet is made up of the molded crushable foam with attached retention system, surrounded by a removable lycra cover. The mini-shell helmets have the denser outer layer molded right to the foam helmet and have no cover. Both of these helmets are light and attractive. There has been some concern that the no-shell helmet might have more sliding friction against the pavement in a crash, and might therefore predispose the wearer to neck injury.[121]

Bicycle helmets are aerodynamically designed to reduce drag[67,69,70,121] and to entrain air under the front edge and through exterior vent holes for a cooling effect.[43,121]

Most bicycle accidents produce relatively low velocity impact to the head. If the rider is wearing a helmet, it is highly likely to protect from major trauma.

Mirrors

There are many mirrors from which cyclists may choose in order to see overtaking traffic. Several models mount on the handlebars, attach to the brake lever housing, or plug into the handlebar tip. These generally work well on upright bicycles, but they may not provide good visibility for bicyclers with dropped handlebars. A better option is a small adjustable mirror, similar to a dental mirror, which can be attached to the side of the helmet or clipped onto the glasses or protective eyewear. Because it moves with the rider's head, this mirror provides good rear vision with the rider in a variety of positions on the bicycle.[33,80]

Protective Eyewear

With the broad range of protective eyewear currently available, cyclists can shield themselves from dust, bugs, stones, and other flying objects that may jeopardize their eyesight as well as avoid the discomfort caused by sun, rain, cold air, and allergens. According to the International Federation of Sports Medicine, protective eyewear can almost completely prevent or minimize eye injuries in sports participation.[31] There is even some evidence that proper eye protection may improve performance in competitions. For general sports activities, wraparound or semi-wraparound models are generally recommended, but goggles are better for more extreme weather. Plastic or polycarbonate lenses and frames avoid potential injury from shattering or sharp edges.[33,80]

Cycling Clothing and Padding

Cycling clothes are designed to attract attention to the rider's presence, to maintain appropriate body temperature, and to be relatively streamlined. Bright colors and reflective materials make the rider highly visible. In summer heat, singlets, mesh materials, lycra, and a variety of new synthetic fabrics allow for cooling. In cooler seasons, polypropylene, other new synthetics, and wool will wick perspiration away from the skin while still insulating the body and preventing extreme heat loss. Cycling clothes are form-fitting to prevent flopping or slapping in the breeze. Their aerodynamic qualities actually enhance racing performance.[11,12,67,68]

Cycling Shorts. Bicycling racing shorts have now become standard "equipment" for most serious riders. They are tight fitting, knee-length shorts made of lycra, wool, or polypropylene stretch material with a padded seamless crotch pad made of synthetic materials or natural chamois. Their main purpose is to protect the inner thighs, groin, and buttocks from chafing and pressure trauma, and they perform extremely well. Women's models are available with crotch pads which conform better to the female anatomy. For those who are embarrassed to appear in public in these flimsy elastic shorts, baggier touring shorts are available. Both styles are worn without underpants because the seams of the underwear may chafe and cause blistering and traumatic ulceration. There are also special cyclists' underpants with crotch liners which can be used with regular shorts. Chamois crotch liners should be treated periodically with lanolin or a synthetic lubricant to maintain their softness. Synthetic crotch pads work equally well, wash easier, and dry faster.[33,80]

Saddle Pads. Some riders find that even with a good pair of shorts they need more seat padding. They may choose from padded seat covers made of an elastopolymer gel material surrounded by closed-cell neoprene, air bladders, or synthetic fleece. Racers may avoid padded saddles because the soft material may absorb some of the racer's energy instead of transmitting all of it to the pedals.[33] Another potential disadvantage of the saddle pad is that it may widen the effective size of the saddle, and thus cause chafing on the inner thighs. A better solution for the serious rider may be a saddle with extra padding built into the surface. The padding in this increasingly popular type of saddle is made of a variety of gels, foam, and air bladders.

Gloves and Handlebar Padding. Bicycle gloves are designed to cushion the rider's palm from the pressure and vibration of the handlebar on the long or intense ride.[80,98] Some of the better gloves contain shock-absorbing elastopolymer or neoprene padding in the palms. Summer gloves are fingerless, with a leather palm and a lycra or string net back. Winter gloves cover the fingers and contain insulation as well as padding.

In addition to padded gloves, many riders choose to wrap the handlebars with a variety of handlebar padded tapes, or to use heavily cushioned slip-on handlebar pads for further protection.

Shoes. One of the most underrated pieces of bicycle safety equipment is the shoe. There are three types—touring shoes, mountain bike shoes, and racing shoes. What they have in common is a stiff midsole that distributes the pedaling forces over the entire foot and helps prevent overuse syndromes in the foot and ankle.

Touring shoes resemble court shoes and have a similar feel. The toe is roomy inside, but small enough to fit in the toe clips that are popular on performance bicycles. Some have transverse grooves on the soles to grip the pedal and generate more power through the entire pedal revolution.

Mountain bike shoes are simply heavier-duty touring shoes. Many of the mountain bike shoes, however, have step-in bindings which may be inset into the sole.

Racing shoes are designed to generate the most possible power through the entire pedal revolution. They are designed to fit tightly around the racer's foot. Traditional racing shoes employ a cleat that fits snugly into a "cage" formed by the racing pedal. It is fastened into place with a toe clip and toe strap. The cleated shoe allows the rider to apply force to the pedal throughout most of the 360° revolution in order to ride faster. Cleats that are not adjusted properly can result in painful knees and ankles.

Most racers have gone from the traditional cleat and pedal into a step-in system which locks the racing shoe into a special quick-release pedal. The rider frees the foot by rotating it out of the pedal. The original step-in cleat/pedal systems provided a tight union without any rotational freedom (laxity). If the cleat was not set properly, repetitive torquing forces could contribute to overuse injuries of the knee and ankle. More recently, "floating" cleats have been designed. These allow 5 to 10° of rotational freedom and reduce overuse injuries.[13,33,140] Replacement cleats are available for many of the earlier fixed step-in bindings to provide this "float."[33]

INJURIES AND OVERUSE

Head Injury

Head trauma carries the threat of significant morbidity and mortality to bicyclists. Over 60% of bicycle-related deaths are caused by head injuries.[18,39,88,92,106,135] Similarly, 60% of serious bicycle injuries are caused by head trauma.[40,77,135,143] Although there is good evidence that most bicycle-related head and facial injuries could be prevented by wearing a protective helmet,[71,77,85,88,92,106,111,125,133,143] the victims of major bicycle accidents have only rarely worn them.[71,77,80,88,92,106,125,126,133,143] Clearly, a prolonged intense educational campaign about helmet use must be undertaken for riders of all ages.

Neck and Back Pain

Symptoms related to the neck and shoulder are quite common, especially in long-distance riding. In one study involving long-distance touring, 66.4% of all riders reported some discomfort, with 20.4% of those reporting significant symptoms.[137] The trapezius muscle was the commonest site of pain, primarily left sided, which was attributed to looking backward to check for traffic. It also occurred in the riders using small review mirrors attached to their glasses or helmet. Backache was the third most common complaint in a major bicycle tour.[65]

Most neck and back problems in cyclists are caused by a combination of an increased load on the arms and shoulders necessary to support the rider and the hyperextension of the cyclist's neck in the horizontal riding position.[14,80,82,116] When a rider is positioned in a "hands low" posture on the bicycle, the load on the arms and shoulders is increased and the neck is hyperextended.[5,80,82] If the reach (see Fig. 7) is too long for the rider, neck hyperextension is increased further. If a rider is using aero bars and is stretched out on the bike in a fully extended position, the amount of neck hyperextension required to look at the road ahead may also be increased even further.[116,141] The impact the rider in the weight-forward, neck-hyperextended position experiences is magnified by road shock transmitted through the handlebars, arms, and shoulders girdle to the neck.[14] If the rider's helmet is positioned too far forward on the forehead, it may partially block vision and force the rider to extend an already hyperextended neck further in order to see.[7,14] Neck pain and adjacent soft tissue trigger-point spasms, most commonly in the levator scapulae muscles, often result.[7] This pair of muscles, which often contract together, serve as "check reins" that hold the neck in the hyperextended position. Prolonged tension in this position may produce a bilateral traumatic levator scapula tendinitis.[35]

Trigger-point spasms in the left levator scapula and upper- and middle-thirds of the trapezius are common in countries where the bicycle is ridden on the right side of the road. They are believed to be related to straining to look for overtaking traffic. Because they often occur even when using a mirror attached to the helmet of or glasses, they may also be a consequence of prolonged head positioning to maintain an adequate view through the mirror.[80]

Another form of disabling neck pain occurs in ultramarathon bicyclists after a series of long, hard rides in the "drops" as the result of "thousands of micro-whiplash motions to the neck each day."[81]

Most lower-back pain in cyclists also occurs when the rider is in an exaggerated, stretched out position because the combined length of the stem and top tube is too great or because the handlebars are set extremely low.[7]

Because increased "reach" is the primary mechanical problem causing most overuse syndromes of the neck and back, changing the cyclist's riding position to reduce the amount of hyperextension is the key mechanical change required. This can be accomplished by raising the handlebars, using handlebars with a smaller drop, using a stem with shorter extension, moving the bicycle seat forward on its rails, or a combination of these strategies.[7,80,82,116] Changing hand positions on the handlebar frequently, wearing padded gloves, using padding on the handlebar, riding with the elbows "unlocked" and using wider tires all help to reduce or absorb road shock. Switching to an upright bicycle may be the only other solution of these mechanical adjustments and riding technique changes fail to relieve the neck or back pain.

Therapeutic exercise, consisting of a strength and flexibility program for the neck, back, and shoulders is the foundation of medical therapy. The techniques of cervicothoracic muscular stabilization[122,123] and dynamic lumbar musculostabilization[99,102,103,104,105] have been adapted for use by cyclists.[81] Special stretching programs have been developed.[1,7,14,81] Ice massage (occasionally alternated with heat), aspirin, and nonsteroidal anti-inflammatory drugs (NSAIDs), and rarely skeletal muscle relaxants, may be useful adjuncts. Pain and spasm which fail to respond to therapy may warrant further evaluation for underlying spine pathology.

Scheuermann's Disease

According to reports from French and Belgian medical literature, Scheuermann's disease is common in adolescent bicycle racers, with one report demonstrating that 40% of a group of 19-and-under racers presented with signs of Scheuermann's disease.[129] Cyclists with immature vertebral bodies may damage the end plates by pulling too hard on the handlebars with the upper body while pedaling too large a gear. The result may be anterior vertebral endplate damage, often categorized as Schmorl's nodes.[83,118,120] A similar process has been reported in rowers[34] and gymnasts.[83,119] It is not clear whether all of these reports are classic Scheuermann's disease or an atypical variant of it in which the criterion of vertebral body wedging is not met. Athletes who develop this problem may resume cycling when they are asymptomatic. They should ride with a higher cadence and lower gears. Raising the handlebars and shortening the reach by using a stem with less extension may be helpful. For the athlete with persistent symptoms, intense riding and racing on the road bike is contraindicated.[60,129]

HANDLEBAR PROBLEMS

Ulnar Neuropathy

One of the most common overuse problems in bicyclists is ulnar neuropathy, more commonly referred to as "cyclist's palsy" or "handlebar palsy." Almost 10% of the riders in an 8-day, 500-mile tour reported uncomfortable hand problems, and 63% of these experienced paresthesias in the ulnar nerve distribution.[137] It is not a new problem; Destot first described it in 1896 as a problem for some of the competitors in the Paris-Brest-Paris bicycle race.[41,56,89,98]

Clinically, the bicyclist will experience the insidious onset of numbness and tingling and/or weakness and difficulty with fine motor control after several days of intensive touring or racing. The pattern may include loss of sensory or motor function, or both.[112]

There is some debate about the location and mechanism of ulnar nerve damage in cyclist's palsy. Enough material has been published to make it safe to say that the exact location is variable. Several authors have adopted a system of three anatomically determined types of lesions for ulnar compression syndromes. Type I involves the ulnar nerve proximal to or within Guyon's canal and involves both the superficial sensory and deep motor branches. Sensation in the distribution of the dorsal cutaneous branch is spared. Type II lesions involve the deep motor branch after the ulnar nerve bifurcates, and sensation is intact. Type III lesions involve the superficial sensory branch without causing motor deficits.[32,89,98,112] The mechanism of injury is generally nerve compression, but it is likely that in some patients riding with the wrists hyperextended causes a traction on the nerve, which, in turn, contributes to the injury.

Almost all cyclist's palsy problems resolve with conservative measures. Cutting back on the length and intensity of rides is helpful in the short term, but some other changes are necessary to prevent recurrences. The rider should wear well-padded riding gloves and use handlebar padding as well. Frame size should be checked because too large or too small a frame may prevent proper handlebar positioning. The position of the bicycle saddle and the handlebars should be checked so that a disproportionate amount of the rider's weight does not rest on the hands (see previous section on fitting the bicycle). The rider should avoid wrist positions with marked hyperextension. Finally, the rider should develop a habit of changing hand positions frequently.[17] Aero bars may be an acceptable alternative to dropped handlebars.[80] Occasionally, the cyclist will need to stop riding for a period to allow healing, but only rarely will surgical decompression be necessary.[17,32,41,56,89,98]

If problems recur in spite of adhering to all the aforementioned suggestions, the rider might be encouraged to use an upright bicycle.

Carpal Tunnel Syndrome. Although ulnar nerve problems are common in cyclists, carpal tunnel syndrome is rarely the result of handlebar trauma alone. Most injury surveys in cyclists do not list carpal tunnel syndrome as a bicycling injury. One study of 89 cyclists covering 4500 miles in 80 days revealed 23 riders with numbness in the ulnar nerve distribution, 10 riders with numbness in median nerve distribution and 2 riders with index finger numbness.[65] No other information was available to establish a diagnosis of carpal tunnel syndrome. There is a single case report of bilateral nerve palsy in a recreational cyclist after a 100-mile ride.[9] With the trauma of mountain bike riding on rough terrain, it is likely that more cases of carpal tunnel syndrome in cyclists will be reported. As a practical matter, the suggestions for riders with ulnar neuropathy would be helpful for those with median nerve symptoms as well.[55,75]

de Quervain's Syndrome. Tenosynovitis of the abductor pollicis longus and extensor pollicis brevis tendons in the first dorsal compartment of the wrist has been reported in a 27-year old mountain biker following a difficult 25-mile off-road ride. The problem was attributed to repeated ulnar deviation and forced flexion-adduction of the right thumb while shifting gears, because a mountain bike rider may shift over 100 times per hour.[113] There have been anecdotal reports of tenderness at the base of the thumb metacarpal related to shifting in road bikes as well, but these have not been documented as de Quervain's syndrome. A practical treatment for these problems has been deep friction massage. De Quervain's syndrome is generally treated conservatively with ice, NSAIDs, a thumb spica splint, active range of motion exercises, and occasional corticosteroid injections. Rarely, surgical decompression is warranted.

Saddle Problems

The most talked about bicycle problems are those which result from the interaction between rider and saddle. The narrow front of the saddle is designed to avoid chafing and to allow freedom of leg movement during rapid pedaling. Modern dropped handlebar bicycles are designed so that most of the rider's weight is borne by the ischial tuberosities. This is true even for racers who tend to use extremely narrow saddles for freer leg movement. For recreational riding and touring, slightly wider saddles are usually more comfortable. Generally, recreational saddles should be 1 to 2" wider than the distance between the ischial tuberosities.[22] Women generally prefer wider saddles than men because the ischial tuberosities are usually more widely spaced in the gynecoid pelvis. Most saddle manufacturers now produce models designed specifically for women.

Noncyclists often wonder about the traditional narrow design of the bicycle saddle. In fact, an experiment by the author demonstrated that the shape is extremely well conceived. A traditional, unmolded leather bicycle saddle was soaked in neat's-foot oil for several days to soften it and then was used for several thousand miles of riding. By 500 miles the seat was beginning to contour comfortably, and after 1,000 miles it had molded into the shape of a modern man's racing saddle.[80] The point, of course, is that saddle designers understand what works best for specific types of riding. A saddle should be chosen with consideration to the rider's anatomy, experience, and projected riding needs.

When a rider has a saddle-related irritation or injury, the usual source of the problem is in the fit or setup of the bicycle.[22,39,45,50,80,95,100,110,131,136,138] Before considering replacing the saddle or adding a saddle pad, it is wise to evaluate the bicycle's fit methodically. No amount of padding will prevent trauma when the rider is sitting in the wrong place.

Ischial Tuberosity Soreness. Many cyclists who have not ridden for a while will report tenderness around the ischial tuberosities for the first days of regular riding. This problem is generally self-limited. Occasionally, however, ischial bursitis can result.[95] In the case of this rare complication, treatment consists of ice, NSAIDs, deep friction massage, phonophoresis, and, rarely, corticosteroid injection.

Skin Problems. Chafing, heat, and perspiration can result in a variety of skin problems in the rider's groin, most of which can be prevented by wearing padded racing shorts that are washed and dried after each ride. Simple chafing can often be prevented by using talcum powder for its drying effect on shorts rides. On longer rides, the opposite approach of using lubricating agents such as Cramer's Skin Lube or Mueller's Lubricant is more effective. For extremely long rides, a heavy application of such a lubricant to the pad in the rider's bicycle shorts is generally very effective. Petroleum jelly is much less effective because it can be warmed by the rider's body heat and then largely washed away by sweat. Corticosteroid creams have been demonstrated to be no better than placebo in preventing bicycle-related seat pain.[138] When groin chafing becomes an established problem, the key issue in treatment and preventing progression is personal hygiene. First, the rider should remove wet bicycle shorts and shower or bathe immediately after a ride. The groin area should be kept as dry as possible.

Mild established chafing lesions may be treated with nonfluorinated corticosteroid cream, but fluorinated corticosteroids should not be applied to the groin. In more severe lesions that have progressed to blistering or ulceration, the adjacent perineum should be shaved and a hydrophilic dressing, such as DuoDerm or Tegasorb applied. The lesion and a 1" border on all sides should be covered; the dressing should conform fairly well to the contour of the skin.

Skin infections of the groin are occasional problems. Warm soaks and incision and drainage are standard therapy for furuncles. If antibiotics are warranted, they should be active against not only the coliforms, which are often involved in folliculitis and furuncles in this area, but also against the more typical staphylococci.[136] These lesions can occasionally necessitate time off the bicycle.

Callus formation may occur over the ischial tuberosities as an adaptive response to the friction and pressure of cycling. They may vary in size from a new keratin layers to thick pads of horny skin that may warrant trimming.

Inflamed 1–2-cm fibrous masses may develop as a similar reaction to trauma and pressure in the deeper fascial tissue between the skin and the ischial tuberosities. If conservative therapy such as rest, sitz baths, NSAIDs, and saddle padding fails to control the pain in these lesions, then excision may be necessary.[26]

Subcutaneous peroneal nodules, generally with a cystic quality, occasionally develop in racers and other serious riders.[55,95,100,110,131] These nodules may look like "accessory testicles" posterior to the natural testicles.[100,110,131,136] Pathologic evaluation in one report revealed that they are local, aseptic areas of "necrosis" with pseudocyst formation involving connective tissue in the superficial fascia of the perineum.[131]

Pudendal Neuropathy. Male bicyclists may experience numbness and tingling in the scrotum and the penile shaft.[6,26,45,78,95,114] This syndrome has been attributed to compression of the dorsal branches of the pudendal nerve between the bicycle seat and the pubic symphysis.[45] The phenomenon usually results from riding on a saddle that has the front angled up too high, or one that is too narrow to support the ischial tuberosities. The saddle top should be horizontal or only minimally angled upward in front. Strategies for prevention include changing the seat angle, wearing padded cycling shorts, using a saddle pad, and changing to a wider saddle.

Pudendal neuropathy has been reported in riders using aero bars. The marked forward leaning posture places increased pressure on the pudendal nerve and can cause compression.[114]

Impotence. Male impotence may develop as a complication of pudendal neuropathy in cyclists.[25,62,84,114,115] The rider may complain of inability to obtain an erection after frequent long or multiday rides. Treatment consists of rest without use of the bicycle and of a complete reevaluation of bicycle fit.[62,84,115] Padded shorts and saddles are mandatory when resuming riding.

Traumatic Urethritis. Bicycle saddles can induce a range of urinary tract outflow problems in men and boys. The mildest of them is a silent hematuria reported with both 10-speed and BMX (bicycle motocross) bicycles.[87,107] In its more severe forms, the urethral trauma may sensitize the outflow tract to infection[50] or obstruction.[26,50,87,90,107] Saddle-related obstruction must be distinguished from benign prostatic hypertrophy in order to avoid unnecessary prostate surgery. The preventive strategies suggested above for pudendal neuropathy are also helpful in these conditions.

Vulva Trauma. Women may experience a variety of vulval lesions ranging from superficial abrasions and lacerations to deeper contusions and hematomata resulting from bicycle trauma. A vulvar hematoma may have the same cord-like consistency of a thrombophlebitis, but the diagnosis is clearly hematoma because there are no large veins in the vulva. Trauma-induced abscesses may also develop in the vulva.[79] They should be treated in the same manner as other saddle sores. Mechanical treatment of vulva trauma consists of lowering the front end of the saddle slightly. Special saddle clamps are available which allow extremely fine adjustment. Occasionally, it is necessary for the rider to change to a broader saddle. Padded bicycle shorts and saddle pads are helpful as well.

Torsion of the Testis. Torsion of the testis has been described in relationship to bicycling, but a distinct cause and effect relationship[58] has not been established.[42,44]

Hip Problems

Greater trochanteric bursitis and iliopsoas tendinitis are the two major problems encountered in the hip of bicyclists.[75] Greater trochanteric bursitis develops from repetitive sliding of the fascia lata over the greater trochanter. This produces pain around the greater trochanter in the abductor muscle groups. Treatment includes intermittent ice applications, anti-inflammatory medications, and occasional injection of corticosteroid into the bursa. Seat height adjustment is important in this condition.

Iliopsoas tendinitis or hip-flexor pain is another problem that presents with pain in the medial and proximal aspect of the thigh. Management includes rest as necessary and anti-inflammatory medication.

Knee Problems

Biker's Knee

"Biker's knee," also called "cyclist's knee," is a general term for a cluster of anteromedial knee problems which frequently affect cyclists. These problems, common to many sports ("runner's knee," "breast stroker's knee"), are the subject of an entire chapter (Tracking Problems of The Patella) and are also discussed in great depth elsewhere in the sports medicine literature.[132] The discussion here will focus on their specific relationship to bicycling. Holmes, Pruitt, and Whalen[52,54] divide knee pain problems in cyclists into four anatomical categories: anterior, medial, lateral, and posterior. Anterior and medial knee problems fall under the what is broadly termed "biker's knee."

Anterior Knee Problems. Anterior knee problems in cyclists include patellofemoral pain syndrome, quadriceps tendinitis, chondromalacia patella, patella tendinitis, and Osgood-Schlatter disease. For practical purposes, the first three entities should be considered together as the patellofemoral pain syndrome. Use of the older term, chondromalacia, indicating softening and degeneration of the cartilage lining of the patella, should be reserved for surgically visualized changes, because chondromalacia is so often absent when expected from clinical examination and so often present in asymptomatic patients. Occasionally quadriceps tendinitis is an isolated finding, but most commonly it occurs in concert with retropatellar pain. Patellar tendinitis may be an isolated finding or may be present in combination with patellofemoral pain syndrome. Osgood-Schlatter disease is common just before or during the pubertal growth spurt, and may be present in serious young cyclists.

These overuse problems are usually the result of training errors, bicycle fit problems, and the anatomy and conditioning of the athlete. Common training errors include inadequate training base for the rider's workload, pedaling up too many hills aggressively, doing too much training in high gears, allowing inadequate rest, and inappropriate work in the weight room including deep squats and overly aggressive leg extension exercises.[22,26,52,54,80]

Technique and training errors often contribute to anterior knee pain. Riding at a low cadence and "muscling" the bike up hills are likely to injure the knees, especially early in the spring after a winter lay-off. As one author has noted: "The rule of the road for many cyclists has come to be, 'If the knee hurts, gear down'; the cyclist is in too high a gear for the terrain and his or her ability."[22] Consequently, gearing down and increasing cadence are recommended for all of these anterior knee problems. Reducing or eliminating hill climbs for time may be necessary. In some extreme cases, it is even necessary for the cyclist to change the bicycle cassette or freewheel in order to have some lower gears available for recuperation.

The most common bicycle fit problem is that the seat is too low or too far forward in relation to the pedals. Seat height and fore-aft position should be rechecked (see figs. 3–6). For riders using cleated shoes, the cleats should be positioned to avoid abnormal biomechanical forces which tend to sublux the patella onto the lateral femoral condyle. In many cases, the cleat position can be checked with the Rotational Adjustment Device of the Fit Kit. Floating cleat systems should be used to allow 5° of float in either direction. Finally, a less common but still extremely important issue is to replace a crank which is too long for the rider.

Anatomic variants also warrant special consideration in setting up the bicycle. Severe hyperpronating feet and rear foot valgus may cause knee pain in cyclists. Standard orthotics are rarely effective on the bicycle. One biomechanical approach is to cement a 1/8 to 3/16" medial wedge to the sole of a touring shoe or to install a wedge or shims between the cleat and sole of a racing shoe medially.[26] Some new models of racing shoes with recessed shoe pedal interfaces will not accommodate an external device. Another option available for any rider, but necessary for those using recessed interfaces, is the cycling orthotic. Runner's orthotics are designed to exert their effect at heel strike and stance phase, but bicyclists have no heel strike or stance phase. A cyclist's orthotic must exert its force at the forefoot; consequently, it must extend further forward and provide support underneath the metatarsal heads.[26,54] The cyclist's orthotic is stiffer than the runner's orthotic, it should be lightweight, and is often constructed of a layer of acrylic sandwiched between two layers of carbon graphite.[22]

Genu varum and genu valgus are particularly important etiologically in quadriceps tendinitis. Significant genu varum can be treated by placing spacers between the pedal and crank arm to improve leg alignment by widening the stance width.[54] Genu valgum can be treated with wedges or cants between the pedal and shoe, as already noted for hyperpronation.[54] Internally and externally rotated feet may be the result of one or more leg variants and may do well with floating cleats.

The cyclist with anterior knee pain will benefit from an aggressive rehabilitation program focusing on strengthening the vastus medialis obliquis and stretching the hamstrings, quadriceps, and heel cords. Adjunctive therapy includes ice, NSAIDs, and dynamic patella bracing.[80] McConnell patella taping is generally useful in recreational and touring riders, but the intense training required of highly competitive cyclists often loosens or tears the tape.[54] Surgery is occasionally necessary even in the well-rehabilitated patient.

Medial Knee Pain. Holmes, Pruitt, and Whalen have noted two common medial knee problems which occur only among cyclist who are training and competing at a high level. They report irritation and fibrosis of the plica and of the medial patellofemoral ligament in these high-intensity riders.[52,54] Conservative treatment is the same as for anterior knee pain; however, arthroscopic surgery may be warranted to excise the plica, release the medial patellofemoral ligament, and perform a partial medial wall synovectomy.[54]

Lateral Knee Pain

Iliotibial Band (ITB) Friction Syndrome. Iliotibial band friction syndrome, first described in runners by Renne in 1975, accounts for the knee pain in 24% of 254 cyclists presenting with cycling-related knee problems.[53,97] It is an inflammatory overuse response caused by repetitive friction of the iliotibial band over the lateral femoral condyle which appears to be more prevalent since the introduction of the rigid step-in cleat systems in 1985.[53] Knee extension beyond 150° draws the posterior fibers of the iliotibial band anteriorly across the lateral femoral condyle, and flexion from this position can abrade these fibers as they move back posteriorly. Aggressive training routines which involve pedalling several hours at an intensity over 5,000 pedal revolutions per hour, combined with anatomical or cleat-related alignment problems, may induce an inflammatory response in the posterior fibers of the iliotibial band where it rubs against the lateral femoral condyle. Hyperpronation of the foot, genu varum, a tight ITB, an overly prominent lateral femoral condyle, and leg-length discrepancy all anatomically predispose to iliotibial band friction syndrome. Improper cleat adjustment and a bicycle seat set too high or too far aft also predispose to ITB friction syndrome.[53,54]

Treatment is directed at eliminating or compensating for the predisposing conditions, as well as specific medical treatment for the problem. A rotational problem should be corrected using floating pedals with a fixed endpoint which matched the patient's anatomical alignment while preventing excessive internal rotation. Hyperpronation should be corrected with cycling orthotics and ITB stretching exercises should be instituted. Saddle height should be maintained so that the rider's knee has 30 to 35° of flexion at dead bottom center. (Compare this with Figure 5, which shows a saddle set for the standard of 25 to 30°.) In resistant cases, the saddle can be lowered to more than 35° of flexion. Spacers between the pedal and the crank arm can be used to reduce the stress on the iliotibial band in riders with genu varum.[53,54]

In riders with a leg-length discrepancy of ¼″ (6 mm) or more, especially if the discrepancy is due to tibial rather than femoral shortening, leg-length discrepancy should be corrected using a combination of shims, orthotics, and foot positioning as indicated in Table 2.[53,54]

Medical treatment should include complete (occasionally prolonged) or relative rest, ice, ITB stretching, phonophoresis, iontophoresis, and NSAIDs. In resistant cases, corticosteroid injections of the ITB are warranted. If intensive rehabilitation, rest and two injections 7 to 14 days apart fail to produce marked improvement, however, surgery is warranted.[53,54] Surgical excision of a semicircular piece of the distal posterior ITB has been particularly effective in cyclists.[53]

Posterior Knee Pain

Biceps Femoris and Semimembranosus Tendinitis; Posterior Capsule Strain. Posterior knee problems in cyclists are infrequent compared to problems in the other portions of the knee and they are generally limited to cyclists in competition. They usually result from overly aggressive training on or off the bike. Overinvolvement of the hamstrings in the upstroke and too much riding out of the saddle, particularly when combined with sudden increases in mileage and intensity, may cause increased stress on the posterior knee structures. Off the bike, the cyclist may have a history of overemphasis on hamstring curls or cross-training activities including running and rollerblading. Bicycle setup can contribute to posterior knee problems if the saddle is set too high or too far aft or if the cleats are excessively toed-in. In a cyclist with a leg-length discrepancy with the bicycle fit to the long leg and with inadequate correction for the short leg, excessive reaching for the pedal can produce posterior knee stress.[52,54]

Treatment consists of complete or relative rest, refitting the bicycle when appropriate, and adjusting it for leg-length discrepancy. Medical treatment involves ice, hamstring, quadriceps and heel cord stretching, phonophoresis, iontophoresis, and NSAIDs. When conservative therapy fails, tenolysis and even excision of irritated fibers of the biceps tendon have been recommended. Occasionally a small bursa forms under the fibers of the biceps tendon and fibula head. Excision of this bursa may also be warranted.[54]

Foot and Ankle Problems

Ankle and foot problems occurred in less than 15% of the riders in a long-distance-tour study.[137] Common problems include paresthesias, metatarsalgia, Achilles tendinitis, plantar fasciitis, and traumatic injuries resulting from spoke problems.

TABLE 2. **The Treatment of Leg Length Discrepancies with Bicycle Fit Adjustments**

Rule 1. Always adjust the bicycle first to the longer leg.
Rule 2. Corrections for length should always slightly undercompensate the total difference since many cyclists adapt by increased "ankling" (dorsiflexion/plantar flexion) while pedaling.

Example A: Tibial length discrepancy of 6 mm

1. Adjust saddle height to allow 25 to 30 degrees of knee flexion at dead bottom center of the pedaling stroke on the long leg.
2. Correct for the length difference on the short leg using approximately 4 millimeters of a lift or leather shim that is placed between the shoe and the cleat.
3. Utilize cycling orthotics to correct for active pronation.

Example B: Femoral length discrepancy of 6 mm

1. Adjust saddle height to allow 25 to 30 degrees of knee flexion at dead bottom center of the pedaling stroke on the long leg.
2. Place a 2- or 3-mm lift or shim between the shoe and the cleat on the short leg.
3. Move the foot of the short leg back 2 mm on the pedal.
4. Move the foot of the long leg forward 2 mm on the pedal.

From Holmes JC, Pruitt AL, Whalen NJ: Lower extremity overuse in bicycling. Clin Sports Med 13:187–203, 1994, with permission.

Paresthesia. Foot paresthesias and numbness are relatively common among bicyclists riding long distances. These conditions generally resolve spontaneously within a few minutes to an hour off the bike. They are often caused by tight toe clip straps. If loosening the straps fails to alleviate the problem, switching to one of the step-in shoe-pedal combinations is recommended.

Metatarsalgia. Metatarsalgia is due to poor foot position or improperly placed shoe cleats; riding in high gears with low cadence may also cause increased pedal pressure. A metatarsal pad, cleat position adjustment, and gearing and cadence changes usually correct the problem. If the cyclist's metatarsalgia is accompanied by marked pes planus with or without hyperpronation, using cycling orthotics which extend to the metatarsal heads may provide relief.

Achilles Tendinitis. Achilles tendinitis commonly results from improper bicycle fit. If the saddle height is too low, pronounced dorsiflexion of the ankle will increase stress on the Achilles tendon. If the toe clip is too short or if the cleat is set so that the foot is too far behind the pedal spindle, excessive "ankling" (flexion/extension) will occur while pedaling and thus cause excessive stress to the Achilles tendon. If the cleats are set with excessive toe-in, the Achilles tendon will be subject to increased torquing stress. All of these problems should be addressed by a thorough re-evaluation of bicycle fit.

Additionally, leg-length inequality should be accommodated with a combination of orthotics, cants, shims, and special bicycle fit techniques (see Table 2). In adjusting the foot position on the pedal, temporarily placing the foot 1 to 3 mm forward of neutral on the pedal spindle to overcompensate for Achilles tendinitis may allow the rider to continue pedaling during treatment and rehabilitation.[54]

Out-of-saddle riding may contribute to Achilles tendinitis on any type of bike, but it is much more likely to do so on a mountain bike because of the "radical shifts in body weight" and "body English" that are necessary for stability and traction off-road.[15] With newer models of mountain bikes, it is now possible to have similar or identical geometry between a cyclist's road bike and mountain bike, thus allowing a similar fit to reduce muscle and tendon stress.[15]

Treatment consists not only of correcting the fit and related technique problems predisposing to the tendinitis, but also conservative medical therapy including hamstring and Achilles tendon stretching, ice, NSAIDs, phonophoresis, and iontophoresis. Corticosteroids should never be injected into the Achilles tendon because they cause tendon weakness and degeneration with possible subsequent rupture. In recalcitrant cases, diagnostic ultrasound or magnetic resonance imaging may reveal an underlying tear in the Achilles tendon.

Plantar Fasciitis. Plantar fasciitis may also occur, commonly seen as pain in the sole at the origin of the plantar fascia on the anterior calcaneus. The pain can be produced by dorsiflexing the toes and by palpation. Management includes seat height elevation, heel cord stretching, NSAIDs, ice, and occasionally local corticosteroid injection into the painful area.

Spoke Injuries. Traumatic injuries of the foot and ankle are commonly caused by spoke injury. Laceration of soft tissue from a knife-like action of the spoke, crushing injuries from impingement between the wheel and frame, and shearing injuries are the major mechanisms. These injuries most often occur when a passenger "riding double" catches a foot in the wheel of a moving bicycle. Most lacerations occur over the malleoli, Achilles tendon, and dorsolateral aspect of the foot. Prevention education should cover proper riding technique, not using the bike to carry passengers improperly, and the danger of riding a bicycle with loose spokes.[48,63,72,108]

A second form of spoke injury may occur when a broken spoke becomes trapped and causes the bicycle to come to a sudden stop. Generally this type of injury can be prevented by tightening or removing loose spokes. If a spoke is removed, the two adjacent spokes should be loosened with a spoke wrench and the rider should travel slowly until the wheel is repaired or replaced.[80]

Mountain Bike Injuries

With the shift in preference from road bikes to mountain bikes, injury patterns have changed. Mountain bikes are ridden off-road in a variety of terrains, producing an increasing incidence of trauma. Few studies have been published documenting these changes, but two well-done reports warrant discussion. In a retrospective study, Chow, Bracker, and Patrick[20] solicited 459 members of two Southern California off-road bicycling organization; 268 (58.4%) responded. Of these, 225 (84%) indicated they had been injured while riding all-terrain bicycles, 51% in the preceding year. Most characterized their injuries as minor, but 26% of the injuries required professional medical care, and 4% were admitted to hospital. Soft-tissue extremity injuries including abrasions, lacerations, and contusions occurred in 201 (90%) of the cyclists, and 27 (12%) sustained a fracture or dislocation. Head and neck trauma were experienced by 12%. The authors concluded that high levels of helmet use (88%) accounted for this low incidence.

Of the injuries, 197 (87.6%) occurred off paved roads, 74.2% occurred while descending a grade,

TABLE 3. Mountain Bike Injuries by Type

	Male: 47 riders, 208 injuries	Female: 14 riders, 91 injuries
Wound (laceration, abrasion, puncture, etc.)	36.5%	35.2%
Bruise	21.6%	33.0%
Strain	16.3%	15.4%
Tendinitis	10.1%	5.5%
Sprain	8.2%	6.6%
Fracture	4.3%	4.4%
Dislocation	2.9%	0.0%

Adapted from Pfeiffer RP: Off-road bicycle racing injuries—the NORBA Pro/Elite category: Care and prevention. Clin Sports Med 13:207–218, 1994.

80 (36%) thought excessive speed contributed to their injury, and 78 (34.7%) attributed it to riding unfamiliar terrain. Inattentiveness was cited as a factor by 22%, and 19.6% admitted riding beyond their ability. Most of the injuries occurred in falls without a preceding collision, but 13 riders collided with stationary objects, 5 collided with other bicycles and 5 incidents involved motor vehicle collisions with 4 of these on paved terrain.

Pfeiffer[94] surveyed 47 male and 14 female National Off-Road Bicycle Association Pro/Elite riders retrospectively for injuries sustained during the 1992 competitive season. The men reported a total of 208 injuries, producing an incidence of 4.43 per rider per year. The women sustained 91 injuries, yielding an incidence of 6.5 per rider per year. The results are tabulated by injury type in Table 3 and by body part in Table 4. Soft tissue trauma categorized as bruises and wounds produced 58.1% of the male injuries and 68.2% of the female injuries. Of the male injuries 26.4%, and of the female injuries 21% were strains and tendinitis, i.e., acute and chronic muscle/tendon injuries. Sprains, fractures and dislocations accounted for 15.4% of male injuries and 11% of female injuries. Over half the reported male injuries involved the lower extremities with the knee accounting for 22.6%. For female riders, the lower extremity injuries accounted for 39.6% which was considerably less than shown a similar study performed the previous year. The decrease was accounted for by a significant increase in lower back injuries in the female riders (16.5%). There were not significant head or neck injuries in either group, but there were a few minor concussions. The cyclists sustaining the minor concussions consistently reported substantial helmet damage.

Clearly off-road bicycle riding has a high incidence of trauma. The amount of head trauma is surprisingly low and may, in part, result from the protective effect of helmets worn by the select group of riders surveyed in both these groups.

Bicycle-Mounted Child Seat Injuries

With the increasing popularity of bicycles has come the increasing use of child seats mounted on bicycles to carry young passengers. "Riding in a bicycle-mounted child seat exposes the child to adult-level forces, risking injury because of the bicycle size, speed and instability in the child's size and development."[109] The head and face were the sites of 65–71% of the injuries; many of these could have been prevented or reduced if the children had been wearing bicycle helmets.[109,124] To prevent injuries

TABLE 4. Percent of Injuries by Body Region for Men and Women (1992 Survey)

Body Region	Men	Women	Body Region	Men	Women
Ankle/Foot	4.3	6.6	Shoulder	7.2	8.8
Lower leg	12.3	9.9	Collarbone	1.9	0.0
Knee	22.6	13.2	Upper arm	0.0	5.5
Thigh	8.2	6.6	Elbow	8.2	12.1
Hamstring	1.9	3.3	Forearm	4.8	4.4
Groin	0.96	0.0	Wrist	5.8	3.3
Pelvis	2.9	0.0	Hand/Fingers	5.3	5.5
Abdomen	0.0	0.0	Neck	1.9	0.0
Low back	3.8	16.5	Face dental	0.96	3.3
Chest	3.4	0.0	Head	0.96	1.1
Upper back	2.4	0.0	Eye	0.0	0.0

From Pfeiffer RP: Off-road bicycle racing injuries—The NORBA Pro/Elite category. Clin Sports Med 13:207–218, 1994, with permission.

to these young cyclists, education about the use of bicycle helmets and improvements in seat design are warranted.[124]

DEHYDRATION

Cyclists tend to have greater problems with dehydration because their sweat evaporates rapidly as they ride, thus causing them to underestimate their fluid losses. Thirst becomes noticeable only after a significant fluid loss has taken place. Because a 3% drop in body weight can result in a 20 to 30% drop in performance, waiting for thirst to develop is an inadequate way to meet the body's need for fluid replacement. With long-distance riding and racing, conscious maintenance of good hydration for several days in advance, as well as several hours before the event, is necessary. In hot weather, the generally accepted guidelines are for riders to drink two water bottles hourly and to pass clear urine at least every one and one-half hours. More detailed information is available in the chapter on "Thermoregulation, Heat Illness, and Safe Exercise in the Heat" and elsewhere.[46] Failure to urinate or passing yellow urine indicates dehydration. It is important for cyclists to know how much fluid is contained in each water bottle. Standard bicycle water bottles hold 20 oz and large bicycle water bottles contain 27 or 28 oz. Quart bottles are available but have never become popular.

Medical coverage should be provided for full-day or multi-day recreational cycling and racing events. Guidelines are available for organizing and providing this support.[51,86]

SUNBURN

Sunburn can be a significant problem, especially in long-distance touring because of the time spent on the bicycle. In one study of a long-distance tour, 40% of the riders reported some sunburn problems, with 5.4% of those riders reporting sunburn to be a significant problem that altered the way they rode.[137] Common areas of sunburning are arms, thighs, and lips in order of decreasing frequency.

Sunscreens effectively block the short ultraviolet burning rays of the sun. In one study testing the effects of sun screen during exercise, however, it was noted that in high heat/low humidity atmosphere, sunscreens tended to block water evaporation, thus raising skin temperature.[139] Sweating increased, but evaporation was impaired because of the sunscreen. The implications of this study in bicycle riders are unknown. This effect could potentially cause problems for riders because of heat transfer problems caused by cycling clothing and helmet use. It would seem prudent to recommend judicious use of sunscreens and to make sure that the rider is drinking enough fluids during an extended ride in hot weather.

REFERENCES

1. Anderson B: Stretching techniques for competitive cyclists. Conditioning for Cycling 1(2):10–17, 1991.
2. Berry MJ, Pollock WE, Van Nienenhuizen K, Brubaker PH: A comparison between aero and standard racing handlebars during prolonged exercise. Med Sci Sport Exerc 25(5 Suppl):S115, 1993.
3. Bicycle Institute of America Bicycling Reference Book. Washington, D.C. Bicycle Institute of America, 1993–94, pp 6–7.
4. Bishop PJ, Briard BD: Impact performance of bicycle helmets. Can J Appl Sport Sci 9:94–101, 1984.
5. Bohlmann JT: Injuries in competitive cycling. Physician Sportsmed 9(5):117–126, 1981.
6. Bond RE: Distance bicycling may cause ischemic neuropathy of the penis. Physician Sportsmed 3(11):54–56, 1975.
7. Bones D: Neck pain: Cured: Advice from those who solved the problem. Bicycling 27(7):28–29, 1986.
8. Boning D, Gonen Y, Maassen N: Relationship between work load, pedal frequency, and physical fitness. Int J Sports Med 5:92–97, 1984.
9. Braithwaite IJ: Bilateral median nerve palsy in a cyclist. Br J Sports Med 26:27–28, 1992.
10. Broker JP, Browning RC, Gregor RJ et al: Effect of seat height on force effectiveness in cycling. Med Sci Sports Exerc 20(2 Suppl):S83, 1988.
11. Brownlie L, Chapman A, Bannister E, Gastshore I: Aerodynamic characteristics of sports apparel. Med Sci Sports Exerc 25(5 Suppl):S197, 1993.
12. Brownlie LW, Gartshore I, Chapman A, Banister EW: The aerodynamics of cycling apparel. Cycling Sci 3(3&4):44–50, 1991.
13. Burke ER: Clipping in. Winning Bicycling Illustrated. 119:72, Dec. 1993.
14. Burke ER: Cycling. In Watkins RG (ed.): The Spine in Sports. Chicago, Mosby-Year Book, 1995.
15. Burke ER: Fitness Q & A: Tendon pain. Bicycling 32(3):48, 1991.
16. Burke ER: Proper fit of the bicycle. Clin Sports Med 13: 1–14, 1994.
17. Burke ER: Ulnar neuropathy in bicyclists. Physician Sportsmed 9(4):53–56, 1981.
18. Cass DT, Gray AJ: Paediatric bicycle injuries. Aust NZ J Surg 59:719–724, 1989.
19. Castro J: Rock and Roll. Time 138(7):42–44, August 19, 1991.
20. Chow TK, Bracker MD, Patrick K: Acute injuries from mountain biking. West J Med 159:145–148, 1993.
21. Coast JR, Cox RH, Welch HG: Optimal pedalling rate in prolonged bouts of cycle ergometry. Med Sci Sports Exerc 18:225–230, 1986.
22. Cohen GC: Cycling injuries. Can Fam Physician Med Fam Can 39:628–632, 1993.
23. Davis MW, Litman T, Crenshaw RW, Mueller JK: Bicycling injuries. Phys Sportsmed 13(5):116–123, 1985.
24. DeMoss V, Sanders D: Shopping for bike fit. Bicycle Guide 11(3):34–37, 1994.
25. Desai KM, Gingell JC: Hazards of long distance cycling. BMJ 298:1072–3, 1989.
26. Dickson TB: Preventing overuse cycling injuries. Physician Sportsmed 13(10):116–123, 1985.
27. Dorsa PG, Brilla LR: Physiological responses in cyclists to drop versus aero handlebars. Med Sci Sports Exerc 21(2 Suppl):S9, 1991.
28. Dorsch MM, Woodward AJ, Somers RL: Do bicycle safety helmets reduce severity of head injury in real crashes? Accid Anal Prev. 19:183–190, 1987.
29. Drake G: The cadence question: Is it time to modify the pedal-fast prescription? Bicycling 34(9):44–46, Oct. 1993.

30. Drake G: How to achieve a perfect position on a drop-bar bike. Bicycling 34(2):66–67, 1993.
31. Easterbrook M, Knuttgen HD, Pashby TJ, et al: Eye injuries and eye protection in sports: Position statement for the International Federation of Sports Medicine. Physician Sportsmed 16(11):49, 1988.
32. Eckman PB, Perlstein G, Altrocchi PH: Ulnar neuropathy in bicycle riders. Arch Neurol 32:130–131, 1975.
33. Ellis TH, Streight D, Mellion MB: Bicycle safety equipment. Clin Sports Med 13:75–98, 1994.
34. Endler M, Haber P, Hofner W: Wirbelsaulenveranderungen und ihre mechanopathologie bei leistungsruderern [Spinal deformities and their mechanopathology in oarsmen]. Z Orthop 118(1):91–100, 1980.
35. Estwanik JJ: Levator scapulae syndrome. Physician Sportsmed 17(10):57–66, 1989.
36. Faria IE: Applied physiology of cycling. Sports Med 1:187–204, 1984.
37. Faria I, Dix C, Frazer C: Effect of body position during cycling on heart rate, pulmonary ventilation, oxygen uptake and work output. J Sports Med Phys Fitness 18:49–56, 1978.
38. Faria I, Sjojaard G, Bonde-Petersen F: Oxygen cost during different pedalling speeds for constant power output. J Sports Med 22:295–299, 1982.
39. Fife D, Davis J, Tate L, et al: Fatal injuries to bicyclists: The experience of Dade County, Florida. J Trauma 23:745–755, 1985.
40. Friede AM, Azzara CV, Gallagher S, Guyer B: The epidemiology of injuries to bicycle riders. Pediatr Clin North Am 32:141–151, 1985.
41. Frontera WR: Cyclist's palsy: Clinical and electrodiagnostic findings. Br J Sports Med 17:91–93, 1983.
42. Gibson OB: Bicycle saddles and torsion of the testis. Lancet 1:1149, 1978.
43. Gisolfi CV, Rohlf DP, Navarude SN, et al: Effects of wearing a helmet on thermal balance while cycling in the heat. Phys Sportsmed 16(1):139–146, 1988.
44. Goodfellow RC: Bicycle saddles and torsion of the testis. Lancet 1:1149, 1978.
45. Goodson JD: Pudendal neuritis from biking. N Engl J Med. 304:365, 1981.
46. Grandjean AC, Ruud JS: Nutrition for cyclists. Clin Sports Med 13:235–247, 1994.
47. Gregor RJ, Rugg SG: Effects of saddle height and pedaling cadence on power output and efficiency. In Burke ER (ed) Science of Cycling. Champaign, IL, Human Kinetics, 1986, pp 69–90.
48. Griffiths M, MacKellar A: Bicycle-spoke and doubling injuries. Med J Aust 149:618–619, 1988.
49. Hagberg JM, Mullin JP, Giese MD, Spitznagel E: Effect of pedaling rate on submaximal exercise responses of competitive cyclists. J Appl Physiol 51:447–451, 1981.
50. Hershfield NB: Pedaller's penis. Can Med Assn J 128: 366–7, 1983.
51. Holland SP: Medical care delivery on a 150-mile bicycle tour. Clin J Sports Med 3:242–50, 1993.
52. Holmes JC, Pruitt AL, Whalen NJ: Cycling knee injuries; Common mistakes that cause injuries and how to avoid them. Cycling Sci 3(2):11–14, 1991.
53. Holmes JC, Pruitt AL, Whalen NJ: Iliotibial band syndrome in cyclists. Am J Sports Med 21:419–424, 1993.
54. Holmes JC, Pruitt AL, Whalen NJ: Lower extremity overuse in bicycling. Clin Sports Med 13:187–205, 1994.
55. Hoyt CS: Averting common biking injuries. Physician Sportsmed 4(4):40–43, 1976.
56. Hoyt CS: Ulnar neuropathy in bicycle riders. Arch Neurol 33:372, 1976.
57. Hull ML, Gonzalez H: Bivariate optimization of pedalling rate and crank arm length in cycling. J Biomech 21:839–849, 1988.
58. Jackson RH, Craft AW: Bicycle saddles and torsion of the testis. Lancet 1:983–4, 1978.
59. Johnson S, Schultz B: The physiologic effect of aerodynamic handlebars. Cycling Sci 2(4):9–12, 1990.
60. Judet H: Pathologie micro-traumatique et inflammatoire. In Judet H, Porte T (Eds): Médecine du cyclisme. Paris, Masson, 1983, pp 106–109.
61. Kiburz D, Jacobs R, Reckling F, Mason J: Bicycle accidents and injuries among adult cyclists. Am J Sports Med 14:416–419, 1986.
62. Koch C: Bike-related impotence. Bicycle Guide 7(4):32–40, 1990.
63. Kravitz HL: Preventing injuries from bicycle spokes. Pediatr Ann 6:713–716, 1977.
64. Kukoda J: Your keys to a comfortable, efficient position on a mountain bike. Bicycling 34(20):68–69, 1993.
65. Kuland DN, Brubaker CE: Injuries in the bikecentennial tour. Physician Sportsmed 6(6):74–78, 1978.
66. Kyle CR: The aerodynamics of handlebars and helmet. Cycling Sci 1(1):22–25, 1989.
67. Kyle CR: Energy and aerodynamics in bicycling. Clin Sports Med 13:39–73, 1994.
68. Kyle CR: How wind affects cycling. Bicycling 19(4):194–204, 1988.
69. Kyle C: Mechanical factors affecting the speed of a cycle. In Burke ER (ed.) Science of Cycling. Champaign, IL, Human Kinetics, 1986, pp 123–136.
70. Kyle CR: The mechanics and aerodynamics of cycling. In Burke ER, Newsom MM (eds): Medical and Scientific Aspects of Cycling. Champaign, IL, Human Kinetics, 1988, pp 235–251.
71. Lindqvist C, Sorsa S, Hyrkas T, Santavirta S: Maxillofacial factures sustained in bicycle accidents. Int J Oral Maxillofac Surg 15:12–18, 1986.
72. Lofthouse GA; Traumatic injuries to the extremities and thorax. Clin Sports Med 13:113–135, 1994.
73. Lollgen H, Ulmer H-V, Gross R, et al: Methodical aspects of perceived exertion rating and its relation to pedalling rate and rotating mass. Eur J Appl Physiol 34:205–215, 1975.
74. Matheny F: Finding perfect saddle height. Bicycling 33(3): 108–109, 1992.
75. Mayer PJ: Helping your patients avoid bicycling injuries: Part 1: What injuries to anticipate this summer. J Musculoskel Med 2(5):31–40, 1985.
76. Mayer PJ: Helping your patients avoid bicycling injuries. Part 2: How to choose, adjust, and use a bicycle properly. J Musculoskel Med 2(6):31–38, 1985.
77. McDermott FT, Klug GL: Injury profile of pedal and motor cyclist casualties in Victoria. Aust NZ J Surg 55:477–483, 1985.
78. McDonald DI: Is there life after genital numbness? N Z Med J 100:465, 1987.
79. McElhinney BE, Horner T, Dinsmore WW, et al: Exercise bicycle-induced bilateral vulva abscesses. Int J STD & AIDS 4:174–175, 1993.
80. Mellion MB: Common cycling injuries: Management and prevention. Sports Med 11:52–70, 1991.
81. Mellion MB: Neck and back pain in bicycling. Clin Sports Med 13:137–164, 1994.
82. Mellion MB, Hill JW: Bicycling. In Mellion MB, Walsh WM, Shelton GL: The Team Physician's Handbook. Philadelphia, Hanley & Belfus, Inc., 1990, pp 609–627.
83. Micheli LJ: Back Injuries in gymnastics. Clin Sports Med 4:85–93, 1985.
84. Midgley AK: Hazards of long distance cycling. BMJ 298: 6684, 1989.
85. Mills NJ: Protective capability of bicycle helmets. Br J Sports Med 24:55–60, 1990.
86. Montalto NJ, Janas TB: Medical coverage of recreational cycling events. Clin Sports Med 13:249–258, 1994.
87. Nichols TW: Bicycle-seat hematuria. N Engl J Med 311:1128, 1984.
88. Nixon J, Clacher R, Pearn J, Corcoran A: Bicycle accidents in childhood. Br Med J 294:1267–1269, 1987.
89. Noth J, Dietz V, Mauritz K-H: Cyclist's palsy: Neurological and EMG study in 4 cases with distal ulnar lesions. J Neurol Sci 47:111–116, 1980.
90. O'Brien KP: Sports urology: The vicious cycle. N Engl J Med 304:1367–1368, 1981.

91. Origenes MM, Blank SE, Schoene RB: Exercise ventilatory response to upright and aero-posture cycling. Med Sci Sports Exerc 25:608–612, 1993.
92. Ostrom M, Bjornstig U, Eriksson A: Pedal cycling fatalities in northern Sweden. Int J Epidemiol 22:483–488, 1993.
93. Patterson RP, Moreno MI: Bicycle pedalling forces as a function of pedalling rate and power output. Med Sci Sports Exerc 22:512–516, 1990.
94. Pfeiffer RP: Off-road bicycle racing injuries—the NORBA pro/elite category. Clin Sports Med 13:207–218, 1994.
95. Powell B: Correction and prevention of bicycle saddle problems. Physician Sportsmed 10(10):60–67, 1982.
96. Redfield R, Hull ML: On the relation between joint moments and pedalling rates at constant power in bicycling. J Biomech 19:317–329, 1986.
97. Renne JW: The iliotibial band friction syndrome. J Bone Joint Surg 57A:1110–1111, 1975.
98. Richmond DR: Handlebar problems in bicycling. Clin Sports Med 13:165–173, 1994.
99. Robinson R: The new back school prescription: Stabilization training: I. Spine: State Art Rev 5:341–355, 1991.
100. Rodier JF, Janser JC, Rodier D: Induration nodulaire perineale. J Chir (Paris) 129:49–50, 1992.
101. Ryschon TW: Physiologic aspects of bicycling. Clin Sports Med 13:15–38, 1994.
102. Saal JA: Intervertebral disc herniation: Advances in nonoperative treatment. Physical Med Rehab: State Art Rev 4:175–194, 1990.
103. Saal JA: The new back school prescription: Stabilization training: II. Spine: State Art Rev 5:357–366, 1991.
104. Saal JA, Saal JS: Initial stage management of lumbar spine problems. Phys Med Rehabil Clin North Am 2:205–221, 1991.
105. Saal JA, Saal JS: Later stage management of lumbar spine problems. Phys Med Rehabil Clin North Am 2:187–203, 1991.
106. Sacks JJ, Holmgreen P, Smith SM, Sosin DM: Bicycle-associated head injuries and deaths in the United States from 1984 through 1988: How many are preventable? JAMA 266: 3016–3018, 1991.
107. Salcedo JR: Huffy bike hematuria. N Engl J Med 315:768, 1986.
108. Sankhala SS, Gupta SP: Spoke-wheel injuries. Indian J Pediatr 54:251–256, 1987.
109. Sargent JD, Peck MG, Weitzman M: Bicycle-mounted child seats. Am J Dis Child 142:765–767, 1988.
110. Sava P, Cattaneo A, Denak A, Boudinet F: Le troisième testicule du cycliste: une affection á ne pas ignorer. Presse Medicale 17:1761, 1988.
111. Seabury JJ, Adams WC, Ramey MR: Influence of pedalling rate and power output on the energy expenditure during bicycle ergometry. Ergonomics 20:491–498, 1977.
112. Shea JD, McClain EJ: Ulnar-nerve compression syndromes at or below the wrist. J Bone Joint Surg 51A:1095–1103, 1969.
113. Shea KG, Shumsky IB, Shea OF: Shifting into wrist pain. Physician Sportsmed 19(9):59–63, 1991.
114. Silbert PL, Dunne JW, Edis RH, Stewart-Wynne EG: Bicycling induced pudendal nerve pressure neuropathy. Clin Exp Neurol 28:191–6, 1991.
115. Solomon S, Cappa KG: Impotence and bicycling. A seldom-reported connection. Postgraduate Med 81(1):99–102, 1987.
116. Spence WR: Sports Medicine Tips for Cyclists. Waco, TX, WRS Publishing, 1991.
117. Suzuki Y: Mechanical efficiency of fast- and slow-twitch muscle fibers in man during cycling. J Appl Physiol 47:263–267, 1979.
118. Sward L: The thoracolumbar spine in young elite athletes: Current concepts on the effects of physical training. Sports Med 13:357–364, 1992.
119. Sward L, Hellstrom M, Jacobsson B, et al: Acute injury of the vertebral ring apophysis and intervertebral disc in adolescent gymnasts. Spine 15:144, 1990.
120. Sward L, Hellstrom M, Jacobsson B, Karlsson L: Vertebral ring apophysis injuries in athletes: Is the etiology different in the thoracic and lumbar spine? Am J Sports Med 21:841–845, 1993.
121. Swart R: Hard facts about bicycle helmets. Cycling Sci 1(1):14–16, 1989.
122. Sweeney T: Neck school: Cervicothoracic stabilization training. Spine: State Art Rev 5:367–378, 1991.
123. Sweeney T, Prentice C, Saal JA, Saal JS: Cervicothoracic muscular stabilization techniques. Physical Med Rehabil: State Art Rev 4:335–359, 1990.
124. Tanz RR, Christoffel KK: Tykes on bikes: Injuries associated with bicycle-mounted child seats. Pediatr Emerg Care 7:297–301, 1991.
125. Thompson DC, Thompson RS, Rivara FP, Wolf ME: A case-control study of the effectiveness of bicycle safety helmets in preventing facial injury. Am J Public Health 80:1471–1474, 1990.
126. Thompson RS, Rivara FP, Thompson DC: A case-control study of the effectiveness of bicycle safety helmets. N Engl J Med 320:1361–1367, 1989.
127. Too D: Biomechanics of cycling and factors affecting performance. Sports Med 10:286–302, 1990.
128. Tucci JJ, Barone JE: A study of urban bicycling accidents. Am J Sports Med 16:181–184, 1988.
129. van Elegem P: Cyclisme et pathologie chronique. Acta Orthop Belg 49(1–2):88–100, 1983.
130. Van der Plas R: The bicycle racing guide: technique and training for bicycle racers and triathletes. San Francisco, Bicycle Books, 1986.
131. Vuong PN, Camuzard P, Schoonaert MF: Perineal nodular indurations ("accessory testicles" in cyclists.) Fine needle aspiration cytologic and pathologic findings in two cases. Acta Cytol 32:86–90, 1988.
132. Walsh WM: Patellofemoral joint. In DeLee JC, Drez D Jr. (eds.): Orthopaedic Sports Medicine: Principles and Practice, Vol. 2. Philadelphia, W.B. Saunders, 1993, pp 1163–1248.
133. Wasserman RC, Buccini RV: Helmet protection from head injuries among recreational bicyclists. Am J Sports Med 18:96–97, 1990.
134. Wasserman RC, Walter JA, Monty MJ, et al: Bicyclists, helmets and head injuries: A rider-based study of helmet use and effectiveness. Am J Public Health 78:1220–1221, 1988.
135. Weiss BD: Bicycle-related head injuries. Clin Sports Med 13:99–112, 1994.
136. Weiss BD: Clinical syndromes associated with bicycle seats. Clin Sports Med 13:175–186, 1994.
137. Weiss BD: Nontraumatic injuries in amateur long distance bicyclists. Am J Sports Med 13:187–192, 1985.
138. Weiss BD: Skin cream for alleviating seat pain in amateur long-distance bicyclists. Sports Med Training Rehab 4:27–32, 1993.
139. Wells T: Effects of sunscreen use during exercise in the heat. Physician Sportsmed 12(6):132–144, 1984.
140. Wheeler JB, Broker JP, Gregor RJ: A comparison of torsional moments across different shoe-pedal interfaces in cycling. Med Sci Sports Exerc 24(5 Suppl):S186, 1992.
141. White J: Aero handlebars: Too fast to handle? Physician Sportsmed 19(10):29, 1991.
142. Widrick JJ, Freedson PS, Hamill J: Effect of internal work on the calculation of optimal pedaling rates. Med Sci Sports Exerc 24:376–382, 1992.
143. Worrell J: Head injuries in pedal cyclists: how much will protection help? Injury 18:5–6, 1987.
144. Zahradnik F: A better biff bucket. Bicycling 34(9):120, 1993.
145. Zinn L: Finding an efficient bike position. VeloNews 21(5): 68–70, 1992.

Index

Page numbers in **boldface** type indicates complete chapters.